20 Update in Intensive Care and Emergency Medicine

Edited by J.-L. Vincent

R. Bellomo C. Ronco (Eds.)

Acute Renal Failure in the Critically Ill

With 55 Figures and 27 Tables

Springer-Verlag
Berlin Heidelberg New York
London Paris Tokyo
Hong Kong Barcelona
Budapest

Series Editor

Prof. Dr. Jean-Louis Vincent
Clinical Director, Department of Intensive Care
Erasme University Hospital
Route de Lennik 808, 1070 Brussels, Belgium

Volume Editors

Dr. med. Rinaldo Bellomo
Intensive Care Unit
Austin Hospital
Victoria 3084, Australia

Dr. med. Claudio Ronco
Dept. of Nephrology and Clinical Dialysis
St. Bartolo Hospital
36100 Vicenza, Italy

ISBN-13: 978-3-642-79246-5 e-ISBN-13: 978-3-642-79244-1
DOI: 10.1007/978-3-642-79244-1

Library of Congress Cataloging-in-Publication Data. Acute renal failure in the critically ill/R. Bellomo, C. Ronco, (eds.). p. cm. – (Update in intensive care and emergency medicine; 20) Includes bibliographical references and index. ISBN-13: 978-3-642-79246-5
1. Acute renal failure. 2. Critical care medicine. I. Bellomo, R. (Rinaldo), 1956– . II. Ronco, C. (Claudio), 1951– . III. Series. [DNLM: 1. Kidney Failure, Acute. 2. Critical Illness. W1 UP66H v. 20 1995/WJ 342 A18954 1995] RC918.R4A3447 1995 616.6′14 – dc20 DNLM/DLC for Library of Congress 94-42307

Softcover reprint of the hardcover 1st edition 1995

Typesetting: Best-set Typesetter Ltd., Hong Kong

SPIN: 10127901 19/3130/SPS – 5 4 3 2 1 0 – Printed on acid-free paper

To Debrah and Hilary, Paola and Federico
for their love, patience, and support

Preface

Over the last 10 years the syndrome of severe acute renal failure has progressively changed in its epidemiology. It is now most frequently seen in critically ill patients, typically in the context of sepsis and multiorgan failure. This epidemiologic change has meant that intensive care physicians and nephrologists must now work in close cooperation at all times and must take many complex issues of prevention, pathogenesis, and management into account that they did not previously have to tackle.

Simultaneously, the last 10 years have seen the development of major technical and conceptual changes in the field of renal replacement therapy. There are now previously unavailable therapeutic options that provide physicians with a flexible and rapidly evolving armamentarium.

The nutrition of these patients, previously limited by the partial efficacy of renal replacement therapies, has also become more aggressive and more in tune with the needs of critically ill patients.

Increased understanding of the pathogenesis of the multiorgan failure syndrome has focused on the role of many soluble "mediators of injury" (cytokines, leukotrienes, prostanoids etc.). These molecules are likely to participate in the pathogenesis of acute renal failure. Their generation and disposal is also affected by different techniques of artificial renal support.

Despite these changes, the approach to acute renal failure in the critically ill remains very close to the conventional renal ward style in many institutions. This partly stems from the difficulties inherent to proving that new therapies change mortality rates in critically ill patients and partly from a lack of knowledge and familiarity with new conceptual and technical developments.

This book, coedited by an intensive care physician and a nephrologist, aims to provide both a model for the integration of critical care skills and nephrological skills and a "state of the art" review of all major aspects of acute renal failure in the intensive care unit. It first explores issues of morhology and pathophysiology in experimental models and patients and then moves to the area of renal recovery and prevention of renal injury. The epidemiology of acute renal failure in the intensive care unit is explored and the difficulties inherent to the assessment of renal function in these patients are discussed.

Having set the necessary background, the book then moves on to the clinical arena, exploring specific disorders and forms of injury. Next it explores therapeutics, focusing on renal replacement, nutritional therapy, and the immunologic aspects of acute renal failure in the intensive care unit.

Inevitably, the book enters the debate of which renal replacement therapy should be used in these patients and why, as it tries to provide sound rationales for the choices necessary in clinical practice. Finally, pharmacokinetics during acute renal failure and various renal replacement therapies are described and explained with a strong emphasis on practical prescription guidelines.

We believe this book to be an important source of scientific information, practical advice, useful references, and modern thinking in this area. We hope that it will not simply inform and guide our interested colleagues, but that it will also stimulate them to challenge our views and pursue much needed additional research.

In closing, we are thankful to all those who have offered their advice and support during this endeavor, in particular Professor Michael Pinsky and other colleagues and friends in the Division of Critical Care Medicine at the University of Pittsburgh Medical Center and in the Division of Nephrology at the San Bortolo Hospital in Vicenza.

Victoria, Australia
Vicenza, Italy
January 1995

R. Bellomo
C. Ronco

Contents

List of Contributors

Bellomo R.
Intensive Care Unit, Austin Hospital, Heidelberg, Victoria 3084, Australia

Bersten A.D.
Intensive Care Unit, Flinders Medical Centre, Bedford Park, Adelaide, South Australia 5042 Australia

Bosch J.P.
Department of Nephrology, Hypertension, George Washington University Medical Center, Burns Building, 2150 Pennsylvania Avenue, NW, Washington, DC 20037, USA

Boyce N.
212 Nelson Road, South Melbourne, Victoria 3205, Australia

Brezis M.
Department of Renal Medicine, Hadassah University Hospital, Mount Scopus, PO Box 24035, Jerusalem 91240, Israel

Chertow G.M.
Department of Nephrology, Brigham Women's Hospital, 75 St. Francis Street, Boston, MA 02115, USA

Camussi G.
Laboratory of Immunopathology, Department of Nephrology, Corso A.M. Dogliotti, 14, 10126 Torino, Italy

Chew S.L.
Department of Nephrology, Hypertension, Algemeen Ziekenhuis Stuivenberg, Lange Beeldekensstraat 267, 2060 Antwerp, Belgium (Current Address: Department of Endocrinology, St. Bartholomew's Hospital, London, United Kingdom)

Daelemans R.
Department of Nephrology, Hypertension, Algemeen Ziekenhuis Stuivenberg, Lange Beeldekensstraat 267, 2060 Antwerp, Belgium

Epstein M.
Room A-1006, V.A. Medical Center, 1201 N.W. 16th Street, Miami, FL 33125, USA

Fabris A.G.
Department of Nephrology, City Hospital, Bassano del Grappa (Vicenza), Italy

Fabris G.
Department of Internal Medicine, City Hospital, Este (Padova), Italy

Golper T.A.
Division of Nephrology, University of Arkansas for Medical Sciences, 4301 West Markham, Mail Slot 501, Little Rock, AR 72205, USA

Grootendorst A.F.
Department of Internal Medicine, Nephrology and Intensive Care, St. Clara Ziekenhuis, Olympiaweg 350, 3078 HT Rotterdam, The Netherlands

Holt A.W.
Intensive Care Unit, Flinders Medical Centre, Bedford Park, Adelaide, South Australia 5042, Australia

Johnson J.P.
Department of Nephrology, University of Pittsburg, Medical Centre, Scaife Hall, Terrace Street 3550, Pittsburgh, PA 15216, USA

Kaloyanides G.J.
Department of Medicine, Division of Nephrology, Hypertension, State University of New York at Stony Brook, Stony Brook, NY 11794-8152, USA

Kierdorf H.
Department of Internal Medicine II, RWTH Aachen, Pauwelstr. 30, 52057 Aachen, Germany

Kroh U.F.
Department of Anesthesiology and Intensive Therapy, Clinicum of the Philipps-University of Marburg, Baldingerstr., 35003 Marburg, Germany

Lazarus J.M.
Division of Nephrology, Brigham Women's Hospital, 75 St. Francis Street, Boston, MA 02115, USA

Lins R.L.
Department of Nephrology, Hypertension, Algemeen Ziekenhuis Stuivenberg, Lange Beeldekensstraat 267, 2060 Antwerp, Belgium

Lieske J.C.
Department of Medicine and Cell Physiology, The University of Chicago, PO Box 453, 5841 S. Maryland Ave. MC 5100, Chicago, IL 60637, USA

Montrucchio G.
Internal Medicine, University of Turin, 10126 Turin, Italy

Owen W.F., Jr.
Division of Nephrology, Brigham Women's Hospital, 75 St. Francis Street, Boston, MA 02115, USA

Racusen L.C.
Department of Physiology, Johns Hopkins Medical Institutions, Ross Research Building, 720 Rutland Avenue, Baltimore, MD 21205-2196, USA

Rokaw M.D.
Department of Nephrology, University of Pittsburg Medical Centre, Scaife Hall, Terrace Street 3550, Pittsburgh, PA 15216, USA

Ronco C.
Department of Nephrology and Clinical Dialysis, St. Bortolo Hospital, 36100 Vicenza, Italy

Sieberth H.G.
Department of Internal Medicine II, RWTH Aachen, Pauwelstr. 30, 52057 Aachen, Germany

Solez K.
Department of Pathology, University of Alberta, Edmonton, Alberta, Canada 5B4 02WC

Symon Z.
Department of Renal Medicine, Hadassah University Hospital, Mount Scopus, PO Box 24035, Jerusalem 91240, Israel

Tetta C.
Clinical Respiratory Department, Bellco S.p.A., Via Camurama 1/A, 41037 Mirandola (Modena), Italy

Toback F.G.
Department of Medicine, Section of Nephrology, The University of Chicago, 5841 S. Maryland Avenue, MC 5100, Chicago, IL 60637, USA

Trpkov K.
Department of Pathology, University of Alberta, Edmonton, Alberta, Canada 5B4 02WC

van Saase J.L.C.M.
Department of Internal Medicine, Nephrology and Intensive Care, St. Clara Hospital, Olympiaweg 350, 3078 HT Rotterdam, The Netherlands

Vincent H.H.
St. Antonius Hospital, Nieuwegein, The Netherlands

Pathology of Acute Renal Failure

L.C. Racusen, K. Trpkov, and K. Solez

Introduction

The pathology of acute renal failure (ARF) as it is encountered in the mid-1990s reflects the changing character of the patients developing this condition. Increasingly, individuals develop ARF as a part of a multiorgan failure syndrome rather than with a single organ disease presentation (Solez and Racusen 1993). As a consequence, ARF patients are more likely to be in the intensive care unit than on the renal medicine ward, and their primary physician is more likely to be an intensive care physician than a nephrologist. These trends reflect improvement in the general medical care of the critically ill patient. Patients who would not have survived their acute event in the past now live long enough to develop multiorgan failure. The high proportion of (concurrent) heart and liver disease means that many more of the patients present with a "prerenal" picture in which the kidney is still capable of reabsorbing sodium and concentrating the urine and morphologic alterations are minimal. Similarly, the increasing complexity and general poor health of the patients makes it less likely that a renal biopsy will be performed. Thus the renal morphologic alterations that accompany some types of ARF in critically ill patients remain largely unknown.

In this chapter, we will review histologic findings in clinical ARF and in animal models of acute tubular necrosis (ATN), including morphologic–functional correlations. The nature of tubular injury in ATN and the terminology used will be discussed. In this overview, we will describe and illustrate the spectrum of cell injury in ATN, including injury with loss of cell adhesion, necrosis, and apoptosis. Renal infarction and cortical necrosis will also be discussed, and we will consider specific morphologic features in hepatorenal syndrome, sepsis, crush injury, and the transplant setting. Finally, we will compare pathologic findings in experimental models of ARF and consider unanswered questions and areas for future investigation.

Morphologic Findings in Clinical Acute Renal Failure

Prerenal Failure

As noted, clinical ARF may result from prerenal factors reducing perfusion pressure in the kidney; this pattern is typical of that seen in early ischemia/hypoperfusion and in the hepatorenal syndrome. In this phase of ARF, renal tubules are still able to reabsorb Na normally, and structural injury to the tubular epithelium is not yet apparent. The morphologic findings in biopsies from this early phase (which are rarely obtained outside the renal allograft setting), may consist only of glomerular collapse with wrinkling of glomerular basement membranes, which may be seen on periodic acid–Schiff (PAS) or silver stains, hyperplasia of the juxtaglomerular apparatus, and/or constriction of arterioles with focal vacuolization of vascular smooth muscle cells. It should be noted, however, that morphologic manifestations of tubular cell injury, to be described below, may be seen at least focally on renal biopsy at a time when FeNa remains within the normal range.

Acute Tubular Necrosis

As in other tissues and organs, cellular changes in the kidney in response to injury, and specifically in the tubular epithelium, may be seen as a continuum, varying from subtle metabolic changes to total breakdown and dissolution of cell structure. Due to some relatively unique structural peculiarities of nephron structure, injury to and/or death of even small numbers of tubular epithelial cells may impact on nephron and ultimately whole kidney function. Tubular epithelial cells form a complete intact epithelium lining long enclosed cylindrical tubular luminal spaces of finite diameter. Swelling of cells in this setting may impinge on the patency of the tubular lumen, especially in narrow parts of the nephron, and/or may impinge on peritubular capillaries. Sloughing of cells and cell debris may obstruct the nephron and reduce function. Renal tubular epithelial cells are also normally exposed to continual fluid flows through the tubular lumina. This fluid may be nutrient/substrate rich, which may have important effects on injured cells, as flow factors and substrate delivery may modify tubular cell injury and its impact on nephron function.

The high metabolic activity and substrate demand of subpopulations of tubular epithelial cells make them especially vulnerable to injury. As a corollary consideration, susceptibility to injury is to some extent segment specific, since cells from different parts of the nephron have different functions and metabolic requirements. With toxic injury, segmental patterns of injury may also be related to the relative concentration of toxin to which the cells are exposed and to differential transport and metabolic processes which tend to concentrate toxins in some cells. However, it is true that the morphologic and functional manifestations of injury at the cellular level and the mechanisms leading to cell injury are similar in many ways among these subpopulations, the differences being largely a matter of degree.

Sites of injury along the nephron may vary, depending on the nature of the insult, underlying hemodynamic factors and adequacy of collateral circulation, and metabolic demand on the cells in the face of energy depletion. Different nephron segments have different types of metabolism and different metabolic rates (Guder and Ross 1984). In addition, there is a gradient of O_2 tension within the kidney, with higher levels in cortex and only marginal O_2 tension in medulla (Brezis et al. 1984a). Venkatachalam et al. (1978) were among the first to point out the increased susceptibility of the proximal tubular S_3 segment to ischemic injury in rats. Using a 25-min unilateral renal artery occlusion model of ischemia in rats, they found that, while S_1 and S_2 segments were reversibly injured and recovered within 4 h, S_3 segments underwent progressive cell injury and death. Brezis et al. (1984) have emphasized the susceptibility of the medullary thick ascending limb to hypoxic injury in the isolated perfused kidney. They point out the marginal vascular perfusion to this region of the kidney and have clearly related the extent of necrosis to the proximity to/distance from perfusing vessels. Wilson and Schrier (1986), using primary cultures of microdissected tubular epithelial cells, have also demonstrated segment-specific susceptibility to hypoxic injury.

Metabolic differences among tubular segments may underlie differential susceptibility (Ross and Guder 1982). Using the isolated perfused kidney and inhibitors of mitochondrial respiration and intermediary metabolism, Brezis et al. (1985) found that, while hypoxic-like changes could be produced in S_1 and S_2 proximal tubular segments with metabolic inhibition alone, both types of inhibitors were needed to produce visible injury to medullary thick ascending limb (mTAL). Even adenosine triphosphate (ATP) depletion produced by combined inhibitors did not reproduce the m-TAL structural injury seen with O_2 deprivation. Thus S_1 and S_2 show largely reversible changes with only moderate ATP depletion, while mTAL tolerates marked ATP depletion without structural change. In the mTAL, persistent mitochondrial function (Brezis et al. 1986) and/or transport work in the face of O_2 deprivation (Brezis et al. 1984; Zager et al. 1983, 1987; Shanley and Johnson 1989) produce the most severe injury. Ruegg and Mandel (1990) have shown that, at least in freshly isolated rabbit nephron segments, proximal convoluted tubule cannot utilize glucose to support oxidative metabolism, a result also reported by others (Ross and Guder 1982; Gullans et al. 1984). However, rabbit proximal straight tubular segments did utilize glucose (Ruegg and Mandel 1990). The S_3 segment of the mouse also utilizes glucose for ATP generation more than the S_1 and S_2 segments (Uchida and Endou 1988).

Variable transport functions along the nephron also may result in differential injury. As noted above, segments with active transport processes may suffer irreversible injury if transport function continues in the face of oxygen deprivation (Brezis et al. 1984; Zager et al. 1983, 1987; Shanley and Johnson 1989). Transport functions also become important in determining sensitivity to drug toxicity. Aminoglycosides, for example, are avidly reabsorbed in the proximal tubule, accumulating to toxic levels in the cells and producing injury localized to this segment; aminoglycosides tend to selectively affect S_1 and S_2 (Houghton et al. 1976). In ischemia, the medullary thick ascending limb may be particularly vulnerable (Brezis et al. 1984), though injury may occur elsewhere as well. While renal biopsy most frequently samples cortex, there is ample evidence that injury in ATN also occurs in distal segments in the medulla.

It has been noted for some time that renal biopsy findings in ATN, the ARF produced by ischemia and/or nephrotoxins, may be subtle and seemingly out of proportion to the level of organ dysfunction. There are a variety of reasons for this, including:

1. More subtle types of tubular cell injury, short of overt necrosis, may have major functional impact on the kidney.
2. Injury of cells in relatively short segments of a majority of nephrons may compromise renal function to the same extent as more extensive injury, but may be more difficult to document on renal biopsy due to sampling error.
3. Typical renal biopsies may not sample medulla, where an important component of tubular injury may take place.
4. Biopsies obtained during recovery may show less cell injury and more reconstitution and regeneration-related changes, at a time when tubular epithelial function and renal function are still compromised.

The type of insult to some extent determines extent and manifestations of injury. In the critically ill hospitalized patient, ATN may be produced by a variety of factors acting alone or in combination. Ischemia/hypotension and nephrotoxins are the most common direct causes of renal injury and renal failure, but in the critically ill sepsis, rhabdomyolysis, and a variety of other metabolic disturbances may exaceberate injury. We will describe the features of typical ATN (with some emphasis on sublethal injury), apoptosis, infarction/cortical necrosis, and a few special features which may be seen in specific clinical settings.

Morphologic changes in renal tubular epithelial cells reflect injury which may be either reversible or irreversible. While severity of injury is a continuum and the precise point at which a cell has been irreversibly injured is not defined, in general cellular changes in ATN may be divided into manifestations of sublethal versus lethal injury. As we will discuss, the former may be much more widespread than the latter.

Sublethal Injury

Sublethal injury is manifested by a variety of changes in tubular epithelial cells, a few of which have been shown to correlate with functional renal failure. These changes reflect alterations in cellular energy stores, fluid and electrolyte concentrations, cell calcium, and ultimately the function of cellular enzyme systems and the cell cytoskelton. An early change is cell swelling and vacuolization, a change seen in a variety of settings including ischemia and toxic injury (see Fig. 1). Isometric vacuolization of tubular cells is a change typical of cyclosporine-associated renal injury (Racusen and Solez 1992) and is seen at its most extreme with (presumed) osmotic insults, including treatment with IV immunoglobulin (Cantu et al. 1994). Other early changes include loss and/or internalization of the apical brush border and blebbing of apical cell cytoplasm (see Fig. 2); these latter changes result

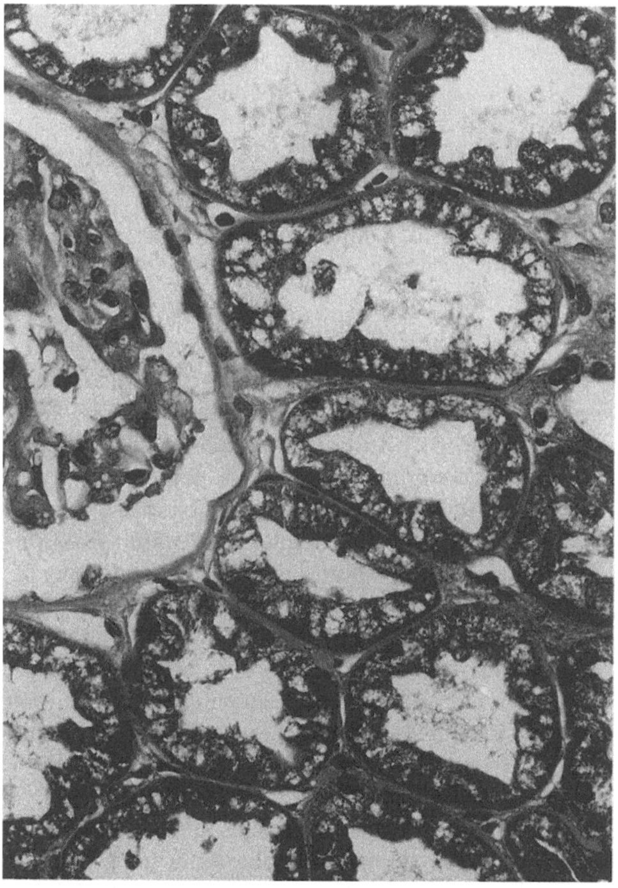

Fig. 1. Tubular cell vacuolization in a biopsy from a patient with acute renal failure (×400)

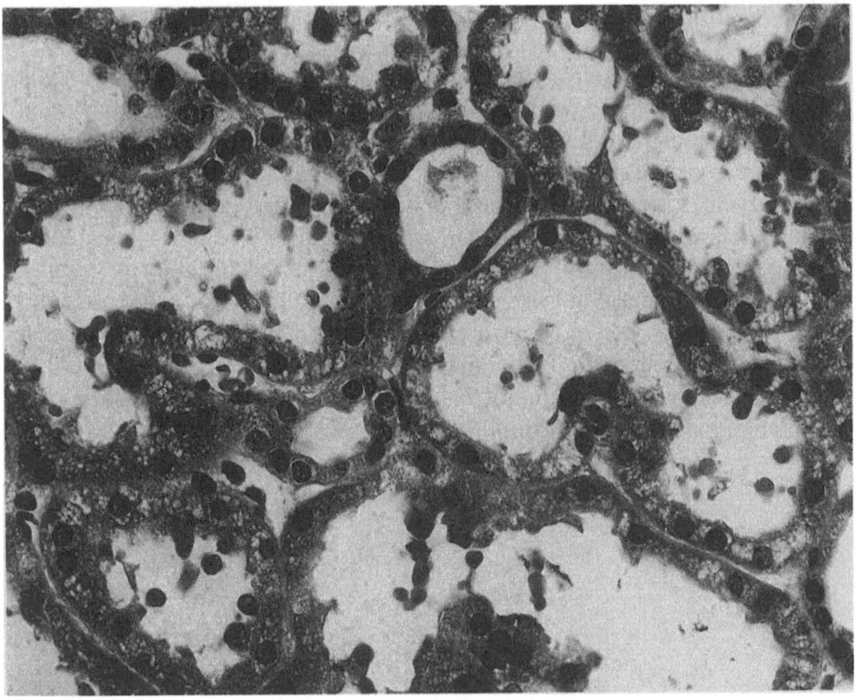

Fig. 2. Biopsy from a patient with toxic shock syndrome and acute renal failure showing loss of brush border, blebbing of apical cytoplasm, and vacuolization of tubular cells (×400)

in large part from alterations in cell calcium (Troyer et al. 1982) and associated changes in the apical microfilaments which maintain the complex apical surface structure in these cells (Kellerman et al. 1990).

Another morphologic change which appears to be due at least in part to alterations in structure and/or function of the cell cystoskelton is the detachment of cells from the tubular epithelium. Loss of tubular cells, either as individual cells or short arrays of cells, is one of the few findings that appears to correlate with renal functional status (Solez et al. 1979). Tubular epithelial cells may be seen in substantial numbers in voided urine in ATN. These cells were initially thought to represent cells which had suffered lethal injury in situ and had then detached and been swept away in the urinary stream. Recent studies have shown, however, that these voided cells may be viable, having detached from the epithelium in response to a sublethal injury (Racusen et al. 1991; Graber et al. 1991). There is evidence that alterations in cell microfilaments and/or surface attachment proteins are involved in the altered cell adhesion leading to exfoliation from the epithelium (Racusen 1994; Kroshian and Lieberthal 1991; Mandel and Bacallao 1991; Gailit et al. 1993). In particular, there is early rearrangement in the actin cytoskeleton, demonstrated both in vivo and in vitro (Racusen 1994; Kellerman and Bogusky 1992; Mandel and Bacallao 1991). In addition, cell surface integrin molecules are rearranged with injury, perhaps contributing not only to decreased in situ adhesion (Gailit et al. 1993; Goligorsky et al. 1993), but ultimately to impaction of cells in the nephron and obstruction (Goligorsky and DiBona 1993). Liver cell adhesion molecule (L-CAM), a major protein of the tight junction, is also internalized with "anoxic" injury in vitro (Bacallao and Mandel 1991), potentially contributing to decreased cell–cell adhesion.

Morphologically on renal biopsy, with exfoliation of tubular cells gaps can be seen along the tubular basement membrane either denuded of cells or covered by only a thin layer of cell cytoplasm (see Fig. 3). Adjacent cells are often flattened and attenuated. Lateral spreading and migration of surviving cells has been described in vitro in response to wounding of epithelial monolayers, including monolayers of renal epithelial cells (Kartha and Toback 1992). The mechanisms of this response have not been fully defined, but altered distribution of cell surface attachment molecules and associated cytoskeletal and attachment proteins has been documented. As a result of this early reactive process of reconstitution combined with a later proliferative/regenerative response, defects representing sites of cell detachment may be covered and/or be relatively inapparent, making the extent of cell loss difficult to evaluate (Racusen 1992). In addition to these alterations in the epithelium with detachment, intact epithelial cells may be seen in

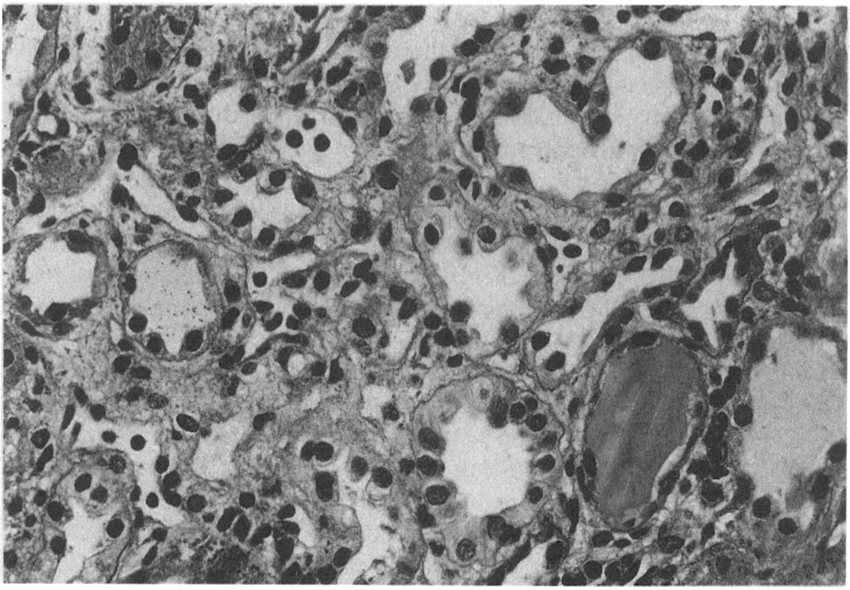

Fig. 3. Flattened tubular epithelium with gaps representing sites of cell loss (×400)

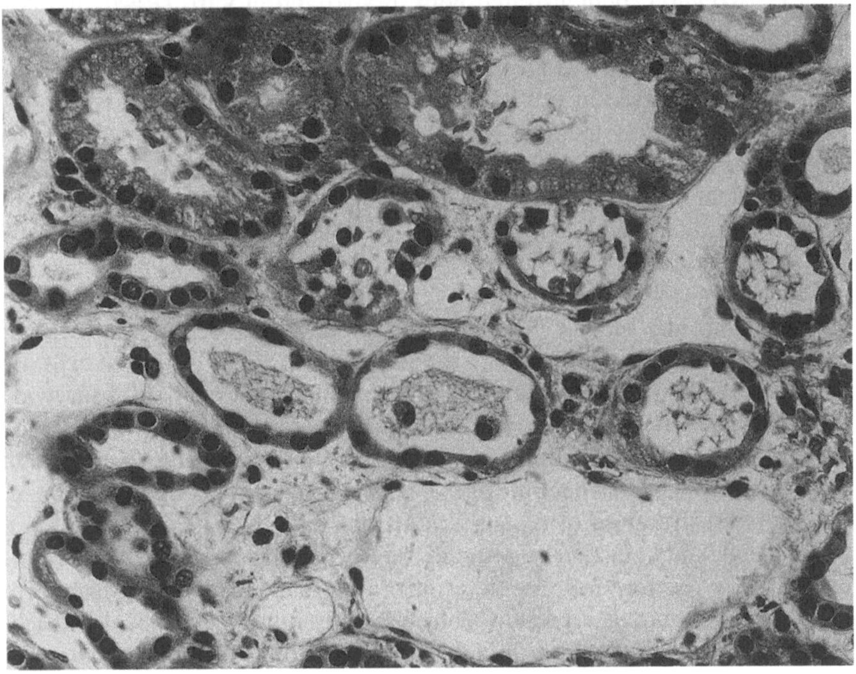

Fig. 4. Exfoliated cells in tubular lumina. While a few exfoliated cells appear necrotic, several are morphologically well preserved (×400)

tubular lumina (see Fig. 4), and these cells may contribute to tubular obstruction (Goligorsky and DiBona 1993).

While less dramatic than frank cellular necrosis, the tubular epithelial cell changes occurring with potentially reversible cell injury may contribute to the pathogenesis of ARF via mechanisms very similar to those invoked when there is extensive cell death (Fig. 5). Brush border loss and marked simplification of the apical surface of the injured cells (or the immature regenerating cells replacing them) leads to faulty tubular reabsorption, which in turn tiggers hemodynamic alterations which reduce the glomerular filtration rate (GFR). Altered cell–cell adhesion and/or overt cell loss provide sites for "backleak" of glomerular filtrate. Sloughed cells and cell debris may impact in the nephron and particularly narrow segments, such as the loop of Henle, obstructing nephron flow. Affected nephron segments may be short and relatively difficult to detect without careful microdissesion (Oliver et al. 1951), leading to underestimation of this feature on biopsy. What may be seen on biopsy, however, is dilation of the tubules proximal to the occluded segment during the period when GFR continues in the face of obstruction (see Fig. 2); tubular dilation may be the most prominent feature in biopsies, especially early in ATN.

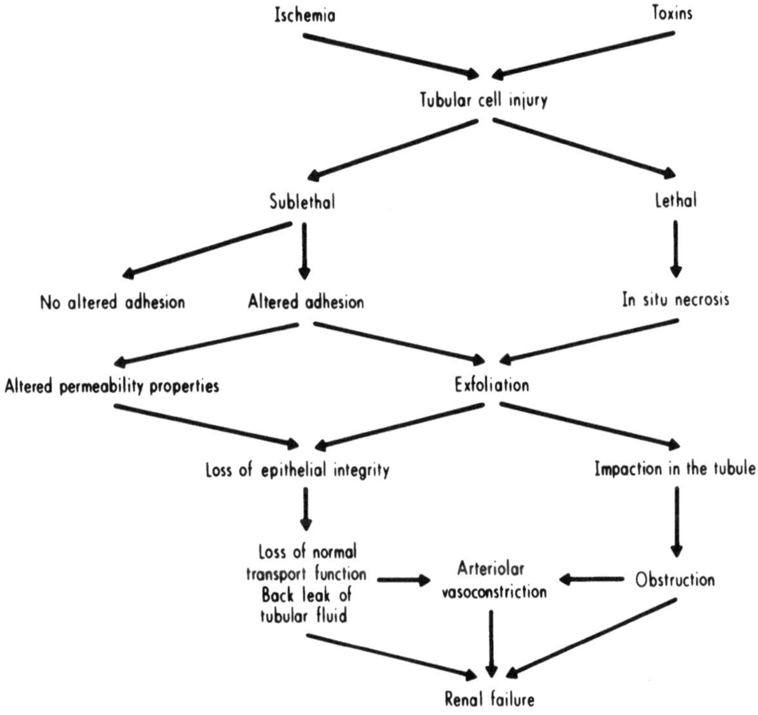

Fig. 5. Potential functional consequences of altered tubular cell adhesion. (From Racusen 1992, with permission)

One particularly useful finding on renal biopsy that is a hallmark of ATN of the ischemic type, and that is also a reliable finding in autopsy kidneys, is the presence of nucleated cells in the vasa recta (see Fig. 6). These cells are likely responding to endothelial injury, and there is evidence that they may themselves represent effector cells amplifying tubular injury. Interstitial inflammation and accumulation of leukocytes in the ascending vasa recta have been reported in clinical and experimental ATN of both ischemic and toxic origin. Solez et al. (1979) have shown that these accumulated cells correlated with renal dysfunction, as well as with tubular casts, tubular brush border loss, and tubular necrosis on histologic examination. There is experimental evidence that leukocytes/neutrophils exacerbate ischemic injury in the isolated perfused rat kidney (Linas et al. 1988), and neutrophil depletion in a nephrectomy/pedicle clamp model increased renal blood flow, lowered creatinine levels, and reduced histologic ATN, and at the same time reduced vasoconstrictor prostaglandin levels (Klausner et al. 1989). Following depletion of polymorphonuclear leukocytes (PMN) by anti-neutrophil serum, intrarenal neutrophils were reduced, as was transtubular leakage of insulin, and treated animals were able to produce a concentrated

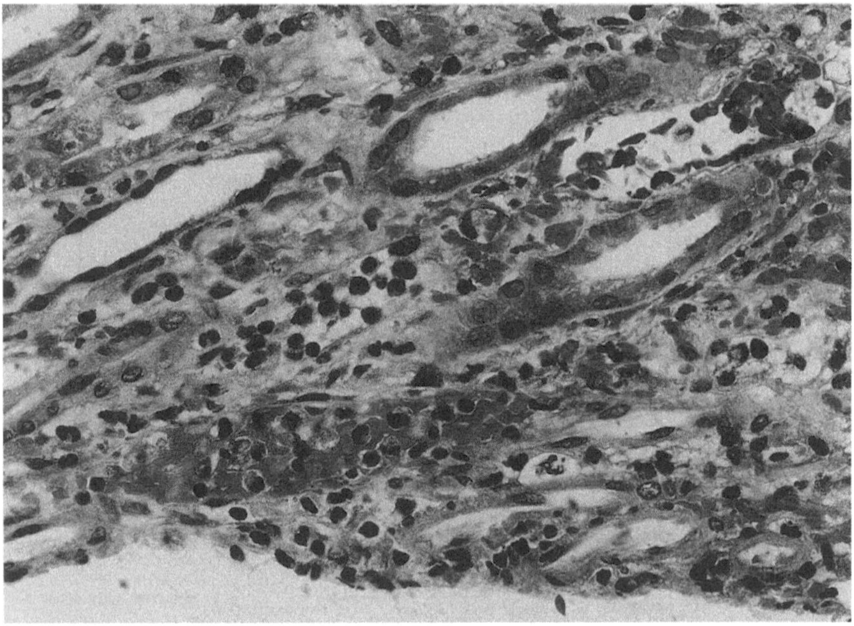

Fig. 6. Biopsy from a patient with acute renal failure showing nucleated cells in the vasa recta (×400)

urine (Klausner et al. 1989). One investigator, while unable to reduce postischemic injury by antineutrophil serum, found that nitrogen mustard was efficacious in improving inulin clearance without correlation with total neutrophil count, suggesting that other leukocytes may be involved in pathogenesis (Paller 1989). The cells in the vasa recta include monocyte/macrophages, and T and B lymphocytes following both clinical and experimental ATN (Solez et al. 1979).

On light microscopy, in addition to the various tubular changes described, mild glomerular changes may be detectable as well. These include wrinkling and collapse of glomerular capillary loops reflecting decreased perfusion. Tubularization of the epithelial cells lining Bowman's capsule may also be seen.

Using immunohistochemistry, it may be possible to identify alterations in cell cytoskeleton, including redistribution and/or altered expression of fodrin, actin, and vimentin with acute reversible injury (Kellerman and Bogusky 1992; Hansson et al. 1987; Witzgall et al. 1993; Younes et al. 1990) as well as redistribution of polarized membrane proteins such as Na:K ATPase (Molitoris et al. 1988). Enhanced expression of proliferation- and/or injury-associated proteins may also be detected as a marker of injury (Witzgall et al. 1993). These immunohistologic findings may ultimately prove useful as additional markers of sublethal cell injury, complementing light microscopy alone, where changes may be subtle.

Expression of injury-related proteins such as heat shock proteins may also be enhanced. Heat shock proteins are a highly conserved family of proteins induced by heat or cold (Tissiere et al. 1974; Muller-Taubenberger et al. 1988), toxins (Muller-Taubenberg et al. 1988; Levinson et al. 1979; Li 1983), drugs (Levinson et al. 1978), and anoxia (Dwyer et al. 1989). Some of these proteins are constitutively expressed in normal cells, and others are only expressed under conditions of cell stress (Lindquist and Craig 1988). These proteins are important in degradation of normal and abnormal proteins in cells, and in the molecular chaperoning for transport of constitutive proteins across internal cell membranes via the modulation of the tertiary structure of proteins (Pelham 1988). The 72-kDa heat shock protein has been detected by immunoblot analysis after at least 15 min of renal ischemia in the rat, reaching a maximum after 60 min; no HSP72 was detected after 90 min of ischemia or in the contralateral nonischemic kidney (Emami et al. 1991). This protein has also recently been demonstrated by immunohistochemistry in tubular cells in human kidneys with ischemic injury, acute tubulointerstitial nephritis, cytomegalovirus (CMV) infection, and analgesic nephropathy (Dodd et al. 1993). Increased synthesis of 70- and 90-kDa proteins also occurs after exposure to mercuric chloride; increased synthesis is dose related (Goering et al. 1992). These proteins may serve to mediate cell repair and/or increase resistance to subsequent injury by a variety of mechanisms (Clerget and Polla 1990; Donati et al. 1990; Polla and Kanatengwa 1991) and appear to be potentially useful biomarkers of renal cell injury.

By electron microscopy (EM), the ultrastructural correlates of light microscopic changes are seen. In addition, there are a number of structural changes only appreciable by EM. On scanning and/or transmission EM (TEM), loss of the microvillous brush border has been documented in experimental and clinical ischemic tubular injury (Jones 1979, 1982; Venkatachalam et al. 1981; Olsen and Hansen 1990). By TEM, the apical microvilli or fragments thereof can sometimes be seen in subapical cytoplasm (Venkatachalam et al. 1981). The simplification of the apical cell surface is mirrored by simplification of the complex basolateral membrane infoldings. Cell vacuoles may be seen to be collections of intracellular lipid, fluid vacuoles, and/or swollen endoplasmic reticulum. Mitochondrial changes, including swelling and some disruption of cristal structure, may also be seen with reversible injury; more severe changes reflect lethal injury (see below). Many of the clinical cases examined by EM in one series included cases with both ischemia and toxic exposure (Jones 1982). Glomeruli may show wrinkling of the glomerular basement membrane (GBM), collapse of capillary loops, and coarsening of epithelial cell foot processes, a finding which has been quantitated on scanning EM (SEM) and may reflect altered protein permeability (Solez et al. 1981).

Lethal Injury

By light microscopy, early changes in cells which have undergone irreversible injury may be indistinguishable from changes due to sublethal injury. Soon, however, cells manifest alterations which are recognizable as cell necrosis. The nucleus undergoes progressive changes from dense condensation (pyknosis), to breakdown of nuclear membranes and dispersion of chromatin karyorrhexis), to disappearance of recognizable nuclear material (karyolysis). The cells typically undergo coagulative necrosis with a sometimes swollen eosinpohilic cytoplasm (see Fig. 7). Some cells become densely eosinophilic. Ultimately, the cell membrane breaks down and the cell disintegrates. This type of necrosis ultimately results from membrane injury and elevated intracellular calcium (Farber 1982).

On EM, in addition to some of the changes described with sublethal injury, the nuclear disintegration described above can be documented in lethally injured cells undergoing coagulative necrosis. The cell cytoplasm becomes more rarefied as osmotic regulation is lost and water accumulates in the cell, and organelles disintegrate. The mitochondria show loss

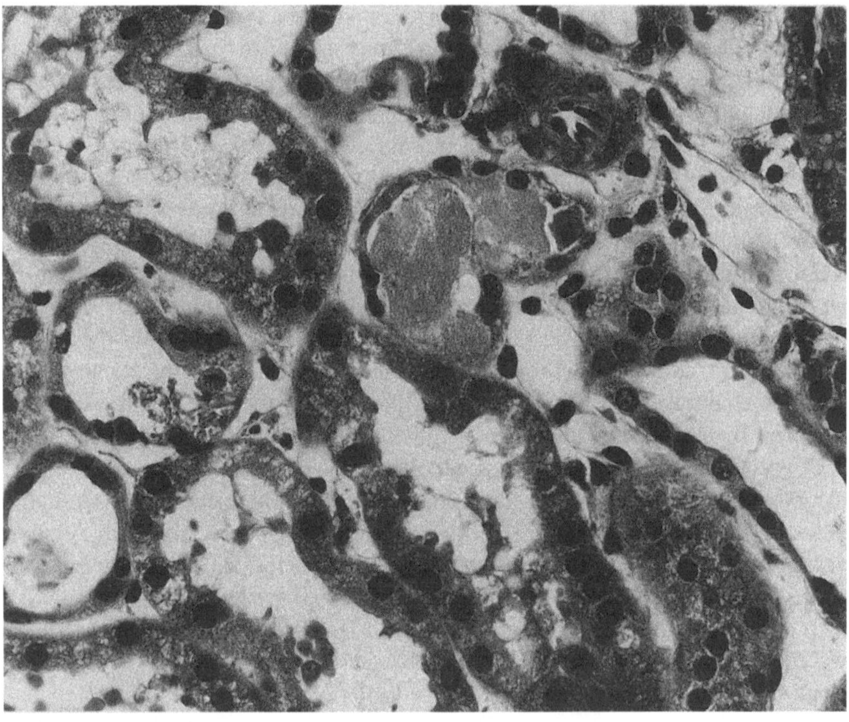

Fig. 7. Focal coagulative necrosis of tubular cells in a biopsy from a patient with toxic shock syndrome. Note also gaps in the epithelium, brush border loss, and surface blebbing (×400)

of cristae and formation of dense calcifications which ultimately fill the mitochondria.

Apoptosis

Apoptosis is a process of cell destruction producing cell death in a number of physiologic settings such as in embryogenesis and regulation of the immune system; in atrophy of tissues after trophic hormone withdrawal or after ischemic, toxic, or radiation injury; and in regression of hypertrophy (Kerr et al. 1972; Wyllie et al. 1980; Arends and Wyllie 1991). The DNA from apoptotic cells shows a characteristic degradation to oligonucleosomal fragments on gel electrophoresis (Wyllie et al. 1980; Arends et al. 1990). Apoptosis is an active process, dependent on protein synthesis in some cells (Wyllie et al. 1984; Shi et al. 1989). Apopotic cells may be removed via phagocytosis, with recognition of "self-senescence" mediated by the vitronectin receptor (Savill et al. 1990).

Morphologic changes with apoptosis in epithelial cells occur in three phases (Wyllie 1988). In the initial phase, chromatin is condensed at the periphery of the nucleus, the nucleolus disintegrates, and the nucleus shrinks. Total cell volume also decreases, cell density increases, and cytoplasmic organelles are compacted. Surface microvilli disappear and desmosomal attachments break down. In the second phase, nucleus and cytoplasm bud and separate into small membrane-bound "apopotic bodies." These bodies may be shed from the cell surface and/or phagocytosed. In the final phase, residual nuclear and cytoplasmic structures degenerate. Mechanisms leading to apoptosis may include influx of calcium ions (McConkey et al. 1989a,b). Altered expression of oncogenes has also been documented (Barnes 1988; Buttyan et al. 1988; Wyllie et al. 1987). Key cell proteins necessary for apoptosis to occur are calcium–magnesium endonuclease and gamma-glutamyltransferases (Wyllie 1980; Arends et al. 1990; Fesus and Thomazy 1988).

Apoptosis has been noted in renal tubular cells in clinical biopsies in ischemic renal injury (Olsen et al. 1989; Bonventre 1993) and experimentally in ischemic atrophy postobstruction and after lead nitrate-induced renal hypertrophy (Gobe and Axelsen 1987; Ledda-Columbano et al. 1989; Gobe et al. 1990). Gobe et al. (1990) induced renal artery stensosis by placing a partially occluding clip around the renal artery. During the first week, there was both necrosis and apoptosis of renal tubular epithelial cells. From 2–4 weeks, cell death continued only as apoptosis as the clipped kidney atrophied. With experimental acute ischemia and reperfusion following very brief renal ischemia (5 min of pedicle clamping), though no overt coagulative necrosis was detected, apoptosis was identified early in reperfusion (12 h) as well as at 24 and 48 h with longer periods (30 or 45 min) of pedicle clamping. With longer intervals of ischemia, overt cell necrosis was also seen (Schumer et al. 1992). The role of apoptosis in ischemic injury remains to be defined; there is some evidence that it may be more common in the transplant setting than in native kidney (Olsen et al. 1989). It may play a role especially in the maintenance phase and in epithelial "remodeling" after proliferative response to injury.

Renal Infarction/Cortical Necrosis

Renal infarction may occur in the critically ill patient and may be extensive enough to produce ARF. Patterns of infarction vary, depending on whether obstruction to flow is arterial or venous (Racusen and Solez 1994). Arterial obstruction may involve: (a) compromised flow in large vessels, generally due to spontaneous or iatrogenic embolization, spontaneous or traumatically induced thrombosis, or ostial occlusion; or (b) decreased flow in small arteries due to atheroembolic disease, thrombotic miroangiopathies, or sickle cell disease. Thrombosis of renal veins occurs in hypercoagulable states and thrombophlebitis and/or may be related to compression of the renal pedicle due to trauma, malignancy, or other causes.

Renal infarction must be extensive and/or bilateral to produce ARF. Emboli, which most often arise in the setting of cardiac diseases (Lessman et al. 1978), may be bilateral and may produce severe oliguria or acute anuria (Peterson and McDonald 1968); marked oliguria may also occur with unilateral embolization, presumably due to vasospasm in the contralateral kidney (Lessman et al. 1978). Thrombosis of the renal arteries, if bilateral, may also present with acute renal failure: the most common antecedents are trauma or preexisting vascular disease involving the renal artery or abdominal aorta (Peterson 1989; Stanley and Whitehouse 1984; Magilligan et al. 1975). Bilateral renal vein thrombosis may also occur and requires intervention to prevent infarction of renal parenchyma.

The pathology in these settings progresses from evidence of widespread tubular injury in affected areas to frank coagulative necrosis of the parenchyma. Two to four hours of warm ischemia in experimental animals seems to be the time point beyond which necrosis is inevitable (Hoffman et al. 1974); however, there are many clinical reports of recovery following delayed revascularization, perhaps related to collateral circulation. (Stables et al. 1976; Barry and Hodges 1978) If flow is restored promptly, evidence of lethal and sublethal tubular cell injury is seen to be followed by regenerative changes; interstitial hemorrhage may be seen in areas where flow resumes through injured vessels, and vascular thrombi may form. With collateral flow and/or in areas in which vessels remain patent, infarction is patchy, and a renal biopsy may reveal only tubular injury, interstitial hemorrhage, and/or an inflammatory infiltrate in zones adjacent to the infarcts. Infarction due to renal vein thrombosis, while similar in appearance, is usually hemorrhagic.

In thrombotic microangiopathy, infarcts occur but are usually small. On histologic examination, complex changes are seen, most of which result from endothelial cell injury in the setting of hemolytic uremic syndrome, thrombotic thrombocytopenic purpura, scleroderma, postpartum acute renal failure, or exposure to toxic drugs, especially cyclosporine or mitomycin (Heptinstall 1992; Remuzzi et al. 1994; Neild 1987). Changes seen include endothelial cell injury and proliferation, subendothelial widening in glomerular capillary loops, and expansion of the intima of smaller arteries by edema and an acid-mucopolysaccharide substance; mesangiolysis may occur, fibrinoid necrosis may be seen in small arteries, and microthrombi may form. Fragmented red blood cells may be seen in glomerular mesangium and in the wall of affected vessels. As noted, small cortical infarcts may also be seen.

Cortical necrosis, focal or global necrosis of renal cortical parenchyma, occurs in a variety of clinical settings (Racusen and Solez 1992; see Fig. 8) These include pregnancy-related conditions, such as abruptio placenta, or severe toxemia; with severe vascular insufficiency as seen in sepsis, hemor-

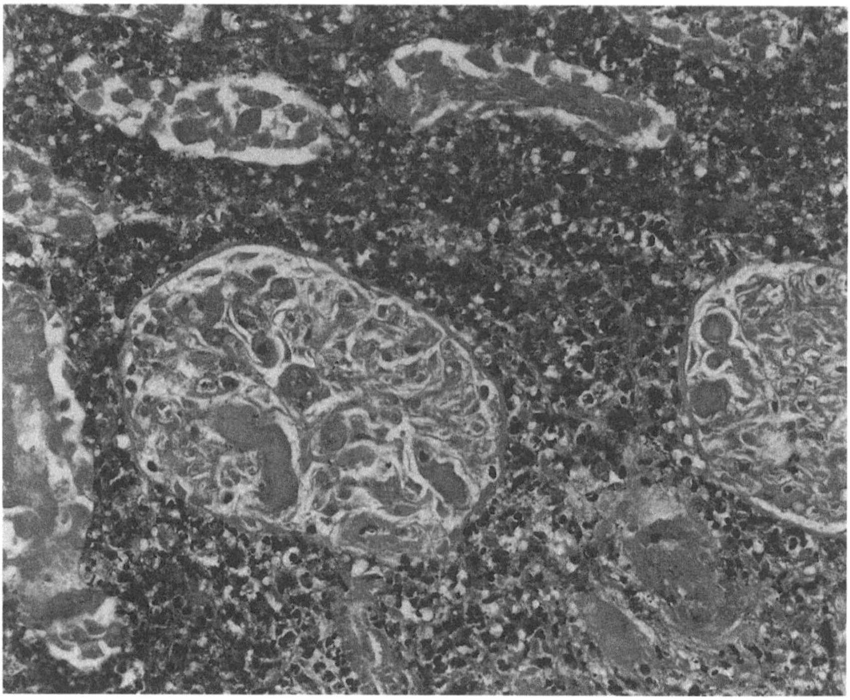

Fig. 8. Biopsy from a patient with cortical necrosis. Note glomerular thrombosis, interstitial hemorrhage and inflammation, and coagulative necrosis of the parenchyma (×220). (From Racusen and Solez 1994, with permission)

rhage, or severe dehydration; due to toxins and/or venoms; and in some cases of thrombotic microangiopathy (Chugh et al. 1983; Kleinknecht et al. 1973; Spiegel et al. 1992; George et al. 1987). While often diffuse, patchy and more focal forms have been recognized. In more focal forms, while proximal tubule injury is widespread, glomerular and vascular necrosis and thrombosis may be focal and distal tubules may be relatively spared; with diffuse involvement, necrosis is extensive though there is often sparing of the renal medulla and juxtamedullary and subcapsular cortex. Calcification develops in the necrotic cortex and provides a reliable radiologic sign of cortical necrosis; calcification may occur within 1–2 weeks.

Morphologic Findings in Specific Clinical Settings

While the general changes described above may be seen as the most typical findings in ARF in the critically ill, there may be additional pathologic features in specific clinical settings. We will here review briefly findings in the hepatorenal syndrome, sepsis, traumatic injury, and in recipients of solid organ allografts. We will also briefly describe changes due to nephrotoxic agents not directly injurious to the renal tubule, but which may contribue to ARF in the critically ill.

Hepatorenal Syndrome. Intense vasoconstriction can be seen on flow studies, and most cases of ARF in this setting appear to represent either severe "prerenal" failure, generally with preserved FeNa, or true ATN, as described above. Interestingly, in a small series of biopsies obtained from patients with hepatorenal syndrome very early postmortem, the changes of acute tubular injury described above were present despite normal FeNa in life. In addition, some findings were present that appear to be unique in this setting, including large leucine crystals in tubules, many bile-stained casts with associated polymorphonuclear leukocytes in the tubules, and coarse vacuoles and/or bile pigment in the cytoplasm of the tubular cells (Solez 1992). Glomerular abnormalities have been reported in many of the patients with native liver disease and hepatorenal syndrome (Eknoyan 1983), but these are minor and not severe enough to produce ARF.

Rhabdomyolysis. This may contribute to ARF in the critically ill. Traumatic injury producing the crush syndrome was first recognized during World War II (Bywaters and Beall 1941) and remains a cause of ARF largely in disaster settings. However, nontraumatic rhabdomyolysis with ARF may also occur as a sequel of coma, seizures, myopathies, or viral illness (Koffler et al. 1976). Alcoholism and drug abuse (Gabow et al. 1982), toxic shock syndrome (Bachhuber et al. 1983), Legionnaire's disease (Hall et al. 1983), or poisoning (Sanz et al. 1989) also may be antecedents. On morphologic examination, one sees acute tubular injury with myoglobin casts in tubules. Cocaine intoxication (Ahijado et al. 1990; Anard et al. 1989; Roth et al. 1988) as well as abuse of other drugs (Gabow et al. 1982; Ahijado et al. 1990; Patel and Connor 1986; Terada et al. 1988) may also produce acute rhabdomyolysis and a morphologic picture of acute tubular injury.

Nephrotoxic Drugs. Critically ill patients are often treated with a variety of nephrotoxic drugs administered as diagnostic or therapeutic agents. A number of these, including aminoglycosides, cephalosporines, and *cis*-platinum, may produce tubular injury analogous to that described above (see Table 1). Some may produce a morphologic picture with somewhat distinctive features. For example, with aminoglycoside nephrotoxicity, myeloid bodies may be seen in tubular cells by EM. Some general anesthetics such as methoxyfluorane and exposure to ethylene glycol can cause deposition of crystals in tubules (Racusen and Solez 1986). As described above, some drugs, including cyclosporine and mitomycin, may produce a picture of hemolytic uremic syndrome.

Other drugs produce a pattern of interstitial nephritis (see Table 2). The inflammatory infiltrate may be patchy or diffuse, and there may be associated tubular injury. Polymorphonuclear leukocytes and/or eosinophils are often

Table 1. Agents associated with acute tubular necrosis of the kidney (modified from Solez 1992)

Drugs	
Gentamicin	Methoxyflurane
Tobramycin	Halothane
Kanamycin	Glafenine
Amphotericin B	Sulfonamides
Polymyxins	Cephaloridine
Rifampicin	Cephalothin
Streptozotocin	Radiographic contrast material
cis-platinum	Ethylenediamine tetracetic acid (EDTA)
Gamma interferon	Quinine
Barbiturates, cocaine	
Germanium	
Gold	
Poisons	
Mercury, inorganic	Ethylene glycol, diethylene glycol, and polyethylene glycol
Bismuth	Insecticides
Carbon tetrachloride and other organic solvents	Diesel oil
Chromium	Multiple bee stings, scorpjon sting, snake bite
Arsenic	Mushroom poisoning, ingestion of poisonous fish or fish gallbladder
Phosphorus	
Potassium dichromate and chlorate	
Uranium	

Table 2. Drugs associated with acute interstitial nephritis (modified from Racusen and Solez 1986)

Common *causes*	*Rare causes*	
Methicillin	Penicillin G	Cotrimoxizole
Ampicillin	Oxacillin	Phenylbutazone
Rifampicin	Nafcillin	Phenazone
Phenindione	Carbenicillin	Diphenylhydantoin
Sulfonamides	Cephalexin	Phenobarbital
	Glafenine	Fenoprofen
	Allopurinol	Naproxen
	Thiazides	Diflunisal
	Furosemide	Ticrynafen
	Cephalothin	Sulindac
	Cimetidine	Azathioprine
	Ibuprofen	Zomepirac
	Tolmetin	

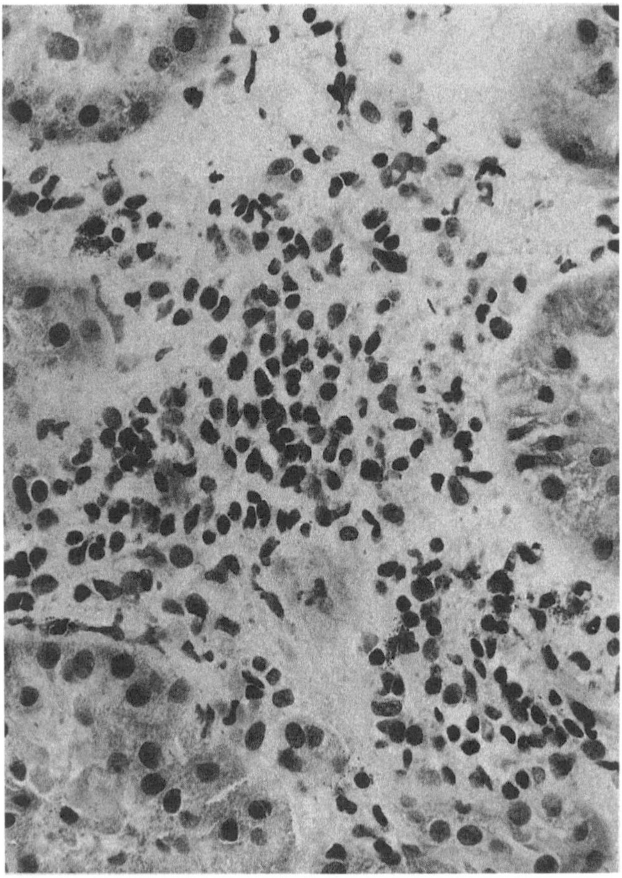

Fig. 9. Acute interstitial nephritis with eosinophils (×250)

present in these infiltrates, helping to differentiate drug-related interstitial nephritis from other causes (see Fig. 9).

Sepsis. In sepsis and especially with septic shock, acute tubular injury of the ATN type may occur. In addition, a variety of other changes may be seen. Systemic infection with septicemia may give rise to an acute interstitial nephritis with focal or diffuse infiltration by inflammatory cells, including numerous polymorphonuclear leukocytes. Localized microabscess may form; it may be possible to demonstrate bacteria or fungi in these abscesses. Other changes which may be seen in the kidney in septic patients include glomerular proliferative changes with immune deposits, intraglomerular thrombi, and/or drug-related charges produced by antibiotic agents used to treat the sepsis. As noted above, frank cortical necrosis may occasionally develop in septic patients.

Renal Transplant. The differential diagnosis of causes of acute renal dysfunction in renal transplant recipients is extensive and the morphologic changes potentially complex; these have been reviewed elsewhere (Porter 1992). The histologic changes of acute rejection have recently been standardized, and a working formulation for rejection grading in the kidney has been published (Solez et al. 1993a). ATN in the renal allograft has some morphologic features different from ATN in native kidneys, including more overt cell necrosis, sometimes involving entire tubular cross-sections, better preservation of apical brush border and basolateral infoldings, greater interstitial inflammation, and more calcium oxalate deposition (Olsen et al. 1989; Solez et al. 1993a). The pathology of nephrotoxic injury due to immunosuppressive agents, another major cause of ARF in this setting, is described below. In addition, thrombosis of the renal artery or vein may occur as a complication of the transplant surgery, and infarction may ensue if early intervention is not undertaken (see above).

Solid Organ Allografts. ARF may also be seen in patients receiving nonrenal solid organ allografts. In addition to findings described above related to poor cardiovascular status, hepatic dysfunction (hepatorenal syndrome), and/or supervening infection, the relatively high doses of immunosuppressive drugs used in these patients often produce altered renal function. Both cyclosporine and FK506, which are widely used in allograft recipients, affect GFR. Both agents affect arterioles, causing vasoconstriction via the vasoactive actions of renin–angiotensin, endothelin, platelet-activating factor, and/or transforming growth factor-β (TGF-β; Racusen and Solez 1992). Morphologically, in additon to ischemia-related changes such as collapse of glomerular capillary loops, there may be vacuolization of smooth muscle cells in the arterioles. Individual smooth muscle cells may become necrotic and hyalinize, resulting in nodular protein deposits in the wall of arterioles and small arteries, most characteristically in a peripheral pattern. Occasionally, vessels are narrowed by a mucoid thickening of the intima (Mihatsch et al. 1985). Occasional patients will develop a syndrome difficult to distingusih from hemolytic uremic syndrome, with marked intimal thickening of small vessels and entrapment of red cells and red cell fragments in the expanded intima, thrombi and fibrinoid necrosis of vessels. Glomeruli may appear ischemic or contain areas of segmental necrosis or be globally infarcted, and there may be parencyhmal infarcts related to this process as well. Tubular cells may show isometric vacuolization, giant mitochondria, and/or calcification (Mihatsch et al. 1985).

Morphologic Findings in Experimental Acute Renal Failure

Ischemic and toxic injury are the most common causes of clinical ARF of the ATN type, and experimental models have been developed for each of these. Many of the models, however, result in much more extensive tubular injury than is usually documented clinically. Moreover, it is not unusual in clinical settings to have injury due to a combination of factors, a scenario which has not been extensively modeled experimentally. Repetitive insults may also occur clinically and have variable impact on the tubular epithelium, since vulnerability to a second insult may be substantially altered by a preceding injury, depending importantly on time and nature of noxious events. Some studies looking at repetitive insults have been done, though more are needed.

The most widely used in vivo models of ischemic injury are renal artery or renal pedicle clamping and norepinephrine-induced vasoconstriction. Several species have been used; though the rat is the most commonly used, other species may actually represent better models of clinical ARF (Solez et al. 1977). Clamping/vasoconstriction, if prolonged, produces injury more severe and extensive than injury found clinically in typical ARF; shorter periods of clamping/vasoconstriction may be more analogous to the clinical state. However, most ischemic injury is due not to total cessation of flow (with some exceptions such as thromboembolic disease or surgical cross-clamping) but to hypoperfusion.

Zager (1987) has developed a hypoperfusion model, which is proposed to mimic clinical ATN more closely, in the rat. In this system, when the right kidney is removed and left renal perfusion pressure is lowered to 15–20 mmHg, there is less ATP depletion during ischemia, fewer casts, less medullary congestion, and less azotemia than is seen with equivalent periods of total artery occlusion. However, there is comparable tubular cell injury, oxidant stress, and postischemic ATP depletion in the two models. Twenty-four hours after 30 min of (unilateral) hypoperfusion, tubular necrosis was seen in a patchy distribution in outer medulla and inner medulla, primarily in S3; only minimal hyaline cast formation was seen. After 45 min, there was severe, widespread tubular necrosis in the outer stripe involving both proximal and distal tubule; patchy necrosis was also seen in the cortex and in the inner stripe, though less extensive than in the outer stripe. Necrotic tubular cell debris was seen in tubular lumina in the medulla. More subtle tubular cell changes such as those described above in typical clinical ATN were not described. This single hypoperfusion insult in an otherwise healthy animal, therefore, produces less renal dysfunction than would be predicted from the tubular injury, a situation opposite that seen in clinical specimens.

In the clinical setting, the etiology of renal tubular cell injury is often multifactoral, and some experimental studies have modeled combined insults. In in vivo studies it is difficult to define combined effects of injurious agents at the cellular level, since a number of critical variables including renal hemodynamics, circulating factors, the function of renal nerves etc. come into play in vivo. However, there is accumulating evidence that an initial injurious process may alter renal tubular cell response to subsequent injury. Previous injury may make renal tubular cells more or less susceptible to subsequent injury, depending on the experimental models being studied.

In vivo, Spiegel et al. (1990) have shown that a brief period of ischemia (15 min of renal pedicle clamping), not sufficient to produce overt cell injury in itself, predisposed the cells of the S_3 segment of the proximal tubule to injury when a single dose of gentamicin (100 mg/kg) was administered 4 h after ischemia, at a time when renal hemodynamics had normalized. The effect was associated with increased cortical uptake of gentamicin, but this effect did not appear to explain the potentiation. Zager (1988) reported a similar potentiation in the S_3 segment in vivo when renal hypoperfusion is combined with high-dose gentamicin. Obversely, sublethal nephrotoxic tubular injury may increase susceptibility to superimposed ischemia (Zager 1983).

Zager et al. (1985) have also shown that a mild ischemic insult (15 min of pedicle clamping) lowers resistance to a second ischemic insult (25 min of pedicle clamping), but only if the interval between the two insults is brief (30 min versus 210 min). This increased susceptibility was associated with tubular cell swelling and injury to the luminal membrane, and failure of ATP synthesis immediately following the second insult. With a more prolonged initial ischemic insult (40 min), there was resistance to a second ischemic insult 18–48 h later, apparently due at least in part to uremic solute loading (Zager et al. 1984).

While a previous insult appears to potentiate injury in some models, acquired resistance to ARF has also been demonstrated in others. While acquired resistance to a second insult may be due to hemodynamic and/or intraglomerular factors, tubular cells, and especially regenerated cells, themselves appear to be directly resistant to reinjury. Cross-resistance has not been demonstrated between ischemic and other models of ARF (Honda et al. 1987). However, cross-resistance has been described with uranium toxicity (MacNider 1929; Honda and Sudo 1982). A similar phenomenon has been described with the myoglobinuric glycerol model (Campbell 1958;

Westenfelder et al. 1982). It has been suggested that this resistance could be due to refractoriness of regenerated tubular cells to the influx of calcium (Honda et al. 1987), though clearly other mechanisms may be involved.

Future Directions

Important data on the morphologic changes in ARF in the critically ill, i.e., from renal biopsy, are not obtained frequently and probably will not be due to ethical considerations. In the absence of additional morphologic material from patients with ARF, especially in this setting, better models, particularly in vivo ones, need to be developed, models that mimic more closely typical clinical scenarios. In particular, better models of repeated and/or combined injuries are needed to define susceptibility and manifestations of cell injury/reinjury in these settings. Additional important factors that may contribute to ongoing injury in ARF patients on hemodialysis are the hemodynamic stress, complement activation, and cytokine release resulting from the dialysis itself, and this also needs to be carefully studied. The repair phase following injury also needs further investigation. Through study of these models, it may be possible to delineate important pathologic and pathophysiologic changes contributing to ARF in the critically ill and design new therapeutic strategies to enhance renal and patient recovery.

Acknowledgment. The authors wish to thank Ms. Kimberly Gill for typing this manuscript.

References

Ahijado F, de Vinuesa G, Luno J (1990) Acute renal failure and rhabdomyolysis following cocaine abuse. Nephron 54:268
Anard V, Siami G, Stone WJ (1989) Cocaine-associated rhabdomyolysis and acute renal failure. South Med J 82:67
Arends MJ, Wyllie AH (1991) Apoptosis. Int Rev Exp Pathol 32:223–254
Arends MJ, Morris RG, Wyllie AH (1990) Apoptosis. The role of the endonulease. Am J Pathol 136:543–608.
Bacallao R, Mandel L (1991) Internalizational of E-cadherin and NaK ATPase in cultured renal cells ocurs rapidly with energy depletion. J Am Soc Nephrol 2:643
Bachhuber R, Parker RA, Bennett WM (1983) Acute renal failure in toxic shock syndrome owing to rhabdomyolysis. Ann Clin Lab Sci 13:25–26
Banfi G, Tarantino A, Fogazzi GB, Mihatsch MJ, Ponticelli C (1985) Significance of vascular lesions in cyclosporine treated renal transplant. Kidney Int 28:392
Barnes DM (1988) Cells without growth factors commit suicide. Science 242:1510–1511
Barry JM, Hodges CV (1978) Revascularization of totally occluded renal arteries. J Urol 119:412–415
Bonventre JV (1993) Mechanisms of ischemic acute renal failure. Kidney Int 43:1160–1178
Brezis M, Rosen S, Silva P, Epstein FH (1984a) Selective vulnerability of the thick ascending limb to anoxia in the isolated perfused kidney. J Clin Invest 73:182–198

Brezis M, Rosen S, Silva P, Epstein FH (1984b) Transport activity modifies thick ascending limb damage in the isolated perfused kidney. Kidney Int 25:65–72

Brezis M, Shanley P, Silva P, Spokes K, Lear S, Epstein FH, Rosen S (1985) Disparate mechanisms for hypoxic cell injury in different nephron segments. J Clin Invest 76:1796–1806

Brezis M, Rosen S, Shanley P, Spokes K, Epstein FH (1986) Mitochondrial activity: a possible determinant of anoxic injury in renal medulla. Experentia 42:570–572

Buttyan R, Zakeri Z, Lockshin R, Wolgemuth D (1988) Cascade induction of c-fos, c-myc and heat shock 70K transcripts during regression of the rat ventral prostate gland. Mol Endocrinol 2:650–657

Bywaters EGL, Beall D (1941) Crush injuries with impairment of renal function. Br Med J 51:427

Campbell JAH (1958) Subcutaneous fat necrosis hemolysis without siderosis and renal tubular atrophy following repeated glycerol injection. J Pathol Bacteriol 126:473–481

Cantu TG, Hoehn-Saric EW, Burgess KM, Racusen LC, Scheel PJ (1994) Renal failure associated with immunoglobulin therapy. Am J Kidney Dis (in press)

Chugh KS, Singhl PC, Kher VK, Gupta VK, Malik GH, Narayan G, Datta BN (1993) Spectrum of acute cortical necrosis in Indian patients. Am J Med Sci 286:10–20

Clerget M, Polla BS (1990) Erythrophagocytosis induces heat shock protein synthesis by human monocytes-macrophages. Proc Natl Acad Sci USA 87:1081–1085

Dodd SM, Martin JE, Swash M, Mather K (1993) Expression of heat shock protein epitopes in renal disease. Clin Nephrol 39:239–244

Donati YR, Slosman DO, Polla BS (1990) Oxidative injury and the heat shock response. Biochem Pharmacol 50:2571–2577

Dwyer BE, Nishimura RN, Brown IR (1989) Synthesis of the major inducible heat shock protein in rat hippocampus after neonatal hypoxia-ischemia. Exp Neurol 104:28–31

Eknoyan G (1983) Glomerular abnormalities in liver disease. In: Epstein M (ed) The kidney in liver disease, 2nd edn. Elsevier, New York, pp 119–146

Emami A, Schwartz JH, Borkan SC (1991) Transient ischemia or heat stress induces a cytoprotectant protein in rat kidney. Am J Physiol 260:F479–F485

Farber JL (1982) Membrane injury and calcium homeostasis in the pathogenesis of coagulative necrosis. Lab Invest 47:114–123

Fesus L, Thomazy V (1988) Searching for the function of tissue transglutaminase: its possible involvement in the biochemical pathway of programmed cell death. Adv Exp Med Biol 231:119–134

Gabow PA, Kaehny WD, Kelleher SP (1982) The spectrum of rhabdomyolysis. Medicine (Baltimore) 61:141–152

Gailit J, Colflesh D, Rabiner I, Simone J, Goligorsky MS (1993) Redistribution and dysfunction of integrins in cultured renal epithelial cells exposed to oxidative stress. Am J Physiol 264:F149–F157

George A, Thasakas VT, Solez K (1987) Viper bite poisoning in India. A review with special reference to renal complications. Ren Fail 10:91–94

Gobe GC, Axelsen RA (1987) Genesis of renal tubular atrophy in the rat: role of apoptosis. Lab Invest 56:273–281

Gobe GC, Axelsen RA, Searle JW (1990) Cellular events in experimental unilateral ischemic renal atrophy and in regeneration after contralateral nephrectomy. Lab Invest 63:770–779

Goering PL, Fisher BR, Chaudhary PP, Dick CA (1992) Relationship between stress protein induction in rat kidney by mercuric chloride and nephrotoxicity. Toxicol Appl Pharmacol 113:184–191

Goligorsky MS, DiBona G (1993) Pathogenic role of Arg-Gly-Asp recognizing integrins in acute renal failure. Proc Natl Acad Sci USA 90(12):5700–5704

Goligorsky MS, Lieberthal W, Racusen L, Simon EE (1993) Integrin receptors in renal tubular epithelium: new insights into pathophysiology of acute renal failure. Am J Physiol 264: F1–F8

Graber M, Lane B, Lamina R, Pastoriza-Munoz E (1991) Bubble cells: renal tubular cells in the urinary sediment with characteristics of viability. J Am Soc Nephrol 1:999–1004

Guder WG, Ross BD (1984) Enzyme distribution along the nephron. Kidney Int 26:101–111

Gullans SR, Harris SI, Mandel LJ (1984) Glucose-dependent respiration in suspensions of rabbit cortical tubules. J Membr Biol 78:257–262

Hall SL, Wasserman M, Dahl L, Schubert T (1983) Acute renal failure secondary to myoglobinuria associated with Legionaire's disease. Chest 84:633–635

Hansson RB, Hansson HA, Jonsson O, Lindholm L, Pettersson S, Schersten T, Waldenstrom J (1987) Protection of renal cells against free radical damage in vitro. Am J Clin Pathol 87:601–607

Heptinstall RH (1992) Hemolytic uremic syndrome, thrombotic thrombocytopenic purpura, and systemic sclerosis. In: Heptinstall RH (ed) Pathology of the kidney, 4th edn. Little and Brown, Boston, p 1163

Hoffman RN, Stieper KW, Johnson RWG, Belzer FO (1974) Renal ischemic tolerance. Arch Surg 109:550–551

Honda N, Sudo M (1982) Resistance to uranylacetate-induced acute renal failure in rabbits: renal function and morphology. In: Eliahou HE (ed) Acute renal failure. Libbey, London, p 105

Honda N, Hishida A, Ikuma K, Yonemura K (1987) Acquired resistance to acute renal failure. Kidney Int 31:1233–1238

Houghton DC, Hartnett M, Campbell-Boswell M, Porter G, Bennett W (1976) A light and electron microscopic analysis of gentamicin nephrotoxicity in rats. Am J Pathol 82:589–612

Jones DB (1979) SEM of human and experimental renal disease. Scanning Electron Microsc 2:679–689

Jones DB (1982) Ultrastructure of human acute renal failure. Lab Invest 46:254–264

Kartha S, Toback FG (1992) Adenine nucleotides stimulate migration in wounded cultures of kidney epithelial cells. J Clin Invest 90:288–292

Kellerman PS, Bogusky RT (1992) Microfilament disruption occurs very early in ischemic proximal tubule cell injury. Kidney Int 42:896–902

Kellerman PS, Clark RAF, Hoilien CA, Linas SL, Molitoris BA (1990) Role of microfilaments in the maintenance of proximal tubule structural and functional integrity. Am J Physiol 259:F279–F285

Kerr JFR, Wyllie AH, Currie AR (1972) Apoptosis: a basic biological phenomenon with wide-ranging implications in tissue kinetics. Br J Cancer 26:239–257

Klausner JM, Paterson IS, Goldma G et al. (1989) Postischemic renal injury is mediated by neutrophils and leukotrienes. Am J Physiol 256:F794–F802

Kleinknecht D, Grunfeld JP, Gomez PC, Moreau JF, Garcia-Torres R (1973) Diagnostic procedures and long term prognosis in bilateral renal cortical necrosis. Kidney Int 4:390–400

Koffler A, Friedler RM, Massry SG (1976) Acute renal failure due to non-traumatic rhabdomyolysis. Ann Intern Med 85:23

Kroshian VM, Lieberthal W (1991) Sublethal injury induced by ATP depletion impairs cell adhesion in mouse proximal tubular cells. J Am Soc Nephrol 2:649

Ledda-Columbano GM, Columbano A, Coni P, Faa G, Pani P (1989) Cell depletion by apoptosis during regression of renal hyperplasia. Am J Pathol 135:657–662

Lessman RK, Johnson SF, Coburn JW, Kaufman JJ (1978) Renal artery embolism: clinical features and long-term followup in 17 cases. Ann Intern Med 89:477–482

Levinson W, Oppermann H, Jackson J (1978) Induction of four proteins in eukaryotic cells by thiosemicarbozone. Biochim Biophys Acta 518:410–412

Levinson W, Idriss J, Jackson J (1979) Metal binding drugs induce synthesis of four peptides in normal cells. Biol Trace Elem Res 1:15–23

Li GC (1983) Induction of thermotolerance and enhanced heat shock protein synthesis in Chinese hamster fibroblasts by sodium arsenite and by ethanol. J Cell Physiol 115:116–122

Linas SL, Shanley PF, Whittenburg D, Berger E, Repine JE (1988) Neutrophils accentuate ishemia-reperfusion injury in isolated perfused rat kidneys. Am J Physiol 255:F728–F735
Lindquist S, Craig EA (1988) The heat shock proteins. Annu Rev Genet 22:631–637
Logue VA, Nufse HM (1989) Cocaine-associated acute myoglobinuric renal failure. Am J Med 86:183
MacNider WDeB (1929) The functional and pathological response of the kidney in dogs subjected to a second subcutaneous injection of uranium nitrate. J Exp Med 49:411–431
Magilligan DJ Jr, DeWeese JA, May AG, Rob CG (1975) The occluded renal artery. Surgery 78:730–738
Mandel L, Bacallao R (1991) Alterations in the cytoskeleton and transepithelial resistance during ATP depletion in cultured renal epithelial cells. J Am Soc Nephrol 2:651
McConkey DJ, Hartzell P, Nicotera P, Orrenius S (1989a) Calcium activated DNA fragmentation kills immature thymocytes. FASEB J 3:1843–1849
McConkey DJ, Nicotera P, Hartzell P, Bolloma G, Wyllie AH, Orrenius S (1989b) Glucocorticoids activate a suicide process in thymocytes through an elevation of cytosolic Ca2+ concentration. Arch Biochem Biophys 269:365–370
Mihatsch MJ, Thiel G, Busler V, Ryffel B, Landmann J, von Overbech J, Zollinger HU (1985) Morphologic patterns in cyclosporin A treated renal transplant recipients. Transplant Proc 17:101–116
Molitoris BA, Hoilien CA, Dahl RH, Ahnen DJ, Wilson PD, Kim J (1988) Characterization of ischemia-induced loss of epithelial polarity. J Membr Biol 106:233–242
Muller-Taubenberger A, Hagmann J, Noegel A, Gerisch G (1988) Ubiquitin gene expression in dictyostelium is induced by heat and cold shock, cadmium, and inhibitors of protein synthesis. J Cell Sci 90:51–58
Neild G (1987) The haemolytic syndrome. A review. Q J Med 63:367–376
Oliver J, MacDowell M, Tracy A (1951) The pathogenesis of acute renal failure associated with truamatic and toxic injury. Renal ischemia, nephrotoxic damage and the ischemuric episode. J Clin Invest 30:1307–1339
Olsen TS, Hansen HE (1990) Ultrastructure of medullary tubules in ischemic acute tubular necrosis and acute interstitial nephritis in man. APMIS 98:1139–1148
Olsen TS, Burdick JF, Keown PA, Wallace AC, Racusen LC, Solez K (1989) Primary acute renal failure ("acute tubular necrosis") in the transplanted kidney: morphology and pathogenesis. Medicine (Baltimore) 68:173–187
Paller MS (1989) Effect of neutrophil depletion on ischemic renal injury in the rat. J Lab Clin Med 113:379–386
Patel R, Connor G (1986) A review of 30 cases of rhabdomyolysis-associated acute renal failure among phencyclidine users. Clin Toxicol 23:547
Pelham H (1988) Heat shock proteins; coming in from the cold. Nature 332:776–777
Peterson NE (1989) Review article. Traumatic bilateral renal infarction. J Truama 29:158–167
Peterson NE, McDonald NF (1968) Renal embolization. J Urol 100:140–145
Polla BS, Kanatengwa S (1991) Heat shock proteins and inflammation. Curr Top Microbiol Immunol 167:93–105
Porter K (1992) Renal transplantation. In: Heptinstall RH (ed) Pathology of the kidney, 4th edn. Little and Brown, Boston, p 1799
Racusen LC (1992) Alterations in tubular epithelial cell adhesion and mechanisms of acute renal failure. Lab Invest 67:158–165
Racusen LC (1994) Alterations in human proximal tubule cell attachment in response to hypoxia – role of microfilaments. J Lab Clin Med 123:357–364
Racusen LC, Solez K (1986) Nephrotoxic tubular and intersititial lesions: morphology and classification. Toxicol Pathol 14:45–57
Racusen L, Solez K (1992) Nephrotoxicity of cyclosporine and other immunosuppressive and immunotherapeutic agents. In: Hook J, Goldstein R (eds) Toxicology of the kidney, 2nd edn. Raven, New York, p 319

Racusen L, Solez K (1994) Renal infarction, cortical necrosis, and atheroembolic disease. In: Tisher CC, Brenner BM (eds) Renal pathology. Lippincott, Philadelphia, p 810

Racusen LC, Fivush BA, Li Y-L, Slatnik I, Solez K (1991) Dissociation of tubular cell detachment and tubular cell death in clinical and experimental "acute tubular necrosis." Lab Invest 64:546–556

Remuzzi G, Ruggenei P, Bertani T (1994) Thrombotic microangiopathy. In: Tisher CC, Brenner BM (eds) Renal pathology. Lippincott, Philadelphia, p 1154

Ross BD, Guder WG (1982) Heterogeneity and compartmentation in the kidney. In: Sies H (ed) Metabolic compartmentation. Academic, New York, p 363

Roth D, Alarcon FJ, Fernandez JA, Preston RA, Bourgoigne JJ (1988) Acute rhabdomyolysis associated with cocaine intoxication. N Engl J Med 319:673–677

Ruegg CE, Mandel LJ (1990) Bulk isolation of renal PCT and PST I. Glucose-dependent metabolic differences. Am J Physiol 259:F164–F175

Sanz P, Corbella J, Nogue S, Munne P, Rodriquez-Pazos M (1989) Rhabdomyolysis in fatal arsenic trioxide poisoning. JAMA 262:3271

Savill J, Dransfield I, Hogg N, Haslett C (1990) Vitronectin-receptor mediated phagocytosis of cells undergoing apoptosis. Nature 343:170–173

Schumer KM, Olsson CA, Wise GJ, Buttyan R (1992) Morphologic, biochemical and molecular evidence of apoptosis during the reperfusion phase after brief periods of renal ischemia. Am J Pathol 140:831–838

Shanley PF, Johnson GC (1989) Adenine nucleotides, transport activity and hypoxic necrosis in the thick ascending limb of Henle. Kidney Int 36:823–830

Shi Y, Sahai BM, Green DR (1989) Cyclosporin A inhibits activation-induced cell death in T-cell hybridomas and thymocytes. Nature 339:625–626

Solez K (1992) Acute renal failure. In: Heptinstall RH (ed) Pathology of the kidney, 4th edn. Little and Brown, Boston, p 1235

Solez K, Racusen LC (1993) Acute renal failure at a crossroads. In: Neild G, Bihari D (eds) Acute renal failure in intensive therapy unit. Springer, New York

Solez K, D'Agostini RJ, Stowowy L, Freedman MT, Scott WW Jr, Sieglman SS, Heptinstall RH (1977) Beneficial effect of propranolol in a histologically appropriate model of post-ischemic acute renal failure. Am J Pathol 88:163–192

Solez K, Morel-Maroger L, Sraer J-D (1979) The morphology of "acute tubular necrosis" in man: analysis of 57 renal biopsies and a comparison with the glycerol model. Medicine (Batimore) 58:362–376

Solez K, Racusen LC, Whelton A (1981) Glomerular epithelial cell changes in early postischemic acute renal failure. Am J Pathol 103:163–173

Solez K, Axelsen RA, Benediktsson H et al. (1993a) International standardization of nomenclature and criteria for the histologic diagnosis of renal allograft rejection: the Banff working classification of kidney transplant pathology. Kidney Int 44:411–422

Solez K, Racusen LC, Marcussen N, Slatnik I, Keown P, Burdick J, Olsen S (1993b) Morphology of ischemic acute renal failure, normal function, and cyclosporine toxicity in cyclosporine-treated renal allograft recipients. Kidney Int 43:1058–1067

Spiegel DM, Shanley PF, Molitoris BA (1990) Mild ischemia predisposes the S3 segment to gentamicin toxicity. Kidney Int 38:459–464

Spiegel RA, Tomori O, Nasidi A, Auerbach S, Noji E (1992) Acute renal failure following ingestion of contaminated paracetamol syrup, Nigeria. Ren Fail 14:107–110

Stables DP, Fouch RF, DeVillers van Niekirk JP, Cremin BJ, Holt SA, Peterson NE (1976) Traumatic renal artery occlusion: twenty-one cases. J Urol 115:229–233

Stanley JC, Whitehouse WM Jr (1984) Occlusive and aneurysmal disease of the renal arterial cirrulation. Dis Mon 30:1–62

Terada Y, Shinohara S, Matui N, Takashi I (1988) Amphetamine-induced myoglobinuric acute renal failure. Jpn J Med 27:305–308

Tissiere A, Mitchell HK, Tracy UM (1974) Protein synthesis in salivary glands of Drosophila melanogaster; relation to chromosome puffs. J Mol Biol 84:389–398

Troyer D, Kreisberg J, Venkatachalam M (1982) Role of calcium in plasma membrane blebbing and cell death in a kidney epithelial cell line after toxin exposure. Kidney Int 21:207

Uchida S, Endou H (1988) Substrate specificity to maintain cellular ATP along the mouse nephron. Am J Physiol 255:F977–F983

Venkatachalam MA, Bernard DB, Donohoe JD, Levinsky NG (1978) Ischemic damage and repair in the rat proximal tubule. Differences among the S1, S2, and S3 segments. Kidney Int 14:31–49

Venkatachalam MA, Jones DB, Rennke HG, Sandstrom D, Patel Y (1981) Mechanism of proximal tubule brush border loss and regeneration following mild renal ischemia. Lab Invest 45:355–365

Westenfelder C, Crawford PA, Hamburger PK, Baranowski RL, Kurtzman NA (1982) Tubular function in glycerol-induced acute renal failure in rats: effects of saline loading and prior acute renal failure. Clin Sci 62:667–676

Wilson PD, Schrier RW (1986) Nephron segments and calcium as determinants of anoxic cell death in renal culture. Kidney Int 29:1172–1179

Witzgall R, Brown D, Schwarz C, Bonventre JV (1993) Localization of PCNA, vimentin, clusterin, and c-fos in post-ischemic kidneys. Evidence for a large pool of mitotically active and dedifferentiated cells. J Am Soc Nephrol 4:747

Wyllie AH (1980) Glucocorticoid-induced thymocyte apoptosis associated with endogenous endonuclease activation. Nature 284:555–556

Wyllie AH (1988) Apoptosis. Immunology 1:192–196

Wyllie AH, Kerr JFR, Currie AR (1980) Cell death: the significance of apoptosis. Int Rev Cytol 68:251–306

Wyllie AH, Morris RG, Smith AL, Dunlop D (1984) Chromatin cleavage in apoptosis: association with condensed chromatin morphology and dependence on macromolecular synthesis. J Pathol 142:67–77

Wyllie AH, Rose KA, Morris RG, Stell CM, Foster E, Spandidos DA (1987) Rodent fibroblast tumors expressing human myc and ras genes: growth, metastasis, and endogenous oncogene expression. Br J Cancer 56:251–259

Younes M, Doce S, Taylor K, True L (1990) Redistribution of fodrin is a marker of acute tubular necrosis. Lab Invest 62:109

Zager RA (1983) Gentamicin increases renal susceptibility to an acute ischemic insult. J Lab Clin Med 101:670–678

Zager RA (1987) Partial aortic ligation – a hypoperfusion model of ischemic acute renal failure and a comparison to renal artery occlusion. J Lab Clin Med 110:396–405

Zager RA (1988) Gentamicin nephrotoxicity in the setting of acute renal hypoperfusion. Am J Physiol 254:F574–F581

Zager RA, Johannes GA, Sharma HM (1983) Organic anion infusions exacerbate experimental acute renal failure. Am J Physiol 244:F48–F55

Zager RA, Baltes LA, Sharma HM (1984) Responses of the ischemic acute renal failure kidney to additional ischemic events. Kidney Int 26:689–700

Zager RA, Jurkowitz MS, Merola AJ (1985) Responses of the normal rat kidney to sequential ischemic events. Am J Physiol 249:F148–F159

Zager RA, Teubrer EJ, Adler S (1987) Low molecular weight proteinuria exacerbates experimental ischemic renal injury. Lab Invest 56:180–188

Experimental Acute Renal Failure

J.P. Johnson and M.D. Rokaw

Introduction

Acute renal failure (ARF) has been studied in the laboratory for many years in an attempt to define its pathophysiologic mechanisms and to define possible therapies to either prevent, reverse, or ameliorate the process. Like its clinical counterpart, experimental ARF is characterized by considerable heterogeneity and model to model variation as well as a number of unifying characteristics. This chapter will review the relevant model systems and describe current thoughts on the mechanisms of vascular and tubular cell injury in experimental ARF with a particular view to highlighting clinically relevant observations. Many agents have been described which moderate injury in the experimental setting, but few have so far moved into practical usage and it is commonly observed that clinical outcomes in ARF have improved little in recent decades. Nevertheless, a number of observations from the experimental literature suggest promising avenues for clinical trials, and these will be reviewed in the final section.

Model Systems

Studies of the pathophysiology and treatment of acute renal failure have been carried out at virtually all levels of complexity, ranging from intact animal models to preparations of isolated mitochondria (Table 1). Each system of study has its own peculiar advantages and disadvantages. Intact animal studies most closely mimic the interplay of local and systemic factors, but are complicated by the need to control many such factors in order to study a single intervention or process. Isolated perfused kidneys preserve the architectural complexity of the organ while giving greater control over systemic factors. Isolated tubule preparations allow for direct study of effects on cellular metabolism and function, but eliminate the ability to examine the relation between vascular and tubular function. Cell cultures derived from tubular epithelial cells permit precise control of cellular environments, but are hampered by the fact that cells in culture often differ from cells in vivo, particularly in their metabolic requirements. Isolated subcellular fractions such as mitochondria give the greatest control over experimental conditions,

Table 1. Model systems for the study of acute renal failure (ARF)

- Whole animal models
  - Ischemic ARF
    - Renal artery cross-clamping
    - Norepinephrine infusion
  - Nephrotoxic ARF
    - Heavy metal (mercuric chloride, uranyl nitrate, *cis*-platinum, potassium dichromate)
    - Antibiotic (aminoglycoside, amphotericin)
  - Pigment
    - Glycerol
    - Hemoglobin or myoglobin infusion
  - Mixed
    - Endotoxin plus sublethal hemorrhage
    - Aminoglycoside plus sublethal hemorrhage
    - Other combinations of the above
- Isolated perfused kidney
  - Perfused with hypoxic perfusate
  - Dye plus hypoxia
- Isolated tubule preparations
- Renal epithelial cells in culture
- Subcellular fractions (membranes, organelles)

but their study involves significant assumptions concerning intracellular conditions in vivo. The ideal study would combine the various model systems and be able to demonstrate a pathologic process or treatment effect over the range of models. This has rarely been achieved.

Animal Models: Pathophysiology

The most common model system for study of experimental acute renal failure is the intact animal (rat, rabbit, and dog). The hallmark of these studies, considered as a whole, is heterogeneity. Nevertheless, as in clinical acute renal failure, certain common features are apparent. All models are characterized by an acute decline in glomerular filtration rate (GFR), histologic evidence of tubular cell necrosis in varying segments, and eventual recovery if the animal does not die. This course is generally conceptualized as existing in three phases (Brezis et al. 1991). The first phase is the induction phase, in which the kidney responds to the ischemic or toxic insult by an acute decline in blood flow and filtration rate. This may extend for hours depending on the model. In the maintenance or established phase, whole organ blood flow returns towards normal, but glomerular filtration remains depressed. Conceptually, tubular cell necrosis in some manner maintains the loss of functional filtration. This phase lasts several days to weeks, depending on the severity of the insult. Finally, there is the recovery

Table 2. Model variations in pathophysiology

Model	Initiation phase	Maintenance
Ischemia	Decreased RBF	Decreased K_f Obstruction, backleak (prolonged)
Pigment	Decreased RBF	Obstruction
Mercuric Chloride	Backleak	Backleak
Uranyl nitrate	Decreased K_f	Backleak, obstruction (?)
Aminoglycoside	Decreased K_f, decreased RBF (high dose)	Backleak (high dose)

RBF, renal blood flow; K_f, glomerular permeability.

phase, in which filtration returns towards normal accompanied by histologic evidence of tubular cell regeneration. This phase is typically rapid lasting several days.

Whole animal ARF models are typically characterized in terms of the mechanisms which occur during their initiation and maintenance phases (Hostetter and Brenner 1988). Broadly speaking, these may be considered as several possible, mutually nonexclusive events. Glomerular filtration may be suppressed due to: (a) decreased glomerular filtration pressure due to diminished blood flow and/or increased preglomerular resistance; (b) decreased glomerular permeability (conceptualized as K_f), due to decreased surface area or decreased conductivity of the membrane; (c) increased tubular pressures due to tubular obstruction from cellular debris; (d) backleak of filtrate due to loss of epithelial integrity of the tubules. Table 2 reviews some of the more classical models of experimental ARF, largely from the rat, and indicates the mechanisms thought to predominate in each during induction and maintenance phases of acute renal failure. Inspection of Table 2 indicates that the same pathophysiologic processes may be involved to a differing extent depending on the model of ARF.

Ischemic Acute Renal Failure

Ischemic ARF, either induced by clamping of the renal arteries or by intrarenal infusion of norepinephrine, is clearly initiated by a reduction in blood flow. Following the initial insult, renal blood flow does not return to normal but remains suppressed by 50% or more for up to 24 h (Daugharty et al. 1974; Arendshorst et al. 1975; Kashgarian et al. 1976; Williams et al. 1981). Subsequently, whole organ blood flow may return towards normal over a period of days while GFR remains depressed (Williams et al. 1981). Efforts to return renal blood flow to normal levels several hours after ischemia by the infusion of vasodilators can produce relatively normal rates of perfusion, but do not alter the course of ARF (Reineck et al. 1980; Riley 1978). Several conclusions may be drawn from these observations. First, though ischemia is (by definition) the initiating event, reductions in whole organ renal blood flow after the insult are significantly less than the reductions in GFR. This suggests that other factors may be involved even during the initiation phase. Reduction in glomerular permeability (K_f) has been demonstrated by several groups (Baylis et al. 1977; Williams et al. 1981) along with morphologic evidence of glomerular ultrastructural changes (Solez et al. 1981; Stein and Sorkin 1976; Cronin et al. 1978). These findings have generally been interpreted to represent a decrease in surface area for filtration due to hormonally mediated glomerular constriction (Daugharty et al. 1974). Alternatively, the regional pattern of blood flow may be of greater significance than the overall reduction of flow to the organ. A number of studies using differing techniques have demonstrated a greater than 50% diminution of blood flow to the medulla and a marked reduction in perfusion of corticomedullary nephrons (Diethelm and Wilson 1971; Summers and Jamison 1971; Frega et al. 1976). This is an area where regional oxygenation is already known to be marginal with respect to metabolic demand, and Brezis and colleagues (Brezis et al. 1984) have suggested that reduction in blood flow to this area in particular is a major factor in the development of tubular necrosis. By contrast, the inner medulla is congested with increased blood flow following reperfusion, and this leads to medullary congestion and stagnation of blood flow, which may ultimately result in further damage (Olof et al. 1991). The observation that return of blood flow to normal 24–48 h following ischemic insult does not reverse the process of ARF suggests that continuing ischemia is probably not a major factor in the maintenance phase.

Convincing evidence for both tubular obstruction and backleak has been demonstrated during the maintenance phase of ischemic ARF. Stop-flow pressures measured by micropuncture techniques have usually, but not always, demonstrated increased intratubular pressures compatible with obstruction (Tanner and Steinhausen 1976; Mason et al. 1977). Morphologic studies repeatedly demonstrate tubule lumens occluded by debris of damaged cells (Reimer et al. 1972; Glaumann et al. 1975; Glaumann and Trump 1975). Studies with microinjected inulin or horseradish peroxidase demonstrate both delays in excretion typical of obstruction (Yagil et al. 1988) and incomplete recovery typical of backleak of filtrate (Donohoe et al. 1978; Tanner and Steinhausen 1976). So in ischemic ARF it appears that although the initial insult is decreased blood flow, very soon after initiation the pattern of injury is dominated by tubular cell damage with some unknown contribution from continuing regional ischemia.

Heavy Metal-Induced Acute Renal Failure

Several models of toxic ARF induced by heavy metals also induce early declines in renal blood flow. Both uranyl nitrate and mercuric chloride result in declines in whole kidney and cortical blood flow during the initiation phase, though this effect is more profound with uranyl nitrate (Flamenbaum et al. 1972a; Kleinman et al. 1975) than with mercuric chloride (Solez et al. 1976; Vanholder et al. 1982). In both models, fall in GFR is out of proportion to decline in blood flow (Kleinman et al. 1975; Vanholder et al. 1982), and restoration of blood flow by vasodilators does not alter the course of ARF (Mauk et al. 1977; Flamenbaum et al. 1976). K_f has been measured in both models and found to be markedly reduced in uranyl nitrate model (Blantz et al. 1985) and minimally reduced in mercuric chloride (Bulger et al. 1983). Although morphologic studies show severe damage to tubular epithelial cells in both models and debris in tubules, functional evidence for intratubular obstruction is not compelling (Flanigan and Oken 1965; Flamenbaum et al. 1972b). Evidence of dose-dependent backleak can be demonstrated in both models, consistent with the degree of tubular cell necrosis (Olbricht et al. 1977; Bank et al. 1967).

Pigment-Induced Acute Renal Failure

These models may be contrasted with myohemoglobinuric models of ARF, either induced by infusion of pigments or, more commonly, by glycerol injection. Glycerol injection into a hind limb produces both rhabdomyolysis and myoglobinuria, but also a severe inflammatory reaction resulting in volume depletion of the animal. The earliest renal effect is a marked reduction in renal blood flow with a nearly parallel decline in GFR (Kurtz et al. 1976; Chedru et al. 1972). Restoration of blood flow by volume expansion results in amelioration of ARF, suggesting that in this model decreased perfusion is of major pathophysiologic significance during initiation. During maintenance phase, however, there is less consistent decrease in renal blood flow, and the pathologic and functional picture is dominated by the appearance of intratubular casts of precipitated pigment and a clear pattern of intratubular obstruction (Oliver et al. 1951).

Aminoglycoside-Induced Acute Renal Failure

Aminoglycoside nephrotoxicity has been widely studied. It is apparent that these nephrotoxins directly affect tubular cell metabolism (Weinberg and Humes 1980) and induce tubular cell damage (Humes 1988). Early in the course of ARF there is also a marked reduction in renal blood flow with an even greater reduction in GFR. Marked declines in K_f have been measured under these circumstances and this appears to play a major role, at least during the initiation phase (Baylis et al. 1977; Chonko et al. 1979). As in humans, aminoglycoside toxicity is dose dependent, and some agents are more nephrotoxic than others.

Mixed Models

Finally, a number of interesting models examine the interactions of multiple insults in the generation of ARF (Zager 1992). Since it is rare to identify a single cause of ARF in most clinical settings, these models may actually be closer to mimicking the true state of ARF than the single insult models reviewed above. A variety of investigators have demonstrated that individual insults to the kidney may be additive or even synergistic in producing ARF. Endotoxemia, developed by infusion of *Escherichia coli* endotoxin, combines with minimal ischemia to produce profound ARF where neither insult results in ARF when given alone (Zager 1986). Similarly, ischemia and endotoxemia both have been shown to exacerbate the course of aminoglycoside-induced ARF (Zager 1983, 1986). Hyperthermia has also been shown to exacerbate ischemic ARF (Zager et al. 1991a). On the whole, these interactions appear to be mediated by enhanced toxicity at the cellular level, through mechanisms described below. These experiments also suggest a significant role for cytokines, elaborated locally or systemically in response to endotoxins, in the pathogenesis of ARF. This fascinating possibility is just beginning to be explored.

The classic formulation of experimental ARF into initiation and maintenance phases dominated by injury due to either vascular or tubular cell events does not result in a clear and unifying understanding of the pathophysiology of ARF. Clearly, the events which produce ARF vary somewhat from model to model and throughout the evolution of ARF in any single model. It is not therefore possible at this time to pinpoint any single, potentially reversible step as the cause of ARF. Vascular events and reduced or redistributed renal blood flow often predominate during the initiation phase of ARF. Tubular cell necrosis and its consequences (backleak, obstruction) seems to predominate during maintenance phases when renal blood flow returns towards normal. Since no single satisfying mechanism can be described, it is necessary to review the multiple mechanisms proposed for mediating the vascular and cellular phenomena in experimental ARF. What should emerge from this review is the central concept that prevention of tubular cell injury or enhancement of tubular cell recovery (or regeneration) offer the best hope for altering the course of experimental ARF.

Mechanisms of Injury

Vascular Factors

Diminished renal blood flow and redistribution of blood flow away from glomeruli associated with increased renal vascular resistance is typical of the initiation phases of most models of ARF. The course of ARF can be related to the extent and severity of renal ischemia (Donohoe et al. 1978), and sublethal ischemia may be additive to other insults (Spiegel et al. 1990; Zager 1992). The mediators of this renal vasoconstriction have been intensely studied.

Renin–Angiotensin System

The renin–angiotensin system is activated in virtually all forms of experimental ARF. Ischemia is known to be a major influence on renin secretion (Ochoa et al. 1970; Brown et al. 1972), but intrarenal and juxtaglomerular apparatus renin concentrations have also been shown to be elevated in toxic models of ARF, including mercuric chloride (Mathews et al. 1974), uranyl nitrate (Flamenbaum et al. 1972b), and glycerol (DiBona and Sawin 1971). Similar elevations in circulating renin and angiotensin II have been described in clinical ARF (Brown et al. 1970). Angiotensin, either systemically or

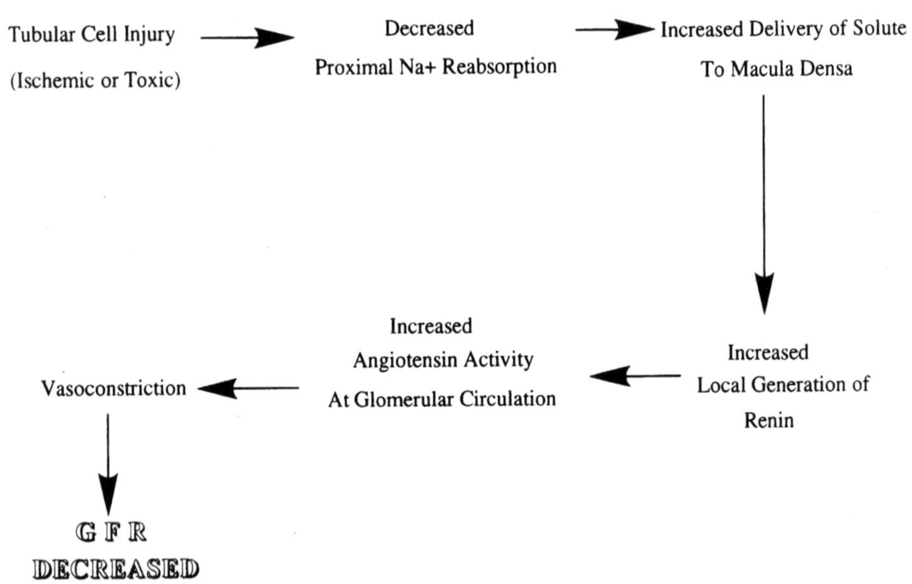

Fig. 1. Tubuloglomerular feedback. GFR, glomerular filtration rate

generated locally, is envisaged as leading to intense glomerular vasoconstriction, resulting in either a fall in GFR due to decreased plasma flow, to mesangial cell contraction leading to decreased K_f, or a combination (Thurau and Boylan 1976). The rise in renin–angiotensin activity could either be a direct result of ischemia or secondary to activation of tubuloglomerular feedback (McDonald et al. 1969). Tubuloglomerular feedback (see Fig. 1) is activated by increased solute delivery to the macula densa as a result of decreased proximal reabsorption by injured tubule segments. Local angiotensin is then released and a vicious circle is initiated which results in further declines in glomerular filtration and more intense local ischemia (Flamenbaum et al. 1973, 1976). In support of this hypothesis, it has been observed in many models of ARF that reduction of intrarenal renin content by prior volume expansion reduces the severity of ARF (Dibona et al. 1971; Ryan et al. 1973; Bidani et al. 1978). This attractive theory, however, has not proven to be entirely satisfactory in explaining the vascular abnormalities in ARF. Attempts to inhibit this pathway with either renin antibodies (Flamenbaum et al. 1972b; Oken et al. 1975) or angiotensin II inhibitors have been generally unsuccessful in terms of reversing ARF or even blocking its generation (Baehler et al. 1978; Bidani et al. 1979; Hollenberg et al. 1988). Although the renin–angiotensin system is clearly activated during ARF, other factors must coexist (Spielman and Osswald 1979).

Adenosine

Adenosine is a potent renal vasoconstrictor whose levels may well be elevated following renal injury. The source of increased adenosine presumably is from the breakdown of purine nucleotides in metabolically damaged cells (Miller et al. 1978). The major evidence that adenosine may be involved in reduced renal blood flow in ARF comes from studies involving inhibitors of adenosine action. Both broad inhibitors of adenosine receptor binding such as theophylline (Lin et al. 1986; Bidani and Churchill 1983) and more specific A_1 receptor antagonists (Bowmer et al. 1988; Kellett et al. 1988) have been shown to blunt the reduction of renal blood flow in early experimental ARF and to decrease the severity of injury. Similar findings have been generated concerning endothelin. This potent vasoconstrictor, locally produced in endothelial cells, is abundant in the kidney (Kon et al. 1989; Zeidel et al. 1989) and can be shown to increase in the kidney following ischemic injury (Shibouta et al. 1990). In addition, several groups have now shown that endothelin receptor antagonists, when given prior to or throughout the course of ischemic ARF, will blunt the severity of the injury (Kon and Badr 1991; Chan et al. 1994), suggesting that this mediator is of importance in the maintenance of local renal ischemia. Unfortunately, these agents are not particularly efficacious when given following the induction of ARF.

Other Vasoactive Substances

Intense renal vasoconstriction during ARF may also be due to loss of vasodilatory action from endogenous vasodilators such as prostaglandins and nitrous oxide. Infusions of prostaglandins have variable efficacy in promoting return of GFR (Mauk et al. 1977; Neumayer et al. 1985; Finn et al. 1987; Lifschitz and Barnes 1984). Tubular as well as vascular effects of prostaglandins have been proposed (Paller and Manivel 1992). It does seem apparent that the normal balance between vasoconstrictor and vasodilator substances within the renal circulation is disrupted during induction of ARF, but no single reversible step has been identified which can be successfully manipulated in multiple models of ARF.

Autoregulatory Responses

Recently a number of investigators have pointed out that the normal autoregulatory response of the renal circulation which serves to maintain glomerular blood flow over broad ranges of perfusion pressure is impaired well into the maintenance phase of acute renal failure (Adams et al. 1980; Williams et al. 1981; Kelleher et al. 1987). The mechanism of this loss of autoregulatory control is not known, but the clinical implications seem clear. A kidney which cannot autoregulate would be particularly susceptible to repeated injury during the fluctuations in blood pressure so commonly seen during the clinical course of ARF. Conger and Hammond (1992) have suggested that this phenomenon may be responsible for the protracted course and variably fresh patterns of injury seen in many cases of human ARF.

Cell swelling of endothelial cells has long been proposed as a possible mechanism of increased vascular resistance during induction of ARF (Flores et al. 1972), and this has been suggested as the site of action of impermeant solutes such as mannitol which appear to blunt the course of ARF when given before the insult (Morris et al. 1972). Cell swelling is, however, also a prominent feature in tubular epithelial cells, and the relevant site of action of impermeant solutes remains a subject of dispute (B. Glaumann et al. 1977; G. Glaumann et al. 1977). Protection afforded by these agents is not complete (Hanley and Davidson 1981; Burke et al. 1980; Schrier et al. 1984; Zager et al. 1991b) and is of limited value when they are given following an ischemic or toxic insult.

Redistribution of Blood Flow

An interesting aspect of blood flow during ischemic episodes is the regional distribution within the kidney. Virtually all methods demonstrate marked reductions in cortical perfusion, but vascular phemonema within the medulla are somewhat less clear (Olof et al. 1991). Careful measurements employing laser-Doppler flowmetry and isotopically labeled red blood cells (RBC) indicate that outer medullary blood flow may be less severely reduced while inner medullary blood flow may be increased relative to the normal state (Mason et al. 1984, 1989). This appears to be due to shunting of blood to the inner medulla as a result of sludging or trapping of RBC in the congested circulation of the outer medulla (Olof 1991; Hellberg et al. 1991; Vetterlein et al. 1986) as medullary blood flow may be returned to normal by hemodilution (Hellberg et al. 1985). The pathophysiological significance of this phenomenon is not clear, however, since hemodilution does not protect against the fall in GFR seen following ischemic insults (Andersson and Jennische 1987). It has been proposed that the slowing of blood flow in the outer medulla consequent to this vascular congestion might contribute to sustained decreases in oxygen delivery in an area of the kidney with the most marginal oxygen delivery, thus aggravating injury in this segment (Rosen et al. 1992).

Tubular Cell Factors

The final common pathway for the maintenance of oliguric ARF in virtually all models is injury and damage to tubular epithelial cells. These factors lead to tubular obstruction and backleak of filtrate and apparently explain why GFR remains depressed even after organ blood flow has returned toward normal. More significantly, it is apparent in most models that recovery from ARF is associated with regeneration of tubular epithelia.

Energy Metabolism

A characteristic of all types of ARF is depletion of ATP and other high-energy intermediates in tubular epithelial cells. Adenosine triphosphate (ATP) levels fall rapidly with the development of ischemia (Gaudio et al. 1986; Stromski et al. 1986; Cunarro et al. 1982; Siegel et al. 1983) and remain severely depressed during the ischemic phase. Following return of blood flow, tissue ATP levels return to about 50% of control levels and then slowly return towards normal. The level of ATP depletion varies somewhat in tubule segments, depending on both work load (ATP requirements) and dependence of the segment on oxidative metabolism (Basten et al. 1987; Brezis et al. 1985). Thus, more distal segments and medullary tubules, which have greater capacity for glycolytic metabolism, will have higher levels of cellular ATP than proximal segments, which correspondingly show greater susceptibility to injury (Weinberg et al. 1991).

Failure of ATP levels to return to normal with restoration of blood flow indicates that intermediary metabolism may be impaired even in the absence of ongoing oxygen deprivation. Several reasons have been advanced as possible explanations of this phenomenon. First, mitochondrial function leading to the phosphorylation of adenosine diphosphate (ADP) may be abnormal. Studies of mitochondrial respiration in isolated mitochondria from ischemic hepatocytes have demonstrated decreased rates of state 3 and state 4 respiration (Aw et al. 1987a,b). This has been correlated with increased mitochondrial calcium concentration (Burke et al. 1984; Malis and Bonventre 1986), although, as mentioned above, it is not clear this is a cause or effect of impaired respiratory function. Numerous studies have demonstrated morphologic abnormalities in mitochondria from ischemic tubules,

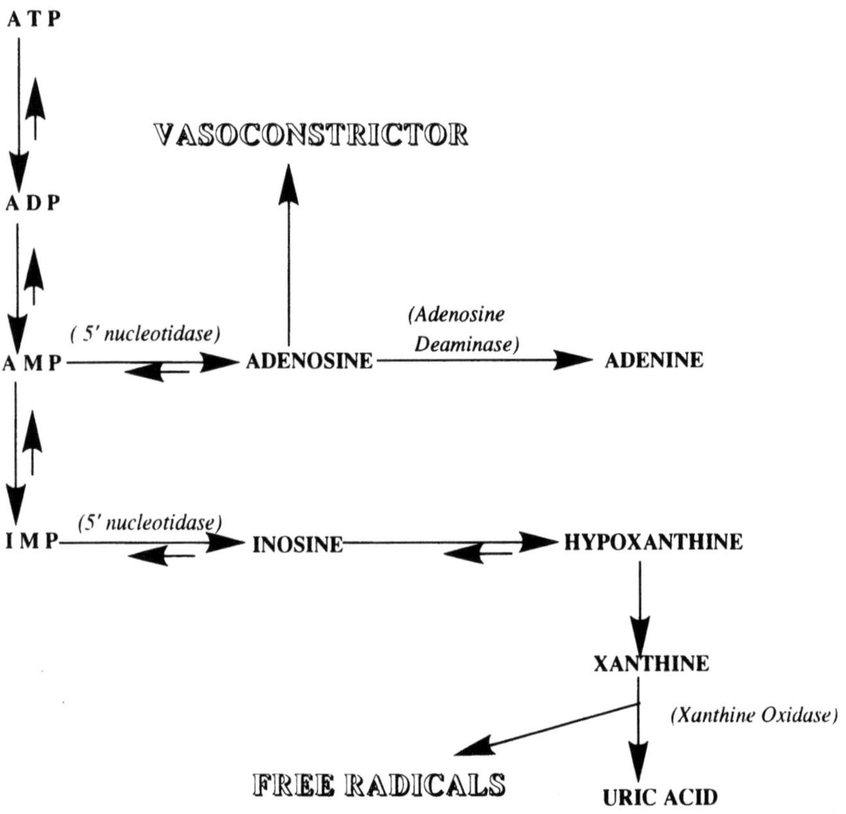

Fig. 2. Purine pathways in acute renal failure. Purine breakdown during ischemia leads to loss of adenylates, generation of the vasoconstrictor adensosine, and free radical production. Infusion of adenylates or blockers of 5′ nucleotidase or adenosine deaminase promotes higher levels of adenosine triphosphate (*ATP*) through reversal of this process (salvage pathway synthesis). *ADP*, adenosine diphosphate; *AMP*, adenosine monophosphate; *IMP*, inosine monophosphate

including swelling and loss of cisternal outlines (Mergner et al. 1977, 1979). Secondly, a considerable body of evidence suggests that with reperfusion there is depletion of adenylate substrates for synthesis of ATP through salvage pathways (see Fig. 2). ATP is broken down to ADP and adenosine monophosphate (AMP). AMP may be acted on by either adenosine deaminase or 5′ nucleotidase to produce adenosine, inosine, and hypoxanthine. Adenosine, as mentioned above, is a potent vasoconstrictor of cortical vasculature. Hypoxanthine is further reduced to uric acid through the action of xanthine oxidase, which is activated in ischemia, and a byproduct of this reaction is the production of oxygen free radicals (see below). Total levels of all adenylate pools are reduced in ARF (Cunarro et al. 1982), and several lines of evidence suggest that this limits ATP synthesis. ATP levels may be enhanced by the postischemic infusion of adenylates, either AMP, ADP, or ATP (Siegel 1980). Blockade of AMP degradation by inhibitors of either adenosine deaminase or 5′ nucleotidase results in an increase in ATP levels (Stromski et al. 1988; Van Waarde et al. 1989). As will be described below, all maneuvers which increase ATP levels are associated with an improved course of ARF, pointing to a central role for energy depletion in tubular cells in the pathophysiology of ARF.

Calcium

While cytosolic free calcium is low in normal renal cells, it is generally agreed that cytosolic free calcium increases during oxygen deprivation potentially leading to cell damage (Young and Humes 1991; Bonventre 1993). A role for increased cytosolic calcium levels in eliciting damage during oxygen deprivation has been inferred from studies demonstrating the appearance of plasma membrane blebs, changes in membrane lipid composition, the protective effects of calcium channel blockers, and the ability of calcium-free media to reduce either anoxic or postanoxic damage in isolated cells (Young and Humes 1991; Bonventre 1993; Wetzels et al. 1992). While cellular calcium overload is clearly the pathogenetic mechanism with certain types of cellular injury, it is considerably less clear whether calcium overload is the cause or the result of plasma membrane damage and cellular dysfunction in ischemic injury.

A number of theoretical considerations, however, have made calcium an attractive etiologic candidate for irreversible cell injury in response to an ischemic insult. High cytosolic calcium levels will activate all energy-consuming reactions of the cell, such as sarcolemmal calcium ATPase and mitochondrial calcium uptake processes, further stressing an already limited supply of ATP in an ischemic cell (Lehninger 1970; Rossi and Lehninger 1964; Cheung et al. 1986; Mandel et al. 1987). Calcium uptake into mitochondria takes precedence over energy production and will ultimately result in the uncoupling of oxidative phosphorylation. Increased calcium will activate phospholipases, which can produce changes in membrane structure and alter membrane enzyme activity and permeability (Nakamura et al. 1991). The increased fatty acids produced as a result of phospholipase activation can become saponified, acting as detergents which will further contribute to membrane damage (Bonventre 1993). Lastly, increased calcium theoretically can cause dysfunction of the cellular cytoskeleton (Molitoris and Nelson 1990).

To implicate increased calcium as a causative factor in anoxic or ischemic cell injury, it is necessary to demonstrate that: (a) cellular calcium increases before irreversible cell injury occurs; (b) cytosolic calcium concentration increases with ischemia and that increase is large enough to account for activation of destructive processes; and (c) prevention of the rise in cellular calcium prevents cell injury.

All these issues have been addressed, and provocative data has been generated in response to each question; unfortunately, each approach has yielded results which are either conflicting or difficult to interpret. Preparations of rabbit proximal tubules subjected to inhibitors of oxidative phosphorylation (chemical hypoxia) were found to suffer plasma membrane damage without increase in free calcium concentration (Weinberg 1985). Other investigators have found only modest increases in cytosolic calcium concentrations in isolated cell systems during prelethal injury (Weinberg et al. 1983; Lefurgey et al. 1986). Given the large capacity of mitochondria and other organelles to sequester calcium without an effect on respiratory function, it is difficult to attribute the severe mitochondrial respiratory defect seen in ARF to minor increases in mitochondrial calcium contents. The role of cellular sequestration continues to require exploration (Young and Humes 1991). Nevertheless, a substantial body of literature exists which links increased cellular and mitochondrial calcium to cellular dysfunction in ARF (Wilson et al. 1984; Wilson and Schrier 1986; Burnier et al. 1988; Schieppati et al. 1985; Weinberg et al. 1991; Burke et al. 1984).

With regard to the premise that prevention of the rise in cellular calcium prevents injury, two experimental approaches have been pursued. The first involves removing extracellular calcium during the period of anoxia, typically in a cultured cell study system; the second involves the use of slow calcium channel blockers to prevent entry of extracellular calcium. Both approaches are associated with difficulties. In the case of cultured cells, the relative dependence of cellular viability on oxidative metabolism is critical to the interpretation of the results and is often lacking in studies. The use of calcium channel blockers involves the obvious, and generally invalidated, assumption that these agents act at the major calcium entry pathway for injured epithelial cells. Wilson and Schrier (1986) demonstrated that primary cultures from multiple tubule sites were protected to some degree against anoxic cell death by growth in calcium-free media. The effects of slow calcium channel blockers has been examined both in vitro and in vivo. Verapamil offers remarkable protection of both structure and function in the norepinephrine model of ischemic acute renal failure when given before and during the insult, though results are considerably less impressive when the agent is given after ischemia (Burke et al. 1984). These impressive studies correlated protection with improved mitochondrial function and lower levels of mitochondrial calcium. Unfortunately, these results did not translate well to a model of ischemia produced by other means. Malis and colleagues (1983) were able to reproduce the protective effects of verapamil in norepinephrine-induced ARF, but could not demonstrate any protective effect in the renal artery clamp model. They proposed that the protection conferred by calcium channel blockers was specific; the vascular effects of norepinephrine and the subsequent correlations described with mitochondrial calcium levels and function were simply the difference between cells exposed to ischemia and those whose ischemic insult was blocked. The exact role of cellular calcium in the genesis to tubular cell injury in ARF remains to be established.

Oxygen Free Radicals

It is commonly observed that tubular epithelial cell injury progresses following reperfusion of the kidney after an ischemic insult. Reperfusion injury is observed in many tissues and is thought to relate to the production of oxygen-derived free radicals which have injurious effects on membranes and cellular enzymes (Halliwell 1987; McCord 1985). A number of observations suggest that reactive oxygen species may be generated in the kidney during reperfusion (Paller et al. 1984; Paller and Hebbel 1986; McCoy et al. 1988; Linas et al. 1987). Free radical species may be generated either through metabolism of purine degradation products by xanthine oxidase (McCord 1985; Paller et al. 1984), by interaction with hemoglobin Fe through the Haber-Wiess reaction (Paller 1988), or by activated neutrophils infiltrating the ischemic interstitium (Linas et al. 1988).

The pathophysiologic significance of these reactive oxygen species has been suggested by multiple studies using agents which interfere with free radical production (Paller et al. 1984) or which take up free radicals (Kedar et al. 1983; Paller et al. 1984; Paller and Hedlund 1988; Paller 1992), resulting in improved renal histology and function in the postischemic period. However, an almost equally large number of studies show little effects of such maneuvers in virtually identical models (Gamelin and Zager 1988; Zager et al. 1994; Thornton et al. 1989), and there is little evidence that reactive oxygen species damage tubular cells in vitro (Doctor and Mandel 1991; Borkan and Schwartz 1989). It seems likely that free radical damage does occur during reperfusion, but it is not sufficiently proximal in the injury cascade to be of major importance in the maintenance of ARF (Weinberg 1991).

Other Mediators of Injury

Cellular acidosis develops during ischemia, and it was initially proposed that this too could lead to enhanced tissue damage (Williamson et al. 1976). Recent studies from several laboratories, however, have suggested that the lowered pH seen in ischemic tissues could actually have an intrinsic protective effect (Weinberg et al. 1991; Bonventre 1993). The mechanism of protection by acidosis is not known, though ATP levels are not markedly changed, suggesting that it is not due to improved energy metabolism (Weinberg 1985). Weinberg et al. (1991) have proposed that it may be related to decreased entry of calcium into the cell, and Bonventre (1993) has suggested that it may be due to inactivation of pH-dependent phospholipases. The exact significance of this protection by low pH is not clear.

Membrane lipid metabolism is markedly altered during acute renal failure. There is an increase in degradation of membrane phospholipids (Matthys et al. 1984). This is probably potentiated by the peroxidation of unsaturated membrane acyl groups of phospholipids by the presence of reactive oxygen species (Malis et al. 1990; Portila et al. 1992). The net result is membrane degradation, a decrease in membrane integrity and in total membrane phospholipid mass (Chien et al. 1978), and an increase in free fatty acids, which themselves may have toxic effects (Katz and Messineo 1981; Smith et al. 1980; Savanian and Kin 1985).

In addition to increased degradation, there is also impaired reacylation of membrane lipids and decreased synthesis, both of which are energy-dependent processes (Weinberg 1991). The net result of increased breakdown and impaired synthesis of membrane lipids is loss of membrane function, perhaps particularly important in mitochondria. The exact significance of these findings in experimental ARF remains, however, unclear, as most of these observations have been made in isolated cellular and mitochondrial preparations (Bonventre 1993; Weinberg 1991).

An interesting form of cellular injury that has recently come under study in the area of experimental ARF is the phenomena of apoptosis. Apoptosis refers to a form of chromosomal damage characterized pathologically by condensation of chromatin and the formation of spherical apoptotic bodies (Wyllie et al. 1980). This pathologic picture corresponds to a characteristic pattern of DNA degradation, with apparently nonrandom fragmentation resulting in a distinctive appearance when analyzed on gel electrophoresis (Kerr and Harmon 1991). Apoptosis has been documented to occur in ischemic ARF (Schumer et al. 1992) and in post-transplant ARF, which may be a unique variant of clinical ARF (Olsen et al. 1989; Bonventre and Weinberg 1992). The nonrandom appearance of apoptotic DNA is in distinct contrast to the random fragmentation seen in cellular necrosis and suggests that it may be the consequence of enzyme activation. A calcium-activated endonuclease has been proposed as the mediator of this phenomenon (Bonventre 1993). Whether apoptosis is simply a marker for cellular injury or plays a significant role in maintenance of ARF remains to be determined.

Cytoskeleton and Polarization

During ischemia and during maintenance of ARF, a number of intriguing abnormalities in cellular function have been studied in various in vitro preparations which may have significance for the full understanding of cellular injury and repair in ARF. These include cell swelling, cellular adhesion, and the loss of the unique polarized phenotype of the epithelial cell. Cell swelling has been studied for many years as a significant phenomenon related to both vascular and tubular obstruction. Ischemic cells swell due to loss of energy-dependent, volume-regulatory mechanisms and this may be prevented, to a significant degree, by the use of impermeant solutes (Flores et al. 1972). This, indeed, is the rationale for the use of impermeant solutes and perfusion solutions resembling intracellular ionic composition in the maintenance of cadaver kidneys prior to transplantation (Bonventre and Weinberg 1992). Considerable evidence suggests that prevention of cell swelling may alter the course of ARF (see below). Whether this is primarily due to an effect on tubular or vascular cells, or both, is a subject of dispute.

A characteristic of epithelial cells which is essential to their normal function is the maintenance of the apical and basolateral membranes as unique domains, both in terms of their lipid composition and their constituent membrane proteins. Considerable evidence now exists that this characteristic polarity is lost during the maintenance phase of ARF (Molitoris 1991). Both membrane lipids and proteins, including the Na^+, K^+ ATPase (Molitoris and Nelson 1990), redistribute globally following ischemic injury. This is associated with loss of ability to carry out vectorial transport of a number of solutes (Spiegel et al. 1989; Molitoris et al. 1989a,b; Molitoris and Kinne 1987) as well as loss of the junctional integrity necessary to prevent backleak (Molitoris 1991). This phenomenon, like others described above, appears to be the consequence of energy depletion, and it appears to be mediated, in part at least, through disruption of the cytoskeleton (Bershadsky and Gelfand 1981, 1983).

Disruption of cytoskeletal function has also been implicated in tubular cell detachment (Racusen 1992). The cytoskeleton is known to interact with multiple cellular adhesion molecules (CAM), which serve to anchor the epithelial cells both to each other and to the basement membrane. Alterations in these interactions due to disruption of the cytoskeleton seen following ischemia lead to sloughing and detachment of tubular epithelial cells and perhaps represent the final common pathway for both tubular obstruction and backleak (Mandel and Bacallao 1991; Molitoris et al. 1989a,b). Studies of these phenomena not only help us understand the cell biology of cellular and organ dysfunction, but may also be the target of therapeutic interventions (see below).

Recovery

Virtually all models of experimental ARF are characterized by recovery. Clinical ARF is also characterized by recovery in the vast majority of survivors. The mechanisms by which the kidney regenerates following tubular necrosis are not known. The process is associated with multiple lines of evidence showing tubular cell regeneration. This includes morphologic evidence of new cell division and cellular proliferation (B. Glaumann et al. 1977; G. Glaumann et al. 1977), biochemical evidence of increased gene activity (Cuppage et al. 1969), increased protein (Mendley and Toback 1989) and lipid (Toback et al. 1977) biosynthesis, and the reestablishing of epithelial cell polarity (Molitoris 1991) and cellular adhesion to basement membrane (Racusen 1992). The stimuli for these processes are not entirely clear. Likely candidates include known growth factors and a wide variety of autocrine and paracrine factors which may promote growth (see Toback 1992 for a review). Therapeutic modalities in experimental ARF may either aim at promoting the normal recovery processes or at inhibiting the injury processes.

Protective Agents

A number of agents have been described which ameliorate or inhibit ARF if given to animals before and during the injury phase. They are listed in Table 3 along with their putative sites of action. These agents may be viewed as primarily protective in nature, as there is little evidence that they are of value once renal failure is established. Their potential clinical value for ARF is therefore minimal.

Treatment of experimental animals subjected to ischemic ARF with mannitol or other impermeant solutes has repeatedly been shown to have a protective effect when the agents are given before and during the ischemic insult (Flores et al. 1972; Morris et al. 1972; Hanley and Davidson 1981; Burke et al. 1980; Schrier et al. 1984). Unfortunately, mannitol provides little protection on its own when given only after the ischemic insult (Lieberthal et al. 1990).

Prior Na^+ loading and the establishment of a solute diuresis, with or without tubular alkalinization, has minimized the extent of renal injury and the course of ARF following a wide variety of insults (McDonald et al. 1969; DiBona et al. 1971; Flamenbaum et al. 1973). This finding is consistent with the well-known clinical observation that patients who are volume depleted

Table 3. Protective agents in experimental acute renal failure (ARF)

Agent	Possible site of action
Mannitol	Cell swelling, free radical scavenger
Na^+ loading	Washout of tubular debris down regulation of TGF
Loop diuretics	Washout of tubular debris, abort TGF, decrease O_2 consumption
Calcium channel blockers	Decrease cell calcium, vascular effect (?)
Fructose diphosphate	Enhance glycolytic metabolism
Bicarbonate	Inhibit cast formation
Thyroidectomy	Decrease free radical formation
Glycine	Cytoprotective
Prostaglandins	Vascular effect, cytoprotective (?)

TGF, Tubulo-glomerular feedback.

seem to be at greater risk for sustaining ARF. The mechanism of protection conferred by solute diuresis is not clear. One theory is that chronic saline loading depletes the kidney of renin and therefore aborts the process of tubuloglomerular feedback which is essential to sustaining ARF (DiBona et al. 1971). Though renin depletion can be observed following Na^+ loading, the protective effects of Na^+ loading have been dissociated from this phenomenon (Baehler et al. 1978), and it seems more likely that the mechanism of protection lies elsewhere. Similar protection is seen when diuresis is established with loop diuretics prior to the insult. Once again, with the exception of establishment of an alkaline diuresis following pigment injury (Better and Stein 1990), this maneuver has little value once ARF is established. Neither nonpermeant solutes, loop diuretics, nor post-ischemic Na loading has been shown to be of clinical value in established ARF.

A number of studies have documented the protective effects of infusions of various vasodilatory prostaglandins prior to and during ischemic injury to the kidney (Koyama et al. 1987; Lifschitz and Barnes 1984; Finn et al. 1987; Mauk et al. 1977; Neumayer et al. 1985; Paller and Manivel 1992). This protection has been assumed to be due to the vasodilatory effects of prostaglandins on the cortical microcirculation, although Paller (1992) has also advanced evidence for a cytoprotective effect. Unfortunately, vasodilatation after ARF is established has little effect on the course of ARF (Siegel et al.

1980), so the value of prostaglandins appears to be protective rather than therapeutic.

Calcium channel blockers also appear to be protective in several models of ARF, probably through a vascular effect as indicated above. They offer considerably less benefit when given following ischemic injury and their effect is most remarkable in norepinephrine-induced ARF (Burke et al. 1984).

Several amino acids, notably glutathione and glycine, have remarkable protective effects in physiological concentrations when hypoxic injury to isolated tubules or cells is studied (Weinberg et al. 1987). Glutathione is proposed to act primarily as a free radical scavenger (Paller 1988), but it appears that most of its activity may be conferred by its constituent amino acid glycine (Weinberg et al. 1987). The mechanism of cellular protection by glycine is unknown. However, studies of glycine infusions subsequent to renal injury in intact animal models, as with other amino acids, have suggested that rather than promoting recovery they may even worsen injury (Zager and Venkatachalam 1983). Their therapeutic potential remains to be explored in detail (Weinberg 1991).

Agents Effective After Induction of Injury

In contrast to the agents described above, a number of therapeutic maneuvers have been described which improve the course of ARF when given

Table 4. Agents effective after initiation of acute renal failure (ARF)

Agent	Possible site of action
Allopurinol	Inhibit free radical formation
Desferrioxamine	Inhibit free radical formation
Superoxide dismutase catalase, DMTU	Free radical scavengers
Aminophylline, A_1 receptor blockers	Inhibit adenosine mediated vasoconstriction in cortex
Clonidine	Decrease capillary congestion
Atrial natriuretic peptides	Decrease vascular resistance, Increase K_f
Adenine nucleotides	Reversal of energy depletion
Thyroid hormone	Promote recovery of critical cellular enzymes, enhance growth factor effects
Growth factors	Promote cellular regeneration
Cellular adhesion molecules	Block cellular sloughing

K_f, glomerular permeability; DMTU, dimethyl thiourea.

after the insult in experimental animals. These agents may be properly considered therapeutic, and a partial list is given in Table 4. Allopurinol, superoxide dismutase, and catalase have all been given in an effort to inhibit oxygen free radical toxicity seen during reperfusion injury (see above). There are a number of reports of amelioration of experimental ARF by these agents, but unfortunately an almost equal number that suggest that they are not effective (see above). The few clinical trials in transplanted kidneys have not been optimistic. Although reperfusion injury mediated by reactive oxygen species undoubtedly occurs, it appears that reversal of this single component of cellular injury is not sufficient to have a major impact on the course of ARF.

Several investigators have described a beneficial effect of infusions of atrial natriuretic peptides, either alone, or in combination with mannitol, following induction of ARF (Shaw et al. 1987; Heidbreder et al. 1988; Lieberthal et al. 1990). The mechanism of this effect is thought to be twofold. First, there is an improved glomerular blood flow; second, there is a diuresis, which may wash out tubular debris. This agent is particularly exciting in that a controlled clinical trial has demonstrated reduction of oliguric time and decreased requirement for dialysis in patients who receive ANF during early established ARF (Rahman et al. 1993).

Adenosine blockers show promise of reducing injury even when given after the insult in ARF (see above). Their mechanism is thought to be through A_1 receptor blockade and reversal of the intense cortical vasoconstriction seen in ARF.

The dramatic effects of postischemic infusions of ATP and other adenine nucleotides on raising cellular ATP levels and moderating the course of ARF have been documented in a series of elegant studies by Seigel and colleagues (Siegel et al. 1980; Siegel et al. 1983; Stromski et al. 1986; Gaudio et al. 1986). These studies point to the central role for energy depletion in ischemic tubular cell injury. These studies are particularly interesting in that the beneficial effects are seen in more than one injury model. Unfortunately, the vasoactive effects of these agents may limit their clinical utility.

Several agents have now been described whose main action appears to be in promoting renal regeneration following injury. These include thyroid hormone (Siegel et al. 1984; Sutter et al. 1988; Cronin et al. 1986), epidermal growth factor (EGF; Humes et al. 1989; Norman et al. 1990), hepatocyte growth factor (Miller et al. 1994), and insulin-like growth factor (Miller et al. 1992). Like adenine nucleotides, these agents are of particular interest because they appear to be effective in a wide variety of injury models, including ischemia, heavy metal toxicity, and gentamicin nephrotoxicity. Thyroid hormone is thought to act either by enhancing levels of essential cellular enzymes (Siegel et al. 1984) or through potentiating the action of growth factors (Seiken et al. 1994).

The kidney is a major source of EGF, a potent cellular mitogen, and it is known that mRNA for the precursor of this protein decreases in kidney during ischemic ARF (Safirstein 1989, 1990). This is associated with a rise in tissue levels of soluble EGF, apparently released from membrane-bound precursors by proteolysis (Schaudies and Johnson 1993; Seiken et al. 1994). Infusions of exogenous EGF are beneficial in severe ARF induced either by ischemia (Humes et al. 1989) or nephrotoxins, but are of less benefit in moderate ARF (Seiken et al. 1994), so it appears that the efficacy of these agents may depend upon the degree of injury. In any case, these mitogens appear to be involved in the recovery so typical of all models of ARF, and clinical trials should be forthcoming.

Conclusion

Experimental studies of ARF in a wide variety of model systems have detailed many of the pathophysiologic mechanisms of vascular and tubular cell injury. In many cases, these studies have led to therapeutic or protective maneuvers which may have clinical relevance in the future. Some effects, no doubt will turn out to be artifacts of the experimental study systems or will represent a step in the injury cascade whose reversal has little clinical value. Nonetheless, considerable progress has been made in these areas and clinical trials of several potentially promising therapies are now under way. The world of experimental ARF is moving into the clinical realm.

New insights continue to emerge from experimental studies. Hakim and colleagues (Schulman et al. 1991) recently demonstrated that rats with ARF who were exposed to biocompatible dialysis membranes improved more rapidly that rats exposed to compliment-activating membranes, and early clinical results (Hakim 1992) suggest that patients with ARF may do better when dialyzed with biocompatible membranes. The emergence of mixed models of ischemia and endotoxemia suggest an explanation for the frequent development of ARF in the septic, volume-compromised host and point to a role for cytokines in mediating some aspects of ARF. Therapy directed towards modifying the effects or concentrations of such agents may prove quite useful in the future. The loss of epithelial polarity and cellular adhesion is now understood as a potentially important event in the pathogenesis of ARF, and therapy directed at cellular adhesion molecules shows significant promise in the laboratory. Bonventre and colleagues, for example, have demonstrated remarkable functional and anatomical protection by an antibody to intracellular adhesion molecule-1 given before or after an ischemic insult (Kelly et al. 1993). Thus, better understanding of the pathophysiology and cellular biology of ARF both in maintenance and recovery has led to a number of promising therapeutic avenues which will soon be explored in clinical trials.

References

Adams PL, Adams PF, Bells PD et al. (1980) Impaired renal blood flow autoregulation in ischemic acute renal failure. Kidney Int 19:68–76

Andersson G, Jennische E (1987) Lack of casual relationship between medullary blood congestion and tubular necrosis in postischaemic kidney damage. Acta Physiol Scand 130:429–432

Arendshort WJ, Finn WF, Gottschalk CW (1975) Pathogenesis of acute renal failure following renal ischemia in the rat. Circ Res 37:558

AW TY, Andersson BS, Jones DP (1987a) Suppression of mitochondrial respiratory function after short-term anoxia. Am J Physiol 252:C362–C368

AW TY, Andersson BS, Jones DP (1987b) Mitochondrial transmembrane ion distribution during anoxia. Am J Physiol 252:C356–C361

Baehler RW, Kotchen TA, Ott CE (1978) Failure of chronic sodium chloride loading to protect against norepinephrine-induced acute renal failure in dogs. Circ Res 42:23–27

Bank N, Mutz BF, Aynedjian HS (1967) The role of "leakage" of tubular fluid in anuria due to mercury poisoning. J Clin Invest 46:605

Basten J, Cambon N, Thompson M et al. (1987) Change in energy reserves in different segments of the nephron during brief ischemia. Kidney Int 31:1239–1247

Bayati A, Hellberg O, Odlind B et al. (1987) Prevention of ischaemic acute renal failure with superoxide dismutase and sucrose. Acta Physiol Scand 130:367–372

Baylis C, Rennke HG, Brenner BM (1977) Mechanisms of the defect in glomerular ultrafiltration associated with gentamicin administration. Kidney Int 12:344

Bershadsky AD, Gelfand VI (1981) ATP-dependent regulation of cytoplasmic microtubule disassembly. Proc Natl Acad Sci USA 78:3610–3613

Bershadsky AD, Gelfand VI (1983) Role of ATP in the regulation of stability of cytoskeletal structures. Cell Biol Int Rep 7:173–187

Better OS, Stein JH (1990) Early management of shock and prophylaxis of acute renal failure in traumatic rhabdomyolysis. N Engl J Med 322:825–829

Bidani AK, Churchill PC (1983) Aminophylline ameliorates glycerol-induced acute renal failure in rats. Can J Physiol Pharmacol 61:567–571

Bidani AK, Fleischmann LE, Churchill P et al. (1978) Natriuresis-induced protection in acute myohemoglobinuric renal failure without renal cortical renin content depletion in the rat. Nephron 22:529–537

Bidani AK, Churchill P, Fleischmann L (1979) Sodium-chloride-induced protection in nephrotoxic acute renal failure: idependence from renin. Kidney Int 16:481–490

Blantz RC, Pelayo JC, Gushwa LC et al. (1985) Functional basis for the glomerular alterations in uranyl nitrate acute renal failure. Kidney Int 28:733

Bonventre JV (1993) Mechanisms of ischemic acute renal failure. Kidney Int 43:1160–1178

Bonventre JV, Weinberg JM (1992) Kidney preservation ex vivo for transplantation. Annu Rev Med 43:523–553

Borkan SC, Schwartz JH (1989) Role of oxygen free radical species in in vitro models of proximal tubular ischemia. Am J Physiol 257:F114–F125

Bowmer CJ, Collis MG, Yates MS (1988) Amelioration of glycerol-induced acute renal failure in the rat with 8-phenyltheophylline: timing of intervention. J Pharm Pharmacol 40:733–735

Brezis M, Rosen S, Silva P et al. (1984) Selective anoxic injury to thick ascending limb. An anginal syndrome of the renal medulla? Adv Exp med Biol 180:239

Brezis M, Shanley P, Silva P et al. (1985) Disparate mechanisms for hypoxic cell injury in different nephron segments: studies in the isolated perfused rat kidney. J Clin Invest 76:1796–1806

Brezis M, Rosen S, Epstein FH (1991) Acute renal failure. In: Brenner BM, Rector FC (eds) The kidney. Saunders, New York, pp 993–1062

Brown JJ, Gleadle RI, Lawson DH et al. (1970) Renin and acute renal failure: studies in man. Br J Med 1:253–258

Brown WCB, Brown JJ, Gavras H (1972) Renin acute circulatory renal failure in the rabbit. Circ Res 30:114–122
Bulger RE, Eknoyan G, Purcell DJ et al. (1983) Endothelial characteristics of glomerular capillaries in normal, mercuric chloride-induced, and gentamicin-induced acute renal failure in the rat. J Clin Invest 72:128
Burke TJ, Cronin RE, Duchin KL et al. (1980) Ischemia and tubule obstruction during acute renal failure in dogs: mannitol in protection. Am J Physiol 238:F305–F314
Burke TJ, Arnold PE, Gordon JA et al. (1984) Protective effect of intrarenal calcium membrane blockers before or after renal ischemia. J Clin Inv 74:1830–1841
Burnier M, Van Putten VJ, Schieppati A et al. (1988) Effect of extracellular acidosis on ^{45}Ca uptake in isolated hypoxic proximal tubules. Am J Physiol 254:C839–C846
Chan L, Chittinandana A, Shapiro JI et al. (1994) Effect of an endothelin-receptor antagonist on ischemic acute renal failure. Am J Physiol 266:F135–F138
Chedru MF, Baethke R, Oken DE (1972) Renal cortical blood flow and glomerular filtration in myohemoglobinuric acute renal failure. Kidney Int 1:232
Cheung JY, Thompson IG, Bonventre JV (1982) Effects of extracellular calcium removal and anoxia on isolated rat myocytes. Am J Physiol 243:C184–C190
Cheung JY, Constantine JM, Bonventre JV (1986) Regulation of cytosolic free calcium concentration in cultured renal epithelial cells. Am J Physiol 251:F690–F701
Chien KR, Abrams J, Serroni A et al. (1978) Accelerated phospholipid degradation and associated membrane dysfunction in irreversible, ischemic liver cell injury. J Biol Chem 253:4809–4817
Chonko A, Savin V, Stewart R et al. (1979) The effects of gentamicin on renal function in the mature vs. immature rabbit. Kidney Int 16:772
Conger JD, Hammond WS (1992) Renal vasculature and ischemic injury. Ren Fail 14(3):307–310
Cronin RE, de Torrrente A, Miller PD et al. (1978) Pathogenic mechanisms in early norepinephrine-induced acute renal failure. Functional and histological correlates of protection. Kidney Int 14:115
Cronin RE, Brown DM, Simonsen R (1986) Protection by thyroxine in nephrotoxic acute renal failure. Am J Physiol 251:F408–F416
Cunarro JA, Schultz SE, Johnson WA et al. (1982) Effects of ischemia on metabolite concentrations in dog renal cortex. Renal Physiol 5:143–155
Cuppage FE, Cunningham N, Tate AL (1969) Nucleic acid synthesis in the regenerating nephron following injury with mercuric chloride. Lab Invest 21:449–457
Daugharty TM, Ueki IF, Mercer PF et al. (1974) Dynamics of glomerular ultrafiltration in the rat. I. Response to ischemic injury. J Clin Invest 53:105
DiBona GF, Sawin LL (1971) The renin-angiotensin system in acute renal failure in the rat. Lab Invest 25:528–532
DiBona GF, McDonald FD, Flamenbaum W et al. (1971) Maintenance of renal function in salt loaded rats despite severe tubular necrosis induced by $HgCl_2$. Nephron 8:205–220
Diethelm AG, Wilson SJ (1971) Obstruction to the renal microcirculation after temporary ischemia. J Surg Res 11:265
Doctor RB, Mandel LJ (1991) Minimal role of xanthine oxidase and oxygen free radicals in rat renal tubular reoxygenation injury. J Am Soc Nephrol 1:959–969
Donohoe JF, Venkatachalam MA, Bernard DB et al. (1978) Tubular leakage and obstruction after renal ischemia: Structural-functional correlations. Kidney Int 13:208–222
Finn WF, Hak LJ, Grossman SH (1987) Protective effect of prostacyclin on postischemic acute renal failure in the rat. Kidney Int 32:479–487
Flamenbaum W, McNeil JS, Kotchen TW et al. (1972a) Experimental acute renal failure induced by uranyl nitrate in the dog. Circ Res 31:682
Flamenbaum W, Kotchen TA, Oken DE (1972b) Effect of renin immunization on mercuric chloride and glycerol-induced renal failure. Kidney Int 1:406–412

Flamenbaum W, Kotchen TA, Nagle R et al. (1973) Effect of potassium on the renin-angiotensin system and $HgCl_2$-induced acute renal failure. Am J Physiol 224:305–311
Flamenbaum W, Hamberger RJ, Huddleston ML et al. (1976) The initiation phase of experimental acute renal failure: an evaluation of uranyl nitrate-induced acute renal failure in the rat. Kidney Int 10:S115
Flamenbaum W, Schwartz JH, Hamburger RJ et al. (1977) The pathogenesis of experimental acute renal failure: the role of membrane dysfunction. Prog Mol Subcell Biol 5:73–115
Flanigan WJ, Oken DE (1965) Renal micropuncture study of the development of anuria in the rat with mercury-induced acute renal failure. J Clin Invest 44:449
Flores J, DiBona DR, Beck CH et al. (1972) The role of cell swelling in ischemic renal damage and the protective effect of hypertonic solute. J Clin Invest 51:118–126
Frega NS, DiBona DR, Guertter B et al. (1976) Ischemic renal injury. Kidney Int 10:S17
Gamelin LM, Zager RA (1988) Evidence against oxidant injury as a critical mediator of postischemic acute renal failure. Am J Physiol 255:F450–F460
Gaudio KM, Stromski M, Thulin G et al. (1986) Postischemic hemodynamics and recovery of renal adenosine triphosphate. Am J Physiol 251:F603–F609
Glaumann B, Trump BF (1975) Studies on the pathogenesis of ischemic cell injury. III. Morphological changes of the proximal pars recta tubules (P_3) of the rat kidney made ischemic in vivo. Virchows Arch [Cell Pathol] 19:303–323
Glaumann B, Glaumann H, Berezesky IK et al. (1975) Studies on the pathogenesis of ischemic cell injury. II. Morphological changes of the pars convoluta (P_1 and P_2) of the proximal tubule of the rat kidney made ischemic in vivo. Virchows Arch [Cell Pathol] 19:281–302
Glaumann B, Glaumann H, Berezesky IK et al. (1977) Studies on cellular recovery from injury. II. Ultrastuctural studies on the recovery of the pars convoluta of the proximal tubule of the rat kidney from temporary ischemia. Virchows Arch [B] 24:1–18
Glaumann G, Glaumann H, Trump BF (1977) Studies of cellular recovery from injury. III. Ultrastructural studies of the recovery of the pars recta of the proximal tubule (P3) segment of the rat kidney from temporary ischemia. Virchows Arch [B] 25:281–308
Hakim RM, Wingard RL, Lawrence P (1992) Use of biocompatible membranes improves outcome and recovery from acute renal failure. J Am Soc Nephrol 3:367
Halliwell B (1987) Oxidants and human disease: some new concepts. FASEB J 1:358–364
Hanley MJ, Davidson K (1981) Prior mannitol and furosemide infusion in a model of ischemic acute renal failure. Am J Physiol 24:F556–F564
Heidbreder E, Schafferhans K, Heyd A et al. (1988) Uranyl nitrate-induced acute renal failure in rats: effect of atrial natriuretic peptide on renal function. Kidney Int 34 Suppl 25:S79–S82
Hellberg POA, Andren T, Bayati A et al. (1985) Pathophysiological significance of rheological factors in the development of acute renal failure. Acta Physiol Scand Suppl 124:542
Hellberg POA, Källskog Ö, Wolgast M (1991) Red cell trapping and postischemic renal blood flow. Differences between the cortex, outer and inner medulla. Kidney Int 40:625–631
Hollenberg NK, Wilkes BM, Schulman G (1988) The renin-angiotensin system in acute renal failure. In: Brenner BM, Lazarus JM (eds) Acute renal failure, 2nd edn. Churchill Livingstone, New York, p 19
Hostetter TH, Brenner BM (1988) Renal circulatory and nephron function in experimental acute renal failure. In: Brenner BM, Lazarus JM (eds) Acute renal failure, 2nd edn. Churchill Livingstone, New York, pp 67–91
Humes HD (1988) Aminoglycoside nephrotoxicity. Kidney Int 33:900–911
Humes HD, Cieslinski DA, Coimbra T et al. (1989) Epidermal growth factor enhances renal tubule cell regeneration and repair and accelerates recovery of renal function in postischemic acute renal failure. J Clin Invest 84:1757–1761
Ishikawa I, Hollenberg NK (1976) Pharmacologic interruption of the renin-angiotensin system in myohemoglobinuric acute renal failure. Kidney Int 10:S183
Johnson JP, Grillo FG (1994) Thyroid hormone induction of ornithine decarboxylase in ischemic acute renal failure. Ren Fail 16(4):433–442

Kashgarian M, Siegel NJ, Ries Al et al. (1976) Hemodynamic aspects in development and recovery phases of experimental post-ischemic acute renal failure. Kidney Int 10:S160
Katz AM, Messineo FC (1981) Lipid-membrane interactions and the pathogenesis of ischemic damage in the myocardium. Circ Res 48:1–16
Kedar I, Jacob ET, Bar-Natan N et al. (1983) Dimethyl sulfoxide in acute ischemia of the kidney. Ann NY Acad Sci 411:131–134
Kelleher SP, Robinette JB, Miller F et al. (1987) Effects of hemorrhagic reduction in blood pressure on recovery from acute renal failure. Kidney Int 31:725–730
Kellett R, Bowmer CJ, Collis MG et al. (1988) Ameloration of glycerol-induced acute renal faiture in the rat with 8-cyclopentyl-1,3-dipropylxanthine. Br J Pharmacol 98:1066–1074
Kelly KJ, Williams WW, Colvin RB et al. (1993) Antibody to intracellular adhesion molecule (ICAM-1) protects the kidney against ischemia. J Am Soc Nephol 4:738
Kerr JFR, Harmon BV (1991) Definition and incidence of apoptosis: an historical perspective. In: Tomei LD, Cope FO (eds) Apoptisus: the molecular basis of cell death. Cold Spring Harbor Laboratory, Cold Spring Harbor, pp 5–29
Kleinman JG, Flamenbaum W, McNeil JS (1975) Uranyl nitrate acute renal failure: early changes in renal function and hemodynamics. Clin Sci Mol Med 48:9
Kon V, Badr KF (1991) Biological actions and pathophysiologic significance of endothelin in the kidney. Kidney Int 40:1–12
Kon V, Yoshioka T, Fogo A et al. (1989) Glomerular actions of endothelin in vivo. J Clin Invest 83:1762
Koyama I, Neya K, Ueda K et al. (1987) Protective effect of lipo-prostaglandin E_1 on post-ischemic renal failure. Transplant Proc 19:3542–3544
Kurtz TW, Maletz RM, Hsu CH (1976) Renal cortical blood flow in glycerol-induced acute renal failure in the rat. Circ Res 38:30
Lefurgey A, Ingram P, Mandel LJ (1986) Heterogeneity of calcium compartmentation: electron probe analysis of renal tubules. J Membr Biol 94:191–196
Lehninger AL (1970) Mitochondria and calcium ion transport. Biochem J 119:129–138
Lieberthal W, Sheridan AM, Valeri CR (1990) Protective effect on atrial natriuretic factor and mannitol following renal ischemia. Am J Physiol 258:F1266–F1272
Lifschitz MD, Barnes JL (1984) Prostaglandin I_2 attenuates ischemic acute renal failure in the rat. Am J Physiol 247:F714–F717
Lin JJ, Churchill PC, Bidani AK (1986) Effect of theophyline on the initiation phase of postischemic acute renal failure in rats. J Lab Clin Med 108:150–154
Linas SL, Shanley PF, White CW et al. (1987) O_2 metabolite-mediated injury in perfused kidneys is reflected by consumption of DMTU and glutathione. Am J Physiol 253:F692–F701
Malis CD, Bonventre JV (1986) Mechanism of calcium potentiation of oxygen free radical injury to renal mitochondria: a model for post-ischemic and toxic mitochondrial damage. JBiol Chem 261(30):14201–14208
Malis CD, Cheung JY, Leaf A et al. (1983) Effects of verapamil in models of ischemic acute renal failure in the rat. Am J Physiol 245:F735–F742
Malis CD, Weber PC, Leaf A et al. (1990) Incorporation of marine lipids into mitrochondrial membranes increases susceptibility to damage by calcium and reactive oxygen species: evidence for enhanced activation of phospholipase A_2 in mitochondria enriched with n-3 fatty acids. Proc Natl Acad Sci USA 87:8845–8849
Mandel LJ, Bacallao R (1991) Alterations in the cytoskeleton and transepithelial resistance during ATP depletion in cultured renal epithelial cells. J Am Soc Nephrol 2:651
Mandel LJ, Takano T, Soltoff SP et al. (1987) Multiple roles of calcium in anoxic-induced injury in renal proximal tubules. In: Mandel LF, Eaton DC (eds) Cell calcium and the control of membrane transport. Rockefeller University Press, New York, pp 277–285
Mason J, Olbricht C, Takabatake T et al. (1977) The early phase of experimental acute renal failure. I. Intratubular pressure and obstruction. Pflugers Arch 370:155
Mason J, Torhorst J, Welsch J (1984) Role of the medullary perfusion defect in the pathogenesis of ischemic renal failure. Kidney Int 26:283–293

Mason J, Joeris B, Welsch J et al. (1989) Vascular congestion in ischemic renal failure: the role of cell swelling. Miner Electrolyte Metab 15:114–124

Mathews PG, Morgan TO, Johnston CI (1974) The renin-angiotensin system in acute renal failure in rats. Clin Sci Mol Med 47:79–88

Matthys E, Patel Y, Kreisberg J et al. (1984) Lipid alterations induced by renal ischemia: pathogenic factor in membrane damage. Kidney Int 26:153–161

Mauk RH, Patak RV, Fadem SZ et al. (1977) Effect of prostaglandin E administration in a nephrotoxic and a vasoconstrictor model of acute renal failure. Kidney Int 12:122–130

McCord JM (1985) Oxygen-derived free radicals in postischemic tissue injury. N Engl J Med 312:159–163

McCoy RN, Hill KE, Ayon MA et al. (1988) Oxidant stress following renal ischemia: changes in the glutathione redox ration. Kidney Int 33:812–817

McDonald FD, Thiel G, Wilson DR et al. (1969) The prevention of acute renal failure in the rat by long term saline loading: a possible role of the renin angiotensin axis. Proc Soc Exp Biol Med 131:610–614

Mendley SR, Toback FG (1989) Autocrine and paracrine regulation of kidney epithelial cell growth. Annu Rev Physiol 51:33–50

Mergner WJ, Smith MW, Trump BF (1977) Studies on the pathogenesis of ischemic cell injury. Virchows Arch [A] 26:17–26

Mergner WJ, Chang SH, Marzella L et al. (1979) Studies on the pathogenesis of ischemic cell injury. VIII. ATPase activity of rat kidney mitochondria. Lab Invest 40:686–694

Miller SB, Martin DR, Kissane J et al. (1992) IGF I accelerates recovery from ischemic acute tubular necrosis in the rat. Proc Natl Acad Sci USA 89:11876–11880

Miller SB, Martin DR, Kissane J et al. (1994) Hepatocyte growth factor accelerates recovery from acute ischemic renal injury in rats. Am J Physiol 266:F129–F134

Miller WL, Thomas RA, Berne RM (1978) Adenosine production in the ischemic kidney. Circ Res 43:390–397

Molitoris BA (1991) New insights into the cell biology of ischemic acute renal failure. J Am Soc Nephrol 1:1263–1270

Molitoris BA, Kinne R (1987) Ischemia induces surface membrane dysfunction. Mechanism of altered Na^+-dependent glucose transport. J Clin Invest 80:647–654

Molitoris BA, Nelson WJ (1990) Alterations in the establishment and maintenance of epithelial cell polarity as a basis for disease processes. J Clin Invest 85:3–9

Molitoris BA, Chan LK, Shapiro JI et al. (1989a) Loss of epithelial polarity: a novel hypothesis for reduced proximal tubule Na^+ transport following ischemic injury. J Membr Biol 107: 119–127

Molitoris BA, Falk SA, Dahl RH (1989b) Ischemia-induced loss of epithelial polarity. Role of the tight junction. J Clin Invest 84:1334–1339

Morris CR, Alexander EA, Bruns FJ et al. (1972) Restoration and maintenance of glomerular filtration by mannitol during hypoperfusion of the kidney. J Clin Invest 51:1555

Nakamura H, Nemenoff RA, Gronich JH et al. (1991) Subcellular characteristics of phospholipase A_2 activity in the rat kidney: enhanced cytosolic, mitochondrial, and microsomal phospholipase A_2 enzymatic activity after renal ischemia and reperfusion. J Clin Invest 87:1810–1818

Needleman JV, Passonneau, Lowry OH (1968) Distribution of glucose and related metabolites in rat kidneys. Am J Physiol 215:655–659

Neumayer HH, Wagner K, Groll J et al. (1985) Beneficial effects of long-term prostaglandin-E_2 infusion on the course of postischemic acute renal failure. Renal Physiol 8:159–168

Norman J, Tsan Y, Bacay A et al. (1990) Epidermal growth factor accelerates functional recovery from ischemic acute tubular necrosis in the rat. Clin Sci 78:445–450

Ochoa E, Finkielman S, Agrest A (1970) Angiotensin blood levels during the evolution of acute renal failure. Clin Sci 38:225–231

Ohkawa H, Ohishi N, Yagi K (1979) Assay for lipid peroxides in animal tissues by thiobarbituric acid reaction. Anal Biochem 95:351–358

Oken DE, Cotes SC, Flamenbaum W et al. (1975) Active and passive immunization to angiotensin in experimental acute renal failure. Kidney Int 7:12–18
Olbricht C, Mason J, Takabatake T et al. (1977) The early phase of experimental acute renal failure. II. Tubular leakage and the reliabitity of glomerular markers. Pflugers Arch 373:251
Oliver J, MacDowell M, Tracy A (1951) The pathogenesis of acute renal failure associated with traumatic and toxic injury: renal ischemia nephrotoxic damage and the ischemic episode. J Clin Invest 30:1305
Olof P, Hellberg A, Källskog Ö et al. (1991) Red cell trapping and postischemic renal blood flow. Differences between the cortex, outer and inner medulla. Kidney Int 40:625–631
Olsen S, Burdick JF, Keown PA et al. (1989) Primary acute renal failure ("acute tubular necrosis") in the transplanted kidney: morphology and pathogenesis. Medicine 68:173–187
Paller MS (1988) Renal work, gluthathione and susceptibility to free radical-mediated postischemic injury. Kidney Int 33:843–849
Paller MS (1992) Free radical-mediated postichemic injury in renal transplantation. Renal Failure 14:257–260
Paller MS, Hebbel RP (1986) Ethane production as a measure of lipid peroxidation after renal ischemia. Am J Physiol 251:F839–F843
Paller MS, Hedlund BE (1988) The role of iron in post-ischemic renal failure in the rat. Kidney Int 34:474–480
Paller MS, Manivel JC (1992) Prostaglandins protect kidneys against ischemic and toxic injury by a cellular effect. Kidney Int 42:1345–1354
Paller MS, Hoidal JR, Ferris TF (1984) Oxygen free radicals in ischemic acute renal failure in the rat. J Clin Invest 74:1156–1164
Portila D, Mandel LJ, Bar-Sagi D et al. (1992) Anoxia induces phospholipase A_2 activation in rabbit renal proximal tubules. Am J Physiol 262:F354–F360
Racusen LC (1992) Biology of disease: alterations in tubular epithelial cell adhesion and mechanisms of acute renal failure. Lab Invest 67(2):158–165
Rahman N, Kim G, Mathews A et al. (1993) Atrial nathuretic peptide increases creatinine clearance and reduces need for dialysis in patients with established acute renal failure. J Am Soc Nephrol 4:323
Reimer KA, Ganote CE, Jennings RB (1972) Alterations in renal cortex following ischemic injury. III. Ultrastructure of proximal tubules after ischemia or autolysis. Lab Invest 26:347–363
Reineck HJ, O'Connor GJ, Lifschitz MD et al. (1980) Sequential studies on the pathophysiology and glycerol-induced acute renal failure. J Lab Clin Med 96:356
Riley AL (1978) Effect of ischemia on renal blood flow in the rat. Nephron 21:107
Rosen S, Epstein FH, Brazis M (1992) Determinants of intrarenal oxygenation: factors in acute renal failure. Ren Fail 14(3):321–325
Rossi CS, Lehninger AL (1964) Stoichiometry of respiratory stimulation, accumulation of Ca^{2+} and phosphate, and oxidative phosphorylation in rat liver mitochondria. J Biol Chem 239:3971–3980
Ryan R, McNeil JS, Flamenbaum W et al. (1973) Uranyl nitrate induced acute renal failure in the rat: effect of varying doses and saline loading. Proc Soc Exp Biol Med 143:289–296
Safirstein R, Zelent A, Price P (1989) Reduced preproEGF mRNA and diminished EGF excretion during acute renal failure. Kidney Int 36:810–815
Safirstein R, Price PM, Subodh JS et al. (1990) Changes in gene expression after temporary renal ischemia. Kidney Int 37:1515–1521
Savanian A, Kin E (1985) Phospholipase A_2 dependent release of fatty acids from peroxide membranes. J Free Radicals Biol Med 1:263–271
Schaudies RP, Johnson JP (1993) Increased soluble EGF after ischemia is accompanied by a decrease in membrane-associated precursors. Am J Physiol 264:F523–F531
Schieppati A, Wilson PD, Burke TJ et al. (1985) Effect of renal ischemia on cortical microsomal calcium accumulation. Am J Physiol 249:C476–C483

Schrier RW, Arnold PE, Gordon JA et al. (1984) Protection of mitochondrial function by mannitol in ischemic acute renal failure. Am J Physiol 247:F365–F369
Schulman G, Fogo A, Gung A et al. (1991) Complement activation retards resolution of acute ischemic renal failure in the rat. Kidney Int 40:1069–1074
Schumer M, Colombel MC, Sawczuk IS et al. (1992) Morphologic biochemical, and molecular evidence of apoptosis during the reperfusion phase after brief periods of renal ischemia. Am J Pathol 140:831–838
Schwertschlag U, Schrier RW, Wilson P (1986) Beneficial effects of calcium channel blockers and calmodulin binding drugs on in vitro renal cell anoxia. J Pharmacol Exp Ther 238: 119–124
Seiken G, Grillo FG, Schaudies RP et al. (1994) Epidermal growth factor in acute renal failure: interaction with thyroid hormone. Kidney Int (in press)
Shah SV, Walker PD (1992) Reactive oxygen metabolites in toxic acute renal failure. Ren Fail 14(3):363–370
Shaw SG, Weidmann P, Hodler J et al. (1987) Atrial natriuretic peptide protects against acute ischemic renal failure in the rat. J Clin Invest 80:1232–1237
Shibouta Y, Suzuki N, Shino A et al. (1990) Pathophysiological role of endothelin in acute renal failure. Life Sci 46(22):1611–1618
Siegel NJ, Glazier WB, Chaudry IH et al. (1980) Enhanced recovery from acute renal failure by the postischemic infusion of adenine nucleotides and magnesium chloride in rats. Kidney Int 17:338–349
Siegel NJ, Avison MJ, Reilly HF et al. (1983) Enhanced recovery of renal ATP with postischemic infusion of ATP-$MgCl_2$ determined by ^{31}P-NMR. Am J Physiol 245:F530–F534
Siegel NJ, Gaudio KM, Katz LA et al. (1984) Beneficial effect of thyroxin on recovery from acute renal failure. Kidney Int 25:906–911
Smith MW, Collan Y, Kating MW et al. (1980) Changes in mitochondrial lipids of rat kidney during ischemia. Biochim Biophys Acta 618:192–201
Solez K, Altman J, Rienhoff H et al. (1976) Early angiographic and renal blood flow changes after $HgCl_2$ or glycerol administration. Kidney Int 10:S153
Solez K, Ideura T, Saito H (1980) Role of thromboxane and outer medullary microvascular injury in post-ischemic acute renal failure. Clin Res 28:461A
Solez K, Racusen LC, Whelton A (1981) Glomerular epithelial cell changes in early postischemic acute renal failure in rabbits and man. Am J Pathol 103:163
Spiegel DM, Wilson PD, Molitoris BA (1989) Epithelial polarity following ischemia: a requirement for normal cell function. Am J Physiol 256:F430–F436
Spiegel DM, Shanley PF, Molitoris BA (1990) Mild ischemia predisposes the S3 segment to gentamicin toxicity. Kidney Int 38:459–464
Spielman WS, Osswald H (1979) Blockade of postocclusive renal vasoconstriction by an angiotensin II antagonist: evidence for an angiotensin-adenosine interaction. Am J Physiol 237(6):F463–F467
Stein JH, Sorkin MI (1976) Pathophysiology on a vasomotor and nephrotoxic model of acute renal failure in the dog. Kidney Int 10:S86
Stromski ME, Cooper K, Thulin G et al. (1986) Postischemic ATP-Mg Cl_2 provides precursors for resynthesis of cellular ATP in rats. Am J Physiol 250:F834–F837
Stromski ME, van Waarde A, Avidon MJ et al. (1988) Metabolic and functional consequences of inhibiting adenosine deaminase during renal ischemia in rats. J Clin Invest 82:1694–1699
Summers WK, Jamison RL (1971) The no reflow phenomenon in renal ischemia. Lab Invest 25:635
Sutter PM, Thulin G, Stromski M et al. (1988) Beneficial effect of thyroxine in the treatment of ischemic acute renal failure. Pediatr Nephrol 2:1–7
Tanner GA, Steinhausen M (1976) Tubular obstruction in ischemia-induced acute renal failure in the rat. Kidney Int 10:565
Thornton MA, Winn R, Alpers CE, Zager RA (1989) An evaluation of the neutrophil as mediator of in vivo renal ischemia-reperfusion injury. Am J Pathol 135:509–515

Thurau K, Boylan JW (1976) Acute renal success: the unexpected logic of oliguria in acute renal failure. Am J Med 61:308–315

Toback FG (1992) Regeneration after acute tubular necrosis. Kidney Int 41:226–246

Toback FG, Havener FL, Dodd RC et al. (1977) Phospholipid metabolism during renal regeneration after acute tubular necrosis. Am J Physiol 232:E216–E222

Uchiyama M, Mihara M (1978) Determination of malondialdehyde precursor in tissues by thiobarbituric acid test. Anal Biochem 86:271–278

Van Waarde A, Stromski ME, Thulin G et al. (1989) Protection of the kidney against ischemic injury by inhibition of 5′-nucleotidase. Am J Physiol 256:F298–F305

Vanholder RD, Praet MM, Pattyn PA et al. (1982) Dissociation of glomerular filtration and renal blood flow in $HgCl_2$-induced acute renal failure. Kidney Int 22:162

Vetterlein F, Pethö A, Schmidt G (1986) Distribution of capillary blood flow in rat kidney during postischemic renal failure. Am J Physiol 251:H510–H519

Walker PD, Shah SV (1990) Reactive oxygen matabolites in endotoxin-induced acute renal failure in rats. Kidney Int 38:1125–1132

Weinberg JM (1991) Oxygen deprivation-induced injury to isolated rabbit kidney tubules. J Clin Invest 76:1193–1208

Weinberg JM (1985) The cell biology of ischemic renal injury. Kidney Int 39:476–500

Weinberg JM, Humes HD (1980) Mechanisms of gentamicin-induced dysfunction of renal cortical mitochondrial respiration. Arch Biochem Biophys 205:222–231

Weinberg JM, Harding PG, Humes HD (1983) Alterations in renal cortex cation homeostasis during mercuric chloride and gentamicin nephrotoxicity. Exp Mol Pathol 39:43–60

Weinberg JM, Davis JA, Abarzua M et al. (1987) Cytoprotective effects of glycine and glutathione against hypoxic injury to renal tubules. J Clin Invest 80:1446–1454

Weinberg JM, Davis JA, Roeser NF et al. (1991) Role of increased cytosolic free calcium in the pathogenesis of rabbit proximal tubule cell injury and protection by glycine or acidosis. J Clin Invest 87:581–590

Wetzels JFM, Burke TJ, Schrier RW (1992) Calcium channel blockers: protective effects in ischemic acute renal failure. Ren Fail 14(3):327–332

Williams RG, Thomas CE, Navar LG et al. (1981) Hemodynamic and single nephron function during the maintenance phase of ischemic acute renal failure in the dog. Kidney Int 19:503–515

Williamson JR, Schaffer SW, Ford C et al. (1976) Contribution of tissue acidosis to ischemic injury in the perfused rat heart. Circ Res 53:13–114

Wilson DR, Arnold PE, Burke TJ et al. (1984) Mitochondrial calcium accumulation and respiration in ischemic acute renal failure in the rat. Kidney Int 25:519–526

Wilson PD, Schrier RW (1986) Nephron segment and calcium as determinants of anoxic cell death in renal cultures. Kidney Int 29:1172–1179

Wolgast M, Bayati A, Hellberg O (1992) Osmotic diuretics and hemodilution in postischemic renal failure. Ren Fail 14(3):297–302

Wyllie AH, Kerr JFR, Currie AR (1980) Cell death: the significance of apoptosis. Int Rev Cytol 68:251–306

Yagil Y, Myers BD, Jamison RL (1988) Course and pathogenesis of postischemic acute renal failure in the rat. Am J Physiol 255:F257–F264

Young EW, Humes HD (1991) Calcium and acute renal failure. Miner Electrolyte Metab 17:106–111

Zager RA (1983) Gentamicin increases renal susceptibility to an acute ischemic insult. J Lab Clin Med 101:670–678

Zager RA (1986) *Escherichia coli* endotoxin injections potentiate experimental ischemic renal injury. Am J Physiol 251:F988–F994

Zager RA (1988) Hypoperfusion-induced acute renal failure in the rat: an evaluation of oxidant tissue injury. Circ Res 62:430–435

Zager RA (1992) Endotoxemia, renal hypoperfusion, and fever: interactive risk factors for aminoglycoside and sepsis-associated acute renal failure. Am J Kidney Dis 20(3):223–230

Zager RA, Prior RB (1986) Gentamicin and gram negtive bacteremia: a synergism for the development of experimental nephrotoxic acute renal failure. J Clin Invest 78:196–204
Zager RA, Venkatachalam MA (1983) Potentiation of ischemic renal injury by amino acid infusion. Kidney Int 24:620–625
Zager RA, Gmur DJ, Bredl CR et al. (1991a) Temperature effects on ischemic and hypoxic renal proximal tubular injury. Lab Invest 64:766–776
Zager RA, Foerder C, Bredl C (1991b) The influence of mannitol on myoglobinuric acute renal failure: functional, biochemical, and morphological assessments. J Am Soc Nephrol 2:848–855
Zager RA, Iwata M, Burkhart KM et al. (1994) Post-ischemic acute renal failure protects proximal tubules from O_2 deprivation injury. Kidney Int 45:1760–1768
Zeidel ML, Brady HR, Kone BC et al. (1989) Endothelin, a peptide inhibitor of Na^+/K^+-ATPase in intact renal tubular epithelial cells. Am J Physiol 257:C1101–C1107

Pathophysiology of Acute Renal Failure

Z. Symon and M. Brezis

Introduction

Acute renal failure (ARF) remains a poorly understood response of the kidney to hypoperfusion or nephrotoxins and often to both. Better understanding is of paramount importance, because ARF generally affects the sickest of our intensive care unit (ICU) patients and is associated with an overall mortality rate of over 50%, despite modern dialysis treatment [1]. Current notions of the pathophysiology of ARF will be reviewed as they affect prevention and therapy of this serious condition.

Basic Physiopathology of Kidney Failure

Glomerular filtration is driven by the hydrostatic pressure gradient (across the glomerular capillary wall) which forms daily approximately 180 l of primary urine into the tubule lumen. While the proximal tubule reabsorbs 50%–70% of filtered water and sodium, fine solute reabsorption and urine concentration occur more distally along the nephron. Countercurrent exchange of solutes within Henle's loop maximizes the process of urine concentration. An increase in distal urine sodium triggers (at the macula densa) glomerular constriction, with reflex reduction in glomerular filtration (tubuloglomerular feedback).

Kidney failure results from glomerular constriction, tubular obstruction, or backleak of urinary filtrate. The loss of urinary concentrating ability, one of the most consistent findings in ARF, derives from failure of the medullary function. Brown tubular casts in the urine, typically observed in ARF, originate from Tamm-Horsfall protein (synthetized by the medullary thick ascending limb) and indicate medullary injury [1].

The fundamental lesion underlying ARF is believed to be hypoxic cellular injury. In response to ischemia, renal cells undergo a series of biologic alterations including depletion of energy stores, collapse of electrolyte gradients, calcium entry, activation of proteases and phospholipases, formation of reactive oxygen metabolites, and cytoskeletal alterations [2, 3]. A major target for these changes appears to be the renal outer medulla, a site normally working on the brink of anoxia, as discussed below.

Renal Medullary Hypoxia: A Potential Key for the Susceptibility of the Kidney to Various Insults

Renal blood flow, nearly a quarter of the cardiac output, is principally directed to the renal cortex, which therefore receives one of the highest rates of tissue perfusion in the body. This apparent overabundance is designed to maximize flow-dependent renal functions such as glomerular filtration and bulk solute reabsorption along the proximal tubule. By contrast, in the medulla, blood flow and oxygen supply are low to preserve osmotic gradients and to enhance urinary concentration.

Within the medulla, tubules and vessels (vasa recta) are arranged in a hairpin pattern to allow countercurrent exchange of solutes between the descending and ascending limbs in order to maximize the process of urine concentration. Oxygen diffuses from the arterial to the venous branches of the vasa recta, leaving the medulla deficient in oxygen. Medullary hypoxia under normal conditions has been consistently observed in mammalian kidneys, including in man [4, 5]. Ambient medullary pO_2 is in the range of 10–20 mmHg, contrasting with cortical pO_2, which is around 50 mmHg [6]. Inhalation of 100% oxygen hardly affects medullary pO_2, evidence for the physiological isolation of this area of the kidney from the systemic oxygenation. The structures present in the outer medulla, the medullary thick ascending limb (mTAL) and the last portion of the proximal tubule (S_3), are indeed remarkably prone to injury in a variety of models associated with ARF [1, 2, 7, 8].

Medullary hypoxia is the obligatory price the mammalian kidney pays for an efficient urinary concentrating mechanism. Medullary blood flow has to remain low in order to avoid a washout of medullary gradients of osmolality; on the other hand, if too low, medullary blood flow may allow hypoxic injury to tubules. Optimal urinary concentration requires a *perfect matching between O_2 supply and demand by the most precise regulation of blood flow and tubular work in the outer medulla* [9].

Renal Medullary Oxygenation Is Under Precise Physiological Control

To avoid medullary hypoxic damage, the kidney has developed an organized system controlling medullary function and oxygenation. The medulla is a site of rich production of *prostaglandins*, which are released by tissue hypoxia. Prostaglandins increase medullary blood flow and reduce tubular reabsorption, thus providing a defense mechanism from medullary hypoxia [10]. *Nitric oxide* is a potent vasodilator released by the endothelium to induce relaxation in adjacent smooth muscles of the vessel wall, and nitric oxide synthase is present at a high activity in the medulla [11]. Recent studies suggest an important role for nitric oxide in the normal balance of medullary oxygenation [12, 13]. *Adenosine*, released from adenosine triphosphate (ATP) in cellular hypoxia, induces cortical vasoconstriction (with reduction of glomerular filtration) and medullary vasodilation (with inhibiton of transport), effects consistent with an intrarenal homeostatic role to attenuate medullary hypoxia [14–16]. Finally, reflex reduction in glomerular filtration (by tubuloglomerular feedback), activated when mTAL malfunctions in hypoxia, efficiently contributes to the balance of medullary oxygen homeostasis [9].

An integrated system of paracrine mediators appears therefore to act in concert to relieve medullary hypoxia. The net result from their activation and release is restoration of medullary oxygen balance at the expense of a reduction in renal function, either by reduction of transport work or by medullary vasodilation. Failure of these mechanisms because of disease, medications, and especially their combination predisposes to medullary injury and ARF [8].

Etiopathology of Human Acute Renal Failure: A Synergism of Insults

The majority of patients with ARF have more than one acute insult identified, and preexisting renal disease or subclinical kidney pathophysiology is often present [1, 17]. Renal hypoperfusion, one of the most frequently associated conditions, is not readily identified clinically because of the lack of a reliable test to measure renal blood flow at the bedside. It is the responsibility of clinicians to identify patients likely to underperfuse their kidneys when they have reduced cardiac output, generalized atheromatosis, or long-standing diabetes mellitus.

Insults often encountered in the ICU include hypovolemia, hypotension or shock, and exposure to exogenous toxins (e.g., aminoglycosides or radiocontrast) or endogenous toxins (e.g., myoglobin). These insults, rather than predictably inducing ARF, augment the risk of its occurrence: it is therefore more appropriate to define these conditions as *risk factors*. For instance, volume depletion in any patient increases the chance of developing ARF tenfold. The combination of risk factors, so common in the ICU, proportionally increases the likelihood of renal failure.

Epidemiologic studies of ARF have clearly indicated the importance of chronic premorbid conditions in the development of kidney failure [1, 8, 17]. Congestive heart failure, chronic hypertension, chronic diuretic use, diabetes mellitus, preexisting renal disease, and advancing age are chronic risk factors for the development of ARF. The synergism between acute and chronic risk factors plays a fundamental role in the pathogenesis of human ARF.

This synergism of insults has important clinical implications:

1. Prevention of ARF is possible by avoiding combinations of situations, such as the administration of radiocontrast material to a patient with volume depletion or diabetic nephropathy.

2. Experimental models of ARF using *single insults* may be misleading. Multiple insult models may more closely reflect human ARF [8].

Radiocontrast Nephropathy: A Paradigm for the Synergism Between Hypoxic and Toxic Insults in the Kidney

In normal animals, as in healthy humans, radiocontrast administration, even in large doses, produces little injury to the kidneys. As illustrated in Fig. 1, clinical nephrotoxicity is specifically seen in the presence of multiple risk factors, such as diabetes mellitus and preexisting kidney damage, often associated with compromised renal circulation [17]. To produce a simple model of radiocontrast nephropathy, rats were pretreated by simultaneous inhibition of two medullary protective devices, i.e., prostaglandin and nitric oxide, before the administration of contrast medium. Combined

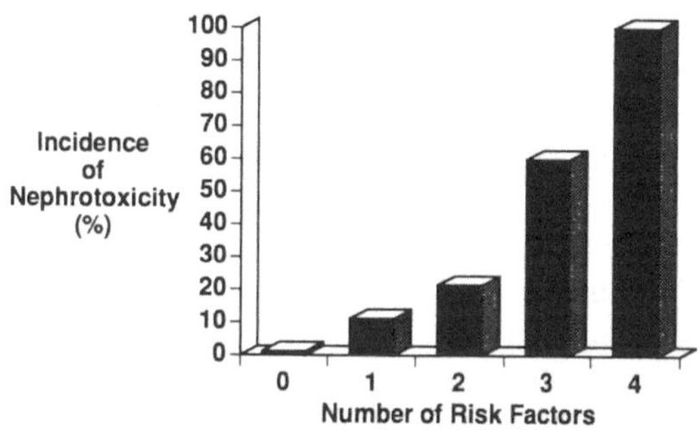

Fig. 1. Incidence of radiocontrast nephrotoxicity as a function of the number of associated risk factors. (Data from [17])

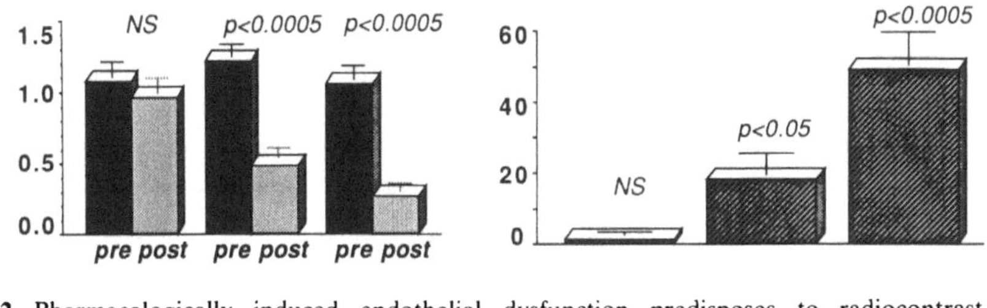

Fig. 2. Pharmacologically induced endothelial dysfunction predisposes to radiocontrast nephrotoxicity. *Left*, creatine clearance (ml/min); *right*, necrosis of medullary thick limbs (%). *NS*, not significant. In the two graphs, *left-hand columns* present data for *N*-nitro-L-arginine methyulester L-NAME alone, *middle columns*, L-NAME with lothalamate, and *right-hand columns*, L-NAME, indomethacin, and lothalamate

pharmacological inhibition of these mechanisms transformed a medullary vasodilator response to radiocontrast into profound vasoconstriction and, as illustrated in Fig. 2, ARF consistently developed, associated with selective necrosis of mTAL [13]. This reversal of the vasoactive response is reminiscent of the effect of endothelial dysfunction in other vascular beds, as for instance in atherosclerotic coronary arteries which paradoxically constrict in response to acetylcholine or serotonin, in contrast to the vasodilation observed in normal arteries. These data suggest a potential role for *endothelial dysfunction* in the pathogenesis of clinical contrast nephropathy.

In fact, imparied endothelium-derived vasorelaxation is often present in diabetes mellitus, hypertension, atherosclerosis, and heart failure, resulting in paradoxical vasoconstriction or reduced vasodilatation with regional hypoxia [18]. Since these diseases are frequently associated with radiocontrast toxicity [1, 17], *endothelial dysfunction* with reduced synthesis of vasodilators in chronic renal/vascular diseases, may predispose patients to medullary injury from contrast medium. Radiocontrast toxicity may be an example for the pathogenic implications of endothelial dysfunction within the kidney. Contrast nephropathy is a paradigm for the synergism between toxic and hypoxic insults to the kidney, illustrating the renal vulnerability to disruption of the delicate O_2 balance within the medulla.

Therapeutic Considerations

Prevention is the most cost-effective management of ARF in the ICU. Particular attention should be directed at preventing volume depletion. Hydration by saline infusion, which reduces the medullary work of urine concentration, is the most rational mode of prophylaxis from injury associated with medullary hypoxia. Cardiac failure, respiratory insufficiency, and brain edema often prohibit volume expansion in the ICU, predisposing patients to renal hypoperfusion and injury from potential nephrotoxins such as radiocontrast or aminoglycosides. Commonly utilized medications may be double edged: furosemide can protect from medullary hypoxic injury, but may induce volume depletion. Since synergism of insults are particularly noxious, clinicians should avoid combination of potential risks, such as volume depletion, nonsteroidal anti-inflammatory drugs, radiocontrast material, or preexisting renal disease.

Growth factors, such as insulin-like growth factor-1, may play a role in enhancing regeneration from ARF, as shown in animals [19], but clinical experience is still lacking. The administration of potent vasodilators (such as atrial natriuretic peptide, dopamine, or endothelin receptor antagonists [20]) in an attempt to improve renal function in ARF has been disappointing. Despite great leaps in our understanding of ARF, new effective therapeutic agents are yet to be implemented. Until such time, salt and water remain our most effective arsenal in preventing ARF.

References

1. Brezis M, Rosen S, Epstein FH (1991) Acute renal failure. In: Brenner BM, Rector F Jr (eds) The kidney, 4th edn. Saunders, Philadelphia
2. Brezis M, Epstein FH (1993) Cellular mechanisms of acute ischemic injury in the kidney. Annu Rev Med 44:27–37
3. Brezis M (1992) Forefront in nephrology: summary of the newer aspects of renal cell injury. Kidney Int 42:523–539
4. Leichtweiss HP, Lubbers DW, Weiss C, Baumgartl H, Reschke W (1969) The oxygen supply of the rat kidney: measurement of intrarenal pO_2. Pflugers Arch 309:328–349
5. Leonhardt KO, Landes RR (1963) Oxygen tension of the urine and renal structures. N Engl J Med 269:115–121
6. Brezis M, Agmon Y, Epstein FH (1994) Determinants of intrarenal oxygenation. I. Effects of diuretics. Am J Physiol (in press)
7. Brezis M, Dinour D, Greenfeld Z, Rosen S (1991) Susceptibility of Henle's loop to toxic and hypoxic insults. In: Grunfeld J, Maxwell MH (eds) Advances in nephrology. Mosby, Chicago, pp 41–56
8. Brezis M, Epstein FH (1993) Pathophysiology of acute renal failure. In: Goldstein RS, Hook JB (eds) Toxicology of the kidney, 2nd edn. Raven, New York, pp 129–152
9. Brezis M, Rosen S, Epstein FH (1989) The pathophysiological implications of medullary hypoxia. Am J Kidney Dis 13:253–258
10. Agmon Y, Brezis M (1993) Effects of nonsteroidal anti-inflammatory drugs upon intrarenal blood flow: selective medullary hypoperfusion. Exp Nephrol 1:357–363
11. Morrissey J, McCracken R, Kaneto H, Vehaskari M, Montani D, Klahr S (1993) Location of an inducible nitric oxide synthase (NOS) in the medullary thick ascending limb. J Am Soc Nephrol 4:560
12. Brezis M, Heyman SN, Dinour D, Epstein FH, Rosen S (1991) Role of nitric oxide in renal medullary oxygenation. J Clin Invest 88:390–395
13. Agmon Y, Peleg H, Greenfeld Z, Rosen S, Brezis M (1994) Nitric oxide and prostanoids protect the renal outer medulla from radocontrast toxicity in the rat. J Clin Invest (in press)
14. Dinour D, Brezis M (1991) Effects of adenosine upon intrarenal oxygenation. Am J Physiol 261:F787–F791
15. Dinour D, Brezis M (1993) Intrarenal adenosine: a regulatory role upon medullary oxygenation? Exp Nephrol 1:152–157
16. Agmon Y, Dinour D, Brezis M (1993) Disparate effects of adenosine A1- and A2-receptor agonists on intrarenal blood flow. Am J Physiol 265:F802–F806
17. Rich MW, Crecelius CA (1990) Incidence, risk factors, and clinical course of acute renal insufficiency after cardiac catheterization in patients 70 years of age or older. A prospective study. Arch Intern Med 150:1237–1242
18. Luscher TF (1993) Mack Forster Award Lecture. Review. The endothelium as a target and mediator of cardiovascular disease. Eur J Clin Invest 23:670–685
19. Ding H, Kopple JD, Cohen A, Hirshberg R (1993) Recombinant human insulin-like growth factor accelerates recovery and reduces catabolism in rats with ischemic acute renal failure. J Clin Invest 91:2281–2287
20. Cantley LG, Spokes K, Clark B, McMahon EG, Carter J, Epstein FH (1993) Role of endothelin and prostaglandins in radiocontrast induced renal artery constriction. Kidney Int 44:1217–1223

Mechanisms of Tissue Damage in Acute Renal Failure

C. Tetta, G. Montrucchio, C. Ronco, and G. Camussi

Introduction

Acute renal failure (ARF) is a rapid decline in renal excretory function. Its clinical hallmark is rapidly progressive azotemia, which is usually, but not necessarily, accompanied by oliguria and overall altered body homeostasis. The significance of the syndrome is accentuated by the fact that ARF is one of the few instances of organ failure that is completely reversible, provided that the cause is rapidly recognized and appropriate treatment is instituted. The major causes of acute renal failure are listed below on the basis of the classical, but still valid classification of prerenal (impaired perfusion), intrarenal (due to damage to renal structures), and finally postrenal causes (obstructive pathologies of the lower urinary tract):

1. Prerenal causes
   a) Hypovolemia
   b) Decreased effective plasma volume
   c) Decreased cardiac output
   d) Renovascular obstruction
   e) Interference with renal autoregulation
2. Renal causes
   a) Glomerular and small vessel diseases
   b) Interstitial nephritis
   c) Tubular lesions
3. Postrenal causes
   a) Bladder outflow obstruction
   b) Ureteral obstruction (bilateral or single kidney)

ARF is rarely seen today as a separate, well-defined entity, although it was frequently seen less than 20 years ago in almost all surgical wards. It has recently become fairly rare to find isolated ARF following shock, bleeding, or trauma.

Being able to prevent milder injuries, we are now faced with the more severely injured patient with multiple injuries. Such patients suffer from failure of many organs simultaneously. They are in shock, in respiratory failure, with signs of liver damage, a low cardiac output, and often disturbed states of consciousness. In a recent overview, every year 172 adults per million inhabitants develop ARF. The causes are cardiovascular insufficiency (13%), postsurgery (14%), obstetrical causes (11%), prostate obstruction (25%), medical causes (34%) including toxins (7%), glomerulonephritis (17%), hematological causes (19%), dehydration or hemorrhage (26%), and miscellaneous (31%) [1–3]. In a recent retrospective study on 118 patients with ARF admitted between 1980 and 1991, Alexopoulos et al. [4] showed a change in the patterns and prognostic factors of ARF in a medical setting in comparison with an earlier series in the 1960s. These authors showed a marked decline in the hypotension-related cases and a concomitant increase in the nephrotoxic causes. The overall mortality rate was 27%, virtually unchanged in comparison to the 1960s. Sepsis and cardiovascular complications are the leading causes of death [4, 5].

ARF is frequently associated with gram-negative sepsis [6]. Bacterial lipopolysaccharides (LPS), released from gram-negative cell walls, possess a wide range of biologic activities and appear to be the main causative factor in sepsis-induced ARF. The mechanism of LPS-induced tissue injury are complex. Hemodynamic changes, namely protracted hypotension, play a primary but not exclusive role in causing the fall in glomerular filtration rate (GFR) [7–10]. In fact ARF may occur in the absence of altered hemodynamics, suggesting that other mechanisms may come into play. Autonomic or hormonal alterations such as increased angiotensin II and norepinephrine have been suggested [8, 11]. Recently, several studies have provided evidence for inflammatory mediators to be of relevance in determining structural and functional changes capable of establishing ARF. Eicosanoids [8, 11], cytokines (tumor necrosis factor, TNF; interleukins, IL, such as IL-1, IL-6, IL-8) [12, 13], endothelin (ET), and platelet-activating factor (PAF) [14] may all contribute to the fall of renal blood flow (RBF) and GFR during sepsis.

The biologic properties of these mediators alone or in combination may account for the metabolic and hemodynamic changes in sepsis-induced ARF.

Many experimental models of ARF have been proposed and studied in detail. However, it is apparent from experimental work in animals that no single mechanisms can account for renal failure [3]. A complex interplay between various mediators and resident or recruited renal cells occurs and may lead to functional alterations in kidney function [15–20]. Different mechanisms operate in different models and at different times (Fig. 1). Transposition into the clinical setting of humans may not be direct, since human ARF is often the consequence of many causes that act synergically and at different times during the history of the disease. This review will discuss our present knowledge of the mechanisms of tissue damage in experimental and human ARF.

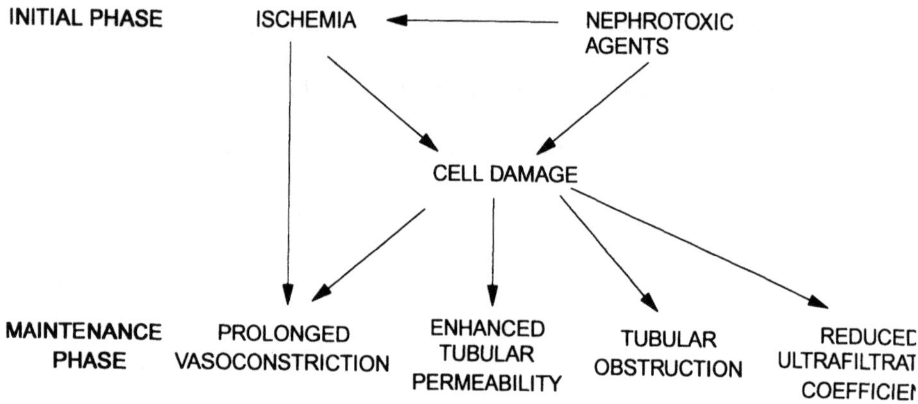

Fig. 1. Pathogenesis of acute renal failure

Role of Metabolic Alterations and Medlators in Acute Renal Failure

Oxygen Free Radicals

Restriction in oxygen availability in ischemic kidney leads to a rapid degradation of tissue adenosine triphosphate (ATP) with an increase in adenosine monophosphate (AMP) that is in turn metabolized into adenosine, inosine, and ipoxantine [21, 22]. Ionic gradients across cell plasma membranes are likewise altered, causing a rise in cytosolic Ca^{2+} that results in activation of proteases capable of triggering the generation of xanthine oxidase (X.O.) from xanthine dehydrogenase [23, 24]. Following reperfusion, restoration of oxygen delivery together with the biochemical events associated with ischemia causes the oxidation of ipoxantine with generation of superoxide anion (O_2^-) according to the following reaction [25]:

$$\text{hypoxanthine} + 2O_2 + H_2O \xrightarrow{XO} \text{xanthine} + 2O_2^- + 2H^+$$

Following the spontaneous or (O_2)-catalyzed dismutation, H_2O_2 is generated. Finally, hydroxyl radicals (OH·) are formed by the interaction between O_2^- and H_2O_2 and transition metals usually iron, acting as catalysts [25]. The formation of O_2^-, H_2O_2 and OH· induces tissue injury through lipid peroxidation. Loss of structural integrity of plasma membranes, mitochondria, and lysosomes then ensues and is accompanied by functional alterations such as derangements in ion transport and increased permeability of lysosomal membranes, leading to the release of proteolytic enzymes that amplify the tissue damage. Regulatory mechanisms of oxygen free radicals normally exist in tissues. Endogenous scavengers such as superoxide dismutase (SOD) may cause anion superoxide to be rapidly removed; catalase and glutathione peroxidase inactivate H_2O_2 [26, 27]. Finally, tryptophan, histidine, ascorbic acid, and vitamin E exhibit scavenging properties on hydroxyl radicals [22, 26–28]. Furthermore, during reperfusion, reactive oxygen species induce the production of heat shock proteins (hsp) [3, 29]. The latter are also protective agents capable of limiting the oxidative damage. This property is related to their ability to function as "chaperones."

Among the known functions of hsp are protein–protein interactions, prevention of aggregation and misassembly of nascent peptides, molecular transport, and translocation across cellular membranes. They also bind ATP, thus maintaining the intracellular levels, inhibit the increase of cytosolic Ca^{2+} following exposition to the reactive oxygen species, inhibit radical formation, increase the tissue concentration of classical scavengers, inhibit phospolipase A_2 activity, and prevent lipid peroxidation [29]. However, in spite of these potent protective mechanisms, ischemia is associated with a remarkable decrease in the scavenging and antioxidant potential, thus leading to unrestrained damaging effects induced by oxygen free radicals. Several studies performed with different scavengers or XO inhibitors have shown that the latter can mediate tissue injury following transient ischemia and reperfusion. In vivo studies have demonstrated a protective effect of SOD infused before ischemia or just before reperfusion, as it reduces both the functional and morphological alterations induced by ischemic kidney [25, 30, 31]. Furthermore, ischemic kidney damage is remarkably more extensive in rats fed with a vitamin E-free or selenium-free diet than in controls, suggesting the important protective role of these antioxidants in modulating the ischemic injury [32].

The generation of oxygen radicals has recently been evaluated in the ischemic-reperfused model of ARF in the rabbit using a modified spin-trap technique [33]. A significant increase in oxygen radical production was observed during reperfusion. Oxypurinol completely abolished such production when administered before ischemia [33]. However, the protective effect of SOD, dimethylurea, or allopurinol is still controversial. Furthermore, in vitro studies on anoxic isolated proximal tubule failed to detect either oxygen radicals or lipid peroxidation [34]. However, cultured epithelial cells may generate oxygen-derived reactive species early during the reoxygenation after anoxia [35]. Nevertheless, a role for oxygen free radicals has been suggested in different experimental models of ARF, i.e., miohemoglobinuric, nephrotoxic (gentamicin, glycerol, or contrast media) [36–40]. Antioxidant therapy may find potential applications in all clinical settings associated with ischemia reperfusion such as transplantation and surgery on the large vessels (aorta, renal arteries).

Phospholipase A_2

A role for phospholipase A_2 in ischemic kidney injury has been suggested [3, 41] Phospholipase A_2 encompasses a family of enzymes capable of hydrolyzing the acyl in position 2 of glycerolphospholipids with formation of free fatty acids and lysophospholipids. Various forms of phospholipase A_2 are present in the cytoplasm and in the mitochondrial and microsomal membranes [41]. Phospholipase A_2 activity in the kidney extract increases after ischemia reperfusion [42]. The increased phospholipase A_2 activity appears to be, at least in part, modulated by intracellular Ca^{2+} concentrations. Phospholipase A_2 contributes to ischemic kidney injury through different mechanisms: (a) phospholipase A_2 can modify phospholipids with generation of free fatty acids and lysophospholipids having toxic effects on plasma and mitochondrial membranes leading to increased permeability, fluidity, and bioenergy; (b) phospholipase A_2 may activate the metabolism of arachidonic acid, resulting in the generation of cyclo- and lipo-oxygenase-dependent products such as prostaglandins, thromboxanes, and leukotrienes with the simultaneous generation of oxygen-derived reactive species [43]; (c) phospholipase A_2 generates precursors that enter the remodeling pathway of PAF synthesis [44]; (d) phospholipase A_2 contributes to mitochondrial injury together with free oxygen radicals and Ca^{2+} [45].

Protease Activation

The exact role of different proteases in ischemic kidney injury still remains to be defined. A role for calpain, a cytoplasmic cistein protease, has been recently suggested in human or rabbit tubules exposed to anoxia or in the presence of cyclosporin A [46]. However, other cysteine proteases present in lysosomes do not seem to be implicated in cell injury [3, 41]. The tubule brush border contains several proteases such as the C3 convertase [47, 48], meprin, and the endopeptidase 24.11. Their possible role in the pathogenesis of tissue injury is likely, but will require confirmation. Finally, it has been suggested that proteases may contribute to the recruitment of blood-borne inflammatory cells in the kidney during ischemia reperfusion [49].

Nitric Oxide

Furchgott and Zawadzki [50] showed that the relaxation induced by acetylcholine was dependent on the presence of an intact endothelium. A humoral factor, distinct from prostacyclin and adenosine, with a short half-life ranging from 6 to 80 s was implicated and tentatively named "endothelium-derived relaxing factor" (EDRF) [51]. Chemical characterization of ERDF led to its identification in nitric oxide (NO) and to the clarification of its synthesis precursors, of the pharmacologic and physiologic alterations that stimulate the release of NO, and of the mechanisms of NO vasodilation [52]. NO is synthesized in endothelial cells from a nitrogen atom contained in the guanidino group of the amino acid L-arginine. The reaction is catalyzed by a constitutive NO synthase, a monoxygenase that induces hydroxylation into N^{G}-hydroxy-L-arginine, which is subsequently converted to N^{G}-oxo-L-arginine by the oxidation of the hydroxylamine group. The amino acid radical generated in this last step is so unstable that it fragments to yield NO and a stable compound that will yield citrulline. The NO synthase, the enzyme that initiates the conversion of L-arginine into citrulline, is a Ca^{2+} and cadmodulin-dependent enzyme. Analogues of L-arginine such as *N*-monomethyl-L-arginine (1-NMMA) and *N*-nitro-L-arginine methylester (L-NAME) completely inhibit the enzyme activity via competitive binding. These analogues have proved extremely useful to implicate NO synthesis in pathophysiological conditions [52–57].

NO plays a key role in the regulation of renal vascular tone, as NO released by either the renal artery or glomerular capillaries regulates the renal vascular resistance. In the vase recta, which are surrounded by a rich net of pericytes containing abundant contractile filaments, the production of NO has been implicated in the increased medullary blood flow and the increased renal interstitial pressure that stimulates natriuresis [58–60]. In animals, the endogenous production of NO might be a factor capable of preventing endotoxin-induced ARF and glomerular thrombosis [61]. Nitro vasodilatation may participate in the balance of renal medullary oxygenation and play an important role in the prevention of tubular hypoxic injury [58]. In humans, some studies have shown an increase in blood pressure in patients with septic shock after the administration of an inhibitor of nitric oxide synthesis [62]. However, the issue is still controversial, since animal studies have demonstrated that such inhibition may increase mortality [63]. The regulation of the renal vascular tone results in the balance of vasodilatory and vasoconstrictor stimuli. If prostacyclin and NO are the most important vasodilatory substances produced by endothelial cells, ET, recently purified from the supernatants of cultured porcine endothelial cells, is the most potent vasoconstrictor ever isolated.

Endothelin

ET is a 21-amino acid peptide presenting two disulfide bonds among amino acids 1–15 and 3–11 [64]. The importance of the disulfide bonds is demonstrated by the loss of biologic activity after reduction. Subsequent to ET-1, two more peptides have been identified, ET-2 and ET-3, However, only ET-1 can be released from endothelial cells, mesangial cells, and several renal cell lines, i.e., tubular epithelial cell lines [65–67]. ET is first produced as a preproET, a 203-amino acid peptide. The latter is cleaved intracellularly to proET. To form ET, proET-1 undergoes proteolytic cleavage by an endopeptidase called endothelin-converting enzyme [64]. ET receptors have been found in many tissues and, of particular interest for renal hemodyamics, in mesangial cells [68]. Interaction within specific receptors triggers increase in cytosolic Ca^{2+} and activation of phospholipases A_2, C, and D.

ET induces contraction of mesangial cells and release of prostaglandins [68]. Several substances, such as thrombin, transforming growth factor-β (TGF-β), IL-1, TNF-α, vasopressin, calcium ionophore, and cyclosporine, or physicochemical stimuli, such as hypoxia and shear stress, induce the expression of preproET mRNA and/or release of ET [64]. Isolated glomeruli and tubule epithelial cells produce significant amounts of ET during renal ischemia [64, 69]. The intrarenal infusion of ET at very low concentrations leads to a marked reduction of RBF and GFR (35% single nephron GFR, SNGFR, reduction) [70, 71]. These data, together with the demonstration that anti-ET antibodies prevent postischemic vasoconstriction and ameliorate SNGFR and RBF in the postischemic period, suggest a role of ET in the pathogenesis of hypoperfusion and hypofiltration associated to ischemic ARF [72].

In humans, significantly increased ET levels have been detected during ARF induced by different causes [73–75]. Recently, Lopez-Farre et al. [69] have shown that the pretreatment with anti-ET antibodies reduces the glomerular production of PAF during renal ischemia. It is likely that ET is an important stimulus for the glomerular synthesis of PAF. However, postischemic production of PAF is not fully abrogated by the administration of anti-ET antibodies, thus suggesting that other ET-independent extraglomerular sites of PAF synthesis may be involved. ET is now recognized as an important mediator in the pathogenesis of ARF. Using an experimental model of bilateral ureteral obstruction in the rat, Reyes and Klahr [72] have shown that rats treated with anti-ET-1 antibodies had a higher GFR and NO than control rats.

A role for ET has also been suggested in sepsis-induced ARF [64]. In sepsis, cytokines such as TNF and IL-1 may be appropriate stimuli for triggering the synthesis of ET-1 [76]. However, the cell targets for ET synthesis are different. TNF induces the synthesis of ET-1 from both glomerular endothelial and epithelial cells [76, 77]. However, only epithelial cells synthesize ET-1 in response to IL-1 [78]. The in vivo administration of endotoxin induces an increase in plasma levels of ET [78].

Finally, ET-1 has been implicated in the vasoconstriction observed in models of glomerular dysfunction induced by cyclosporine [79]. Studies in humans also support the possibility that ET may be relevant in the pathogenesis of ARF.

Platelet-Activating Factor

PAF is a lipid-inflammatory mediator that belongs to the the family of acetylated alkyl phosphoglycerides [44]. PAF is involved in the pathogenesis of both ischemic and toxic ARF. Ischemic rat kidney or isolated glomeruli produce PAF that is, at least in part, due to ET generation [69]. Endotoxin also stimulates PAF synthesis and release from human and rat glomeruli and cultured mesangial cells. The latter synthesize PAF also in response to porins, IL-1, and TNF, suggesting a possible role of PAF in ARF associated to septic shock [80, 81]. PAF acts directly on isolated glomeruli, leading to the reduction of planar surface area ensuing in reduced GFR. The direct action of PAF is related to the contraction of mesangial cells [82]. Moreover, TNF and IL-1 contract mesangial cells via PAF production and its direct action on these cells. Mesangial cell contraction induced by PAF is enhanced following inhibition of prostaglandins and is partially reversed after readdition of exogenous PGE_2. Schlondorff et al. [16] have suggested that the generation of PGE_2 induced by PAF may be a negative feedback on PAF-induced mesangial contraction. PAF stimulates the synthesis of thromboxane A_2 from isolated perfused kidney of the rat and the rabbit and induces the generation of oxygen radicals from cultured mesangial cells, leading to the potential amplification of tissue injury [83, 84].

In in vivo conditions, PAF causes a decline of GFR and RBF as a consequence of arteriolar vasoconstriction and/or of mesangial contraction [82]. Continuous intravenous administration of PAF causes the fall of SNGFR and RBF followed by increased arteriolar resistance and a decreased glomerular ultrafiltration coefficient [85]. These effects are also present

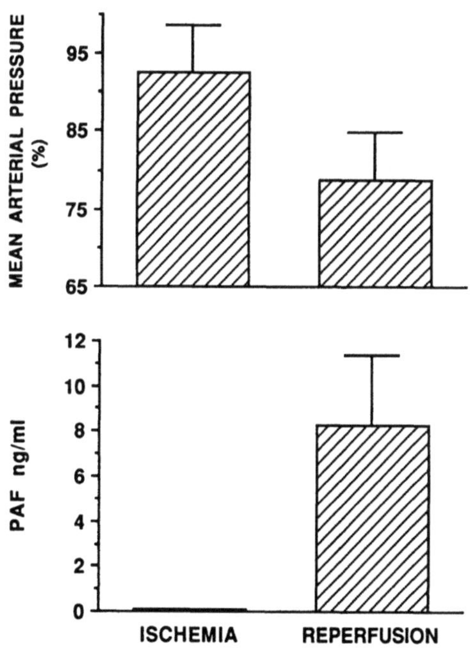

Fig. 2. Renal platelet-activating factor (*PAF*) production (*bottom*) and mean arterial blood pressure (*top*) in rabbit after 30 min clamping of renal artery followed by reperfusion

during the selective infusion of PAF into the renal artery and are associated with a reduction of urine output [86], and Na^+ excretion, and with an increase in glomerular permeability [87, 88].

The potential role of PAF in the pathogenesis of ischemic and toxic ARF has been suggested by evidence of its neosynthesis as well as of the beneficial effect of specific PAF receptor antagonists. Clamping of the renal artery in the rabbit for 30 min leads to the synthesis of high amounts of PAF detectable in the homolateral renal vein following reperfusion and to a significant decrease in mean arterial pressure and reduction in urine output (Fig. 2). These results are in agreement with the data obtained by Lopez-Farre et al. [69], who reported the glomerular synthesis of PAF in renal ischemia/reperfusion injury in the rat associated with oliguria, increased plasma creatinine levels, and reduction of blood creatinine clearance and GFR. These effects are significantly reduced by pretreatment with BN 52021, a specific PAF receptor antagonist.

Wang and Dunn [89] and Tolins et al. [90] have demonstrated that two structurally unrelated PAF receptor antagonists ameliorate the renal function during endotoxemia. PAF is also implicated in ARF caused by gentamicin and *cis*-platinum [91]. The acute or chronic administration of *cis*-platinum or gentamicin causes nonoliguric ARF. A PAF receptor antagonist abrogates the fall of SNGFR or transcapillary hydraulic pressure and the RBF following *cis*-platinum, and ameliorates by about 20% the decline in SNGFR and RBF after gentamicin administration [91].

Prostaglandins and Thromboxane A_2

The renal cortex that comprises arteries, arterioles, and glomerular tufts is the site of prostaglandin synthesis in the kidney. Glomerular endothelial, mesangial, and epithelial cells possess the enzymatic systems necessary for the biosynthesis of prostaglandins and thromboxane A_2 [92]. Mesangial an epithelial cells, when appropriately stimulated, synthesize arachidonic acid-derived metabolites (endoperoxides), (PGG_2 and PGH_2) via the cyclo-oxygenase or the lipo-oxygenase pathways after remodeling of membrane phospholipids due to the activity of phospholipase A_2. PGH_2 is then converted by a specific thromboxane synthetase into TXA_2, a potent vasoconstricting agent of vascular smooth muscle and mesangial cells [93–96].

The glomerulus also synthesizes other products of the cyclo-oxygenase pathway with generation of PGE_2 and PGI_2 with vasodilating properties [97–99]. The amounts of prostaglandins and TXA_2 depends on the animal species, but above all, on the nature of the stimulus [100]. Human glomeruli predominantly synthesize PGI_2 rather than PGE_2, $PGF_{2\alpha}$, and TXA_2 [101, 102]. Furthermore, while angiotensin II induces mainly the synthesis of PGI_2 and PGE_2 [103], other stimuli such as IL-1 [104], oxygen free radicals [105, 106], LPS [107], PAF [82, 85, 108], and ET [109, 110] induce the glomerular neosynthesis of prostaglandins and TXA_2, their relative synthesis being different on the basis of the nature and dose of the stimuli. In contrast, the proximal tubule and the loop of Henle produce only a little amount of eicosanoids, which is consistent with the absence of histochemical and immunohistochemical detection of cyclo-oxygenase peroxidase activity [83]. In connecting tubules, prostaglandin synthesis is also very low, but progressively increases in the cortical and medullary connecting tubules. The predominant prostaglandin generated is PGE_2 [111]. Medullary interstitial cells, which are in close contact with both vasa recta and the ascending loop of Henle, synthesize mainly PGE_2, which has been proposed to affect the handling of sodium chloride by the thick ascending limb of Henle's loop [93, 112, 113]. In addition, PGE_2 generated by intersitial cells may play a role in maintaining blood flow in the poorly oxygenated and hypertonic medullary region [92].

An altered synthesis of prostaglandins and/or TXA_2 has been implicated in drug-induced [114, 115], ischemic, and septic ARF [116–119]. Anti-inflammatory nonsteroidal drugs may cause ARF in hypovolemic states such as cardiac insufficiency and hepatic cyrrhosis in which prostaglandins have an important vasodilatory role in the maintainance of RBF [114, 115]. In fact, in such hypoperfusion conditions, the reduction of RBF causes an increment in renin–angiotensin synthesis, leading to arteriolar vasoconstriction and mesangial contraction as well as the increase in PGE_2 and PGI_2 synthesis. The latter, with their vasodilatory effect, balance the vasoconstricting effects of both renin and angiotensin [119–122].

The inhibition of cyclo-oxygenase by anti-inflammatory nonsteroidal drugs may lead to reduced synthesis of PGE_2 and PGI_2 and cause ARF [92, 114]. Prompt recognition of such situation is imperative, since ARF is fully reversible. An increased synthesis of TXA_2 has been correlated with a rise in vascular resistance and a reduction in GFR and RBF during ARF induced by the administration of LPS in the rat [116–118]. These events on the renal function are abrogated by TXA_2 inhibitors, thus suggesting that TXA_2 influences the afferent and efferent arteriolar tone [116–118]. An increased production of TXA_2 has been implicated in experimental glycerol-induced ARF [123] and in the glomerular vasoconstriction associated with persistent ureteral obstruction [124].

Tubulointerstitial Response to Acute Injury

Several types of cells, including tubular epithelium, a variety of interstitial cells (type I and II in the cortex, types I–III in the medulla), interstitial fibroblasts, vascular endothelium, macrophages, and several phenotypes of lymphocytes, constitute the cellular registry of the tubulointerstial microenvironment. Interstitial fibroblasts form a distinct population of cells adapted to the tubulointerstitial environment. The renal tubule is a polarized, structurally and functionally complex epithelial cell. Situated between the internal and external milieu, tubular epithelia in the nephron perform functions critical to internal homeostasis, including readsorption of filtered solutes and water, secretion of metabolic byproducts, maintainance of acid-base balance, and regulation of fluid volume [125].

The high metabolic rate and transport demands on tubular cells, especially in specific nephron segments in the cortex and outer medulla, make these cells particularly vulnerable to injury. Furthermore, the high normal renal blood flow (3.5 ml/min per g versus an average of 1.0 ml/min per g) results in the rapid delivery of toxins to the tubulointerstitial environment. Despite this generous blood supply, certain regions of the tubule operate under conditions of continuously poor oxygen delivery and are thus susceptible to damage by substances that increase metabolic demand. Substances which are filtered by the glomeruli may be concentrated along the luminal surface of the tubule, from where they enters the cell and are transported intracellularly. The inverse direction is followed by substances that are excreted by the tubules.

For many years, renal injury from ischemia/hypoxia and toxic agents has been often labeled "acute tubular necrosis." However, it is commonly recognized that tubular necrosis is far from being the hallmark of most cases of animal models or human conditions associated with ARF [126, 127]. Rather, the most striking features are sublethal cell injury with loss of apical brush border in the proximal tubule, formation of apical cytoplasmic blebs, cell swelling, and cell vacuolization as well as denuded areas along the tubular basement membrane with loss of the tubular epithelial cell lining. Several molecules are involved in the response to acute tubular injury such as cytokines and adhesion molecules.

Cytokines

Epithelial cells may interact with T cells and macrophages, thus initiating tissue damage. Clinical counterparts of such interaction are seen in acute rejection or in ARF in sepsis. In rejection, renal tubular cells may participate since (a) they can express both major histocompatibility complex (MHC) class I and II as well as intercellular adhesion molecule (ICAM)-1 when stimulated by γ-interferon [128, 129], (b) they can secrete and express membrane-bound cytokines [130], and (c) they are exposed to molecules present in the ultrafiltrate that they may process either to potentially immunogenic compounds or to biologically active fragments [131]. The expression of MHC genes coding for class II antigen is inducible. Tubular cells have the capacity to do so in physiopathological conditions associated with immune stimulation. Kinetic studies of γ-interferon stimulation of proximal tubular epithelial cells indicate that surface expression occurs within 24–48 h and reaches maximal levels in 3–4 days [132]. Removal of γ-interferon results in a gradual loss of class II expression in these cells.

Proximal tubular cells normally produce low levels of secreted and membrane forms of TNF. The production of TNF can be upregulated by LPS and IL-1α in a dose- and time-dependent fashion [130]. Although the physiological relevance of steady production of TNF by renal tubular cells has not been conclusively elucidated, it may facilitate cell communication with T cells or macrophages. TNF production may likely increase in conditions associated with endotoxemia. TNF is a multifunctional cytokine recognized as the primary mediator of septic shock [133]. Thus, TNF may trigger secondary mediators such as thromboxanes and PAF from inflammatory cells recruited in the renal interstitium and contribute to tissue injury [134]. Production of TNF occurs in situ at sites of mononuclear cell infiltrate. The ability of tubular cells to produce IL-6 and IL-8 has also recently been established [135–137].

Adhesion Molecules

Cell attachment normally includes molecules that assure cell–cell and cell–substrate adhesion [138–144]. Moreover, adhesion molecules are connected with cytoskeleton components such as talin and vinculin that are important to maintain cell polarity as well as structural and functional integrity of the epithelium [145, 146]. Integrins have been proposed to mediate the interaction between the extracellular matrix and the cytoskeleton [144, 147]. Integrins are heterodimeric transmembrane receptors constituted by two noncovalently bound α- and β-subunits. The integrin superfamily is subdivided into protein families on the basis of the β-subunits. The β_1 family of integrins includes the collagen receptor ($\alpha_1\beta_1$ and $\alpha_2\beta_1$), the receptor for fibronectin, laminin, and collagens ($\alpha_3\beta_1$), the lymphocyte-homing receptor ($\alpha_4\beta_1$), the fibronectin receptor ($\alpha_5\beta_1$), and the laminin receptor ($\alpha_6\beta_1$). The β_2 family of integrins includes the leukocyte adhesion proteins, and the β_3 family comprises the vitronectin receptor ($\alpha_v\beta_3$) and the platelet glycoprotein IIb/IIIa complex.

Studies on the distribution of the integrin superfamily in human fetal and adult kidney have shown that integrins of the β_1 subtype are found basally and colocalized with talin [147]. However, integrins appear to be absent laterally and therefore represent a novel type of polarized protein distribution in epithelial cells [148]. In this case, a receptor–ligand interaction might be responsible for such compartmentalization and there should be no diffusion barrier between these domains [148].

A major cell adhesion molecule found in the rodent renal tubule is the liver cell adhesion molecule (L-CAM; uvomorulin; E-cadherin) and is also expressed in epithelial cells cultured from isolated mammalian tubules [149]. Others have reported the expression of adherence junction-specific CAM (A-CAM), a member of the *N*-cadherin subclass, as the major ICAM in adult human kidney, present on the basal aspect of tubular cells along the entire length of the nephron [150]. The impact of injury on the expression and distribution of normal adhesion molecules is now beginning to be appreciated [148]. E-cadherin is partially internalized following energy depletion in cultured cell lines derived from the renal tubule [151]. This occurs within 20 min of injury and increases with time. The $\alpha_3\beta_1$-subunits of integrins undergo redistribution over the cell surface rather than a net reduction, probably as a result of disruption of the tight junction barrier and/or alterations in the cell cytoskeleton [152]. The role of cytoskeleton appears critical in maintaining cell–cell and cell–substrate adhesion in renal tubule epithelium [138, 139, 142, 145, 153–157].

Several studies have demonstrated that following experimental injury, vimentin and actin undergo conspicuous alterations (widespread redistribution from disorganization to complete loss of stress fibers). More particularly, in human proximal tubule cell cultures, cells under anoxic conditions undergo shape change with rounding and retraction reflecting at least in part alterations in cell adhesion [158, 159]. This is associated with redistribution of actin filaments from the terminal web to the basal margins of the retracted cells and with aggregation of short filaments around the nuclei of the cells. These alterations and cell shape changes are remarkably inhibited by phalloidin, which is known to stabilize microfilaments. That cytoskeleton changes may be critical in the early cell alterations is also suggested by the redistribution from basolateral membranes to a diffuse pancytoplasmic pattern in both proximal and distal tubules in ischemic pig kidneys following renal artery ligation [160].

Integrins may also be important in mediating increased adherence of desquamated epithelial cells, thus favoring tubular obstruction [161]. Reorientation of the α_3-subunit of integrins from predominantly basal to the apical cell surface of cultured tubule epithelial cells occurs following oxidant stress and complement activation [48, 161]. Stressed epithelial cells exhibited specific recognition and binding of laminin-coated latex beads. These processes were inhibited with the peptide Gly-Arg-Gly-Asp-Asn-Pro, suggesting a role of Arg-Gly-Asp (RGD-) recognizing integrins in augmented adhesion to stressed cells [161].

Drug Nephrotoxicity

Membrane damage is the key event in cell injury caused by many drugs capable of injuring the renal tubular cells directly. Acute tubular damage is a relatively common complication of a prolonged therapy of aminoglycoside antibiotics, occurring in 5%–15% of patients [162, 163]. The renal damage associated with the aminoglycosides is cumulative due to their accumulation in the proximal tubular cells. The mechanism of action appears to rely on the charge interaction (NH_3^+) and the anionic phospholipid receptors in the luminal and subcellular membranes [164]. This interaction at the luminal membrane facilitates the movement of the drug from the lumen into the tubular cell. Within the cell, the drug accumulates within lysosomes, an effect that may be mediated by a similar charge interaction. The number of cationic groups (NH_3^+) per molecule appears to correlate closely with clinical nephrotoxicity [4]. Thus, neomycin (6 NH_3^+/molecule) produces the most renal damage and streptomycin (3 NH_3^+/molecule) the least. *Cis*-diaminedichloroplatinum (cisplatin, DDP), an effective chemotherapeutic agent, is also a frequent nephrotoxin. It acts by interacting with nucleophilic sites on DNA [165], preferably of the proximal tubule cells. Both cisplatin and aminoglycosides also lead to decreased GFR due to reduced RBF and effective filtration pressure. A role for PAF in the altered intrarenal hemodynamics has recently been suggested from the ameliorating effects of PAF receptor antagonists [91].

Mechanisms of Repair and Regeneration

Following the acute insult, a complex series of mechanisms are responsible for regeneration and repair. In recent years, increasing knowledge in the field of interacting signals of cell communication has allowed us to hypothesize new links between cytokines and growth factors to particular forms of acute renal injuy. Growth control mechanisms now appear to be critical in the understanding not only of disturbances of renal function, but also in their resolution [166]. Denudation of the tubular basement membrane reflects the temporary inability of the kidney to accelerate the slow continuous turnover of tubular epithelial cells. Very rare detachment sites are observed in normal controls or in subjects with minimal glomerular lesions without evidence of tubular injury. However, with ischemic and toxic injury, significant increases in thymidine incorporation in both cortical and medullary tubules are observed [167].

The commitment to DNA synthesis following ischemic and nephrotoxic ARF is accompanied by a pattern of gene expression that bears a striking resemblance to that exhibited by growth factor-stimulated cells in culture. Following ischemia, there is a burst in renal DNA synthesis that rapidly reaches a peak and that slowly regresses over a period of days. In the presence of growth factors such as PDGF, epidermal growth factor (EGF), or insulin-like growth factor (IGF), the receptor–ligand interaction commits the cell to a new phase of the cell cycle termed G_1. The expression of so-called early genes is a prominent feature of this phase [167]. Expression of early genes does not depend on new protein syntesis, lasts briefly, and is a necessary step, since some code for well-known DNA-binding transcription factors that presumably initiate a genetic cascade ending in cell division, while others code for small, secreted, proinflammatory polypeptides and proteases [168].

After a time delay, the cells start to synthesize new protein and RNA and to increase in size. The new proteins and RNA are necessary for progression through the remainder of the G_1 and S phases, when DNA synthesis occurs. Following ischemic renal damage, a striking parallel occurs between the changes in gene expression and those induced by growth factor stimulation of quiescent cells in culture. For some genes such as the c-*fos* mRNA, the prototype of the nucleus-binding members of the immediate early genes, and *Egr*-1 mRNA, increased expression is seen almost immediately after the release of renal hilar clamping and precedes the peak of renal DNA synthesis. Another group of immediate early genes, the members of the small cytokine-like genes, is also expressed during renal ischemic injury. The expression of KC and JE that code for small glycoproteins with potent chemotactic and mitogenic properties occurs at a very early stage. Therefore, cellular processes rather than a mere response to hemodynamic alterations might be responsible for cellular hypertrophy in compensatory renal enlargement. The cellular response to an acute injury may thus encompass changes in gene expression.

Among the various growth factors, the EGF would seem one of the likeliest candidates in triggering the cell response to proliferation following renal injury, since EGF gene is normally highly expressed in the normal kidney [169] and EGF is mitogenic for the proximal tubule [170], where the most prominent damages are known to occur. Mouse EGF is synthesized as a prepropreсursor molecule of 1217 amino acids [171]. The active factor (53 amino acids) is released following the proteolytic activity of specific proteases. The thick ascending limb of Henle, but not the proximal tubule or the glomerulus, is the main site of EGF synthesis, which accounts for more than 90% of urinary EGF activity. Although the proximal tubule cells as well as a variety of different cell lines derived from the proximal tubule are unable to synthesize EGF, they express specific receptors in the basolateral membrane [172, 173]. The EGF receptor is a 170-kDa protein with intracellular tyrosine kinase activity. EGF is mitogenic for tubular epithelial cells in culture. Moreover, EGF can inhibit gluconeogenesis in proximal tubules. Following ischemic injury, the epithelial cells lining the thick ascending limb of Henle undergo both positive and negative tregulation of gene transcription. In fact, they stop expressing the gene for EGF while gaining the ability to express the nuclear-binding protein early growth response gene 1 product (EGR1) [174].

Renal ischemia reduces the levels of preproEGF mRNA [175], but increases the expression of EGF receptors by the proximal tubule [176–178]. The enhanced expression of EGF receptors is, however, transient, probably due to its downregulation. The enhanced expression of EGF receptors rather than enhanced synthesis may be crucial in the proliferative response induced by EGF. In fact, administration of EGF in normal rats is not followed by enhanced renal DNA synthesis [179].

EGF excretion is low in pathologic states associated with widespread tubular damage such as diabetic nephropathy [180], polycystic kidney disease [181], and renal transplantation [182]. The repression of preproEGF gene expression during renal injury could be necessary in the regenerative response. Furthermore, endocrine hormones may modify the action of local growth factors. Growth factors and thyroid hormones can induce EGF receptors at least in hepatic tissue. In contrast, α-interferon downregulates EGF receptors on bovine kidney cells [166]. Human PDGF, a heterodimer of two disulfide-linked A (14–18 kDa) and B (16 kDa) chains, is normally released from α-granules of activated platelets as well as from epithelial kidney cells, monocytes/macrophages, and endothelium [183–188]. PDGF exhibits mitogenic properties on kidney endothelial and epithelial cells and interstitial fibroblasts [186]. PDGF can also stimulate the release of other growth factors such as IGF-1 from fibroblasts [186].

IGF, 50% homologous with proinsulin, are a family of monomeric polypeptides of approximately 70 amino acids (IGF-1, or somatomedin C, and IGF-II, or somatomedin A) [186]. The synthesis of IGF is under hormonal control (pituitary growth hormone) or under the action of local hormones such as PDGF or the fibroblast growth factor. Cells of the collecting duct as well as mesangial cells can synthetize IGF. The secretion and response of cells occur in an autocrine/paracrine manner, indicating the potential of complex interactions between tubular epithelium and fibroblasts.

Hepatocyte growth factor (HGF), first identified in sera of partially hepatectomized rats [189], was later purified from rat platelets [190] and from human plasma [191]. The purified rat HGF is a heterodimer glycoprotein composed of a 69-kDa α-subunit and a 34-kDa β-subunit [192]. Besides its remarkable mitogenic activity in mature parenchymal hepatocytes, HGF exhibits pleiomorphic properties, as it can stimulate DNA synthesis in epithelial cells including renal tubule cells [193], shows antiproliferative activity in malignant cells [194], stimulates cell motility, and promotes tubule formation [195–197]. Increased renal expression of HGF has been demonstrated after ischemic and nephrotoxic injury [198]. HGF may function as a renotopic factor for compensatory renal growth after unilateral nephrectomy [199]. In this model a marked and rapid increase of HGF mRNA and HGF activity occurs in the remnant kidney, followed by a marked downregulation of the HGF receptor in the remaining kidney [198]. In ischemia or after $HgCl_2$ administration, both HGF mRNA and HGF activity markedly increased prior to proliferation of the tubular cells [190].

TGF-α, a 50-amino acid peptide, shares 40% sequence homology with EGF [200]. TGF may be an agonist of EGF, since it can bind to EGF receptors. Besides macrophages, TGF-α may be secreted by the cortical collecting ducts. The intra-aortic infusion of TGF-α accelerates renal repair and recovery after experimental injury. While the evidence for a role of TGF-α in the physiological modulation in the renal response to injury is still scarce, more information is now becoming available on TGF-β. TGF-β is unrelated to TGF-α and is a two disulfide-linked chain peptide of 12 kDa [201]. Two types of receptors for TGF-β are known [202]. TGF-β can either stimulate or inhibit proliferation depending on the cell type, growth conditions, and presence of other growth factors. In cultured proximal tubule cells, addition of TGF-β leads to proliferation promoting the change from the normally morphologic appearance of cells in monolayers into solid clusters of cells. The appearance of cell clusters is also accompanied by the enhanced production of procollagens type I, II, IV and fibronectin [203]. TGF-β also inhibits the proteases that normally cleave the extracellular matrix components. Finally, TGF-β increases the adhesion of cells to extracellular matrix components by enhancing specific receptor expression. The latter, coupled with augmented secretion of extracellular matrix components, leads to facilitated hypertrophic enlargement and the arrest of proliferation [204].

Conclusion

ARF remains an important cause of hospital morbidity and is still accompained by a high mortality rate. Convincing evidence for important roles of different mediators in various experimental models has been provided. Along this line, specific inhibitors or inactivators have confirmed the role of the given mediator. However, transposition into the clinical setting of humans must be done with caution. Nevertheless, in some instances of high risk for developing ARF such as in renal artery surgery or in vascular surgery, the use of inhibitors and/or antagonists may be useful. Current research in renal regeneration aims at maximizing the renal regenerative program. This will hopefully be achieved when it is possible to induce only kidney-specific proliferative responses. Molecular biology of the gene response seems promising to provide therapeutic tools to manipulate the regenerative process, to upregulate expression of benefical genes, or to downregulate potentialy deleterious ones.

References

1. Eliahou HE, Marcusohn G, Knecht A, Blau A, Shulman L, Gruzman C, Gavendo S, Yuhas Y (1991) Multiple systems organ failure is gradually replacing isolated acute tubular necrosis in severe trauma. Cardionephrology 1:395–403
2. Feest TG, Round A, Hamad S (1993) Incidence of severe acute renal failure in adults: results of a community-based study. Br Med J 306:481–483
3. Brezis M (1992) Forefronts in nephrology: summary of the newer aspects of renal cell injury. Kidney Int 42:523–539
4. Alexopoulos E, Vakianis P, Kokolina E, Koukoudis P, Sakellariou G, Dimitrios M, Papadimitriou M (1994) Acute renal failure in a medical setting: changing patterns and prognostic factors. Ren Fail 16(2):273–284
5. Zager RA (1992) Endotoxemia, renal hypoperfusion and fever: interactive risk factors for aminoglycoside and sepsis-associated acute renal failure. Am J Kidney Dis 20(3):223–230
6. Pethersdorf RG, Dane DC (1980) Gram negative bacteremia and septic shock. In: Isselbacher KJ, Adams RD, Braunwaud E, Petersdorf RG, Wilson JD (eds) Principles of internal medicine, 19th edn. McGraw-Hill Book, New York, p 563

7. Henrich WL, Hamasaky Y, Said SI, Campbell WB, Cronin RE (1982) Dissociation of systemic and renal effects of endotoxemia. Prostaglandin inhibition uncovers an important role of renal nerves. J Clin Invest 69:691–699
8. Kikeri D, Pennell JP, Hwang KH, Jacob AI, Richman AV, Burgoigne JJ (1986) Endotoxemic acute renal failure in avtike rats. Am J Physiol 250:F1098–F1106
9. Zager RA (1986) Escherichia coli endotoxin injections potentiate experimental ischemic renal injury. Am J Physiol 251:F988–F994
10. Lugon JR, Boim MA, Ramos OL, Ajzen H, Schor N (1989) Renal function and glomerular hemodynamics in male endotoxemic rats. Kidney Int 36:570–575
11. Badr KF, Kelley VE, Rennke HG, Brenner BM (1986) Role for thromboxane A_2 and leukotrienes in endotolin-induced acute renal failure. Kidney Int 30:474–480
12. Baud L, Oudinet JP, Bens M, Noe L, Peraldi MN, Rondeau E, Etienne J, Ardaillou R (1989) Production of tumor necrosis factor by rat mesangial cells in response to bacterial lipopolysaccharide. Kidney Int 35:1111–1118
13. Caverzasio J, Rizzoli R, Dayer JM, Bonjour JP (1987) Interleukin-1 decreases renal sodium reabsorption: possible mechanism of endotoxin-induced natriuresis. Am J Physiol 252:F943–F946
14. Wang J, Dunn J (1987) Platelet-activating factor mediates endotoxin-induced acute renal failure insufficiency in rats. Am J Physiol 253:F1283–F1289
15. Stork JE, Rahman MA, Dunn MJ (1986) Eicosanoid in experimental and human renal disease. Am J Med 80 Suppe 1A:34
16. Schlondorff D, Satriano JA, Hagege J, Perez J, Baud L (1984) Effects of platelet activating factor and serum-treated zymosan on prostaglandin E2 synthesis, arachidonic acid release and contraction of cultured mesangial cells. J Clin Invest 73:1227–1231
17. Camussi G, Tetta C, Baglioni C (1990) The role of platelet-activating factor in inflammation. Clin Immun Immunopathol 57:331–338
18. Camussi G, Mariano F, Biancone L, Montrucchio G, Vercellone A (1993) Effect of cytokines on the cytoskeleton of resident glomerular cells. Kidney Int 43 Suppl 39:S32–S36
19. Camussi G, Turello E, Tetta C, Bussolino F, Baglioni G (1990) Tumor necrosis factor induces contraction of mesangial cells and alters their cytoskeletal organization. Kidney Int 38:795–802
20. Vane JR, Anggard EE, Botting RM (1990) Regulatory functions of the vascular endothelium. N Engl J Med 323:27–36
21. Hems DA, Brosnan JT (1970) Effects of ischemia on content of metabolism in rat liver and kidney in vivo. Biochem J 120:105–111
22. Oswald H, Schmitz HJ, Kemper R (1977) Tissue content of adenosine, inosine and hypoxanthine in the rat kidney after ischemia and postischemic recirculation. Pflugers Arch 371:45–49
23. Miller WL, Thomas RA, Berne M, Rubio R (1978) Adenosine production in the ischemic kidney. Circ Res 43:390–397
24. Malis CK, Bonventre JV (1986) Mechanism of calcium potentation of oxygen free radicals injury to renal mitochondria. A model for postischemic and toxic mitochondrial damage. J Biol Chem 261:14201–14208
25. Greene EL, Paller MS (1991) Oxygen free radicals in acute renal failure. Miner Electrolyte Metab 17:124–132
26. Fridrovich I (1986) Biological effects of the superoxide radical. Arch Biochem Biophys 247:1–11
27. Halliwell B, Gutteridge JMC (1989) Free radicals in biology and medicine. Clarendon, Oxford
28. Grishman MB, McCord JM (1986) Chemistry and cytotoxicity of reactive oxygen metabolites. In: Taylor AE, Matator S, Ward P (eds) Physiology of oxygen radicals. American Physiological Society, Bethesda, pp 1–18
29. Lovis C, Mach F, Donati YRA, Bonventre JV, Polla BS (1994) Heat shock proteins and the kidney. Ren Fail 16(2):179–192

30. Paller MS, Hoidal JR, Ferris TF (1984) Oxygen free radicals in ischemic acute renal failure in the rat. J Clin Invest 74:1156–1164
31. Hansson R, Jonsson O, Lundstam S, Pettersson S, Schersten T, Waldenstrom J (1983) Effects of free radical scavengers on renal circulation after ischemia in the rabbit. J Clin Sci 65:605–610
32. Nath KA, Paller MS (1990) Dietary deficiency of antioxidants exacerbates ischemic injury in the rat kidney. Kidney Int 38:1109–1117
33. Haraldsson G, Nilsson U, Bratell S, Pettersson S, Schersten T, Akerlund S, Jonsson O (1992) ESR-measurement of production of oxygen radicals in vivo before and after renal ischemia in the rabbit. Acta Physiol Scand 146:93–105
34. Doctor RB, Mandel LJ (1991) Minimal role of xanthine oxidase and oxygen free radicals in rat renal tubular reoxygenation injury. J Am Soc Nephrol 1:959–969
35. Paller MS (1990) Formation of reactive oxygen species by proximal tubular epithelial cells during anoxia and reoxygenation (Abstr). Clin Res 38:402a
36. Shah SV, Walker PD (1988) Evidence suggesting a role for hydroxyl radical in glycerol-induced acute renal failure. Am J Physiol 255:F438–F443
37. Walker PD, Shah SV (1988) Evidence suggesting a role for hydroxyl radical in gentamicin-induced acute renal failure in rats. J Clin Invest 81:334–341
38. Bakris GL, Lass N, Gaber AO, Jones JD, Bornett JC Jr (1990) Radiocontrast medium induced declines in renal function: a role for oxygen free radicals. Am J Physiol 258: F115–F120
39. Salahudeen AK, Clark EC, Nath KA (1991) Hydrogen peroxide-induced renal injury. A protective role for pyruvate in vitro and in vivo. J Clin Invest 88:1886–1893
40. Guidet B, Shah SV (1989) Enhanced in vivo H_2O_2 generation by rat kidney in glycerol-induced renal failure. Am J Physiol 257:F440–F445
41. Bonventre JV (1993) Mechanisms of ischemic acute renal failure. Kidney Int 43: 1160–1178
42. Smith MW, Collan Y, Kating MW, Trump BF (1980) Changes in mitochondrial lipids of rat kidney during ischemia. Biochim Biophys Acta 618:192–201
43. Mason J, Torhorst J, Welsch J (1984) Role of the medullary perfusion defects in the pathogenesis of ischemic renal failure. Kidney Int 26:283–293
44. Snyder F (1990) Platelet-activating factor and related acetylated lipids as potent biologically acting cellular mediators. Am J Physiol 259:697–708
45. Nakamura H, Nemenoff RA, Gronich JH, Bonventre JV (1991) Subcellular characteristics of phospholipase A2 activity in rat kidney. Enhanced cytosolic, mitochondrial, and microsomal phospholipase A2 enzymatic activity after renal ischemia and reperfusion. J Clin Invest 87:1810–1818
46. Mellgren RL (1987) Calcium-dependent proteases: an enzyme system active at cellular membranes. FASEB J 1:110–115
47. Camussi G, Rotunno M, Segoloni G, Brentjens JR, Andres GA (1982) In vitro alternative pathway activation of complement by the brush border of proximal tubules of normal rat kidney. J Immunol 128:1659–1663
48. Biancone L, David S, Della Pietra V, Montrucchio G, Cambi V, Camussi G (1994) Alternative pathway activation of complement by cultured human proximal tubular epithelial cells. Kidney Int 45:451–460
49. Baricos WH, Shah SV (1991) Proteolytic enzymes as mediators of glomerular injury. Kidney Int 40:161–173
50. Furchgott RF, Zawadzki JV (1980) The obligatory role of endothelial cells in the relaxation of arterial smooth muscle by acetylcholine. Nature 299:373–376
51. Palmer RMJ, Ferrige AG, Moncada S (1987) Nitric oxide release accounts for the biological activity of endothelium-derived relaxing factor. Nature 327:524–526
52. Moncada S, Palmer RMJ, Higgs EA (1991) Nitric oxide: physiology, pathophysiology, and pharmacology. Pharmacol Rev 43(2):109–134

53. Rees DD, Palmer RM, Schulz R, Hodson HF, Moncada S (1990) Characterization of three inhibitors of endothelial nitric oxide synthase in vitro and in vivo. Br J Pharmacol 101:746–752
54. Vallance P, Leone A, Calver A, Collier J, Moncada S (1992) Accumulation of an endogenous inhibitor of nitric oxide synthesis in chronic renal failure. Lancet 339:572–575
55. MacAllister RJ, Whitley GSJ, Vallance P (1994) Effects of guanidino and uremic compounds on nitric oxide pathways. Kidney Int 45:737–742
56. Baylis C, Mitruka B, Deng A (1992) Chronic blockade of nitric oxide synthesis in the rat produces systemic hypertension and glomerular damage. J Clin Invest 90:278–281
57. Esposito C, Fuiano G, Dal Canton A (1993) Endothelial cells. In: Tetta C (ed) Immunopharmacology of the renal system. Academic, New York, pp 35–46
58. Brezis S, Heyman SN, Dinour D, Epstein FH, Rosen S (1991) Role of nitric oxide in renal medullary oxygenation. Studies in isolated and intact rat kidneys. J Clin Invest 88:390–395
59. Gang V, Berneburg H, Hennemann H, Hevendehl G (1976) Diamine oxidase (histaminase) in chronic renal disease and its inhibition in vitro by methylguandine. Clin Nephrol 3:171–177
60. Kon V, Harris RC, Ichikawa L (1990) A regulatory role for large vessels in organ circulation. J Clin Invest 85:1728–1733
61. Schultz PJ, Raji L (1992) Endogenously synthetized nitric oxide prevents endotoxin-induced glomerular thrombosis. J Clin Invest 90:1718–1725
62. Petros A, Bennett D, Wallance P (1991) Effect of nitric oxide synthase inhibitors on hypotension in patients with septic shock. Lancet 338:1557–1558
63. Cobb JP, Natanson C, Salomon MA (1991) N^G-amino-L-ariginine, an inhibitor of nitric oxide synthase, increases lethality in canine endotoxic shock (Abstr). Clin Res 39:321A
64. Marsen TA, Schramek H, Dunn MJ (1994) Renal actions of endothelin: linking cellular signaling pathways to kidney disease. Kidney Int 45:336–344
65. Yanagisawa M, Kurihara H, Kimura S (1988) A novel potent vasoconstrictor peptide produced by endothelial cells. Nature 332:411–415
66. Sakamoto H, Sasaki S, Hirata Y, Imai T, Ando K, Ida T, Sakuri T, Yanagisawa M, Masaki T, Marumo E (1990) Production of endothelin-1 by rat cultured mesangial cells. Biochem Biophys Res Commun 169:462–468
67. Uchida S, Naruse M, Ogata E, Yanagisawa M, Masaki T, Kurokawa K (1990) Gene expression and synthesis of endothelin in renal tubular epithelial cells in culture (Abstr). Kidney Int 37:380
68. Simonson MS, Jones JM, Dunn MJ (1992) Cytosolic and nuclear signalling by endothelin peptides: mesangial response to glomerular injury. Kidney Int 41:542–545
69. Lopez-Farre A, Gomez-Garre D, Bernabeu F, Lopez-Novoa JM (1991) A role for endothelin in the maintainance of post-ischemic renal failure in the rat. J Physiol (Lond) 444:513–522
70. Kon V, Yoshioka T, Fogo A, Ichikawa I (1989) Glomerular actions of endothelin in vivo. J Clin Invest 83:1762–1767
71. Katoh T, Chang H, Uchida S, Okuda T, Kurokawa K (1990) Direct effects of endothelin in the rat kidney. Am J Physiol 258:F397–F402
72. Reyes AA, Klahr S (1992) Renal function after release of ureteral obstruction: role of endothelin and the renal artery endothelium. Kidney Int 42:632–638
73. Saito Y, Nakao K, Mukoyama M, Imura H (1990) Increased plasma endothelin level in patients with essential hypertension. N Engl J Med 322:205
74. Branch DW, Dudley DJ, Michell MD (1991) Preliminary evidence for homeostatic mechanism regulating endothelin production in pre-eclampsia. Lancet 337:943–945
75. Firth JD, Ratcliffe PH, Raine AEG, Ledingham IGG (1988) Endothelin: an important factor in acute renal failure? Lancet 8261:1179–1182

76. Ohta K, Hirata Y, Imai T, Kanno K, Emori T, Shichiri M, Marumo F (1990) Cytokine-induced release of endothelin-1 from porcine renal epithelial cell line. Biochem Biophys Res Commun 169:578–584
77. Lee ME, Temizer DH, Clifford JA, Quertermous T (1991) Cloning of GATA-binding protein that regulates endothelin-1 gene expression in endothelial cells. J Biol Chem 266:16188–16192
78. Sugiura M, Inagami T, Knon V (1989) Endotoxin stimulates endothelin release in vivo and in vitro as determined by radioimmunoassay. Biochem Biophys Res Commun 161: 1220–1227
79. Fogo A, Hellings SE, Inagami T, Kon V (1992) Endothelin receptor antagonism is protective in in vivo acute cyclosporine toxicity. Kidney Int 12:770–774
80. Biancone L, Tetta C, Turello E, Montrucchio G, Iorio EL, Servillo L, Balestrieri C, Camussi G (1992) Platelet-activating factor biosynthesis by cultured mesangial cells is modulated by proteinase inhibitors. J Am Soc Nephrol 2:1251–1261
81. Camussi G, Biancone L, Iorio EL, Silvestro L, Da Col R, Capasso C, Rossano F, Servillo L, Balestrieri C, Tufano MA (1992) Porins and lipopolysaccharide stimulate platelet activating factor synthesis by human mesangial cells. Kidney Int 42:1309–1313
82. Schlondorff D, Neuwirth R (1986) Platelet activating factor and the kidney. Am J Physiol 251:F1–F11
83. Schwertschlag U, Scherf M, Gerber JG, Mathias M, Nico AG (1986) PAF-induced changes on renal vascular resistance (RVR) vascular reactivity and renin release (RR) in the isolated perfused rat kidney (Abstr). Kidney Int 29:388a
84. Weisman SM, Felse D, Vaughan ED (1985) Platelet-activating factor is a potent stimulus for renal prostaglandin synthesis: possible significance in unilateral ureteral ligation. J Pharmacol Exp Ther 235:10–15
85. Badr KF, DeBoer DK, Takahashi K, Harris RC, Fogo A, Jacobson HR (1989) Glomerular responses to platelet activating factor in the rat: role of thromboxane A2. Am J Physiol 256:F35–F43
86. Scherf M, Nies AS, Schwertschlag U, Hugnes M, Gerber JG (1986) Hemodynamic effects of PAF in the dog kidney in vivo. Hypertension 8:737–741
87. Camussi G, Tetta C, Coda R, Segeloni G, Vercellone A (1984) Platelet-activating factor-induced loss of glomerular anionic charges. Kidney Int 25:73–81
88. Perico N, Delaini F, Tagliaferri M et al. (1988) Effect of platelet-activating factor (PAF) and its specific receptor antagonist on glomerular permeability in isolated perfused rat kidney. Lab Invest 58:163–171
89. Wang J, Dunn MJ (1987) Platelet activating factor mediated endotoxin induced acute renal insufficiency in rats. Am J Physiol 253:1–7
90. Tolins JP, Vercellotti GM, Wilkowske M, Ha B, Jacob HS, Raij L (1989) Role of platelet activating factor in endotoxemic acute renal failure in the male rat. J Lab Clin Med 113:316–324
91. Pavao dos Santos OF, Boim MA, Barros EJG, Schor N (1991) Role of platelet activating factor in gentamicin and cisplatin nephrotoxicity. Kidney Int 40:742–747
92. Schlondorff D (1986) Renal prostaglandin synthesis: sites of production and specific actions of prostaglandins. Am J Med 81(2B):1–11
93. Schlondorff D, Ardaillou R (1986) Prostaglandins and other arachidonic acid metabolites in the kidney. Kidney Int 29:108–119
94. Lands WEM (1979) The biosynthesis and metabolism of prostaglandins. Annu Rev Physiol 41:633–642
95. Ellis EF, Oelz O, Roberts LJ II et al. (1976) Coronary arterial smooth muscle contraction by a substance relased from platelets: evidence that it is thromboxane A2. Science 193: 1135–1137
96. Mene P, Dunn MJ (1986) Contractile effects of TxA, and endoperoxide analogues on cultured rat glomerular mesangial cells. Am J Physiol 251:F1029–F1035

97. Bolger PM, Einster GM, Ramwell PW et al. (1978) Renal action of prostacyclin. Nature 271:467–469
98. Terragno NA, Terragno A, Early JA et al. (1978) Endogenous prostaglandin synthesis inhibitor in the renal cortex. Effect on production of prostacyclin by renal blood vessels. Clin Sci 55 Suppl:199–215
99. Edwards RM (1985) Effects of prostaglandins on vasocontrictor action in isolated renal arterioles. Am J Physiol 248:F779–F784
100. Remuzzi C, Fitzgerald GA, Patrono C (1992) Thromboxane synthesis and action within the kidney. Kidney Int 41:1483–1493
101. Stahl RA, Paravicini M, Schollmeyer P (1984) Angiotensin II stimulation of PGE2 and 6-keto-PGF formation by isolated human glomeruli. Kidney Int 26:30–34
102. Sraer J, Ardaillou N, Sraer JD, Ardaillou R (1983) In vitro prostaglandin synthesis by human glomeruli and papillae. Prostaglandins 23:855–864
103. Scharschmidt LA, Dunn MJ (1983) Prostaglandin synthesis by rat glomerular mesangial cells in culture. Effects of angiotensin II and arginine vasopressin. J Clin Invest 73: 1756–1764
104. Lovett DH, Resch K, Gemsa D (1987) Interleukin 1 and the glomerular mesangium. II. Monokine stimulation of mesangial cell prostanoid secretion. Am J Pathol 129:543–551
105. Baud L, Nivez MP, Chansel D, Ardaillou R (1981) Stimulation by oxygen radicals of prostaglandin production by rat renal glomeruli. Kidney Int 20:322–339
106. Adler S, Stahl AK, Baker PJ, Chen YP, Pritz PM, Couser WG (1987) Biphasic effect of oxygen radicals on prostaglandin production by rat mesangial cells. Am J Physiol 252:F743–F749
107. Wang J, Dunn MJ (1987) Endotoxin stimulates prostaglandin release by cultured rat glomerular mesangial cells (Abstr). Kidney Int 31:291
108. Stork JE, Shen TY, Dunn MJ (1985) Stimulation of prostglandin E2 and thomboxane B2 production in cultured rat mesangial cells by platelet activating factor: inhibition by a specific receptor antagonist (Abstr). Kidney Int 27:267
109. Simonson MS, Dunn MJ (1990) Endothelin-1 stimulates contraction of rat glomerular mesangial cells and potentiates β-adrenergic-mediated cyclic adenosine monophosphate accumulation. J Clin Invest 85:790–797
110. Zoja C, Benigni A, Renzi D, Piccinelli A, Perico N, Remuzzi G (1990) Endothelin and eicosanoid synthesis in cultured mesangial cells. Kidney Int 37:927–933
111. Bohman SO (1977) Demonstration of prostaglandin synthesis in collecting duct cells and other cell types of the rabbit renal medulla. Prostaglandins 14:729–744
112. Zusman RM, Keiser HR (1977) Prostaglandin biosynthesis by rabbit renomedullary interstitial cells in tissue culture. Stimulation by angiotensin II, bradykinin and arginine vasopressin. J Clin Invest 60:215–223
113. Beck TR, Hassid A, Dunn MJ (1980) The effect of arginine vasopressin and its analogs on the synthesis of prostaglandin E2 by rat renal medullary interstitial cells in culture. J Pharmacol Exp Ther 215:15–19
114. Carmichael J, Shankel SW (1985) Effects of nonsteroidal antiinflammatory drugs on prostaglandins and renal function. Am J Med 78:992–1000
115. Shankel SW, Johnson DC, Clark PS, Shankel TL, O'Neil WM Jr (1992) Acute renal failure and glomerulopathy caused by nonsteroidal antiinflammatory drugs. Arch Intern Med 152:986–990
116. Badr KE, Kelley VE, Rennke HG, Brenner BM (1986) Roles of thromboxane A2 and leukotrienes in endotoxin-induced acute renal failure. Kidney Int 30:474–480
117. Tempel GE, Cook JA, Wise WC et al. (1986) Improvement in organ blood flow by inhibition of thromboxane synthetase during experimental endotoxic shock in the rat. J Cardiovasc Pharmacol 8:514–519
118. Burnier M, Waeber B, Aubert JF et al. (1988) Effects of nonhypotensive endotoxiemia in conscious rats: role of prostaglandins. Am J Physiol 254:H509–H516

119. Lifschitz MD (1981) Prostaglandins and renal blood flow: in vitro studies. Kidney Int 19:781–785
120. Carr AA (1970) Hemodynamic and renal effects of a prostaglandin PGA, in subjects with essential hypertension. Am J Med Sci 259:21–26
121. Johnston HH, Herzog JP, Lauler DP (1967) Effect of prostaglandin E, on renal hemodynamics, sodium and water excretion. Am J Physiol 213:939–946
122. Weber P, Larson C, Anggard E et al. (1976) Stimulation of renin release from rabbit renal cortex by arachidonic acid and prostaglandin endoperoxides. Circ Res 39:868
123. Sraer JD, Moulonguet-Doleris L, Delarue F, Sraer J, Ardaillou R (1981) Prostaglandin synthesis by glomeruli isolated from rats with glycerol-induced acute renal failure. Circ Res 49:775–783
124. Morrison AR, Nishikawa K, Needleman P (1977) Unmasking of thromboxane A2 synthesis by ureteral obstruction in the rabbit kidney. Nature 267:259–260
125. Ratcliffe PJ (1992) Pathophysiology of acute renal failure. In: Cameron S, Davison AM, Grunfeld JP, Kerr D, Ritz E (eds) Oxford textbook of clinical nephrology, vol 2. Oxford Medical, Oxford, pp 982–1006
126. Kreisberg H, Matthys E, Venkatachalam MA (1983) Morphologic factors in acute renal failure. In: Brenner BM, Lazarus JM (eds) Acute renal failure. Saunders, Philadelphia, p 21
127. Olsen S (1989) Acute tubular necrosis and toxic renal injury. In: Tisher C, Brenner B (eds) Renal Pathology. Lippincott, Philadelphia, p 656
128. Benson EM, Colvin RB, Russel PS (1985) Induction of la antigen murine renal transplant. J Immunol 134:7–9
129. Sinclair GD, Wadgymar A, Halloran PF, Delovitch T (1984) Graft-vs.-host reaction induce H-2 class II gene transcription host kidney cells. Immunogenetics 20:503–511
130. Yard BA, Daha MR, Kooymans-Couthino M, Bruijn JA, Paare ME, Schrama E, van Es LA, van der Woude FJ (1992) IL-1α stimulated TNFa production by cultured human proximal tubular epithelial cells. Kidney Int 42:383–389
131. Neilson EG (1989) Pathogenesis and therapy of interstitial nephrosis. Kidney Int 35: 1257–1270
132. Seelen MAJ, Brooimans RA, van der Woude FJ, van Es LA, Daha MR (1993) IFN-γ mediates stimulation of complement C4 biosynthesis in human proximal tubular epithelial cells. Kidney Int 44:50–57
133. Beuttler B, Cerami A (1989) The biology of cachectin/TNF: a primary of host response. Annu Rev Immunol 7:625–655
134. Camussi G, Bussolino F, Salvidio G, Baglioni C (1987) Tumor necrosis factor/cachectin stimulates peritoneal macrophages, polymorphonuclear neutrophils, and vascular endothelial cells to synthesize and release platelet-activating factor. J Exp Med 166:1390
135. Abbot F, Ryan JJ, Ceska M, Matsushima K, Sarraf CE, Rees AJ (1991) Interleukin-1β stimulates human mesangial cells to synthesize and release interleukin-6 and -8. Kidney Int 40(4):597–605
136. Pirotzky E, Delattre RM, Hellegouarch A, Lonchampt MO, Aarden L, Braquet P, Galanaud P (1990) Interleukin-6 production by tumor necrosis factor and lipopolysaccharide-stimulated rat renal cells. Clin Immunol Immunopathol 56:271–279
137. Schmouder RL, Stieter MR, Wiggins RC, Chensu W, Kunkel SL (1992) In vitro and in vivo interleukin-8 production in human renal cortical epithelia. Kidney Int 41:191–198
138. Boyer B, Thiery JP (1989) Epithelial cell adhesion mechanisms. J Membr Biol 112:97–108
139. Burridge K, Fath K, Kelly T, Nuckolls G, Turner C (1988) Focal adhesion transmembrane junctions between the extracellular matrix and the cytoskeleton. Annu Rev Cell Biol 1:487–525
140. Gallin WJ, Edelman GM, Cunningham BA (1983) Characterization of L-CAM, a major cell adhesion molecule from embryonic liver cells. Proc Natl Acad Sci USA 80:1038–1042

141. Gumbiner B, Stevenson B, Grimaldi A (1988) The role of the cell adhesion molecule uvomorulin in the formation and maintenance of the epithelial junctional complex. J Cell Biol 107:1575–1587
142. Hirano S, Nose A, Hatta K, Kawakami A, Takeichi M (1987) Calcium-dependent cell-cell adhesion molecules (Cadherin's): subclass specificities and possible involvement of actin bundles. J Cell Biol 105:2501–2510
143. Nagafuchi A, Takeichi M (1988) Cell binding function of E cadherin is regulated by the cytoplasmic domain. EMBO J 7:3679–3684
144. Ruoslahti E (1991) Integrins. J Clin Invest 87:1–5
145. Carraway KL, Carraway CAC (1989) Membrane-cytoskeleton interactions in animal cells. Biochim Biophys Acta 988:147–171
146. Racusen LC (1992) Biology of disease. Alterations in tubular epithelial cell adhesion and mechanisms of acute renal failure. Lab Invest 67(2):158–163
147. Korhonen M, Ylanne J, Laitinen L, Virtanene I (1990) Distribution of β1 and β3 integrins in human fetal and adult kidney. Lab Invest 62(5):616
148. Molitoris BA (1991) Ischemia induced loss of epithelial polarity: potential role of the actin cytoskeleton. Am J Physiol 260(29):F769–F778
149. Vestweber D, Kemler R, Ekblom P (1985) Cell adhesion molecule uvomorulin during kidney development. Dev Biol 112:213–221
150. Biddlestone LR, Fleming S (1991) Morphological evidence that A-CAM is a major intercellular adhesion molecule in human kidney. J Pathol 164:9–15
151. Bacallao R, Mandel L (1991) Internalization of E-cadherin and Na-K ATPase in cultured renal cells occurs rapidly with energy depletion. J Am Soc Nephrol 2:643
152. Goligorsky MS, Gailit J (1991) Alpha-3 integrin receptor in stressed renal epithelial cells. J Am Soc Nephrol 2:575
153. Geiger B (1989) Cytoskeleton-associated cell contacts. Curr Opin Cell Biol 1:103
154. Morrow JS, Cianci CD, Ardito T, Mann AS, Kashgarian M (1989) Ankyrin links fodrin to the alpha subunit of Na-K ATPase in Madin-Dachy canine kidney cells and in intact renal tubule cells. J Cell Biol 198:155–165
155. Nelson WJ, Hammerton RW, McNeil H (1991) Role of the membrane cytoskeleton in the spatial organization of the NaK ATPase in polarized epithelial cells. Soc Gen Physiol Ser 46:77–87
156. Niggli V, Burger MM (1987) Interaction of the cytoskeleton with the plasma membrane. J Membr Biol 100:97–121
157. Rodriquez-Boulan E, Nelson W (1989) Morphogenesis of the polarized epithelial cell phenotype. Science 245:718–725
158. Kellerman PS, Clark RAF, Hoilien CA, Linas SL, Molitoris BA (1990) Role of microfilaments in maintenance of proximal tubule sturctural and functional integrity. Am J Physiol 259:G279–F285
159. Racusen LC (1990) Anoxia-induced shape changes in cultured human renal proximal tubular cells-role of microfilaments. J Am Soc Nephrol 1:602
160. Younes M, Doce S, Taylor K, True L (1990) Redistribution of fodrin is a marker of acute tubular necrosis (Abstr). Lab Invest 62:109
161. Goligorsky MS, Leiberthal W, Racusen L, Simon EE (1993) Integrin receptors in renal tubular epithelium: new insights into pathophysiology of acute renal failure. Am J Physiol 33:F1–F8
162. Moore RD, Smith CR, Lipsky JJ, Mellits ED, Lietman PS (1984) Risk factors for nephrotoxicity in patients treated with aminoglycosides. Ann Intern Med 100:352
163. Meyer RD (1986) Risk factors and comparisons of clinical nephrotoxicity of aminoglycosides. Am J Med 80 Suppl 6B:119
164. Humes WD (1988) Aminoglycoside nephrotoxicity. Kidney Int 33:900
165. Ries F, Klastersky J (1986) Nephrotoxicity induced by cancer chemotherapy with special emphasis on cisplatin toxicity. Am J Kidney Dis 8:368

166. Safirstein R (1994) Gene expression in nephrotoxic and ischemic acute renal failure. J Am Soc Nephrol 4:1387–1395
167. Bravo R (1990) Genes induced during the G0/G1 transition in mouse fibroblasts. Cancer Biol 1:37–46
168. Greenberg ME, Ziff EB (1984) Stimulation of 3T3 cells induced transcription of the c-fos proto-oncogene. Nature 311:433–438
169. Rall LB, Scott J, Bell BI et al. (1985) Mouse preproepidermal growth factor synthesis by the kidney and other tissues. Nature 313:228–231
170. Norman J, Bradie-Dezfooly B, Nord EP et al. (1987) EGF-induced mitogenesis in proximal tubule cells: potentiation by angiotensin. II. Am J Physiol 253:F299–F309
171. Daughaday WH (1989) Growth hormone, normal synthesis, secretion, control, and mechanism of action. In: De Groot LJ (ed) Endocrinology, vol 1. Saunders, Philadelphia, pp 318–329
172. Goodyer PR, Kachra Z, Bell C, Rozen R (1989) Renal tubular cells are potential targets for epidermal growth factor. Am J Physiol 24:F1191–F1196
173. Norman J, Tsan YK, Bacay A et al. (1990) Epidermal growth factor (EGF) accelerates functional recovery from ischemic acute tubular necrosis: role of the EGF-receptor. Clin Sci 78:445–449
174. Bonventre JV, Ouellette AJ, Sukhatme VP, Brown D (1990) Localization of the EGR-1 protein product to the distal nephron after renal ischemia and reperfusion. Clin Res 38:442A
175. Safirstein R, Zalent A, Price P (1989) Reduced preproEGF mRNA and diminished EGF excretion during acute renal failure. Kidney Int 36:810–815
176. Safirstein R, Price PM, Saggi SJ, Harris RC (1990) Changes in gene expression after temporary renal ischemia. Kidney Int 37:1515–1521
177. Nonclerg D, Toubeau G, Lambricht P, Heuson-Steinnou J, Laurent G (1991) Redistribution of epidermal growth factor immunoreactivity in renal tissue after nephrotoxin-induced tubular injury. Nephron 57:210–215
178. Richmond A, Balentien E, Thomas HG et al. (1988) Molecular characterization and chromosomal mapping of melanoma growth stimulatory factor structurally related to β-thromboglobulin. EMBO J 7:2025–2033
179. Humes DH, Cieslinski DA, Coimbra TM et al. (1989) Epidermal growth factor enhances renal tubular cell regeneration and repair and accelerates the recovery of renal function on postischemic acute renal failure. J Clin Invest 84:1757–1761
180. Mathiesen ER, Nexo E, Hommel E, Parving H-H (1989) Reduced urinary excretion of epidermal growth factor in incipient and overt diabetic nephrology. Diabetic Med 6:121–126
181. Gattone VH II, Andrews GK, Niu FW et al. (1990) Defective epidermal growth factor gene expression in mice with polycystic kidney disease. Dev Biol 138:225–258
182. Kvist N, Nexo E (1989) Epidermal growth factor in urine after kidney transplantation in humans. Urol Res 17:225–258
183. Tranqui I, Duperray A, Chebnais F, Alix JL, Cordonnier D (1985) Influence of human platelet factors on the proliferation of rat mesangial glomerular cells. Thromb Res 39: 245–251
184. Rodemann P, Muller GA, Knecht A, Normal JT, Fine L (1991) Fibroblasts of the rabbit kidney in culture. I. Characterization of growth properties and identification of cell-specific markers. Am J Physiol 261:F238–F291
185. Knecht A, Fine LG, Rodemann P, Muller G, Woo DDL, Normal JT (1991) Fibroblasts of the rabbit kidney in culture. II. PDGF-mediated paracrine stimulation of papillary fibroblasts by inner medullary collecting duct cells. Am J Physiol 261:F292–F299
186. Fine LG, Hammerman MR, Abboud HE (1992) Evolving role of growth factors in the renal responser to acute and chronic disease. J Am Soc Nephrol 2:1163–1170
187. Silver BJ, Jaffer FE, Abboud HE (1989) Platelet-derived growth factor synthesis in mesangial cells: induction by mitogenic peptides. Proc Natl Acad Sci USA 86:1056–1060

188. Schena FP, Montinaro V, Gesualdo L (1993) Glomerular mesangial and epithelial cells. In: Tetta C (ed) Immunopharmacology of the renal system. Academic, New York, pp 49–86
189. Nakamura T, Nawa K, Ichihara A (1984) Partial purification and characterization of hepatocyte growth factor from serum of hepatectomized rats. Biochem Biophys Res Commun 122:1450–1459
190. Nakamura T, Teramoto H, Ichihara A (1986) Purification and characterization of a growth factor from rat platelets for mature parenchymal hepatocytes in primary cultures. Proc Natl Acad Sci USA 83:6489–6493
191. Gohda E, Tsubouchi H, Nakayama S, Hirono O, Daikuhara Y (1988) Purification and partial characterization of hepatocyte growth factor from plasma of a patient with hepatic failure. J Clin Invest 81:414–419
192. Seki T, Sugimura A, Shimonishi S, Nishizawa Asami T, Hagiya M, Nakamura T, Shimizu S (1990) Isolation and expression of cDNA for different forms of hepoatocyte growth factor from human leukocytes. Biochem Biophys Res Commun 172:321–327
193. Igawa T, Kanda S, Kanetake H, Saitoh Y, Ichihara A, Tomita Y, Nakamura T (1991) Hepatocyte growth factor is a potent mitogen for culture rabbit epithelial cells. Biochem Biophys Res Commun 174:831–838
194. Shiota G, Rhoads DB, Wang T, Nakamura T, Schmidt EV (1992) Hepatocyte growth factor inhibits growth of hepatocellular carcinoma cells. Proc Natl Acad Sci USA 89: 373–377
195. Gherardi E, Stoker M (1991) Hepatocyte growth factor-scatter factor: mitogen, motogen, and morphogen, and met. Cancer Cells 3:227–232
196. Matsumoto K, Hashimoto K, Yoshikawa K, Nakamura T (1991) Marked stimulation of growth and motility of human keratinocytes by hepatocyte growth factor. Exp Cell Res 196:114–120
197. Montesano R, Matsumoto K, Nakamura T, Urci L (1991) Identification of a fibroblast-derived epithelial morphogen as hepatocyte growth factor. Cell 67:901–908
198. Nagaike M, Hirao S, Tajima H, Noji S, Taniguchi S, Matsumoto K, Nakamura T (1991) Renotropic functions of hepatocyte growth factor in renal regeneration after unilateral nephrectomy. J Biol Chem 266:22781–22784
199. Igawa T, Matsumoto K, Kanda S, Saito Y, Nakamura T (1993) Hepatocyte growth factor may function as a renotropic factor for regeneration in rats with acute renal injury. Am J Physiol 265:F61–F69
200. Sporn MB, Robert AB, Wakefield LM, Assoian RK (1986) Transforming growth factor-β. Biological function and chemical structure. Science 233:532–534
201. Massague J (1987) The TGF-β family of growth and differentiation factors. Cell 49: 437–438
202. MacKay K, Striker LJ, Stauffer JW, Doi T, Agodoa LY, striker GE (1989) Transforming growth factor-β. Murine glomerular receptors and responses of isolated glomerular cells. J Clin Invest 83:1160–1167
203. Nakamura T, Miller D, Ruoslahti E, Border WA (1992) Production of extracellular matrix by glomerular epithelial cells is regulated by transforming growth factor-betal. Kidney Int 41:1213–1221
204. Jaffer F, Saunders C, Shultz P, Throckmorton D, Weinshell E, Abboud HE (1989) Regulation of mesangial cell growth by polypeptide mitogens. Am J Pathol 135:261

Renal Epithelial Repair After Acute Tubular Necrosis

J.C. Lieske and F.G. Toback

Introduction

The mortality rate of acute renal failure (ARF) remains unchanged despite the advent of dialysis, and it is the most costly condition amongst patients hospitalized with kidney disease [1]. Thus, measures to speed recovery of the injured kidney could have a significant impact on medical care. Cellular proliferation is often a prominent feature in the regenerating nephron, despite the systemic catabolic milieu [2–5]. Studies during the past 40 years have identified some of the factors that could mediate recovery and proliferation of epithelial cells in this setting. Better definition of these factors may eventually provide the physician with knowledge necessary to alter the local environment of tubular epithelial cells to speed recovery of renal function. This chapter will review some of what is known about factors that regulate cellular repair and regeneration after acute renal injury.

Kidney Cell Injury and Recovery in Acute Renal Failure

The relationships between kidney cell dysfunction, morphological damage, and impairment of glomerular filtration and renal blood flow (RBF) in ARF are poorly understood [6]. In some patients with this condition, and in certain animal models, extensive tubular cell necrosis is associated with functional renal failure. Often, however, this is not the case. Kidney tissue from many patients does not exhibit significant abnormalities despite oliguria, which suggests that injury to renal cells often causes their dysfunction rather than necrosis. When structural injury is apparent, it probably serves more as a guide to the severity of the lesion than as a marker of disrupted biochemical pathways responsible for loss of specific cell functions. Important biochemical abnormalities in ARF are a reduction in the cytosolic concentration of adenosine triphosphate (ATP) and an increase in calcium, alterations in the cytoskeleton, generation of free radicals, and reduced protein synthesis [7]. How a specific ischemic or toxic insult induces biochemical perturbations in renal cells that result in a marked reduction in glomerular filtration, a lesser decrement in RBF, and oliguria is not clear. If the injury is mild, structural changes may not be apparent at the light

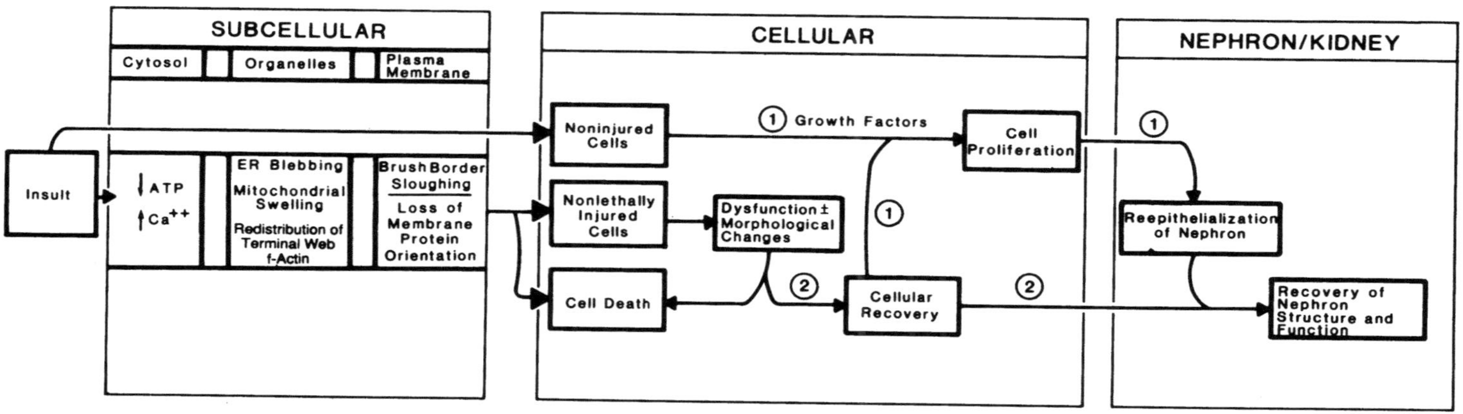

Fig. 1. Renal epithelial cell repair after acute injury. A renal insult (such as hypoxia) affects the cytosol, organelles, and plasma membrane. Cells may be killed, nonlethally injured, or not injured. Dead cells couldˊ be repaced by proliferation of noninjured cells and/or nonlethally injured cells that have recovered (pathway *1*). Nonlethally injured cells that are dysfunctional may die or subseuqently recover function and structure (pathway *2*). Growth factors are likely to play a role in the proliferative response along pathway 1 and possibly in recovery of nonlethally injured cells (pathway) 2). *ATP*, adenosine triphosphate

microscopic level; if the insult is more severe, alterations such as sloughing of proximal tubular brush border microvilli may occur that are rapidly reversed following return of adequate blood flow; and if the injury is of sufficient intensity and/or duration, cell death ensues. In most patients with well-developed acute glomerular filtration failure, cellular dysfunction appears to predominate because the two most consistently found structural lesions in humans, loss of microvilli and necrosis of individual tubular epithelial cells, are relatively infrequent findings [8].

When a renal insult induces nonlethal cell injury and necrosis, recurrent episodes probably continue after the onset of the ARF syndrome and during the regenerative process [9]. A schematic response to renal injury is presented in Fig. 1. At the subcellular level, mitochondrial swelling and endoplasmic reticulum blebbing occur, and the proximal tubular brush border can undergo sloughing. In the plasma membrane, loss of protein orientation and alterations in phospholipid content occur such that Na/K-ATPase is displaced from its normal basolateral position to the apical surface of the cell, and fence function of the membrane is lost [10]. At the cytoskeletal level, gaps in the terminal web of actin microfilaments develop, and actin redistributes in the cytoplasm [10]. If the intensity and/or duration of the insult is limited, the cell may become dysfunctional. Injury that is more severe probably leads to detachment of the cell from the tubular basement membrane, before or after necrosis. Cell detachment could be related to disruption of the cytoskeleton, loss of plasma membrane integrin receptors on the basolateral surface of the cell which mediate binding to the extracellular matrix, or both [11]. This analysis suggests two therapeutic strategies: one to stimulate proliferation of noninjured and surviving injured cells to replace those that detached, and a second to facilitate recovery of cells after nonlethal injury. Polypeptide factors that induce hyperplasia of renal epithelial cells have been identified [12], and may play a role in the repair of nephrons after acute injury and necrosis (Fig. 1, pathway 1). Although recovery of nonfatally injured cells is of major importance in the healing process, mechanisms that repair this population of cells (Fig. 1, pathway 2) are not well defined and could involve protective molecules such as heat shock proteins (HSP) [13]. How repair of injured cells and proliferation to replace necrotic ones result in restoration of normal glomerular filtration and RBF remains uncertain.

Supportive Measures: Dialysis and Nutrition

Prescott [14] has shown that under physiological conditions nearly 2×10^6 tubular epithelial cells slough into the urine each day, about one cell per human nephron. The number of sloughed cells, many of which are still viable, increases dramatically after acute tubular necrosis [15]. Proliferation is required, therefore, to replace the detached cells and maintain structural integrity of the kidney. In ARF, injury increases the rate of cell loss beyond the capacity of basal physiological proliferative mechanisms that keep the nephron intact. To restore renal structure and function, recovery must take place despite retention of toxins and nitrogen, acidosis, electrolyte imbalance, anemia, hypervolemia, and a severely curtailed intake of nutrients. That repair does occur demonstrates the extraordinary capacity of renal cells to regenerate. It is important to recognize that renal repair and regeneration are anabolic processes that must be carried out in this setting of systemic catabolism. The often unstated therapeutic principle that underlies management of ARF is that the kidney will heal by itself if supportive care such as dialysis is provided. However, another strategy exists: acceleration of the pace of regeneration by administration of nutrients, such as amino acids, and growth factors [16]. The rationale for this approach lies in the observation that the rate of renal regeneration is ordinarily suboptimal because hypercatabolism increases the demand for calories and nutrients, while at the same time adverse effects of the renal failure syndrome on kidney excretory and gastrointestinal function decrease their supply. The role of dialysis is to correct acid-base, electrolyte, and volume imbalances and remove retained toxins so that the extracellular environment for renal cellular repair is more favorable. Provision of nutrients, calories, and growth factors could reverse the catabolic state, permit accelerated repair of injured renal tissue, and thereby speed recovery.

In rats with mercuric chloride-induced ARF there is enhanced synthesis of cellular protein, nucleic acids, and phospholipid followed by rapid proliferation of tubular epithelial cells on the second day of the syndrome [17–19]. These observations indicate that anabolic mechanisms overcome the unfavorable effects of systemic catabolism and the azotemic environment that ordinarily inhibit cell growth. Amino acids infused into rats with nephrotoxic ARF can act directly on regenerating kidney cells to stimulate synthesis of phosphatidylcholine and protein – essential for the biogenesis of organelles and surface structures required for normal cell function – and to ameliorate the loss of renal function [20, 21]. These results suggest that in patients with ARF, amino acids delivered after the injury could act directly on kidney cells to speed recovery of renal structure and function. Provision of nutrients and effective dialysis may also promote regeneration by facilitating the action of growth factors released by surviving renal cells in the injured nephron.

Growth Factors

Growth factors are polypeptide messengers that stimulate dormant cells in the G_0 phase of the cell cycle to initiate DNA synthesis and subsequently undergo mitosis. Growth factor proteins affect target cells by binding to specific surface receptors. This ligand–receptor interaction can activate an intracellular effector mechanism, such as the tyrosine kinase domain of the receptor protein or the phosphatidylinositol signaling pathway [22, 23]. Signal transduction is followed by a cascade of biochemical events that initiate DNA synthesis. Recent work in many laboratories has identified the amino acid sequence of growth factor proteins and the nucleotide sequence of the genes that encode them [12]. Growth factors are derived from larger precursor molecules by proteolytic processing [12]. Epidermal growth factor (EGF), hepatocyte growth factor (HGF), and insulin-like growth factors (IGF) act on renal cells to enhance exit from the premitotic or resting (G_0/G_1) phase of the cell cycle, whereas transforming growth factor-β (TGF-β) is a growth inhibitor that impedes the exit of renal cells from G_1. These observations and the low mitotic index (0.1%) of kidney cells in vivo [24] suggest that growth inhibitory factors predominate under physiological conditions, although the set point could be shifted when regeneration after injury is required.

Figure 2 illustrates four different mechanisms whereby cell–cell communication can be mediated by peptide messengers. Endocrine signaling occurs when a protein is secreted into blood or lymph for transport to distant cell target sites, as is the case with erythropoietin. A paracrine signaling cell secretes proteins that affect only adjacent target cells that have functional growth factor receptors on their surface. In autocrine signaling, cells respond to protein factors they released, so that cells participating in this mechanism both secrete the growth factor and express receptors for it on the plasma membrane [25]. A juxtacrine mechanism has been described for TGF-α in which the growth factor domain of the plasma membrane-bound precursor molecule acts as a ligand for a receptor on an adjacent

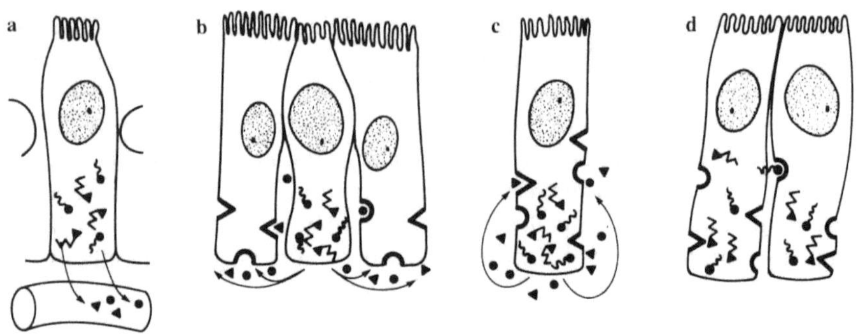

Fig. 2a–d. Mechanisms of cell–cell communication by growth factors. The cells synthesize precursor molecules depicted in the cytosol that can be processed and released to act growth factors on cells that produced them (autocrine, **c**), neighboring (paracrine, **b**), or distant cells (endocrine, **a**). Alternatively, the precursor may be incorporated into the plasma membrane and act upon adjacent cells (juxtacrine, **d**). The thickened curved and angular regions of the plasma membrane indicate receptor sites for growth-promoting and growth-inhibitory mlecules, respectively. *Circles*, stimulatory; *triangles*, inhibitory; [symbol], [symbol], precursor molecules

target cell that is thereby stimulated to enter mitosis [26]. Consideration of the juxtacrine mechanism could provide fresh insight into the as yet unknown role of the large amount of preproEGF protein present in the distal nephron of the murine kidney [27]. Receptor number, affinity, biosynthesis and recycling, and the integrity of signal transduction mechanisms at the level of the plasma membrane, cytosol, cytoskeleton, and nucleus are also critical determinants of how cells respond to growth factors. It is important to note that these molecules may have physiological effects that are unrelated to their mitogenic properties.

Renal Epithelial Cells Release Growth Factors When Exposed to Diverse Signals

Here we review evidence that kidney epithelial cells release growth factors in response to physiological signals and can also respond to them [28, 29]. Study of these interactions in culture provides a paradigm to better understand how renal cells in vivo may signal one another and respond to alterations in their environment. These factors have been studied in cultures of nontransformed renal epithelial cells derived from the African green monkey (*Cercopithecus aethiops*, BSC-1 line) [30] because this model circumvents many of the problems inherent in studies of organ growth in a tissue as complex as kidney. High-density, quiescent cultures have been employed to simulate the low proliferative activity of highly differentiated kidney cells in vivo [31, 32]. Under these conditions the epithelial monolayer forms small domes which suggests that the cells have the capacity for transepithelial transport [33]. The nephron segment from which BSC-1 cells originated is unknown.

Small reductions in the extracellular K or Na concentration induce DNA synthesis and cell multiplication of BSC-1 cells [34, 35]; adenosine diphosphate (ADP) is the most powerful mitogen yet defined for these cells [36]; and a cytokine of mesangial cell origin, interleukin-1β, also promotes their growth [37]. These diverse mitogenic signals, i.e., changes in extracellular cation concentration, a nucleotide, and a cytokine, also have in common the fact that they induce production of autocrine or paracrine growth factors by these renal cells.

Lowering Extracellular Potassium Concentration Stimulates Growth of Renal Cells by an Autocrine Mechanism

More than 50 years ago, systemic K depletion achieved experimentally by feeding rats a diet deficient in K was found to induce kidney growth [38]. Sustained mild hypokalemia in rats is associated with doubling of renal mass due to both hyperplasia and hypertrophy [39, 40]. An in vitro model to study this phenomenon was developed by lowering the extracellular K concentration from 5.4 m*M* (control) to 3.2 m*M* in confluent cultures of BSC-1 cells which induced accelerated growth [34]. Proliferation in response to low-K medium is mediated by release of a growth-promoting factor from the cells with an apparent relative molecular mass (M_r) of 12–30 kDa. This activity differs from previously described growth factors and is antagonized by purified TGF-β_2, the autocrine inhibitor of BSC-1 cell growth [41].

These observations provided the first evidence that renal cell growth induced by an alteration in the ion concentration of the extracellular fluid could be mediated by an autocrine mechanism. It remains to be determined if this growth factor(s) is produced by renal cells in animals rendered hypokalemic by a K-deficient diet. In vivo, the factor(s) could act to recruit unstimulated cells along the nephron to replicate, maintain the mitogenic signal, and/or serve a purpose related to cell transport which is not yet defined.

Reduced Extracellular Sodium Concentration Induces Renal Cell Growth and Production of Growth Factors

Since augmented influx of Na ions occurs during the onset of proliferation in mammalian cells [42, 43], one would expect that exposure of BSC-1 cells to medium containing a reduced concentration of Na would inhibit mitogenesis. Surprisingly, cell multiplication was stimulated when the Na concentration of the medium was reduced from 155 m*M* (control) to 130 m*M* [35]. The capacity of low-Na medium to enhance cell proliferation was due specifically to the decrease in Na concentration and not a fall in osmolarity, because growth stimulation was equivalent when equiosmolar amounts of choline chloride or sucrose were used to replace NaCl deleted from the medium.

After exposure of confluent cultures for only 3–5 min to low-Na medium (130 m*M*), the cells release two growth-stimulatory factors (apparent M_r, 6200 and 9000) whose appearance is not dependent upon new protein synthesis. The growth response to a reduction in extracellular Na concentration appears to be cell-type specific, since low-Na medium does not stimulate proliferation of fibroblasts. Release of growth factor activity is also cell-type specific, as conditioned medium from fibroblasts exposed to a reduced extracellular Na concentration is not stimulatory for epithelial cells. The low-Na growth factors appear chemically and functionally different from other growth factors.

Low-Potassium and Low-Sodium Growth Factors

Brief alterations in the ionic environment cause the release of autocrine products from kidney epithelial cells in culture and possibly in vivo. As alterations in the serum concentration of Na and/or K are common in ARF, it is tempting to speculate that these derangements in the extracellular cation concentration could signal intact nonlethally injured and regenerating cells to release autocrine growth factors to speed the recovery process. These observations also suggest that modest reductions in the extracellular concentration of K and Na may result in the rapid appearance of physiological mediators that could communicate information to other cells along the nephron. These factors might act as messengers between glomerular and tubular cells in response to changes in peritubular or luminal ion concentrations. Although the factors released in response to low-K and low-Na media induce proliferation in cell culture, their physiological role may be different in the intact kidney. Since many mitogens stimulate fluxes of ions and nutrients [44–48], another possible role could be to modify epithelial transport in response to changes in the extracellular environment. Release of autocrine or paracrine factors with this property suggests a mechanism for regulation of ion and nutrient transport in adjacent and nonadjacent epithelial cells. Additional studies will be required to determine whether these factors contribute to the control of kidney epithelial cell growth and/or transport in vivo.

Adenosine Diphosphate Is a Potent Mitogen for Renal Epithelial Cells and Stimulates Production of Paracrine and Autocrine Growth Factors

Each of the adenine nucleotides stimulates DNA synthesis in confluent cultures of BSC-1 cells [36]. ADP and adenosine monophosphate (AMP) are more potent mitogens than ATP, adenosine, or guanine or inosine and their nucleotides. Furthermore, ADP stimulates DNA synthesis threefold more than any known growth-promoting agent for BSC-1 cells. Importantly, ADP and AMP are mitogenic under serum-free conditions, and their stimulatory effect was apparently not mediated by cyclic AMP (cAMP)-dependent mechanisms [36]. In addition, known metabolites such as adenosine, hypoxanthine, or inosine do not appear to mediate ADP or AMP stimulation of DNA synthesis. The mitogenic effect of ADP or AMP do not appear to be mediated through the adenosine receptor, because the predicted stimulation of DNA synthesis is observed in the presence of two adenosine receptor antagonists, theophylline or 5′-deoxy 5′-methylthioadenosine. ATP also stimulates [^{3}H]thymidine incorporation in primary cultures of rabbit proximal tubular cells [49], whereas exogenous adenine nucleotides fail to stimulate DNA synthesis in fibroblasts [36].

The mitogenic response to ADP in BSC-1 cells is associated with activation of specific genes. These include *Egr*-1, c-*fos*, c-*myc*, and c-Ha-*ras*, which are maximally induced at 10 min, 30 min, 1 h, and 12 h, respectively [5o, 51]. Enhanced expression of the genes that encode fibronectin and tenascin, proteins found in the extracellular matrix (ECM), as well as the gene for

TGF-β, which encodes a protein that inhibits growth of BSC-1 cells, is also observed. In summary, ADP can mimic the action of a growth factor, stimulate expression of cell-cycle specific genes (*Egr*-1 and proto-oncogenes), and also stimulate expression of the gene for the negative autocrine growth factor TGF-β which could serve to limit cell proliferation.

Quiescent BSC-1 cells constitutively release platelet-derived growth factor (PDGF)-like activity [52]. The presence of a PDGF-like protein is unexpected, because expression of PDGF was thought to be confined to cells of mesodermal origin such as fibroblasts and smooth muscle cells [53]. This growth factor is released from platelets and macrophages during clotting and wound healing and is a mitogen for cells of mesenchymal origin, a chemoattractant for smooth muscle cells and monocytes, and a promoter of collagen, proteoglycan, and elastic fiber protein synthesis [54]. PDGF is a dimeric glycoprotein with a M_r of 30 kDa comprised of A and/or B chains linked by disulfide bonds [53]. It is most commonly found as a heterodimer (AB), although biologically active homodimers (AA and BB) are known. The amino acid sequence of the B chain is nearly identical to the putative transforming protein of the simian sarcoma virus which is encoded by the v-*sis* oncogene; the cellular homologue is termed c-*sis* [55, 56]. Three classes of PDGF receptors have been defined which are each comprised of two subunits located in the plasma membrane [57, 58]. The α and β receptor subunits are brought together by the presence of one of the three isoforms of PDGF to form the mature receptor dimer. The receptor α-subunit can bind PDGF-A chain or PDGF-B chain homodimers, whereas the β-subunit can bind only PDGF-B chains.

Conditioned medium from quiescent BSC-1 cells is mitogenic for NRK fibroblasts and chemoattractant for bovine aortic smooth muscle cells, and both activities can be blocked by human anti-PDGF immunoglobin G (IgG) [52]. The gene for the B chain of PDGF (c-*sis*) is constitutively expressed in these cells, whereas no PDGF-A chain mRNA can be detected. Thus the cells appear to synthesize and secrete a PDGF-like protein that is a BB homodimer. ADP increases threefold the amounts of PDGF-B chain mRNA and secreted immunoreactive PDGF-like protein. Importantly, ADP rapidly induces release of PDGF-like activity, so that 1 h after exposure of cells to the nucleotide the amount of growth factor increases by more than tenfold. BSC-1 cells do not exhibit a mitogenic response to authentic PDGF, nor do they express the gene encoding the PDGF receptor. These results imply that if a PDGF-like protein is released by renal epithelial cells in vivo, it could act by a paracrine mechanism to initiate proliferation of adjacent stromal (fibroblastic) and/or vascular (smooth muscle) cells within the organ.

Some transformed cells can release PDGF-like proteins and express PDGF receptors [59, 60], which suggests that an autocrine mechanism contributes to their proliferation. Both human fetal kidney and Wilms' tumor cells have been shown to produce PDGF [61], so that production of the

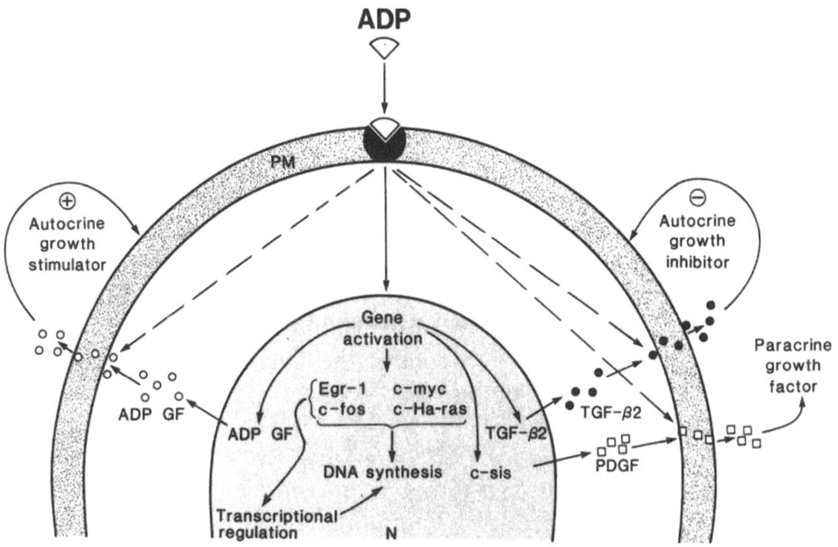

Fig. 3. Growth-regulatory events in BSC-1 cells follwoing exposure to adenosine diphosphate (*ADP*). The adenine nucleotide binds to the plasma membrane (*PM*) and subsequently acts in the nucleus (*N*) to stimulate the expression of genes that encode growth-stimulatory and -inhibitory factors, as well as transcriptional regulators. ADP also stimulates rapid release (*broken line*) of growth factors (*GF*) such as platelet-derived GF (PDGF)-B chain-like protein, transforming GF (TGF)-β, and a novel autocrine growth stimulator

growth factor by Wilms' tumor cells may be a marker for their embryonic origin rather than the malignant phenotype. Like the BSC-1 line, cells derived from Wilms' tumor and fetal kidney bind little PDGF, suggesting a paracrine function for the growth factor in vivo.

Figure 3 provides a schema that summarizes some of the mechanisms by which ADP can initiate growth of renal epithelial cells. ADP is presumed to bind to a specific plasma membrane receptor and activate the early response genes *Egr*-1, c-*fos*, c-*myc*, and NAK1 [62]. There is rapid release of PDGF-B chain homodimer, a paracrine factor; TGF-β_2 a negative autocrine factor; and an apparently novel positive autocrine growth factor under study in this laboratory. Activation of proto-oncogenes (c-*sis* and c-Ha-*ras*) and genes encoding growth factors is also a consequence of ADP action. Thus ADP induces release of paracrine and autocrine growth factors, both positive and negative, providing an example of a single type of renal epithelial cell generating diverse physiological messengers in response to one signal.

When cells detach or die along the nephron not only do nearby cells divide to replace them, but migration of cells into the gap formed in the tubular epithelium can also occur. When a greater number of cells die and slough into the lumen creating a large gap, the process of migration could be even more crucial for repair of the nephron. Little is known about factors which control the migratory behavior of renal epithelial cells. Therefore, recent evidence that ADP can stimulate BSC-1 cells in culture to migrate into denuded areas of a monolayer culture is of particular interest [63]. The concentration of ADP that enhances migration is several-fold less than that which stimulates DNA synthesis. It is not known whether ADP directly increases migration of BSC-1 cells or does so through release of other factors, although the effect does appear to be mediated by binding of the nucleotide to a cell surface receptor [63]. Other factors can also stimulate (EGF, basic FGF, IGF-I) or inhibit (TGF-β, heparin, the tetrapeptide arginine-glycine-aspartic acid-serine, RGDS) the movement of these cells into scrape-wounded areas of a monolayer culture [63]. Therefore, a complex network of signals may exist to control the migratory behavior of renal epithelial cells within the nephron.

Interleukin-1β Stimulates Cell Growth and Induces Expression of the gro/*Melanocyte Growth-Stimulating Activity Gene*

Interleukin-1 is a protein released by mesangial cells, macrophages, and monocytes that has diverse biological effects [64, 65]. It stimulates proliferation of mesangial cells, lymphocytes, fibroblasts, and glioblastoma cells, inhibits the growth of certain tumor cells in vitro, and contributes to the immune response, inflammation, and hematopoiesis. This cytokine also stimulates DNA synthesis in BSC-1 cells [37]. Interleukin-1β rapidly induces expression of the *gro*/melanocyte growth-stimulating activity (MGSA) gene, whereas two other mitogens, ADP, and serum do not. The *gro*/MGSA gene product has diverse growth-regulatory activities and has been identified in three different settings: as the *gro* gene, which is expressed in tumorigenic but not nontumorigenic hamster fibroblasts [66], as MGSA secreted by melanoma cells in culture [67], and as the KC gene product, which is expressed rapidly in PDGF-stimulated fibroblasts [68]. Purified MGSA initiates DNA synthesis in quiescent cultures of BSC-1 cells (unpublished results). These observations suggest that the mesangial cell autocrine growth factor interleukin-1β [65] induces renal epithelial cells to express the gene for MGSA which encodes a protein that is also an autocrine growth factor.

In summary, studies in kidney epithelial cells indicate that perturbations as diverse as reductions in the extracellular concentration of K or Na or exposure to a nucleotide (ADP) or a cytokine (interleukin-1β) each induce the release of autocrine and/or paracrine growth factors.

Renal Growth Factors

Growth factors identified in renal tissue that could contribute to regeneration after ARF via autocrine, paracrine, or juxtacrine mechanisms are described

Table 1. Growth factors that may participate in renal regeneration

Factor	Site of production	Site of action	Action	Comment
EGF	Thick Henle's loop Distal nephron	Basolateral membrane Proximal tubule Collecting duct	Mitogenesis Increased type I collagen synthesis	PreproEGF synthesis decreases in ARF Speeds recovery of ARF in rats
TGF-α	Mesonephric tubules Renal carcinoma cells	Diverse cell types	Transformed phenotype	Binds to EGF receptor
TGF-β	Collecting duct (cow) Distal tubule (mouse)	Diverse cell types	Mitogenesis, fibroblasts Antimitogenic for renal epithelial cells Transforms with TGFα or EGF Increased ECM synthesis	Hyperplastic response becomes hypertrophic
IGFI	Protein in medullary collecting duct (rat); mRNA also in mesangial cells and some PCT cells	Basolateral surface throughout kidney	Hypertrophy of PCT cells in culture	Increased mRNA synthesis after uninephrectomy Increased GFR and RBF Increased protein and mRNA synthesis in early DM in rats Speeds recovery of ARF in rats
IGF-II	Throughout kidney; 100 times more in fetal kidney	?	Activates PLC	
PDGF	Mesangial cells BSC-1 cells Fibroblasts SMC Platelets	Mesangial cells Fibroblasts SMC Macrophages	Mitogenesis of mesangial cells, SMC, fibroblasts Chemotactic for fibroblasts, SMC, macrophages	Possible role in glomerular cell growth

Table 1. *Continued*

Factor	Site of production	Site of action	Action	Comment
FGF	Isolated from renal tissue; cell of origin uncertain	Fibroblasts Myoblasts Endothelial cells	Mitogenesis Chemotactic for vascular endothelial cells Induces release of collagenases	Embedded in ECM (?) if in tubular basement membrane in kidney
Low K^+ GF	BSC-1 cells	BSC-1 cells	Mitogenesis	Isolated from BSC-1 conditioned medium
Low Na^+ GF	BSC-1 cells	BSC-1 cells	Mitogenesis	Isolated from BSC-1 conditioned medium
HGF	Endothelial cells; also liver, spleen lung, thymus	Proximal tubule and other organs	Mitogenesis Migration	Also named scatter factor, tumor cytotoxic factor May act as endocrine factor via circulation as well as locally
Renin/AII	J-G cells Liver	Proximal tubule cells in culture	Low dose: hypertrophy and increased Na^+ transport	
IL-1	Mesangial cells Lymphocytes	Mesangial cells	Mitogenesis	IL-1 mRNA in BSC-1 cells

AII, angiotensin II; ARF, acute renal failure; DM, diabetes mellitus; ECM, extracellular matrix; GFR, glomerular filtration rate; GF, growth factor; IL, interleukin; JG, juxtaglomerular; PLC, phospholipase C; PCT, proximal convoluted tubule; RBF, renal blood flow; SMC, smooth muscle cells.

in Table 1. Administration of purified growth factors as pharmacological agents alone or in combination may eventually prove useful in treatment of patients with this condition.

Epidermal Growth Factor

EGF is a potent renal epithelial cell mitogen comprised of 53 amino acids [69]. The preproEGF mRNA in murine kidney is translated to preproEGF protein, whose function is not certain, whereas intracellular processing to the mature growth factor apparently does not occur [27]. Urinary EGF is probably derived by proteolytic cleavage of preproEGF protein located in the plasma membrane. In mouse kidney, preproEGF mRNA is found in the distal nephron and loop of Henle. The EGF receptor is found in the basolateral membrane of the proximal tubule and collecting duct and to a lesser extent in distal tubules and glomeruli of rabbit nephrons [70]. The EGF membrane receptor protein likely represents the cellular analogue of the protein product of the viral *erb*-B oncogene [71]. In BSC-1 cells the number of EGF receptors is about tenfold higher in sparse cultures than at high cell density, although there is no apparent change in receptor affinity [72]. In vivo, a renal insult could unmask EGF receptors on injured or intact renal cells when adjacent cells detach from the tubular basement membrane. Presumably these surviving cells would be more responsive to the mitogenic effect of EGF produced at the site of injury. Following cell proliferation and reepithelialization of the nephron, the receptors would again be downregulated.

The role of EGF in regeneration after acute renal injury and as a pharmacologic agent has been investigated in recent studies. The renal synthesis of EGF falls rapidly after acute ischemic injury in the rat so that expression of preproEGF mRNA is reduced by 60% at 2h [73]. By 24h, the mRNA is undetectable, and urinary excretion of EGF protein has declined by 97%. In contrast, expression of the early response genes (c-*fos*, *Egr*-1, and c-*myc*) increases. Importantly, binding of [^{125}I]EGF increased 3.6-fold in renal cortical tissue and 2.5-fold in the medulla 24h after injury. In a *cis*-platinum model of acute tubular injury, decreased preproEGF mRNA expression was found in cells of the distal collecting tubule and thick ascending limb 12–72h after injury, whereas salivary gland preproEGF mRNA expression was unaffected [4]. Thus acute tubular injury initiates a specific decline in renal EGF gene expression, but surviving cells exhibit increased binding of the growth factor.

Three recent publications provide strong evidence that pharmacologic administration of EGF accelerates recovery from experimental acute renal injury in the rat. An 8-day intrarenal infusion of EGF or a single subcutaneous injection of the growth factor each ameliorated the rise in serum creatinine following hypoxic renal injury and stimulated [^{3}H]thymidine incorporation into DNA in renal tubular cells 24 h after the insult [75, 76]. A similar augmentation of the repair process following subcutaneous administration of EGF was demonstrated in a model of mercuric chloride-induced ARF [77]. Histologic examination showed that EGF treatment did not alter the extent of tubular necrosis at 24 h. Thus in three different models of acute tubular injury, EGF given soon after an hypoxic or nephrotoxic insult enhanced regeneration of renal epithelial cells and recovery of glomerular filtration.

If autocrine production of EGF plays a role in human renal regeneration, it might do so by binding to an increased number of EGF receptors, as has been demonstrated in rat kidney tissue after ischemic injury [73]. Another source of EGF in vivo could be the systemic circulation; the plasma concentration is approximately 20 pg/ml [69]. This relatively low concentration may become physiologically important in the setting of ARF, because the number of EGF receptors per cell is increased.

The physiologic function of urinary EGF remains undefined, as does the mechanism by which it enters the urine. Even though mRNA encoding preproEGF is detected in the thick loop of Henle and distal nephron in mice, and EGF can be detected immunohistochemically in the apical regions of these cells, little EGF can be extracted from kidney tissue [69]. The amount of EGF excreted in human urine each day (approximately 50 μg) is too large to be accounted for by efficient renal clearance of the growth factor. At present it is thought that preproEGF is inserted in the luminal plasma membrane where it is subsequently cleaved by urinary proteases to release the mature growth factor [69]. The potential actions of EGF in distal tubular fluid are a matter of speculation. One possibility is that EGF stimulates proliferation of epithelial cells to replace those that have detached or died as a result of the acidic pH or the relatively high concentration of toxic metabolites in the lumen of the distal nephron, ureters, and bladder.

There may be a practical problem with administration of pharmacological doses of EGF to patients after acute renal failure. TGF-α, which like EGF binds to the EGF receptor, stimulates calcium resorption from mouse calvaria in culture, and subcutaneous EGF and TGF-α administered over a 2-day period to mice induced mild hypercalcemia [78, 79]. The mechanisms of bone resorption and hypercalcemia remain to be defined, but may be consequences of the interaction of EGF with the parathyroid hormone (PTH) receptor [80]. Hyperphosphotemia is often found in ARF; thus the risk of dystrophic and metastatic calcification caused by elevation of the calcium-phosphorous product after EGF administration may ultimately limit the clinical utility of this growth factor.

Transforming Growth Factor-β

The autocrine release of growth-inhibitory activity was first inferred from observations made on crowded cultures of BSC-1 cells by Holley and coworkers in 1978 [81]. They noted stimulation of [^{3}H]thymidine incorporation into DNA when conditioned medium containing serum was aspirated and replaced by fresh serum-free medium. As no serum growth factors were added to the medium, it appeared that DNA synthesis was initiated by removal of a cell-derived growth inhibitor. Subsequent purification of the inhibitor protein indicated that it could arrest sparse cultures of growing cells in the G_1 phase of the cell cycle, but proliferation resumed when it was removed [82]. This reversible effect on cell growth, and the low concentration required for inhibition, suggested a physiological role for the inhibitor in the control of proliferation. Since the growth-inhibitory effect could be overcome by addition of EGF to the culture medium, proliferation of renal cells in culture can be regulated by factors with opposing effects [83]. In 1984, the growth inhibitor was shown to be biologically and chemically similar to TGF-β [84]. The complete amino acid sequence of the BSC-1 cell growth inhibitor has been determined from the nucleotide sequence of the cDNA and shown to correspond to TGF-β_2 [41]. Human TGF-β_1 is a polypeptide with an apparent M_r of 25 kDa composed of two chains linked by disulfide bonds. There is 71% identity between the amino acid sequences of monkey TGF-β_2 and human TGF-β_1 [41, 85], closely related proteins with similar properties.

TGF-β mRNA is constitutively expressed in most cells, although renal production of the protein detected by immunohistochemistry appears limited to the cortical distal tubule in the mouse and to the collecting duct in bovine kidney [86, 87]. In primary cultures of rabbit proximal tubular cells, TGF-β_2 is able to convert the mitogenic effect usually exerted by insulin and hydrocortisone into a hypertrophic one, which suggests a role for this growth factor in compensatory renal growth after uninephrectomy [88]. TGF-β also induces synthesis of fibronectin and its incorporation into ECM by lung epithelial cells and fibroblasts in culture [89]. In a rat model of wound healing, TGF-β_2 increased synthesis of type I procollagen by fibroblasts and the rate of healing [90]. Since an antiserum to TGF-β_1 appears to be efficacious in the treatment of a mouse model of mesangial proliferative glomerulonephritis [91], this growth factor may play a critical role in the accumulation of basement membrane components in specific glomerulonephritides.

Transforming Growth Factor-α

TGF-α is 50-amino acid polypeptide that exerts its biological effects by binding to the EGF receptor [26]. Recent evidence that the precursor form of TGF-α is biologically active suggests that both the processed soluble and membrane-bound precursor form of the growth factor may serve as mitogens, by autocrine and juxtacrine mechanisms respectively (Fig. 2). TGF-α protein is secreted by developing mouse mesonephric tubules, and the major physiological role of the growth factor is thought to be in embryonic development [92]. Renal carcinomas and other human tumors produce TGF-α, which can sometimes be recovered from the urine of these patients [92]. The growth factor is not produced by kidney epithelial cells of the BSC-1 line (unpublished observations), although a small amount of mRNA for this growth factor is detected in normal adult kidney [93]. Its role in kidney repair after injury has not been defined. Since this growth factor utilizes the EGF receptor, it is anticipated that infusion of TGF-α would be as effective as EGF following acute tubular necrosis.

Insulin-Like Growth Factors

The IGFs, also termed somatomedins, are peptide growth factors, first isolated from human plasma fractions, which share the following biological activities: stimulation of sulfate incorporation into cartilage, insulin-like activity on glucose metabolism, and a mitogenic effect on different cell types [94]. IGF-I, also known as somatomedin C, is a basic, single-chain polypeptide of 70 amino acids with an apparent M_r of 7649 Da [95]. IGF-II is a slightly acidic peptide of 67 amino acids with an apparent M_r of 7471 Da; there is 62% identity between IGF-I and II, and both have a high degree of homology with human proinsulin [96]. Two types of IGF receptor have been described [97]. Type I receptors appear to mediate the mitogenic effect of both IGF-I and II in the kidney, are homologous to the insulin receptor, and are located on the basolateral surface of tubule cells.

The site of production of IGF-I was originally considered to be the liver, from which it is released in response to growth hormone [94]. However, it is now known that IGF-I is produced by most, if not all tissues, and acts as an autocrine or paracrine effector [98]. Moreover, the alterations in its serum level have less significance than changes within a tissue [99]. IGF-I production (and its growth hormone dependence) has been demonstrated in rat kidney as well as other rat tissues [100]. IGF-I mRNA is also present in adult human kidney [101]. In rat kidney, immunoreactive IGF-I is localized primarily in the medullary collecting duct and is not found in the proximal or distal tubules [102]. IGF-II is less directly under GH control and is believed to be an important fetal growth factor [103]. IGF-II mRNA is present in both fetal and adult human kidney; however, it is ten to 100-fold more abundant in the fetal organ.

IGF-I appears to play a role in renal growth: it can induce hypertrophy of proximal tubular cells in culture [104] and increased immunoreactive protein has been demonstrated in kidneys after ischemic injury [105]. Recently, IGF-I administered subcutaneously to rats after ischemia-induced ARF was shown to reduce the severity of renal failure and hasten recovery [106, 107]. Improved renal function was associated with decreased histologic injury [106] and increased DNA synthesis [107] in those rats that received the growth factor. How IGF-I reaches proximal tubular cells in vivo remains uncertain, because its major site of production is the terminal collecting duct. Acutely, IGF-I alters renal hemodynamics by decreasing afferent and efferent arteriolar tone and increasing the ultrafiltration coefficient, all of which can improve renal function [108, 109]. With time IGF-I also increases protein synthesis in the kidney resulting in hypertrophy [109]. Thus IGF-I potentially can improve renal function after injury via multiple mechanisms in addition to promoting cell division.

Platelet-Derived Growth Factor

Mesangial cells secrete a PDGF-like protein and express PDGF receptors [110]. Glomerular endothelial and mesangial cells each proliferate in response to PDGF so that the factor could play a central role in growth responses in the glomerulus [110]. Renal epithelial cells (BSC-1 line) in culture release a factor with PDGF-like activity [52]. Although PDGF is not a mitogen for these renal cells, it could contribute to regeneration after ARF in vivo by attracting infiltrating inflammatory cells and stimulating adjacent fibroblasts to release factors that are ligands for receptors on the surface of tubular cells. In this way PDGF might coordinate tubular and glomerular proliferation after renal injury.

Fibroblast Growth Factors

The two major FGFs are two closely related polypeptides with different isoelectric points, designated as acidic FGF (aFGF) and basic FGF (bFGF). cDNA clones encoding each protein have been isolated and the predicted amino acid sequences indicate 55% structural homology between these two growth factors [111]. FGFs are mitogenic for most, if not all, nonterminally differentiated cells of mesodermal or neuroectodermal origin. FGFs are also potent inducers of blood vessel growth. They are chemotactic for vascular endothelial cells and induce expression of plasminogen activators and collagenases, proteolytic enzymes that presumably mediate tissue remodeling.

FGFs bind to heparan sulfates, which are important components of ECM in tissues and cells in culture [112]. Their presence in ECM suggests they can mediate proliferation of cells adjacent to the basement membrane. In this manner FGF deposited in the ECM could act as a local growth regulator and induce regeneration after detachment of the overlying cell layer. This may explain some of its capacity to promote wound healing. It has been difficult to define the mechanism by which FGF is deposited into the ECM, as both aFGF and bFGF lack a classical leader sequence required for cellular secretion [111, 113]. It is not known whether FGF is released only from damaged or dying cells, is delivered to sites of injury or inflammation by stimulated macrophages, or is secreted by an as yet uncharacterized mechanism [113].

Both aFGF and bFGF are mitogenic for rat proximal tubular cells in culture [114]. Maximal rates of DNA synthesis can be induced with either FGF, obviating the requirement for IGF-I or EGF [114]. Messenger RNA encoding aFGF but not bFGF has been detected in rat kidney, and by western analysis aFGF protein but little bFGF has been found. Therefore, although both aFGF and bFGF can serve as mitogens for proximal tubular epithelial cells in culture, it appears that aFGF would be the candidate to play a physiological role in vivo. Studies in embryonic kidney suggest a role for FGF in renal angiogenesis [115]. During embryonic development, kidney differentiation is driven by the interaction of cells of different types. Contact with the epithelial ureteric bud induces the nephrogenic mesenchyme to differentiate, which then leads to stimulation of blood vessel ingrowth. FGF may have some role in renal neoplasia, as both aFGF and bFGF can promote anchorage-independent growth of SV40-transformed rat proximal tubular cells [116]. Whether FGF participates in renal cell regeneration after injury is not clear.

Hepatocyte Growth Factor

Hepatocyte growth factor (HGF), the most potent mitogen identified for cultured hepatocytes, was initially isolated from the peripheral circulation of rabbits after partial hepatectomy [117]. Subsequently, HGF was shown to be the same molecule as scatter factor and tumor cytotoxic factor [117, 118]. HGF consists of two chains: one of 70 kDa (α-chain) and the other of 30 kDa (β-chain). The α-chain contains four kringle domains, in which a small polypeptide loop is held together by disulfide bonds within a larger loop [117]. Kringle domains are thought to play a key role during intercalation of HGF with other proteins; three of the kringle domains bear sequence similarity to prothrombin. Although the β-chain structurally resembles a serine protease, the intact molecule does not appear to have this function [117]. Native HGF is synthesized as a 728-amino acid precursor which is then cleaved to form the heterodimer, although uncleaved HGF is biologically active. Messenger RNA encoding HGF has been localized in adult liver, kidney, lung, and thymus. In the liver, HGF is produced by nonparenchymal Ito cells. HGF has also been localized in tissues lacking gene expression for the factor such as central nervous system (CNS) cortical neurons, suggesting that certain cells can accumulate HGF from the circulation. In addition to its mitogenic effects, HGF causes "scatter" (dissociation and migration) of several epithelial and endothelial cell lines in culture, but not fibroblasts. The HGF receptor, encoded by the protooncogene c-*met*, is a transmembrane protein with an intracellular tyrosine kinase domain that is widely distributed in the body including the kidney. Norepinephrine (NE) potentiates the mitogenic effect of HGF, and decreased hepatic clearance of NE and HGF after liver injury may lead to high plasma levels of each and thereby enhance liver cell proliferation.

HGF is a mitogen for cultured rabbit proximal tubular cells and two renal epithelial cell lines (LLC-PK_1 and OK cells), but not a third (MDCK) [119, 120]. Both LLC-PK_1 and OK lines are thought to originate from cells of the proximal nephron, whereas MDCK cells are of distal origin, suggesting that HGF may act as a mitogen primarily in the proximal nephron. Interestingly, HGF does promote migration and stimulate Na/K-ATPase activity of MDCK cells [120]. After contralateral nephrectomy, HGF mRNA content increases in the remaining kidney as well as in spleen, suggesting that HGF derived both locally and from a distant organ may contribute to compensatory renal growth after injury [121]. Increased HGF mRNA has been localized in renal endothelial cells after ischemic or toxic injury [122]. Whereas production of HGF protein increases during the first 12 h after renal injury, the amount of receptor for HGF on the plasma membrane of epithelial cells dramatically falls, perhaps due to internalization of HGF–receptor complexes [122]. On the other hand, mRNA encoding the HGF receptor (c-*met*) increases rapidly after renal ischemia or unilateral nephrectomy [123]. The mitogenic effect of HGF is strongly inhibited by increasing cell density and the autocrine factor TGF-β_1 [119]. Therefore, after periods of renal cell death or injury HGF may serve as a potent mitogen. HGF can be eluted from rat liver by a highsalt buffer, suggesting that the growth factor may be stored in the ECM and like FGF could therefore stimulate replication and migration of surviving cells after injury [124].

Although only recently described and characterized, HGF may be an important factor mediating repair and regeneration after renal injury.

Angiotensin II

Angiotensin-converting enzyme (ACE) inhibitors block compensatory kidney hypertrophy after partial renal ablation in rats [125]. Although this observation has been ascribed to changes in intrarenal hemodynamics, direct cellular effects of angiotensin II (AII) have been defined. AII can induce hypertrophy of smooth muscle cells in culture [126] and stimulate sodium transport in both intact nephrons and cultures of proximal tubular cells, possibly via enhanced Na/H antiporter activity [127, 128]. In mouse proximal tubular cells of the MCT line, exposure to $10^{-8}\,M$ AII increases cell size and protein synthesis, effects that can be blocked specifically by saralasin [129]. In MCT cells pretreated with EGF, the hypertrophic action of AII became a proliferative one.

Plasma renin activity is increased in humans and animals with ARF, and elevated intrarenal AII levels may contribute to abnormal autoregulation of blood flow in the recovering kidney [130, 131]. The direct renal cellular effects of AII on sodium transport and hypertrophy suggest that this protein could also have physiologic significance during tubular regeneration after injury.

Sublethal Cellular Injury in Acute Renal Failure: Cytoskeletal Alterations, Cell Polarity, and Cell Detachment

Polar organization of renal tubular cells is essential for their physiological function, whereas altered membrane organization is associated with acute renal injury [132]. Enzymes, receptors, and carriers show an asymmetrical distribution between the apical and basolateral surfaces of polarized epithelial cells, and the lipid content and physical properties of these two plasma membrane domains is distinctly different [10]. The establishment of asymmetry may initially involve cell–cell contacts mediated by cell surface adhesion glycoproteins such as uvomorulin. Also important in the development of cell polarity are contacts between the cell and the ECM. Cellular receptors for ECM laminin, collagen, and fibronectin belong to the integrin supergene family [133]. Laminin is secreted into the basement membrane of cells destined to become renal epithelium [134]. The gene encoding the A chain of laminin is constitutively expressed, whereas expression of B chain mRNA precedes commitment to an epithelial cell morphology in organ culture [135]. Furthermore, antibodies to the A chain can prevent development of polarity in these cells. Type IV collagen production also appears to be linked to development of renal epithelial cell polarity, as undifferentiated mesenchyme produces only collagen types I and III [136]. Syndecan, a cell surface proteoglycan, behaves as an ECM receptor. It associates intracellularly with actin and is localized to the basolateral surface of epithelial cells [137]. The extracellular domain of the syndecan molecule contains heparan sulfate chains, which can reversibly bind bFGF. Mammary epithelial cells made syndecan deficient with antisense cDNA lose epithelial polarity and assume a fibroblastic morphology.

Intact cytoskeletal actin microfilaments and microtubules appear necessary to maintain polarity of renal epithelial cells. Alterations in cytoskeletal components may result from renal injury not severe enough to cause cell death. Permeability of tight junctions in microperfused ischemic tubules, measured by ruthenium red penetration, increases in a stepwise manner for 30 min after the insult [132]. This is accompanied by an abnormal redistribution of Na/K-ATPase from the basolateral to the apical membrane, indicating loss of fence function ordinarily mediated by tight junctions that separate apical and basolateral membrane domains. Other changes of the cytoskeleton with ischemia include loss of brush-border terminal-web actin filaments after 15 min and redistribution of actin throughout the cytoplasm after 50 min [138]. Disrupting microfilaments of perfused tubules with cytochalasin D decreases their capacity for sodium reabsorption [138], which suggests that morphologic alterations of the cytoskeleton after ischemia are correlated with functional derangements of the nephron.

Exposure of BSC-1 cells to an oxidative stress (H_2O_2) for 30 min is associated with cell detachment as well as loss of integrin α_3 receptors from the basolateral surface [15]. Interestingly, there is a corresponding increase of immunostainable integrin α_3 on the apical surface associated with a greater tendency for cell–cell adhesion, a phenomenon that can be blocked by RGD-containing peptides [11, 15]. Therefore, aggregates of desquamated cells could occlude tubular lumens after acute tubular necrosis, leading to increased tubular pressure and backleak of ultrafiltrate, which could contribute to the decline in glomerular filtration. Infusion of RGD-containing peptides into rats ameliorates the observed increment in bubular pressure after ischemia-induced ARF [11]. Thus redistribution of cell surface integrins associated with sublethal cellular injury in ARF, by leading to cell detachment and aggregation, can occlude tubules and thereby impair renal function.

Strategies to ameliorate or repair cytoskeletal alterations in ARF have not yet been developed, although four growth factors – EGF, TGF-β, PDGF, and FGF – each can enhance synthesis of ECM proteins through different mechanisms [69, 89, 139, 140]. As there are direct connections between the ECM and cytoskeleton via the cell proteins ankyrin and fodrin, growth factors could, perhaps indirectly, facilitate repair of the cytoskeleton.

Sublethal Cellular Injury in Acute Renal Failure: Cytoprotection and Programmed Cell Death

Recovery of cells from nonlethal injury may involve participation of heat shock proteins (HSP). These proteins are highly conserved in eukaryotic cells and are induced by a wide variety of agents in addition to heat, including anoxia and toxins [13]. The major HSP in vertebrates have a M_r of approximately 70 kDa (HSP-70) and have recently been characterized in kidney tissue [13, 141]. HSP-70 may function as a molecular chaperone in stressed cells to bind denatured and aggregated proteins, aiding in refolding them to a normal conformation. In a rat model of renal ischemia, HSP-70 mRNA was induced after 15 min, reached a maximal value at 2 h, and returned to the basal level by 24 h after reflow. Immunocytochemical examination revealed localization of HSP-72 protein in the apical region of proximal cells 15 min after injury, with a diffuse cytoplasmic increase in staining 2–6 h later. By 24 h after ischemia, HSP-72 remained diffusely increased in the cytoplasm, but was no longer located in the apical region of cells. Increased cytoplasmic HSP-73 staining has also been detected in rat proximal tubular cells from 2 to 12 days after exposure to a known nephrotoxin, gentamicin [141]. Although their precise function remains to be defined in detail, HSP may be instrumental in the poorly understood process of cellular remodeling and recovery after sublethal cellular injury in ARF.

Sublethally injured cells may subsequently die by a specific pathway known as apoptosis. Apoptotic cells degrade DNA into oligonucleosomal fragments by an active process dependent on DNA synthesis [142, 143]. Apoptotic cells have been observed in ischemic kidneys [144, 145], although the extent and significance of such programmed cell death in renal tubular dysfunction remains to be defined. In the future, therapeutic strategies may be developed to prevent cell death by apoptosis, thereby limiting the extent of renal injury and facilitating recovery from the ARF syndrome [146].

Conclusions and Speculations

Kidney cells release autocrine and paracrine growth factors in response to extracellular signals that could mediate repair of the nephron after acute injury (Table 1, Fig. 2). Examples of such signals are reductions in the extracellular K and Na concentration, liberation of adenine nucleotides by injured or dying cells, and growth factors and cytokines released by intact neighboring cells. As growth factors alter ion and nutrient transport and other aspects of cell metabolism, these effector molecules could mediate repair of biochemical and/or subcellular injuries. After recovery, an injured cell could subsequently respond to autocrine, paracrine, or juxtacrine proliferative signals. Epithelial cells at both ends of a necrotic segment of the nephron, and other surviving isolated cells along its denuded surface are responsible for regenerating the tubular epithelial cell lining [18]. Proliferation of these cells which can subsequently slide along the basement membrane permits rapid restitution of the tubule. Growth factors could enhance the transition of these cells from the G_0 to G_1 phase of the cell cycle, possibly speed protein and phospholipid synthesis for the formation of brush-border and basolateral membranes (Fig. 4), and promote migration of cells into denuded areas. The intact basement membrane plays an important role in the healing process by providing a structural scaffolding for cell migration and proliferation. Alterations in the ECM and its connections to the cytoskeleton occur with acute tubular injury and likely result in profound disruption of cellular function. Since several growth factors stimulate cells to synthesize and release ECM components such as collagens, fibronectin, and tenascin, repair of the damaged basement membrane might also be mediated by molecules of kidney cell origin. At present the factors which govern repair of the ECM and cytoskeleton following acute tubular injury remain to be defined.

Growth factors delivered to renal epithelial cells from local and systemic sources, which can act through more than one mechanism, may orchestrate migration and proliferative repair of the nephron after cellular necrosis. IGF-I and EGF, which are produced by renal epithelial cells, as well as

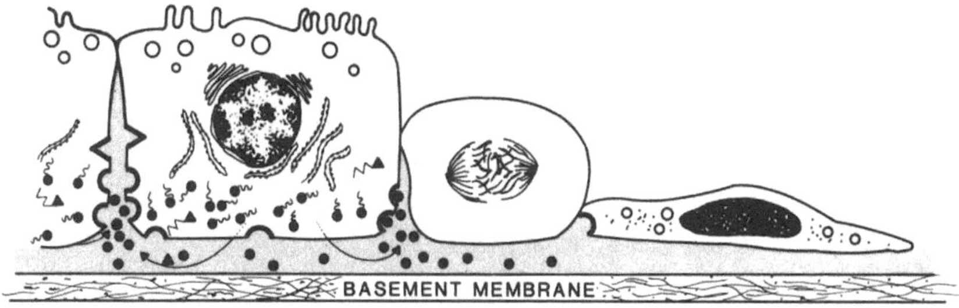

Fig. 4. Growth regulation in regenerating kidney epithelial cells. Cells at the edge of an injured segment of the nephron are shown during early renal regeneration following acute tubular necrosis. Pictured are non-necrotic cells, a dividing cell, and a migrating squamoid cell. Proliferation may be mediated in part by synthesis of growth-stimulatory factors followed by cellular processing and release of the active molecules. Symbols for growth factors, precursors, and receptors are as in Fig. 2

factors made by endothelial cells (HGF), mesangial cells (PDGF and interleukins), and other distant organs (HGF) may also contribute to tissue repair. Evidence now exists that pharmacological administration of IGF-I and EGF can speed recovery from experimentally induced ARF [75–77, 106, 107]. FGF and HGF, which appear to be stored in the ECM, may thereby be available for future use to facilitate recovery of injured cells. TGF-β, which can convert a proliferative signal into a hypertrophic one, may facilitate development of the nascent cells into a mature epithelium and act as a negative feedback signal to limit proliferation as repair of the nephron nears completion.

Renal growth factors may also act on a population of renal cells arrested in the G_2 phase of the cell cycle. Described by Pederson and Gelfant in 1970 [147], these cells could be rapidly mobilized to divide by paracrine or autocrine factors and thereby begin replacement of cells that detached from the tubular basement membrane. Mesangial, endothelial, and/or infiltrating inflammatory cells at the site of renal injury represent additional sources of growth factors that could act on cells of the injured nephron [148, 149]. Growth factors and adenine nucleotides released by regenerating and injured kidney epithelial cells could also stimulate fibroblast cell growth. In addition, tubular and fibroblastic cells may be stimulated by autocrine and/or paracrine mechanisms to synthesize and secrete ECM proteins which could repair rents in the tubular basement membrane.

The National Kidney and Urologic Diseases Advisory Board 1990 Long-Range Plan [1] concluded that ARF is the most costly kidney condition requiring hospitalization, that the number of cases has increased recently as a consequence of complicated surgical procedures in older patients, and that the mortality rate has not changed. Thus there is a considerable need to speed renal regeneration and reduce mortality. This chapter suggests that growth factors may be useful agents to treat this condition. Initially it would be important for a patient with ARF to be well dialyzed, so that any administered agents do not contribute to volume overload. Nutrition is another critical issue. It is important to provide sufficient calories, determined by the nutritional status of the patient and the presence or absence of infection. Provision of amino acids is important to minimize gluconeogenesis and to serve as precursors for protein synthesis. In fact, total parenteral nutrition containing sufficient amino acids has been shown to enhance recovery from ARF in humans [21]. Since these issues have already been addressed experimentally, it is now time to focus attention on specific growth factors and contemplate their use. Infusions of adenine nucleotides with magnesium chloride, EGF, and IGF-I have each been shown to hasten recovery after ARF in animals, but their utility in humans remains to be determined [75, 76, 106, 107, 150]. HGF, which is found in the circulation and is a renal cell mitogen, also awaits study as a potential therapeutic agent [117]. The use of a specific growth factor alone or in combination with others may speed renal regeneration and improve the outcome of patients with this condition.

Acknowledgments. Studies cited in the text were performed in collaboration with Dr. Sreedharan Kartha, Dr. Margaret Walsh-Reitz, Dr. Naga Aithal, and Dr. Vivek Rangnekar. Support for work in this laboratory was provided by NIH Clinical Investigator Award K08 DK 02272 and National Research Service Award DK 08618 to JCL and NIH grants DK 39689, DK 18413, DK 37227, DK 07510, and DK 47631.

References

1. National Kidney and Urologic Diseases Advisory Board (1990) Long-range plan: window on the 21st century. NIH Publ 90(583):47–48
2. Oliver J, MacDowell M, Tracy A (1951) The pathogenesis of acute renal failure associated with traumatic and toxic injury. Renal ischemia, nephrotoxic damage and the ischemuric episode. J Clin Invest 30:1305–1440
3. Cuppage FE, Tate A (1967) Repair of the nephron following injury with mercuric chloride. Am J Pathol 51:405–429
4. Siegel FL, Bulger RE (1975) Scanning and transmission electron microscopy of mercuric chloride-induced tubular necrosis in rat kidney. Virchows Arch [Cell Pathol] 18:243–262
5. Haagsma BH, Pound AW (1980) Mercuric chloride-induced tubulonecrosis in the rat kidney: the recovery phase. Br J Exp Pathol 61:229
6. Solez K, Whelton A (1984) Acute renal failure: correlations between morphology and function. Dekker, New York
7. Weinberg JM (1991) The cell biology of ischemic renal injury. Kidney Int 39:476–500
8. Solez K, Marel-Maroger L, Sraer J-D (1979) The morphology of "acute tubular necrosis" in man: analysis of 57 renal biopsies and a comparison with the glycerol model. Medicine (Baltimore) 58:362–376
9. Darmady EM, Strank F (1975) Microdissection of the nephron in disease. Br Med Bull 13:21–26

10. Molitaris BA, Nelson WJ (1990) Alterations in the establishment and maintenance of epithelial cell polarity as a basis for disease processes. J Clin Invest 85:3–9
11. Goligorsky MS, DiBona GF (1993) Pathogenetic role of Arg-Gly-Asp-recognizing integrins in acute renal failure. Proc Natl Acad Sci USA 90:5700–5704
12. Mendley SR, Toback FG (1989) Autocrine and paracrine regulation of kidney epithelial cell growth. Annu Rev Physiol 51:33–50
13. Van Why SK, Hildebrandt F, Ardito T, Mann AS, Siegel NJ, Kashgarian M (1992) Induction and intracellular localization of HSP-72 after renal ischemia. Am J Physiol 263:F769–F775
14. Prescott LF (1966) The normal urinary excretion rates of renal tubular cells, leukocytes, and red blood cells. Clin Sci 31:425–435
15. Gailit J, Colfesh D, Rabiner I, Simone J, Goligorsky MS (1993) Redistribution and dysfunction of integrins in cultured renal epithelial cells exposed to oxidative stress. Am J Physiol 264:F149–F157
16. Toback FG (1985) Control of renal regeneration after acute tubular necrosis. Nephrology I:748–763
17. Toback FG, Havener FL, Dodd RC, Spargo BH (1977) Phospholipid metabolism during renal regeneration after acute tubular necrosis. Am J Physiol 232:E216–E222
18. Cuppage FE, Cunningham N, Tate AL (1969) Nucleic acid synthesis in the regenerating nephron following injury with mercuric chloride. Lab Invest 21:449–457
19. Toback FG, Dodd RC, Maier ER, Havener LJ (1983) Amino acid administration enhances renal protein metabolism after acute tubular necrosis. Nephron 33:238–243
20. Toback FG (1980) Amino acid treatment of acute renal failure. Contemp Issues Nephrol 6:202–228
21. Toback FG (1987) Amino acid enhancement of renal regeneration after acute tubular necrosis. Kidney Int 12:193–198
22. Yarden Y, Ullrich A (1988) Molecular analysis of signal transduction by growth factors. Biochemistry 27:3113–3119
23. Berridge MJ (1987) Inositol triphosphate and diacylglycerol: two interacting second messengers. Annu Rev Biochem 56:159–193
24. McCreight CE, Sulkin NM (1959) Cellular proliferation in the kidney of young and senile rats following unilateral nephrectomy. J Gerontol 14:440–443
25. Sporn MB, Todaro GJ (1980) Autocrine secretion and malignant transformation of cells. N Engl J Med 303:878–880
26. Massagué J (1990) Transforming growth factor-α. J Biol Chem 265:21292–21396
27. Rall LB, Scott J, Bell GI, Crawford RJ, Penshow JD, Niall HD, Coghlan JP (1985) Mouse prepro-epidermal growth factor synthesis by the kidney and other tissues. Nature 313:228–231
28. Toback FG, Walsh-Reitz MM, Mendley SR, Kartha SR (1990) Kidney epithelial cells release growth factors in response to extracellular signals. Pediatr Nephrol 4:363–371
29. Mendley SR, Toback FG (1990) Cell proliferation in the end stage kidney. Am J Kidney Dis 16:80–84
30. Hopps HE, Bernheim BC, Nisalak A, Tijo JH, Smadel JE (1963) Biologic characteristics of a continuous kidney cell line derived from the African green monkey. J Immunol 91:416–424
31. Rollason HD (1949) Compensatory hypertrophy of the kidney of the young rat with special emphasis on the role of cellular hyperplasia. Anat Rec 104:263–285
32. Toback FG (1980) Induction of growth of kidney cells in culture by Na^+. Proc Natl Acad Sci USA 77:6654–6656
33. Leighton J, Brada A, Estes LW, Justh G (1969) Secretory activity and oncogenicity of a cell line (MDCK) derived from dog kidney. Science 163:472–473
34. Walsh-Reitz MM, Toback FG (1984) Kidney epithelial cell growth is stimulated by lowering extracellular potassium concentration. Am J Physiol 247:C14–C19

35. Walsh-Reitz MM, Gluck SL, Waack S, Toback FG (1986) Lowering extracellular Na^+ concentration releases autocrine grwoth factors from renal epithelial cells. Proc Natl Acad Sci USA 83:4764–4768
36. Kartha SR, Toback FG (1985) Purine nucleotides stimulate DNA synthesis in kidney epithelial cells in culture. Am J Physiol 249:F967–F972
37. Rangekar VV, Waheed S, Davies TJ, Toback FG, Rangekar VM (1991) Antimitogenic and mitogenic actions of interleukin-1 in diverse cell types are associated with induction of *gro* gene expression. J Biol Chem 266:2415–2422
38. Schrader GA, Prickett CO, Salmon WD (1937) Symptomatology and pathology of potassium and magnesium deficiencies in the rat. J Nutr 14:85–110
39. Oliver J, MacDowell M, Welt LG, Holliday MA, Hollander W Jr, Winters RW, Williams TF, Segar WE (1957) The renal lesions of electrolyte imbalance. I. The structural alterations in potassium-depleted rats. J Exp Med 106:563–574
40. Spargo BH (1954) Kidney changes in hypokalemic alkalosis in the rat. J Lab Clin Med 43:802–814
41. Hanks SK, Amour R, Baldwin JH, Maldonado F, Spiess J, Holley RW (1988) Amino acid sequence of the BSC-1 cell growth inhibitor (polyergin) deduced from the nucleotide sequence of the cDNA. Proc Natl Acad Sci USA 85:79–82
42. Cone CD Jr, Tongier M Jr (1973) Contact inhibition of division: involvement of the electrical transmembrane potential. J Cell Physiol 82:373–386
43. Smith JB, Rozengurt E (1978) Serum stimulates the Na^+/K^+ pump in quiescent fibroblasts by increasing Na^+ entry. Proc Natl Acad Sci USA 75:5560–5564
44. Holley RW, Armour R, Baldwin JH (1978) Density-dependent regulation of growth of BSC-1 cells in culture: control of growth by low-molecular weight nutrients. Proc Natl Acad Sci USA 75:339–341
45. Koch KS, Leffert HL (1979) Increased sodium ion influx is necessary to initiate rat hepatocyte proliferation. Cell 18:153–163
46. Rozengurt E, Heppel LA (1975) Serum rapidly stimulates ouabain-sensitive $^{86}RB^+$ influx in quiescent 3T3 cells. Proc Natl Acad Sci USA 72:4492–4495
47. McKeehan WL, McKeehan KA, Calkins D (1981) Extracellular regulation of fibroblast multiplication. Quantitative differences in nutrient and serum factor requirements for multiplication and normal SV40 virus transformed human lung cells. J Biol Chem 256: 2973–2981
48. Weber MJ, Evans PK, Johnson MA, McNair TF, Nakamura KD, Salter DW (1984) Transport of potassium, amino acids, and glucose in cells transformed by Rous sarcoma virus. Fed Proc 43:107–112
49. Ciesinski DA, Messana JM, Humes HD (1987) Adenosine triphosphate stimulates thymidine incorporation but does not promote cell growth in primary cultures of rabbit proximal tubule cells. Kidney Int 33:389a
50. Kartha S, Sukhatme VP, Toback FG (1987) ADP activates protooncogene expression in renal epithelial cells. Am J Physiol 252:F1175–F1179
51. Sukhatme VP, Kartha S, Toback FG, Taub R, Hoover RV, Tsai-Morris C (1987) A novel early growth response gene rapidly induced by fibroblast, epithelial cell and lymphocyte mitogens. Oncogene Res 1:343–355
52. Kartha S, Bradham DM, Grotendorst GR, Toback FG (1988) Kidney epithelial cells express the c-*sis* proto-oncogene and secrete PDGF-like protein: evidence for a paracrine mechanism. Am J Physiol 255:F800–F806
53. Deuel TF, Pierce GF, Hsiu-Jeng Y, Shawver LK, Milner PG, Kimura A (1987) Platelet-derived growth factor/*sis* in normal and neoplastic cell growth. J Cell Physiol Suppl 5:95–99
54. Mustoe TA, Pierce GF, Thomason A, Gramates P, Sporn MB, Deuel TF (1987) Accelerated healing of incisional wounds in rats induced by transforming growth factor-beta. Science 237:1333–1336

55. Johnson A, Heldin C-H, Wasteson A, Westermark B, Deuel TF (1984) The c-*sis* gene encodes a precursor of the B chain of platelet-derived growth factor. EMBO J 3:921–928
56. Josephs SF, Grio C, Ratner L, Wong-Staal F (1984) Human protooncogene nucleotide sequences corresponding to the transforming region of simian arcoma virus. Science 223:487–490
57. Seifert RA, Hart CE, Phillips PE, Forstrom JW, Ross R, Murray MJ, Bowen-Pope DF (1989) Two different subunits associate to create isoform-specific PDGF receptors. J Biol Chem 265:8771–8778
58. Matsui T, Heidaran M, Miki T, Popescu N, LaRochelle W, Kraus M, Pierce J, Aaronson S (1989) Isolation of a novel receptor cDNA establishes the existence of two PDGF receptor genes. Science 243:800–804
59. Leof EB, Proper JA, Goustin AS, Shipley GD, DiCorleto PE, Moses HL (1986) Induction of c-*sis* mRNA and activity similar to platelet derived growth factor by transforming growth factor beta: a proposed model for indirect mitogenesis involving autocrine activity. Proc Natl Acad Sci USA 83:2453–2457
60. Makela TP, Alitalo R, Paulsson Y, Westermark B, Heldin C-H, Alitalo K (1987) Regulation of platelet-derived growth factor gene expression by transforming growth factor beta in human leukemia cell lines. Mol Cell Biol 7:3653–3662
61. Frazier GE, Bowen-Pope DF, Vogel AM (1987) Production of platelet-derived growth factor by cultured Wilms' tumor cells and fetal kidney cells. J Cell Physiol 133:169–174
62. Nakai A, Kartha S, Sakurai A, Toback FG, DeGroot L (1990) A human early response gene homologous to murine nur77 and rat NGFI-B, and related to the nuclear receptor superfamily. Mol Endocrinol 4:1438–1443
63. Kartha S, Toback FG (1992) Adenine nucleotides stimulate migration in wounded cultures of kidney epithelial cells. J Clin Invest 90:288–292
64. Dinarello CA (1988) Interleukin-1. Rev Infect Dis 6:51–95
65. Lovett DH, Szamel M, Ryan JL, Sterzel RB, Gemsa D, Resch K (1986) Interleukin 1 and the glomerular mesangium. I. Purification and characterization of a mesangial cell-derived auto-growth factor. J Immunol 136:3700–3705
66. Anisowicz A, Bardwell L, Sager R (1987) Constitutive overexpression of a growth-regulated gene in transformed Chinese hamster and human cells. Proc Natl Acad Sci USA 84:7188–7192
67. Richmond A, Balentein E, Thomas HG, Flaggs G, Barton DE, Spiess J, Bardoni R, Francke U, Derynck R (1988) Molecular characterization and chromosomal mapping of melanoma growth stimulatory activity, a growth factor structurally related to beta-thromboglobulin. EMBO J 7:2025–2033
68. Cochran BH, Reffel AC, Stiles CD (1983) Molecular cloning of gene sequences regulated by platelet-derived growth factor. Cell 33:939–947
69. Fisher DA, Salido EC, Barajas L (1989) Epidermal growth factor and the kidney. Annu Rev Physiol 51:67–80
70. Breyer MD, Redha R, Breyer JA (1990) Segmental distribution of epidermal growth factor binding sites in rabbit nephron. Am J Physiol 259:F553–F558
71. Spur NK, Solomon E, Jansson M, Sheer D, Goodfellow PN, Bodmer WF, Vennstrom B (1984) Chromosomal localization of the human homologues to the oncogenes erb A and B. EMBO J 3:159–163
72. Holley RW, Amour R, Baldwin JH, Brown KD, Yeh Y-C (1977) Density-dependent regulation of growth of BSC-1 cells in cell culture: control of growth by serum factors. Proc Natl Acad Sci USA 74:5046–5050
73. Saferstein R, Price PM, Saggi SJ, Harris RC (1990) Changes in gene expression after temporary renal ischemia. Kidney Int 37:1551–1521
74. Saferstein R, Zelent AZ, Price PM (1989) Reduced prepro-epidermal growth factor mRNA and decreased EGF excretion in ARF. Kidney Int 36:810–815

75. Humes HD, Cielinski DA, Coimbra TM, Messana JM, Galvao C (1989) Epidermal growth factor enhances renal tubular cell regeneration and repair and accelerates the recovery of renal function in postischemic acute renal failure. J Clin Invest 84:1757–1761
76. Norman J, Tsau Y-K, Bacay A, Fine LG (1990) Epidermal growth factor accelerates functional recovery from ischemic acute tubular necrosis in the rat: role of the epidermal growth factor receptor. Clin Sci 78:445–450
77. Coimbra TM, Cieslinski DA, Humes HD (1990) Epidermal growth factor accelerates renal repair in mercuric chloride nephrotoxicity. Am J Physiol 259:F438–F443
78. Stern PH, Krieger NS, Nissenson RA, Williams RD, Winkler MS, Derynck R, Strewler GJ (1985) Human transforming growth factor-alpha stimulate bone resorption in vitro. J Clin Invest 76:2016–2019
79. Tashijan AH, Voelkel EF, Lloyd W, Derynck R, Winkler ME, Levine L (1986) Actions of growth factors on plasma calcium. J Clin Invest 78:1405–1409
80. Insogna KL, Stewart AF, Morris CA, Hough LM, Milstone LM, Centrella M (1989) Native and a synthetic analogue of the malignancy-associated parathyroid hormone-like protein have in vitro transforming growth factor-like properties. J Clin Invest 83: 1057–1060
81. Holley RW, Armour R, Baldwin JH (1978) Density-dependent regulation of growth of BSC-1 cells in cell culture: growth inhibitors formed by the cells. Proc Natl Acad Sci USA 75:1864–1866
82. Holley RW, Böhlen P, Fava R, Baldwin JH, Kleeman G, Armour R (1980) Purification of kidney epithelial cell growth inhibitors. Proc Natl Acad Sci USA 77:5989–5992
83. Walsh-Reitz MM, Toback FG, Holley RW (1984) Cell growth and net Na^+ flux are inhibited by a protein produced by kidney epithelial cells in culture. Proc Natl Acad Sci USA 75:1864–1866
84. Tucker RF, Shipley GD, Moses HL, Holley RW (1984) Growth inhibitor from BSC-1 cells closely related to platelet type β transforming growth factor. Science 226:705–707
85. Dernyck R, Jarrett JA, Chen EY, Eaton DH, Bell JR, Assoian RK, Roberts AB, Sporn MB, Goeddel DV (1985) Human transforming growth factor-β complimentary DNA sequence and expression in normal and transformed cells. Nature 316:701–705
86. Ellingsworth LR, Brennan JE, Fok K, Rosen DM, Bentz H, Piez KA, Seyedin SM (1989) Antibodies to the N-terminal portion of cartilage-inducing factor-A and transforming growth factor β. J Biol Chem 261:661–669
87. Thompson NL, Flanders KC, Smith JM, Ellingworth LR, Roberts AB, Sporn MB (1989) Expression of transforming growth factor β1 in specific cells and tissues of adult and neonatal mice. J Cell Biol 108:661–669
88. Fine LG, Holley RW, Nasri H, Badie-Dezfooly B (1985) BSC-1 growth inhibitor transforms a mitogenic stimulus into a hypertrophic stimulus for renal proximal tubular cells: relationship to Na^+/H^+ antiport activity. Proc Natl Acad Sci USA 82:6163–6166
89. Ignotz R, Massagué J (1986) Transforming growth factor-beta stimulates the expression of fibronectin and collagen and their incorporation into the extracellular matrix. J Biol Chem 261:4337–4345
90. Pierce GF, Mustoe TA, Lingelbach J, Masakowski VR, Griffin GL, Senior RM, Deuel TF (1989) Platelet derived growth factor and transforming growth factor-β enhance tissue repair activities by unique mechanisms. J Cell Biol 109:429–440
91. Border WA, Okuda S, Languino LR, Sporn MB, Ruoslahti E (1990) An antiserum against transforming growth factor β1 suppresses experimental glomerulonephritis. Nature 346:371–374
92. Wilcox JH, Dernyck R (1988) Developmental expression of transforming growth factors alpha and beta in mouse fetus. Mol Cell Biol 8:3415–3422
93. Gomella LG, Sargent ER, Wade T, Anglard P, Linehan WM, Kasis A (1989) Expression of transforming growth factor α in normal human adult kidney and enhanced expression of transforming growth factors α and β1 in renal cell carcinoma. Cancer Res 49:6972–6975

94. Baxter RC (1986) The somatomedins: insulin-like growth factors. Adv Clin Chem 25: 49–115
95. Rinderknecht E, Humbel RE (1978) The amino acid sequence of human insulin-like growth factor II. FEBS Lett 89:2769–2776
96. Rinderknecht E, Humbel RE (1978) Primary structure of human insulin-like growth factor II. FEBS Lett 89:283–286
97. Rechler MM, Nissley SP (1986) Insulin-like growth factor (IGF)/somatomedin receptor subtypes: structure, function, and relationships to insulin receptors and IGF carrier proteins. Horm Res 24:152–159
98. D'Ercole AJ, Siles AD, Underwood LE (1984) Tissue concentrations of somatomedin C: further evidence for multiple sites of synthesis and paracrine or autocrine mechanisms of action. Proc Natl Acad Sci USA 81:935–939
99. Hammerman MR, Rogers S (1987) Distribution of IGF receptors in the plasma membrane of proximal tubular cells. Am J Physiol 253:F841–F847
100. Murphy LJ, Bell GI, Duckworth ML, Friesen HG (1987) Identification, characterization, and regulation of a rat complimentary deoxyribonucleic acid which encodes insulin-like growth factor-I. Endocrinology 121:684–691
101. Bell GI, Gerhard DS, Fong NM, Sanchez-Pescador R, Rall LB (1985) Isolation of the human insulin-like growth factor genes: insulin-like growth factor II and insulin genes are contiguous. Proc Natl Acad Sci USA 82:6450–6454
102. Bortz JD, Rotwein P, DeVol D, Bechtel PJ, Hansen BA, Hammerman NR (1988) Focal expression of insulin-like growth factor I in the rat kidney collecting duct. J Cell Biol 107:811–819
103. Scott J, Cowell J, Robertson ME, Priestly LM, Wadley R, Hopkins B, Pritchard J, Bell GI, Rall LB, Graham CF, Knott TJ (1985) Insulin-like growth factor-II gene expression in Wilm's tumour and embryonic tissues. Nature 317:260–262
104. Segal R, Fine LG (1989) Polypeptide growth factors and the kidney. Kidney Int 36 Suppl 27:S2–S10
105. Andersson G, Jennische E (1988) IGF-I immunoreactivity is expressed by regenerating renal tubular cells after ischemic injury in the rat. Acta Physiol Scand 132:453–457
106. Miller SB, Martin DR, Kissane J, Hammerman MR (1993) Insulin-like growth factor I accelerates recovery from ischemic acute tubular necrosis in the rat. Proc Natl Acad Sci USA 89:11876–11880
107. Ding H, Kopple JD, Cohen A, Hirschberg R (1993) Recombinant human insulin-like growth factor-I accelerates recovery and reduces catabolism in rats with ischemic acute renal failure. J Clin Invest 91:2281–2287
108. Kopple JD, Hirschberg R (1990) Physiological effects of growth hormone and insulin-like growth factor-I on the kidney. Miner Electrolyte Metab 16:82–88
109. Hammerman MR, Miller SB (1993) The growth hormone insulin-like growth factor axis revisited. Am J Physiol 265:F1–F14
110. Abboud HE, Poptic E, DiCorleto P (1987) Production of platelet-derived growth factor like protein by rat mesangial cells in culture. J Clin Invest 80:675–683
111. Abraham JA, Mergia A, Whang JL, Tumulo A, Friedaman J, Hjerrild KA, Gospodarowicz D, Fiddes JC (1986) Nucleotide sequence of a bovine clone encoding the angiogenic protein, basic fibroblast growth factor. Science 233:5451–548
112. Baird A, Ling N (1987) Fibroblast growth factors are present in the extracellular matrix produced by endothelial cells in vitro: implications for a role of heparinase-like enzymes in the neovascular response. Biochem Biophys Res Commun 142:428–435
113. Jaye M, Howk R, Burgess W, Ricca GA, Chiu I-M, Ravera MW, O'Brien SJ, Modi WS, Maciag T, Drohan WN (1986) Human endothelial cell growth factor: cloning, nucleotide sequence and chromosomasl localization. Science 233:541–545
114. Zhang G, Ichimura T, Wallin A, Kan M, Stevens JL (1991) Regulation of rat proximal tubule epithelial cell growth by fibroblast growth factors, insulin-like growth factor-1 and

transforming growth factor-β, and analysis of fibroblast growth factors in rat kidney. J Biol Chem 148:295–305
115. Gautschi-Sova P, Jiang Z-P, Frater-Schroder M, Böhlen P (1987) Acidic fibroblast growth factor is present in nonneural tissue: isolation and chemical characterization from bovine kidney. Biochemistry 26:5844–5847
116. Zhang G, Stevens JL (1991) Altered growth regulation of rat proximal tubule epithelial cells transformed in vitro by SV40 viral DNA: fibroblast growth factors (heparin-binding growth factors) are potent inducers of anchorage-independent growth. Mol Carcinog 4:1–11
117. Michalopoulos GK, Zarnegar R (1992) Hepatocyte growth factor. Hepatology 15:149–155
118. Furlong RA, Takehara T, Taylor WG, Nakamura T, Rubin JS (1991) Comparison of biological and immunochemical properties indicates that scatter factor and hepatocyte growth factor are indistinguishable. J Cell Sci 100:173–177
119. Igawa T, Kanda S, Kanetake H, Saitoh Y, Ichihara A, Tomito Y, Nakamura T (1991) Hepatocyte growth factor is a potent mitogen for cultured rabbit renal tubular epithelial cells. Biochem Biophys Res Commun 174:831–838
120. Ishibashi K, Sasaki S, Sakamoto H, Nakamura Y, Hata T, Nakamura T, Marumo F (1992) Hepatocyte growth factor is a paracrine factor for renal epithelial cells: stimulation of DNA synthesis and Na, K-ATPase activity. Biochem Biophys Res Commun 182: 960–965
121. Kono S, Nagaike M, Matsumoto K, Nakamura T (1992) Marked induction of hepatocyte growth factor mRNA in intact kidney and spleen in response to injury of distant organs. Biochem Biophys Res Commun 186:991–998
122. Nagaike M, Hirao S, Tajima H, Noji S, Taniguchi S, Matsumoto K, Nakamura T (1991) Renotrophic functions of hepatocyte growth factor in renal regeneration after unilateral nephrectomy. J Biol Chem 266:22781–22784
123. Ishibashi K, Sasaki S, Sakamoto H, Hoshino Y, Nakamura T, Marumo F (1992) Expressions of receptor gene for hepatocyte growth factor in kidney after unilateral nephrectomy and renal injury: Biochem Biophys Res Commun 187:1454–1459
124. Masumoto A, Yamamoto N (1991) Sequestration of a hepatocyte growth factor in extracellular matrix in normal adult rat liver. Biochem Biophys Res Commun 174:90–95
125. Anderson S, Renneke HG, Brenner BM (1986) Therapeutic advantage of converting enzyme inhibitors in arresting progressive renal disease associated with systemic hypertension in the rat. J Clin Invest 77:1993–2000
126. Powell JS, Mueller RKM, Rouge M, Kuhn H, Hefti F, Baumgartner HR (1990) The prolifeative response to vascular injury is suppressed by angiotensin-converting enzyme inhibition. J Cardiovasc Pharm 16 Suppl 4:S24–S48
127. Xie M-H, Liu F-Y, Wong PC, Timmermans PBMWM, Cogan MG (1990) Proximal nephron and renal effects of DuP 753, a nonpeptide angiotensin II receptor antagonist. Kidney Int 38:473–479
128. Saccomani G, Mitchell KD, Navar LG (1990) Angiotensin II stimulation of Na^+-H^+ exchange in proximal tubule cells. Am J Physiol 258:F1188–F1195
129. Wolf G, Nielson EG (1990) Angiotensin II induces cellular hypertrophy in cultured murine proximal tubular cells. Am J Physiol 259:F768–F777
130. Robinnette JB, Conger JD (1990) Angiotensin and thromboxane in the enhanced renal adrenergic nerve sensitivity of acute renal failure. J Clin Invest 86:1532–1539
131. Moran SM, Myers BD (1985) Pathophysiology of protracted acute renal failure in man. J Clin Invest 76:1440–1448
132. Molitoris BA, Falk SA, Dahl RH (1989) Ischemia-induced loss of epithelial polarity. J Clin Invest 84:1334–1339
133. Hynes R (1987) Integrins: a family of cell surface receptors. Cell 48:549–554
134. Ekblom P, Alitalo A, Vaheri R, Timpl R, Saxen L (1980) Induction of a basement membrane glycoprotein in embryonic kidney: possible role of laminin in morphogenesis. Proc Nat Acad Sci USA 77:485–489

135. Klein G, Laugegger R, Timpl R, Ekblom P (1988) Role of laminin A chain in the development of epithelial cell polarity. Cell 55:331–341
136. Ekblom P, Miettineu A, Virtanen I, Wahlstrom T, Dawnay A, Saxen L (1981) In vitro segregation of the metanephric nephron. Dev Biol 84:88–95
137. Bernfield M, Sanderson RD (1990) Syndecan, a developmentally regulated cell surface proteoglycan that binds extracellular matrix and growth factors. Philos Trans R Soc Lond [Biol] 327:171–186
138. Kellerman PS, Clark RAF, Hoilien CA, Linas SL, Molitoris BA (1990) Role of microfilaments in maintenance of proximal tubular structural and functional integrity. Am J Physiol 259:F279–F285
139. Greenhalgh DG, Sprugel KH, Murray MJ, Ross R (1990) PDGF and FGF stimulate wound healing in the genetically diabetic mouse. Am J Pathol 136:1235–1246
140. Pierce GF, Mustoe TA, Lingelbach J, Masakowski VR, Gramates P, Deuel TF (1989) Transforming growth factor beta reverses the glucocorticoid-induced wound-healing deficit in rats: possible regulation in macrophages by platelet-derived growth factor. Proc Natl Acad Sci USA 86:2229–2233
141. Komatsuda A, Wakui H, Satoh K, Yasuda T, Imai H, Nakamoto Y, Miura AB, Itoh H, Tashima Y (1993) Altered localization of 73-kilodalton heat shock protein in rat kidneys with gentamicin-induced acute tubular injury. Lab Invest 68:687–695
142. Arends MJ, Morris RG, Wyllie AH (1990) Apoptosis: the role of the endonuclease. Am J Pathol 136:543–608
143. Wyllie AH, Morris RG, Smith AL, Dunlop D (1984) Chromatin cleavage in apoptosis: association with condensed chromatin morphology and dependence on macromolecular synthesis. J Pathol 142:67–77
144. Bonventre JV (1993) Mechanisms of ischemic acute renal failure. Kidney Int 43: 1160–1178
145. Olsen S, Burdick JF, Keown PA, Wallace AC, Racusen LC, Solez K (1989) Primary acute renal failure ("acute tubular necrosis") in the transplanted kidney: morphology and pathogenesis. Medicine (Baltimore) 68:173–187
146. Racusen LC (1993) Tubular injury in human kidneys. Pathologic findings and pathogenic mechanisms. Clin Invest 71:858–860
147. Pederson T, Gelfant S (1970) G2-population cells in mouse kidney and duodenum and their behavior during the cell division cycle. Exp Cell Res 59:32–36
148. Daniel TO, Gibbs VC, Milfay DF, Garovoy MR, Williams LT (1986) Thrombin stimulates c-*sis* gene expression in microvascular endothelial cells. J Biol Chem 261:9570–9582
149. Rappolee DA, Mark D, Banda MJ, Werb Z (1988) Wound macrophages express TGF-alpha and other growth factors in vivo: analysis by mRNA phenotyping. Science 241: 708–712
150. Siegel NJ, Gaudio KM (1988) Amino acids and adenine nucleotides in acute renal failure. In: Brenner BM, Lazarus JM (eds) Acute renal failure, 2nd edn. Churchill Livingstone, New York, pp 857–873

Prevention of Acute Renal Failure in the Critically Ill Patient

A.D. Bersten and A.W. Holt

Introduction

Renal dysfunction is common in critical care practice, as are measures to reverse or support acute renal failure (ARF). The mortality from ARF remains high [1–4], particularly in the presence of other organ failures [2, 4, 5]. For example, Bell et al. [4] found that ARF markedly increased mortality from the adult respiratory distress syndrome from 20% to 69%. This highlights the widespread multisystem tissue injury found in many critically ill patients, and while this review will focus solely on the kidney, strategies to prevent ARF need to fit within a global approach to the entire patient.

Renal injury may arise from a somewhat predictable, discrete insult such as aortic surgery which allows pre-injury, prophylactic intervention; however, more often, renal injury occurs over hours to days, as in septic shock. Once initiated, therapeutic intervention may attempt to minimise the insult resulting in less injury and dysfunction. Finally, patients may present following a renal insult with an established injury where the remaining therapeutic option is to attenuate the resulting dysfunction. A comprehensive approach to the prevention of ARF needs to take into account these differing therapeutic windows.

The spectrum of ARF has changed from the occasional report of non-oliguric renal failure [6], to the emergence of substantial numbers of patients with non-oliguric renal failure, over 50% of reported cases in some series [7]. This trend should be of substantial benefit, as non-oliguric renal failure generally represents a less severe renal injury than oliguric renal failure, and patients have fewer complications, require dialysis less frequently and have a lower mortality rate [8, 9]. Advances in circulatory resuscitation appear to have resulted in a less severe renal injury, as laboratory studies using fluid replacement, shorter periods of ischaemia, or smaller doses of nephrotoxic agents result in non-oliguric ARF in otherwise oliguric models [10]. However, many promising laboratory interventions fail to make the step to proven clinical benefit. In particular, interventions that generate urine flow without modification of renal injury do not appear to confer any clinical benefit.

This review will examine therapeutic options for renal protection within the current understanding of the pathophysiology of ARF. Many of the conclusions drawn await prospective randomised studies in critically ill patients.

Pathophysiology

Renal blood flow (RBF) is normally 1.2 l/min, about 20% of cardiac output, with little vasodilator reserve compared to most other organs [11]. Unlike other organs, RBF does not normally subserve renal oxygen delivery. Glomerular filtration and the excretion of flow-dependent waste is determined by RBF, while renal oxygen consumption is primarily determined by tubular solute reabsorption. Globally, the kidney has a luxurious blood flow with an oxygen extraction ratio of only 8%–10% and a mixed renal vein PO_2 of about 70 mmHg; however, the basis for the sensitivity of the kidney to ischaemia is not explained by total organ blood flow.

Distribution of Renal Blood Flow and O_2 Consumption Within the Kidney

The kidney has a unique arrangement of blood vessels. The glomerular afferent arterioles give rise to the glomerular capillaries, which then coalesce to form the efferent arterioles, which in turn give rise to a peritubular capillary network. In the juxtamedallary region only, these branches contribute to the vasa recta. The majority of RBF is therefore supplied to the renal cortex with little flow to the renal medulla. The vasa recta, along with tubules of the medulla, form a hairpin loop to enable a countercurrent exchange of solutes and the development of a mechanism that allows the efficient concentration of urine. Analogous to the countercurrent effect on solutes, O_2 diffuses from the arterial to the venous branches of the vasa recta leading to reduced delivery of O_2 to the medulla (Fig. 1). Limited medullary blood flow is also important in preventing the washout of the hyperosmolar interstitium. As this is coupled with the active reabsorption of solute by the medullary thick ascending limb of Henle's loop, medullary hypoxia is seen as the cost of concentrated urine.

Medullary PO_2 is normally around 10 mmHg, critically close to a level at which mitochondrial respiration is affected [12], and the outer stripe of the medulla, corresponding to the medullary thick ascending limb of Henle's loop, is consistently injured in the isolated perfused kidney [13]. Mitochondrial swelling and cell death is seen distant to vascular bundles and is exaggerated by hypoxic perfusion and prevented by an oxygenated red cell perfusate [13]. When careful morphologic studies are performed, selective medullary injury is found in nephrotoxic (indomethacin plus radiocontrast) ARF [14]. Taken together these data suggest that medullary hypoxia may be central to the pathogenesis of ARF.

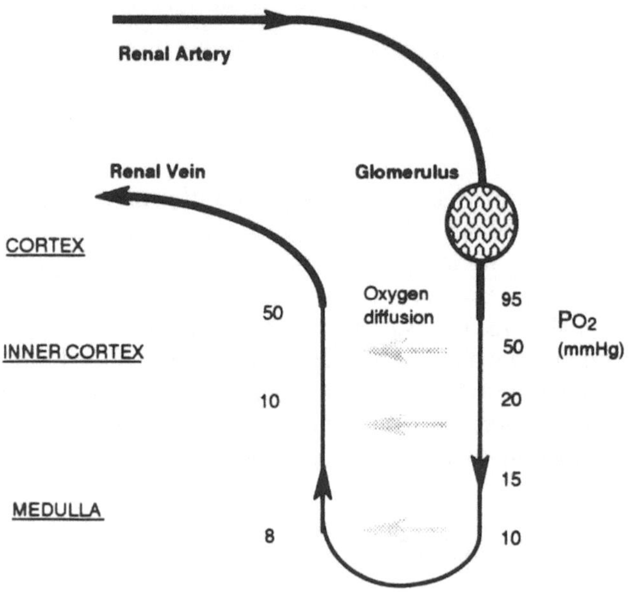

Fig. 1. Countercurrent diffusion of oxygen produces low oxygen tensions within the renal medulla. (From [92], with permission)

Pathophysiology of the Reduction in Glomerular Filtration Rate

Tubular obstruction and backleak of filtrate, secondary to widespread tubular necrosis and sloughing, are commonly implicated in the reduction in glomerular filtration rate (GFR) in laboratory models of ARF [15, 16]; however, renal biopsies from patients with ARF show far less impressive changes. Tubular epithelial cell necrosis is often absent and if present is in the form of single cell necrosis only [17]. There is also some prominence of the juxtaglomerular apparatus, tubularisation of Bowman's capsule and diffuse change along the brush border [15]. Consequently, morphologic data from patients with ARF suggest there is little basis for postulating an important role for tubular backleak. Further, occlusion of tubules with casts is not uniform, and when present there is no morphologic evidence of proximal luminal dilatation or obstruction [17]. The reduction in GFR seen in patients with ARF would appear to be largely functional, involving a decrease in RBF, glomerular capillary hydrostatic pressure and ultrafiltration coefficient, and seems to be better represented by the modest medullary injury model [13] than models such as intrarenal noradrenaline infusion which produce widespread necrosis [16]. The precise mechanism of these changes remains unclear, but is likely an exaggeration of the normal tubuloglomerular feedback mechanism.

Tubuloglomerular Feedback

Tubuloglomerular feedback is a complex, protective, intrarenal mechanism that couples GFR with tubular reabsorptive capacity, and while the precise mediators are unclear, adenosine appears to have a central role. An increase in distal tubular solute load, presented to the macula densa cells, results in the metabolic burden of solute reabsorption, releasing adenosine. This produces an adenosine-mediated (A_1 receptor) afferent arteriolar vasoconstriction and a reduction in GFR [18]. By reducing reabsorption of solute by the cells of the medullary thick ascending limb, work is reduced. This feedback mechanism also acts to defend medullary oxygenation by linking tubular oxygen supply and demand. Consequently, this reduction in GRF makes good taeliological sense in the ischaemic kidney and has been termed "acute renal success" [19]. Renal ischaemia also produces a rapid rise in tissue adenosine [20], producing exaggerated or pathologic tubuloglomerular feedback. This adenosine-mediated A_1 vasoconstriction of interlobular and afferent arterioles and A_2-mediated vasodilatation of efferent arterioles would appear to be an important component of the pathogenesis of ARF, as adenosine antagonists prevent renal injury in a number of models of ARF.

Endothelin-1

Endothelin-1 is a potent peptide vasoconstrictor, particularly within the kidney, which produces both afferent and efferent arteriolar vasoconstriction and a reduction in the glomerular capillary ultrafiltration coefficient [21]. Despite the rapid clearance of endothelin-1, mainly by the lung [21], its exogenous administration, intravenously [22] or intra-arterially [23, 24], produces a functional disturbance similar to ARF which may persist for 24 h following a bolus dose [22]. Further, both hypoxia [25] and endotoxaemia [26], insults known to produce ARF, result in release of endothelin-1. Indeed, patients with ARF have an elevated level of plasma endothelin which falls with recovery [27]. The possible role of endothelin-1 in the initiation of ARF is strengthened by recent laboratory studies that demonstrate both functional and morphologic protection from ischaemic insults with endothelin antagonists.

Nephrotoxins

Both ischaemic and nephrotoxic injuries produce similar morphologic changes and clinical syndromes. In rats infused with myoglobin, Zager [28] noted marked congestion of the outer medulla suggestive of an ischaemic injury [29], while gentamicin nephrotoxicity is greatly exaggerated by concomitant hypoperfusion, with morphologic injury isolated to the outer medullary stripe [30]. Both radiocontrast [31] and cyclosporine [32] produce outer medullary injury, with endothelin-1 release implicated in their nephrotoxicity, and administration of an endothelin antagonist appears to protect against a cyclosporine-induced reduction in RBF and GFR [33]. Furthermore, medullary ischaemia is induced by both indomethacin and radiocontrast dye [34], and this can be reversed by reducing O_2 consumption with frusemide [34]. With other nephrotoxins, such as the heme proteins, coexisting ischaemia appears to be a necessary priming factor for nephrotoxicity [35]. Therefore, besides the elimination of nephrotoxins, our approach to prevention of ARF is similar with ischaemic and nephrotoxic insults.

Strategies to Prevent Acute Renal Failure

The avoidance, rapid cessation of, or effective minimisation of a renal insult, while obvious, is the cornerstone of prevention of renal injury and ARF. In addition to these measures there are four possible strategic directions:

1. Restoration and/or augmentation of RBF (particularly medullary flow)
2. Reduction of renal O_2 consumption during the insult
3. Administration of cytoprotective agents during the insult
4. Antagonism of the mediators of ARF

General Measures

Solute Loading

Solute loading, prior to a renal insult, has been one of the most consistent protective measures described, while salt depletion (perhaps through enhancement of tubuloglomerular feedback [36]) is essential to many laboratory models of ARF. Bidani and co-workers [37] examined the effect of pretreatment with normal saline or water before either mercuric chloride-or uranyl nitrate-induced ARF in the rodent. Solute loading reduced the severity of the insult and led to a more rapid recovery of renal function independent of plasma renin activity, and a strong inverse correlation was noted between the urinary excretion of sodium in the 24 h prior to the insult and the extent of the renal injury (Fig. 2). In man, both Barry et al. [38] and Bush et al. [39] found that preoperative fluid therapy attenuated the fall in RBF and GFR associated with general anaesthesia and abdominal aortic surgery, respectively. Interestingly, in a study of 137 patients undergoing abdominal aortic surgery, Alpert et al. [40] found no correlation of intra-operative urine output with renal dysfunction, despite patients receiving either further solute loading, mannitol or frusemide if they were oliguric. When moderate fluid loading was used during renal transplantation, there was a marked

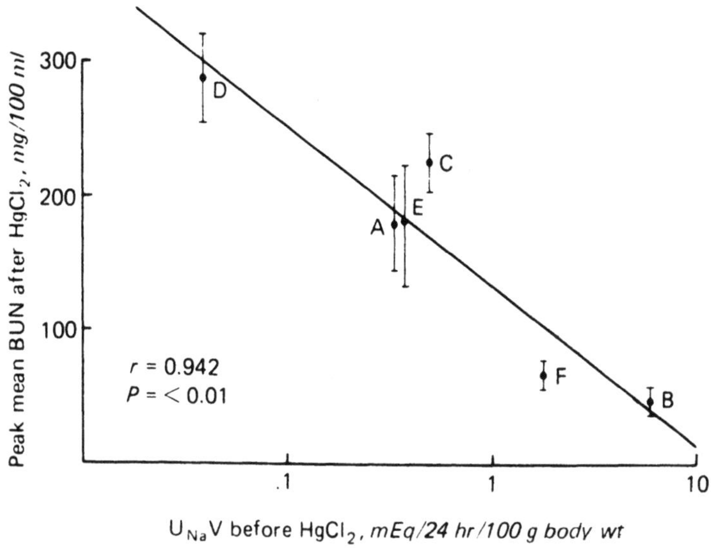

Fig. 2. In mercuric chloride-induced acute renal failure (ARF), an inverse relationship was noted between the severity of ARF and urinary sodium excretion ($U_{Na}V$) in the 24 h prior to the insult. Group *D* was on a low sodium diet and groups *B* and *F* were on high sodium diets. *BUN*, blood urea nitrogen. (From [37], with permission)

reduction in the incidence of ARF from 53% to 4.8% [41], and cisplatin nephrotoxicity was markedly reduced by fluid loading before, during, and following its administration [42]. In addition to solute loading of the kidney, fluid therapy plays a central role in the resuscitation of the circulation and the optimising of RBF and will be now be considered in this more general framework.

Haemodynamic Resuscitation

As renal hypoperfusion is often an important contributing factor to ARF, resuscitation of the circulation will frequently be a key factor in the prevention of renal dysfunction. The two major clinical end-points of circulatory resuscitation are: (1) systemic oxygen delivery and consumption, generally through augmentation of cardiac output, and (2) perfusion pressure.

Although most evidence points to the importance of renal perfusion pressure, it is likely both end-points go hand-in-hand. Schlichtig and coworkers [43] examined the effects of progressive haemorrhage in the anaesthetised dog and found a linear correlation of renal O_2 delivery with systemic O_2 delivery, and a redistribution of O_2 delivery away from the kidney and liver as systemic O_2 delivery fell [44]. Further, despite similar perfusion pressures, it is the lack of improvement from an initially low cardiac output that differentiates patients with renal dysfunction from those who develop ARF following cardiopulmonary bypass [45]. Oxygen delivery is optimised primarily through augmentation of cardiac output through the use of volume loading, catecholamines or vasodilators, as appropriate, and this is most conveniently done using haemodynamic measurements. Of particular interest is the observation that the optimal haematocrit for O_2 delivery to the kidney is greater than 40 [46], much greater than aimed for in many critically ill patients. In turn, the optimal perfusion pressure for the kidney may be greater than achieved in many critically ill patients.

Renal Perfusion Pressure

Autoregulation of Renal Blood Flow and Glomerular Filtration Rate

Both RBF and GFR are normally constant unless perfusion pressure falls below their autoregulatory thresholds. Using a graded reduction in mean arterial pressure (MAP), the autoregulatory threshold for RBF in the dog is 80 mmHg [47]. It is somewhat unclear what the autoregulatory threshold is in healthy man; however, Stone and Stahl [48] found that RBF fell by 20% and GFR fell by 30% during haemorrhage from a MAP of 80 mmHg to 67 mmHg in healthy volunteers, also suggesting an autoregulatory threshold of about 80 mmHg. Of interest, these data were not altered by the administration of mannitol. Careful studies in the dog demonstrate that the autoregulatory threshold for GFR is about 15 mmHg higher than the

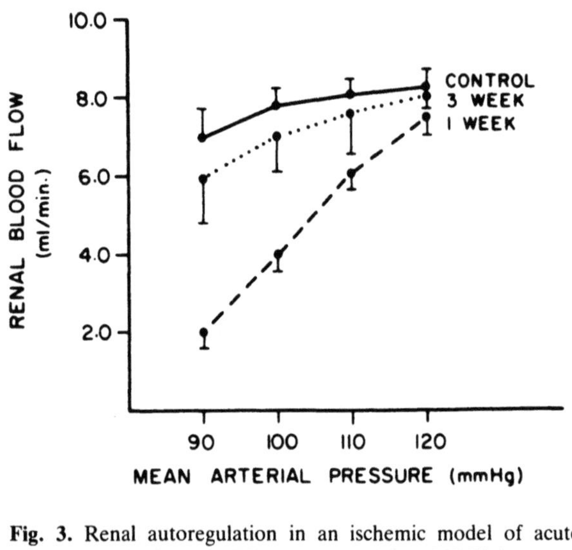

Fig. 3. Renal autoregulation in an ischemic model of acute renal failure (ARF); 1 week following induction of ARF, renal blood flow (RBF) is pressure dependent, but after 3 weeks renal autoregulation and function have improved. (From [51], with permission)

autoregulatory threshold for RBF [49] and that pre-existing hypertension appears to right shift the autoregulatory threshold. In ischaemic models of ARF, Adams et al. [50] and Kelleher et al. [51] found that autoregulation was abolished (Fig. 3), and we have found similar data in a hyperdynamic model of sepsis which does not cause ARF (unpublished findings): Finally, biopsy specimens from patients with ARF often show fresh necrotic lesions some time after the initiating insult [15], suggesting that episodes of hypotension following the injury, e.g., associated with intermittent haemodialysis, readily lead to further ischaemia in a non-autoregulating kidney. These data suggest that higher levels of blood pressure than are often aimed for, or achieved in critically ill patients, may be associated with an augmentation of RBF and GFR, particularly in the setting of a renal insult.

Augmentation of Renal Perfusion Pressure

Volume resuscitation alone is rarely sufficient to adequately augment the MAP in critically ill patients; consequently, vasopressor catecholamines are frequently required. As argued below, there does not appear to be a strong reason to choose dopamine in this setting, and our first-line drug is adrenaline, although noradrenaline may be needed in some patients. Although the use of these agents at first seems illogical and likely to reduce RBF through α-adrenoceptor stimulation producing renal vasoconstriction, the final effect

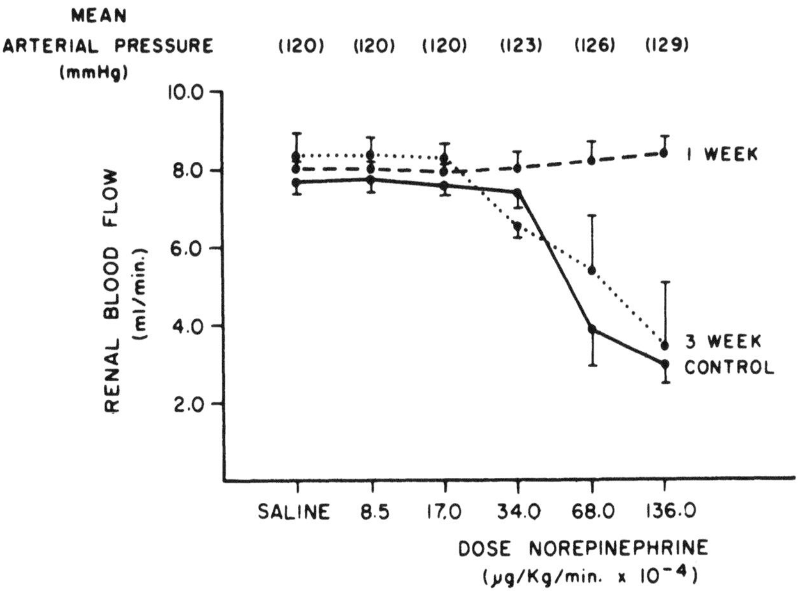

Fig. 4. One week following induction of acute renal failure (ARF) there is loss of renal vasoconstriction with intrarenal noradrenaline; however, by 3 weeks a normal response has returned. (From [51], with permission)

on RBF will depend on the interplay between their direct vascular effects and the increase in perfusion pressure. As renal insults impair renal autoregulation, RBF becomes dependent on perfusion pressure. Further, in an ischaemic model of ARF, RBF was unaffected by the intra-arterial administration of noradrenaline until renal function started to recover [51] (Fig. 4). Clearly, these data suggest that augmentation of perfusion pressure with a vasopressor catecholamine will increase RBF. A number of clinical series in patients with septic shock support this notion. Desjars et al. [52] and Hesselvik and Broolin [53] reported an increase in urine output and MAP in septic patients administered noradrenaline, and Redl-Wenz et al. [54] studied 56 patients infused with noradrenaline to increase the MAP above 60 mmHg and found an increase in creatinine clearance from 75 to 102 ml/min. They continued to infuse dopamine at a low dose, as Schaer et al. [55] had shown this increased RBF when administered concurrently with noradrenaline in the anaesthetised dog, however, we have not been able to show a similar effect in either healthy or septic sheep [56]. In earlier studies, we were unable to demonstrate a sustained reduction in RBF with adrenaline infused over the range 5–40 μg/min, and although renal vascular resistance was initially elevated it fell towards baseline within 15–30 min [57].

Although the use of catecholamines to augment perfusion pressure appears a logical approach and is supported by clinical series, it is important to recognise that there are no prospective randomised data showing a renal protective effect. Further, infusion of these agents may right shift the renal autoregulation curve [58], thereby demanding a greater perfusion pressure for a given RBF. In the conscious, healthy sheep, relatively low doses of adrenaline (5 μg/min, i.e., 0.1 μg/kg per min) tend to shift the renal autoregulation curve to the left, and a right curve shift is only seen with infusion rates of 40 μg/min. Consequently, our haemodynamic approach is to augment both systemic O_2 delivery and perfusion pressure using both appropriate volume expansion and catecholamines. The precise level of MAP aimed for is dependent on both the premorbid blood pressure and the patients response, but is often 90–100 mmHg.

Intra-abdominal Hypertension

Increases in intra-abdominal pressure are common in critically ill patients following abdominal surgery with poorly controlled haemorrhage and may be found in patients with massive ascites. At an intra-abdominal pressure greater than 20 mmHg, flow falls to the renal, splanchnic and hindlimb vascular beds with a fall in cardiac output and stroke volume [59]. Over the past few years, intra-abdominal hypertension has been increasingly recognised to contribute to oliguria and renal dysfunction and consequently may be an indication for abdominal decompression [60, 61]. While a relatively accurate measurement of intra-abdominal pressure can be made by instilling

50–100 ml sterile fluid into the bladder and measuring the pressure through a urinary catheter [61], clinical assessment and an appreciation of the widespread cardiovascular effects of intra-abdominal hypertension may be sufficient.

Specific Measures

Mannitol

Mannitol is frequently suggested as a renal protective agent based on its actions as: (a) an osmotic diuretic with a reduction in tubular obstruction [16, 62] and endothelial cell swelling [63], (b) a free radical scavenger and (c) as a renal vasodilator through the intrarenal production of prostaglandins [64].

However, mannitol is mainly excreted by the kidney and has been implicated as a cause of hyponatraemia and confusion when an osmolar gap has been identified in patients with ARF [65]. In addition, large doses of mannitol have been associated with the development of ARF [66, 67], with suggested mechanisms being elevated colloid osmotic pressure [68] or exaggerated tubuloglomerular feedback [67].

Laboratory Studies

Using the intra-arterial infusion of noradrenaline to induce ARF, Cronin et al. [62] found that the prior administration of mannitol attenuated the fall in GFR. This effect was equivalent with both hypertonic and isotonic mannitol, excluding an osmolar effect, and correlated with the rate of solute excretion. More recent studies with this model have shown that mannitol prevents excessive mitochondrial accumulation of calcium and abnormal mitochondrial function; however, these actions were thought by the authors to be due to a reduction in cell swelling and the consequent relief of tubular obstruction [63]. Hanley and Davidson [69] compared mannitol with frusemide before clamping the renal artery for 60 min in the rabbit and found a greater protective effect with mannitol that correlated with integrity of the proximal nephron, and Zager [70] reported similar findings in the rat following renal artery clamping or mercuric chloride-induced ARF. However, in the dog, administration of mannitol resulted in a fall in GFR with no protective effect from mercuric chloride [71]. More importantly, saline loading increased GFR and, when matched to the diuresis produced by mannitol, prevented any fall in GFR due to mercuric chloride [71]. Further, mannitol following glycerol-induced ARF led to a 28% fall in GFR [72], and mannitol following renal artery clamping also tended to reduce GFR [50]. An important criticism of all these studies is that they do not reflect the mechanism of renal insults in man.

Studies in Man

A number of authors have reported benefit from the use of mannitol prior to surgery in jaundiced patients [73], in patients undergoing aortic surgery, following myoglobinuria [74], and in oliguric ARF [75, 76]; however, these reports are not supported by prospective randomised studies. Gubern and co-workers [77] prospectively randomised 31 patients with obstructive jaundice to receive either no mannitol or mannitol, starting with 50 g in the hour prior to surgery and continuing for a further 48 h, with careful fluid loading in both groups. Creatinine clearance fell significantly in the patients receiving mannitol and was unaltered in controls, while there was no difference in the incidence of ARF (two and one in the mannitol and the control group, respectively). In saline-loaded patients, mannitol and renal-dose dopamine prior to infrarenal aortic cross-clamping did not attenuate the fall in GFR compared to saline loading alone [78], while Pass et al. [79] found no beneficial effect of mannitol prior to thoracic aortic cross-clamping in the dog.

As cadaveric kidney transplantation resembles some of the ischaemic models of ARF, it may be expected that a beneficial effect of mannitol may be demonstrable. In a prospective randomised study, 50 g mannitol was administered prior to graft revascularisation in 25 patients, with a further 25 patients acting as controls [80]. Only three patients receiving mannitol developed ARF compared to 12 controls ($p < 0.01$); however, in a similar study design Tiggeler et al. [41] also controlled fluid status. In patients who were relatively fluid restricted, the incidence of ARF was unchanged by mannitol (43% versus 53%); however, mannitol combined with fluid loading increased the systolic blood pressure intraoperatively and reduced the incidence of ARF to 4.8%. As an earlier study had also shown the importance of fluid loading and the haemodynamic state of the recipient [81], it is likely that solute loading has a more important role than mannitol in the prevention of ARF following kidney transplantation.

Mannitol is also commonly used in the management of crush injuries and myoglobinuria [74, 82], and although not based upon prospective randomised studies these authors present impressive data, with very few patients requiring dialysis. It is unclear which components of fluid resuscitation (an average of 570 ml/h for 60 h in one description [83]), urinary alkalinisation, use of mannitol and non-operative approach to crush injuries, are essential to their success. Alkalinisation of the urine appears to be protective by increasing the solubilty of myoglobin [28]; however, in rats infused with myoglobin solute loading to match administered bicarbonate conferred the same protective effeet [28]. Further, as urinary alkalinisation and mannitol are only initiated after adequate fluid resuscitation and once urine output is established [82], it is likely that compensation for the massive fluid sequestration that occurs is the most important component of this regimen.

In summary, most laboratory data show a protective effect when mannitol is administered prior to a renal insult; however, these data are generally from models showing tubular obstruction and backleak which may not reflect the renal injury found clinically. Prospective randomised studies in man have not shown a clear beneficial effect and tend to underline the importance of circulatory resuscitation and solute loading.

Dopamine

Dopamine is an endogenous catecholamine with numerous roles during normal homeostasis. In addition to its role as a precursor for the synthesis of noradrenaline, dopamine acts as a neurotransmitter and appears to have an important role in sodium balance. Dopamine is barely measureable in normal plasma, but relatively large amounts are excreted in the urine [84]. The source of urinary dopamine may be from neural release, but most evidence supports its intrarenal production from circulation L-dopa [84, 85]. The cytosol of the proximal tubular cells is rich in the enzyme L-amino acid decarboxylase, which converts L-dopa to dopamine, with resultant stimulation of dopamine-1 receptors (DA_1), which in turn produces inhibition of proximal tubular Na^+-K^+-ATPase [86], leading to a diuresis. An increase in dietary sodium results in an increase in tubular L-amino acid decarboxylase with inhibition of Na^+-K^+-ATPase and a reduction in tubular oxygen consumption [86], further suggesting an important role for dopamine in sodium homeostasis. This tubular effect of dopamine has been found in a number of species independent of effects on RBF or GFR [87, 88] and may contribute to or explain the diuretic effect of dopamine in man [89, 90]. As this will result in an increase in sodium presented to the tubular cells of the medullary thick ascending loop generating the metabolic burden of sodium reabsorption, this effect of dopamine may worsen medullary ischaemia.

Dopamine has become a commonly used exogenous catecholamine in critically ill patients; however, its ubiquitous use in critically ill patients has been recently questioned [91, 92]. Infusion of dopamine may augment cardiac output and perfusion pressure, and some studies show specific vascular effects including renal and splanchnic vasodilatation. Dopamine acts as an agonist at both α- and β-adrenoceptors and at DA_1 and DA_2 receptors. At least part of its positive inotropic action appears to be due to an indirect action with displacement of neuronal noradrenaline. The inotropic action of dopamine is markedly diminished in heart failure, and this appears to be due to myocardial depletion of noradrenaline [93]. At DA_1 receptors, dopamine elicits vasorelaxation, while at presynaptic DA_2 receptors there is inhibition of neurotransmitter release.

Central to the use of dopamine as part of any renal protection regimen is the evidence that at low doses dopamine decreases renal vascular resistance, resulting in an increase in RBF; however, this data needs to be carefully examined, as dopamine infusion often augments cardiac output and renal perfusion pressure, while a diuresis may just reflect the tubular effects of this drug. In addition, it cannot be assumed that a low infusion rate will result in low plasma levels with only DA_1 receptor stimulation, as the kidney, liver and lung are important sites for the metabolism of catecholamines. In a study of critically ill infants, Zaritsky et al. [94] found no correlation of infusion rate with plasma level during the constant infusion of dopamine, and infants with liver or renal dysfunction had markedly elevated plasma levels. Consequently, the concept of low-dose dopamine may not be valid in critically ill patients. Nevertheless, a number of laboratory [95, 96] and clinical studies [90, 97] studies have demonstrated renal vasodilatation and an increase in RBF with the infusion of low-dose dopamine. As some studies in other species than the dog do not demonstrate specific renovascular effects of dopamine [87, 88], and most of the studies in man are accompanied by large increases in cardiac output (McDonald et al. [90] reported a mean increase of 47%), a specific renovascular effect of dopamine can be questioned. Most importantly, it does not necessarily follow that dopamine will prevent ARF. Metoclopramide, a dopamine antagonist, increases renal vascular resistance and decreases RBF in healthy man [98, 99], while pretreatment with metoclopramide prevents a dopamine-mediated increase in RBF [100]. As these effects of metoclopramide are seen with clinically used doses (10 mg), it seems likely that renal dysfunction would be a recognised complication of metoclopramide use if the renal effects of dopamine were protective.

Laboratory Studies

Dopamine in combination with frusemide [101] or urodilatin [102] prevents the fall in GFR seen in animal models of ARF; however, low-dose dopamine alone was ineffective [101, 102]. We have recently found that intraperitoneal sepsis prevents the renal vasodilatation that occurs in normal animals during the infusion of dopamine at 2 μ/kg per min [56]. As dopamine appears to cause renal vasodilatation through the intrarenal release of prostacyclin [100], and renal arachidonic acid metabolism is altered during sepsis [103] and ischaemia [104], it is probable that this loss of vascular reactivity was due to impaired release of prostacyclin. Although Manoogian et al. [100] found that inhibition of cyclo-oxygenase blocked the renal vasodilator effects of dopamine and the consequent intrarenal production of prostacyclin, Fink and co-workers [105] found that dopamine preserved RBF in endotoxin-shocked dogs administered ibuprofen.

Studies in Man

Low-dose dopamine is frequently recommended for the prevention of ARF; however, this is mainly supported by anecdotal experience rather than prospective randomised studies. Both De La Cal et al. [106] and Parker et al. [107] described an increase in urine output, fractional excretion of sodium and GFR with the use of dopamine in critically ill patients; however, neither study was randomised, and both blood pressure and stoke volume were significantly increased in the study of De La Cal et al. [106] and not reported by Parker et al. [107]. More recently, two prospective randomised studies have failed to find a specific renal sparing effect of dopamine [108, 109]. Myles and co-workers [108] prospectively randomised 52 patients undergoing elective coronary artery surgery to receive either saline or dopamine at 200 μg/min for 1 day following induction of anaesthesia. They found no difference in urine output, free water clearance, GFR or incidence of transient renal impairment between the two groups, although the patients receiving dopamine had a greater cardiac output and lower peripheral resistance immediately following cardiopulmonary bypass. In an effort to offset the potential systemic effects of dopamine, Duke et al. [109] prospectively examined the effects of dopamine (200 μg/min), dobutamine (175 μg/min) and 5% dextrose infused for 5 h each in a random and blinded fashion in 18 critically ill patients (mean APACHE II score of 18). Dopamine produced an increase in urine output but creatinine clearance was unchanged, while dobutamine infusion led to an increase in creatinine clearance without any change in urine output.

Low-dose dopamine has also been proposed for the prevention of ARF in patients undergoing liver transplantation. Polson et al. [110] descibed a reduction of ARF from 67% to 9.5% when compared to historical controls; however, in prospective, randomised study comparing low-dose dopamine with placebo in 48 patients undergoing liver transplantation, Swygert et al. [111] found no difference in urine output. GFR or the incidence of ARF. These latter data, and the finding of an earlier onset of gut ischaemia during haemorrhagic shock [112], argue against the use of dopamine during liver transplantation. Although cyclosporine-induced renal vaoconstriction and renal dysfunction can be acutely offset by concurrent infusion of dopamine [113], this study was performed in healthy volunteers, and dopamine has not been shown to reduce cyclosporine nephrotoxicity following transplantation. Perhaps this also reflects the inabilty of dopamine to increase renal prostaglandin synthesis in clinical settings where the kidney is already "prostaglandin driven."

In summary, although dopamine is a renal vasodilator and may increase RBF, these actions have not been demonstrated in disease states, and its action as a proximal tubular diuretic may theoretically worsen renal ischaemia by increasing medullary sodium reabsorption. Prospective randomised studies in patients undergoing cardiac surgery and liver transplantation and in critically ill patients have not dmonstrated a beneficial action.

Frusemide

Frusemide is often prescribed to oliguric patients in an effort to promote urine flow and convert oliguric ARF to non-oliguric ARF. Although there is little data in support of these hopes, the reduction in medullary O_2 consumption with frusemide is associated with a dramatic decrease in morphologic damage in the isolated perfused kidney [114] and an improvement in medullary oxygenation during nephrotoxin-induced injury [34]. As this protection is not afforded by the diuretic acetazolimide [114], the key issue appears to be medullary work rather than tubular flow. In addition, frusemide increases RBF, probably through intrarenal prostaglandin release [115, 116]; however, the increase in RBF is short lived and associated with a loss of renal autoregulation in the dog [115], and Epstein and co-workers [117] found no change in RBF or in its intrarenal distribution when frusemide was administered directly into the renal artery in eight patients with ARF.

Laboratory Studies

Frusemide is protective in both noradrenaline [118] and clamping-induced ARF [69] when administered prior to the insult, although mannitol was more effective in the latter study [69]. In contrast, Lindner et al. [101] found that frusemide alone was ineffective in ameliorating uranyl nitrate-induced ARF, but that furosemide plus dopamine increased RBF and attenuated the fall in GFR.

Studies in Man

Although Cantarovich et al. [119] described an increase in urine volume and a reduction in the number of dialyses when they compared retrospective controls with the administration of 2 g frusemide daily to patients with ARF, this has not been confirmed by prospective randomised studies. Kleinknecht and coworkers [120] randomised 66 patients with established oliguric ARF to receive 1.5–6 mg/kg frusemide 4-hourly or to act as controls. They found no difference in the number of dialyses or the mean period of renal failure, and several frusemide-treated patients developed tinnitus or transient deafness. Similar results were found by Brown et al. [121], who prospectively randomised 58 patients with ARF to receive either 1 g frusemide (control group) or an additional 3 g every 24 h until a urine output in excess of 200 ml/h was produced. Despite preventing or reversing oliguria in 24 out of 28 versus two out of 28 control patients, there was no difference in the number of dialyses, the duration of ARF, or mortality rate. Finally, Lucas et al. [122] examined the renal haemodynamic effects of frusemide in 54 critically ill patients and found that despite a marked increase in urine output RBF, including its intrarenal distribution, and GFR were unchanged. These data suggest that although a diuresis can be induced with frusemide, there will be little benefit in established ARF.

In summary, frusemide is of theoretical benefit through a reduction in medullary work and through an increase in RBF. Although prospective randomised clinical studies do not show any beneficial effects, they have aimed at increasing urine output when a renal insult has already produced severe renal dysfunction. Future studies need to examine the effects of early or prophylactic administration of frusemide given to minimise the renal injury.

Calcium Channel Blockade

The cytosolic accumulation of calcium is an early finding following an ischaemic insult, and the administration of agents such as verapamil and diltiazem before initiation of an injury results in functional and morphologic protection [123]. Proposed mechanisms include a number of direct vascular effects with preservation of renal autoregulation, a smaller fall in RBF and enhanced recovery of RBF for a given insult and the attenuation of calcium accumulation in tubular epithelial cells [123]. Renal transplantation is a setting of controlled renal ischaemia with very encouraging data from clinical studies utilising calcium channel antagonists. In a prospective randomised study, Duggan et al. [124] found that 20 mg verapamil administered to the donor prior to nephrectomy resulted in a higher urine volume and creatinine clearance on the day of transplantation than the control group. Similarly, Wagner et al. [125] prospectively randomised 20 graft recipients to receive diltiazem (added to Eurocollin's solution at nephrectomy and administered to the recipient for 2 days postoperatively) or control. The diltiazem-treated recipients had a lower incidence of ARF (two out of 20 versus nine out of 22; $p < 0.05$) and a higher GFR in grafts with primary function; however, the underlying incidence of ARF in this study is fairly high compared with 4.8% achieved by Tiggeler et al. [41]. Before extrapolating this data to other settings, it is important to remember that many critically ill patients may not tolerate the high doses of calcium channel antagonist used in these studies and that these drugs have only been shown to be of benefit prior to an insult.

In summary, calcium channel antagonists are protective when administered prior to and during renal transplantation; however, prospective clinical studies are required in a variety of other renal insults, and their negative inotropic effects may not be tolerated by many critically ill patients.

Potential New Agents

Adenosine Antagonists

Adenosine appears to play a major role in tubuloglomerular feedback, and its release due to renal ischaemia has suggested a role in the functional disturbance of the pathological tubuloglomerular feedback of ARF. This has led to laboratory studies of various adenosine antagonists, e.g., theophylline and 8-phenyl-theophylline, and adenosine enhancers, e.g., dipyridamol, throughout the various evolutionary stages of ARF.

Theophylline is a competitive adenosine (A_1 and A_2) receptor antagonist at plasma levels substantially lower than that required for phosphodiesterase inhibition. Doses of theophylline used to antagonize the renal effects of adenosine in the setting of ARF have varied among different laboratory models with loading doses of 0.02–1 mg/kg and maintenance doses of 15–200 µg/kg per min [126–128], and while not all studies have measured plasma levels they are generally low and range from 0.3 to 0.6 mg/l [126]. Adminstration of theophylline prior to an ischaemic, hypoxic or nephrotoxic insult attenuates [126] or prevents [127, 128] the fall in RBF and GFR. Further, in models of established renal dysfunction following an insult, theophylline increases RBF and GFR [128]; however, the greatest benefit is seen when theophylline is administered prior to an insult and continued into the maintenance phase [128]. In addition to theophylline, other adenosine antagonists have also conferred benefit in the setting of ARF [129].

As well as its role in tubuloglomerular feedback, adenosine redistributes RBF towards the vasa recta and when released within the kidney increases medullary PO_2 [130]. Coadministration of 8-phenyltheophylline prevented this effect [130], and adenosine protects against hypoxic medullary injury in the perfused kidney [131], suggesting that the place of adenosine anatagonists is uncertain. It will be important for careful studies to examine the balance of their potential to increase ischaemic medullary injury and their role in decreasing renal dysfunction by inhibiting tubuloglomerular feedback.

In summary, the role of adenosine in the pathogenesis of ARF requires further delineation. Adenosine antagonists, particularly theophylline, have been of consistent benefit in laboratory studies, and the low dose required and mechanism of action appear attractive for their clinical use; however, their potential to increase renal injury raises some concerns.

Prostaglandins

The intrarenal actions of the prostaglandin series are integral to the control of RBF and renal function. In clinical practice it is common to see acute deteriorations in renal function associated with the administration of non-steroidal anti-inflammatory drugs, and in laboratory studies renal autoregulation is abolished [132]. In an ischaemic model of ARF, Kaufman et al. [133] found large increases in PGE_2, 6-keto-$PGF_{1\alpha}$, and TCB_2, with a strong inverse relationship between renal function and the prostaglandin to thromboxane ratio, while pretreatment with a thromboxane synthetase inhibitor was protective and produced the highest prostaglandin to thromboxane ratio [133]. Badr et al. [134] also studied the effects of thromboxane synthetase inhibition, using an endotoxin model of ARF, and found that pretreatment with dazoxiben prevented both the rise in TXB_2 and fall in RBF and attenuated the reduction in GFR. More recently, Cumming et al. [135] reported similar results with thromboxane synthetase inhibition following the induction of intraperitoneal sepsis in sheep. Other researchers have shown attenuation of the fall in RBF and GFR with the use of PGE_2 during ischaemic renal failure [136], and with PGE_1 during both ischaemic and mercuric chloride-induced ARF [137]. In this latter study, PGE_1 was also protective in vitro against hypoxic injury, and in both in vivo and in vitro studies lipid peroxidation was unaffected, suggesting a cytoprotective effect similar to that produced by the prostaglandins in the gastrointestinal tract. Finally, in laboratory studies prostaglandin analogues have also been shown to prevent acute cyclosporine nephrotoxicity [138, 139].

In summary, manipulation of the renal prostaglandin to thromboxane ratio is protective in laboratory models of ARF and appears to act by increasing RBF and through a separate cytoprotective action. Prospective randomised studies in man appear to be justified.

Atrial Natriuretic Peptide

The renal effects of atrial natriuretic peptide (ANP) include: (a) an increase in glomerular capillary hydrostatic pressure due to afferent arteriolar vasodilatation and efferent arteriolar vasoconstriction and (b) an increase in the glomerular capillary ultrafiltration coefficient.

Laboratory studies suggest that ANP reduces the functional disturbance following renal injury. In a rodent model of ischaemic ARF, Shaw et al. [140] found that a 4-h infusion of α-human ANP started immediately following the insult not only preserved GFR, but medullary hyperaemia was reduced and tubular cell necrosis was prevented. Similar functional and morphologic effects of ANP or ANP analogues have been found following ischaemic insults [141, 142], during ischaemic ARF [143] and following nephrotoxic injury [144, 145] in laboratory models. Deleterious systemic haemodynamic effects of ANP (reduction in plasma volume and perfusion pressure) may offset the potential beneficial effects of ANP on the kidney; however, the defence of perfusion pressure with dopamine does not appear to confer added benefit in laboratory studies [141, 143]. Clinical studies of ANP following cadaveric kidney transplantation have failed to demonstrate any benefit [146, 147].

In summary, the renal effects of ANP are of theoretical benefit following renal injury. Laboratory studies show consistent benefit when the adverse systemic haemodynamic effects of ANP are avoided, but early clinical trials have been disappointing.

Endothelin Antagonists

The hypothesis that release of endothelin-1, by hypoxia, endotoxin and some nephrotoxins, has a central role in the initiation of ARF and that subsequent endothelial damage results in persistent release of endothelin-1 has led to the evaluation of endothelin antagonists in the prevention of renal injury. Laboratory studies have used rabbit polyclonal antibodies [23], mouse monoclonal (IgG) endothelin antibodies [22] and the selective endothelin receptor (ET_A) antagonist BQ-123 [148]. The administration of an endothelin antagonist before and following ischaemic ARF in the rodent prevented a decrease in GFR, corticomedullary necrosis and haemorrhagic congestion [148], and similar effects have been found using endothelin antibodies [22]. Finally, endothelin antibodies given 48 h after ischaemic injury also increased single nephron GFR and glomerular plasma flow [23], suggesting that endothelin is not only involved in the initiation of renal injury, but that it also acts to maintain dysfunction.

Conclusion

Renal dysfunction and ARF continue to be major problems in critically ill patients. While our understanding of their pathophysiology has markedly improved over the last decade, it remains very incomplete and as yet has not been accompanied by clinically proven preventative therapies. Until clinical trials with some of the newer antagonists, e.g., adenosine or endothelin, are completed, adequate haemodynamic resuscitation and the avoidance of nephrotoxins remain the most effective measures.

References

1. Rasmussen HH, Ibels LS (1982) Acute renal failure: multivariate analysis of causes and factors. Am J Med 73:211
2. Knaus WA, Draper EA, Wagner DP et al. (1985) Prognosis in acute organ failure. Ann Surg 202:685–693
3. Hou SH, Bushinsky DA, Wish JB et al. (1983) Hospital acquired renal insufficiency: a prospective study. Am J Med 74:243–248
4. Bell RC, Coalson JJ, Smith JD et al. (1983) Multiple organ failure and infection in adult respiratory distress syndrome. Ann Intern Med 99:293–299
5. Miller SB, Anderson RJ (1987) The kidney in acute respiratory failure. J Crit Care 2:45–48
6. Vertel RM, Knochel JP (1967) Non-oliguric acute renal failure. JAMA 200:118–122
7. Planas M, Wachtel T, Frank H et al. (1982) Characterization of acute renal failure in the burned patient. Arch Intern Med 142:2087–2091
8. Back S-M, Makabali GG, Shoemaker WC (1975) Clinical determinants of survival from post-operative renal failure. Surg Gynecol Obstet 140:685–689
9. Anderson RJ, Linas SL, Berns AS et al. (1977) Nonoliguric renal failure. N Engl J Med 296:1134–1138
10. Honda N, Hishida A (1993) Pathophysiology of experimental nonoliguric acute renal failure. Kidney Int 43:513–521
11. Mellander S, Johansson B (1968) Control of resistance and capacitance function in the peripheral circulation. Pharmacol Rev 20:117–196
12. Brezis M, Rosen SN, Epstein FH (1989) The pathophysiological implications of medullary hypoxia. Am J Kidney Dis 13:253–258
13. Brezis M, Rosen S, Silva P, Epstein FH (1984) Selective vulnerability of the medullary thick ascending limb to anoxia in the isolated perfused rat kidney. J Clin Invest 73:182–190

14. Heyman SN, Brezis M, Reubinoff CA et al. (1988) Acute renal failure with selective medullary injury in the rat. J Clin Invest 82:401–412
15. Solez K, Morel-Maroger L, Sraer J-D (1979) The morphology of "acute tubular necrosis" in man: analysis of 57 renal biopsies and a comparison with the glycerol model. Medicine (Baltimore) 58:362–376
16. Burke TJ, Cronin RE, Duchin KL, Peterson LN, Schrier RW (1980) Ischemia and tubule obstruction during acute renal failure in dogs: mannitol in protection. Am J Physiol 238:F305–F314
17. Bohle A, Christensen J, Kokot F et al. (1990) Acute renal failure in man: new aspects concerning pathogenesis. Am J Nephrol 10:374–388
18. Osswald H, Muhlbauer B, Schenk F (1991) Adenosine mediates tubuloglomerular feedback response: an element of metabolic control of kidney function. Kidney Int 39:S128–S131
19. Thurau K, Boylan JW (1976) Acute renal success. The unexpected logic of oliguria in renal failure. Am J Med 61:308–315
20. Miller WL, Thomas RA, Berne RM, Rubio R (1978) Adenosine production in the ischemic kidney. Circ Res 43:390–397
21. Kon V, Badr KF (1991) Biological actions and pathophysiologic significance of endothelin in the kidney. Kidney Int 40:1–12
22. Shibouta Y, Suzuki N, Shino A et al. (1990) Pathophysiological role of endothelin in acute renal failure. Life Sci 46:1611–1618
23. Kon V, Toshimasa Y, Fogo A, Ichikawa I (1989) Glomerular actions of endothelin in vivo. J Clin Invest 83:1762–1767
24. Firth JD, Ratcliffe PJ, Raine AEG, Ledingham JGG (1988) Endothelin: an important factor in acute renal failure? Lancet 2:1179–1182
25. Rubanyi GM, Vanhoutte PM (1985) Hypoxia releases a vasoconstictor substance from the canine vascular endothelium. J Physiol (Lond) 364:45–56
26. Sugiura M, Inagami T, Kon V (1989) Endotoxin stimulates endothelin-release in vivo and in vitro as determined by radioimmunoassay. Biochem Biophys Res Commun 161:1220–1227
27. Tomita K, Ujiie K, Nakanishi T et al. (1989) Plasma endothelin levels in patients in acute renal failure. N Engl J Med 321:1127
28. Zager RA (1989) Studies of mechanisms and protective maneuvers in myoglobinuric acute renal failure. Lab Invest 60:619–629
29. Hellberg POA, Kallskog O, Wogast M (1991) Red cell trapping and postischemic renal blood flow. Differences between the cortex, outer and inner medulla. Kidney Int 40:625–631
30. Zager RA (1988) Gentamicin nephrotoxicity in the setting of acute renal hypoperfusion. Am J Physiol 254:F574–F581
31. Heyman SN, Clark BA, Cantley L et al. (1993) Effects of ioversol versus iothalamte on endothelin release and radiocontrast nephropathy. Invest Radiol 28:313–318
32. Rosen S, Greenfield Z, Brezis M (1990) Chronic cyclosporine-induced nephropathy in the rat: a medullary ray and inner stripe injury. Transplantation 49:445–452
33. Fogo A, Hellings SE, Inagami T, Kon V (1992) Endothelin receptor antagonism is protective in in vivo cyclosporine toxicity. Kidney Int 42:770–774
34. Heyman SN, Brezis M, Epstein FH et al. (1991) Early medullary hypoxic injury from radiocontrast and indomethacin. Kidney Int 40:632–642
35. Braun SR, Weiss FR, Keller AI et al. (1970) Evaluation of the renal toxicity of heme proteins and their derivatives: a role in the genesis of acute tubular necrosis. J Exp Med 131:443–460
36. Brezis M, Epstein FH (1993) Cellular mechanisms of acute ischemic injury in the kidney. Annu Rev Med 44:27–37
37. Bidani A, Churchill P, Fleischmann L (1979) Sodium-chloride-induced protection in nephrotoxic acute renal failure: independence from renin. Kidney Int 16:481–490

38. Barry KG, Mazze RI, Schwartz FD (1964) Prevention of surgical oliguria and renal-hemodynamic supression by sustained hydration. N Engl J Med 270:1371–1377
39. Bush HL, Huse JB, Johnson WC et al. (1981) Prevention of renal insufficiency after abdominal aortic aneurysm resection by optimal volume loading. Arch Surg 116:1517–1524
40. Alpert RA, Roizen MF, Hamilton WK et al. (1984) Intraoperative urinary output does not predict postoperative renal function in patients undergoing abdominal aortic revascularization. Surgery 95:707–711
41. Tiggeler RGW, Berden JHM, Hoitsma AJ, Koene RAP (1984) Prevention of acute tubular necrosis in cadaveric kidney transplantation by the combined use of mannitol and moderate hydration. Ann Surg 201:246–251
42. Blachley JD, Hill JB (1981) Renal and electrolyte disturbances associated with cisplatin. Ann Intern Med 95:628–632
43. Schlichtig R, Kramer DJ, Boston JR et al. (1991) Renal O_2 consumption during progressive hemorrhage. J Appl Physiol 70:1957–1962
44. Schlichtig R, Kramer DJ, Pinsky MR (1991) Flow redistribution during progressive hemorrhage is a determinant of critical O_2 delivery. J Appl Physiol 70:169–178
45. Hilberman M, Derby GC, Spencer RJ et al. (1980) Sequential pathophysiological changes characterizing the progression from renal dysfunction to acute renal failure following cardiac operation. J Thorac Cardiovasc Surg 79:838–844
46. Fan F-C, Chen RY, Schuessler GB et al. (1980) Effects of hematocrit variatios on regional hemodynamics and oxygen transport in the dog. Am J Physiol 238:H545–H552
47. Shipley RE, Study RS (1951) Changes in renal blood flow, extraction of inulin, glomerular filtration rate, tissue pressure and urine flow with acute alterations in renal artery pressure. Am J Physiol 167:676–688
48. Stone AM, Stahl WM (1970) Renal effects of hemmorhage in normal man. Ann Surg 172:825–836
49. Kircheim HR, Ehmke H, Hackenthal E, Lowe W, Persson P (1987) Autoregulation of renal blood flow, glomerular filtration rate and renin release in conscious dogs. Pflugers Arch 410:441–449
50. Adams PL, Adams FF, Bell PD, Navar LG (1980) Impaired renal blood flow autoregulation in ischemic acute renal failure. Kidney Int 18:68–76
51. Kelleher SP, Robinette JB, Conger JD (1984) Sympathetic nervous system in the loss of autoregulation in acute renal failure. Am J Physiol 246:F379–F386
52. Desjars P, Pinaud M, Potel G et al. (1987) A reappraisal of norepinephrine therapy in human septic shock. Crit Care Med 15:134–137
53. Hesselvik JF, Brodin B (1989) Low dose norepinephrine in patients with septic shock and oliguria: effects on afterload, urine flow, and oxygen transport. Crit Care Med 17:179–180
54. Redl-Wenzl EM, Armbruster C, Edelmann G et al. (1993) The effects of norepinephrine on hemodynamics and renal function in severe septic shock. Intensive Care Med 19:151–154
55. Schaer GL, Fink MP, Parillo JE (1985) Norepinephrine alone versus norepinephrine plus low-dose dopamine: enhanced renal blood flow with combination pressor therapy. Crit Care Med 13:492–496
56. Bersten AD, Rutten AJ, Summersides G et al. (1993) Interaction of sepsis, adrenaline and dopamine in awake sheep. Anaesth Intensive Care 21:704
57. Bersten AD, Rutten AJ, Summersides G et al. (1994) Epinephrine infusion in the sheep: systemic and renal hemodynamic effects. Crit Care Med (in press)
58. Persson PB, Ehmke H, Nafz B et al. (1990) Resetting of renal autoregulation in conscious dogs: angiotensin II and alpha$_1$-adrenoceptors. Pflugers Arch 417:42–47
59. Barnes GE, Laine GA, Giam PY et al. (1985) Cardiovascular responses to elevation of intra-abdominal hydrostatic pressure. Am J Physiol 248:R208–R231
60. Richards WO, Scovill W, Shin B et al. (1983) Acute renal failure associated with increased intra-abdominal pressure. Ann Surg 197:183–187

61. Kron IL, Harman PK, Nolan SP (1984) The measurement of intra-abdominal pressure as a criterion for abdominal re-exploration. Ann Surg 199:28–30
62. Cronin RE, De Torrente A, Miller PD, Bulger RE, Burke TJ, Schrier RW (1978) Pathogenic mechanisms in early norepinephrine-induced acute renal failure: histological correlates of protection. Kidney Int 14:115–125
63. Schrier RW, Arnold PE, Gordon JA, Burke TJ (1984) Protection of mitochondrial function in ischemic acute renal failure. Am J Physiol 247:F365–F369
64. Johnston PA, Bernard DB, Perrin NS, Levinsky NG (1981) Prostaglandins mediate the vasodilatory effect of mannitol in the hypoperfused kidney. J Clin Invest 68:127–133
65. Borges HF, Hocks J, Kjellstrand CM (1982) Mannitol intoxication in patients with renal failure. Arch Intern Med 142:63–66
66. Whelan TV, Bacon ME, Madden M, Patel TG, Handy R (1984) Acute renal failure associated with mannitol intoxication. Arch Intern Med 144:2053–2055
67. Goldwasser P, Fotino S (1984) Acute renal failure following massive mannitol infusion: appropriate response of tubuloglomerular feedback. Arch Intern Med 144:2214–2216
68. Rozich JD, Paul RV (1988) Acute renal failure precipitated by elevated colloid osmotic pressure. Am J Med 87:358–360
69. Hanley MJ, Davidson K (1981) Prior mannitol and furosemide infusion in a model of ischemic acute renal failure. Am J Physiol 241:F556–F564
70. Zager RA (1983) Glomerular filtration rate and brush border debris excretion after mercuric chloride and ischemic acute renal failure: mannitol versus furosemide diuresis. Nephron 33:196–201
71. Vanholder R, Leusen I, Lameire N (1984) Comparison between mannitol and saline infusion in $HgCl_2$-induced acute renal failure. Nephron 38:193–201
72. Klein H, Greven J (1979) Renal effects of mannitol in the early stage of glycerol-induced acute renal failure in the rat. Nephron 23:255–261
73. Dawson JL (1965) Post-operative renal function in obstructive jaundice: effect of a mannitol diuresis. Br Med J 1:82–86
74. Eneas JF, Schoenfeld PY, Humphreys MH (1979) The effect of infusion of mannitol-sodium bicarbonate on the clinical course of myoglobinuria. Arch Intern Med 139:801–805
75. Barry KG, Malloy JP (1962) Oliguric renal failure: evaluation and treatment by the intravenous infusion of mannitol. JAMA 179:510–513
76. Luke RG, Linton AL, Briggs JD, Kennedy AC (1965) Mannitol therapy in acute renal failure. Lancet 1:980–982
77. Gubern JM, Sancho JJ, Simo J, Sitges-Serra A (1988) A randomised trial on the effect of mannitol on postoperative renal function in patients with obstructive jaundice. Surgery 103:39–44
78. Paul MD, Mazer D, Byrick RJ, Rose DK, Goldstein MB (1986) Influence of mannitol and dopamine on renal function during elective infrarenal aortic clamping in man. Am J Nephrol 6:427–434
79. Pass LJ, Eberhart RC, Brown JC, Rohn GN, Estrera AS (1988) The effect of mannitol and dopamine on the renal response to thoracic aortic cross-clamping. J Thorac Cardiovasc Surg 95:608–612
80. Weimar W, Geerlings W, Bijnen AB et al. (1983) A controlled study on the effect of mannitol on immediate renal function after cadaveric donor kidney transplantation. Transplantation 35:99–101
81. Carlier M, Squifflet JP, Pirson Y et al. (1982) Maximal hydration during anesthesia increases pulmonary artery pressures and improves early function of human renal transplants. Transplantation 34:201–204
82. Better OS, Stein JH (1990) Early management of shock and prophylaxis of acute renal failure in traumatic rhabdomyolysis. N Engl J Med 322:825–829
83. Ron D, Taitelman U, Michaelson M et al. (1984) Prevention of acute renal failure in traumatic rhabdomyolysis. Arch Intern Med 144:277–280

84. Ball SG, Gunn IG, Douglas IHS (1982) Renal handling of dopa, dopamine, norepinephrine and epinephrine in the dog. Am J Physiol 242:F56–F62
85. Seri I, Kone BC, Gullans SR et al. (1988) Locally formed dopamine inhibits Na^+-K^+-ATPase activity in rat renal cortical tubule cells. Am J Physiol 255:F666–F673
86. Seri I, Kone BC, Gullans SR et al. (1990) Influence of Na^+ intake on dopamine-induced inhibition of renal cortical Na^+-K^+-ATPase. Am J Physiol 258:F52–F60
87. Wasserman K, Huss R, Kullmann R (1980) Dopamine-induced diuresis in the cat without changes in renal hemodynamics. Naunyn Schmiedebergs Arch Pharmacol 312:77–80
88. McGrath B, Bode K, Luxford A, Howden B, Jablonski P (1985) Effects of dopamine on renal function in the rat isolated perfused kidney. Clin Exp Pharmacol Physiol 12:343–452
89. Goldberg LI, McDonald RH, Zimmerman AM (1963) Sodium diuresis produced by dopamine in patients with congestive heart failure. N Engl J Med 269:1060–1064
90. McDonald RH, Godberg LI, McNAy JL et al. (1964) Effects of dopamine in man: augmentation of sodium excretion, glomerular filtration rate, and renal plasma flow. J Clin Invest 43:1116–1124
91. Szerlip HM (1991) Renal-dose dopamine: fact and fiction. Ann Intern Med 115:153–154
92. Duke GJ, Bersten AD (1992) Dopamine and renal salvage in the critically ill patient. Anaesth Intensive Care 20:277–302
93. Port JD, Gilbert EM, Larrabee P et al. (1990) Neurotransmitter depletion compromises the ability of indirect-acting amines to provide inotropic support in the failing heart. Circulation 81:929–938
94. Zaritsky A, Lotze A, Stull R et al. (1988) Steady-state dopamine clearance in critically ill infants and children. Crit Care Med 16:217–220
95. McNay JL, Goldberg LI (1966) Hemodynamic effects of dopamine in the dog before and after alpha adrenergic blockade. Clin Res 18(S):110–119
96. Kapusta DR, Robie NW (1988) Plasma dopamine in regulation of canine renal blood flow. Am J Physiol 255:R379–R387
97. Hollenberg NK, Adams DF, Mendell P et al. (1973) Renal vascular responses to dopamine: haemodynamic and angiographic observations in normal man. Clin Sci Mol Med 45:733–742
98. Israel R, O'Mara V, Austin B et al. (1986) Metoclopramide decreases renal plasma flow. Clin Pharmacol Ther 39:261–264
99. Manara AR, Bolsin S, Monk CR et al. (1991) Metoclopramide and renal vascular resistance. Br J Anaesth 66:129–130
100. Manoogian C, Nadler J, Ehrlich L et al. (1988) The renal vasodilating effect of dopamine is mediated by calcium flux and prostacyclin release in man. J Clin Endocrinol 66:678–683
101. Lindner A, Cutler RE, Goodman WG et al. (1979) Synergism of dopamine plus furosemide in preventing acute renal failure in the dog. Kidney Int 16:158–166
102. Shaw S, Weidmann P, Zimmerman A (1992) Urodilatin, not nitropusside, combined with dopamine reverses ischemic acute renal failure. Kidney Int 42:1153–1159
103. Badr KF, Kelley VE, Rennke HG et al. (1986) Roles for thromboxane A_2 and leukotrienes in endotoxin-induced acute renal failure. Kidney Int 30:474–480
104. Kaufman RP, Klausner JM, Anner H et al. (1988) Inhibition of thromboxane (Tx) synthesis by free radical scavengers. J Trauma 28:458–464
105. Fink MP, Nelson R, Roethel R (1985) Low-dose dopamine preserves renal blood flow in endotoxin shocked dogs treated with ibuprofen. J Surg Res 38:582–591
106. De La Cal MA, Miravalles E, Pascual T et al. (1984) Dose-related hemodynamic and renal effects of dopamine in septic shock. Crit Care Med 12:22–25
107. Parker S, Carlon GC, Isaacs M et al. (1981) Dopamine administration in oliguria and oliguric renal failure. Crit Care Med 9:630–632
108. Myles PS, Buckland MR, Schenk NJ et al. (1993) Effect of renal-dose dopamine on renal function following cardiac surgery. Anaesth Intensive Care 21:56–61

109. Duke GJ, Bredis JH, Weaver RA (1994) Renal support in critically ill patients: low dose dopamine or dobutamine. Crit Care Med (in press)
110. Polson RJ, Park GR, Lindop MJ et al. (1987) The prevention of renal impairment in patients undergoing orthotopic liver grafting by infusion of low dose dopamine. Anaesthesia 42:15–19
111. Swygert TH, Roberts LC, Valek TR et al. (1991) Effect of intraoperative low-dose dopamine on renal function in liver transplant patients. Anesthesiology 75:571–576
112. Segal JM, Phang PT, Walley KR (1992) Low-dose dopamine hastens onset of gut ischemia in a porcine model of hemorrhagic shock. J Appl Physiol 73:1159–1164
113. Conte G, Dal Canton A, Sabbatini M et al. (1989) Acute cyclosporine renal dysfunction reversed by dopamine infusion in healthy subjects. Kidney Int 36:1086–1092
114. Brezis M, Rosen S, Silva P, Epstein FH (1984) Transport activity modifies thick ascending limb damage in the isolated perfused kidney. Kidney Int 25:65–72
115. Duchin KL, Peterson LN, Burke TJ (1977) Effect of furosemide on renal autoregulation. Kidney Int 12:379–386
116. Patak RV, Fadem SZ, Rosenblatt SG et al. (1979) Diuretic-induced changes in renal blood flow and prostaglandin E excretion in the dog. Am J Physiol 236:F494–F500
117. Epstein M, Schneider NS, Befeler B (1975) Effect of intrarenal furosemide on renal function and intrarenal hemodynamics in acute renal failure. Am J Med 58:510–516
118. De Torrente A, Miller PD, Cronin RE et al. (1978) Effects of furosemide and acetylcholine in norepinephrine-induced acute renal failure. Am J Physiol 235:F131–F136
119. Cantarovich F, Galli C, Benedetti L et al. (1973) High dose frusemide in established acute renal failure. Br Med J 4:449–450
120. Kleinknecht D, Ganeval D, Gozalez-Duque LA et al. (1976) Furosemide in acute renal failure – a controlled trial. Nephron 17:51–58
121. Brown CB, Ogg CS, Cameron JS (1981) High dose frusemide in acute renal failure: a controlled trial. Clin Nephrol 15:90–96
122. Lucas CE, Zito JG, Carter KM et al. (1977) Questionable value of furosemide in preventing renal failure. Surgery 82:314–320
123. Schrier RW, Arnold PE, Van Putten VJ et al. (1987) Cellular calcium in ischemic acute renal failure: role of calcium entry blockers. Kidney Int 32:313–321
124. Duggan KA, Macdonald GJ, Charlesworth JA et al. (1985) Verapamil prevents post-transplant oliguric renal failure. Clin Nephrol 24:289–291
125. Wagner K, Albrecht S, Neumayer H-H (1987) Prevention of posttransplant acute tubular necrosis by the calcium antagonist diltiazem: a prospective randomized study. Am J Nephrol 7:287–291
126. Gouyon G-B, Guignard J-P (1988) Theophylline prevents the hypoxemia-induced renal hemodynamic changes in rabbits. Kidney Int 33:1078–1083
127. Lin J-P, Churchill PC, Bidani AK (1986) Effects of theophylline on the initiation phase of postischemic acute renal failure in rats. J Lab Invest 108:150–154
128. Lin J-P, Churchill PC, Bidani AK (1988) Theophylline in rats during maintenance phase of postischemic acute renal failure. Kidney Int 33:24–28
129. Oken DE, Reilly KM (1989) Total prevention of glycerol-induced acute renal failure (ARF) with adenosine-receptor blockade. Kidney Int 35:415
130. Dinour D, Brezis M (1991) Effects of adenosine on intrarenal oxygenation. Am J Physiol 261:F787–F791
131. Epstein FH, Rosen S, Galicka-Piskorska G et al. (1990) Relation of adenosine to medullary injury in the perfused rat kidney. Miner Electolyte Metab 16:185–190
132. Banks RO (1988) Vasoconstrictor-induced changes in renal blood flow: role of prostaglandins and histamine. Am J Physiol 254:F470–F476
133. Kaufman RP, Anner H, Kobzik L et al. (1987) A high plasma prostaglandin to thromboxane ratio protects against renal ischemia. Surg Gynevol Obstet 165:404–409

134. Badr KF, Kelley VE, Rennke HG et al. (1986) Roles for thromboxane A2 and leukotrienes in endotoxin-induced acute renal failure. Kidney Int 30:474–480
135. Cumming AD, McDonald JW, Lindsay RM et al. (1989) The protective effect of thromboxane synthetase inhibition on renal function in systemic sepsis. Am J Kidney Dis 13:114–119
136. Neumayer H-H, Wagner K, Groll J et al. (1985) Beneficial effects of long-term prostaglandin E_2 infusion on the course of postischemic acute renal failure: long-term studies in chronically instrumented conscious dogs. Renal Physiol 8:159–168
137. Paller MS, Manivel JC (1992) Prostaglandins protect kidneys against ischemic and toxic injury by a cellular effect. Kidney Int 42:1345–1354
138. Paller M (1988) Effects of the prostaglandin E_1 analog misoprostol on cyclosporine nephrotoxicity. Transplantation 45:1126–1131
139. Makowa L, Lopatin W, Gilas T et al. (1986) Prevention of cyclosporine (CyA) nephrotoxicity by synthetic prostaglandins. Clin Nephrol 25:S89–S94
140. Shaw SG, Weidmann P, Hodler J et al. (1987) Atrial natriuretic peptide protects against acute ischemic renal failure in the rat. J Clin Invest 80:1232–1237
141. Pollock DM, Opgenorth TJ (1992) Beneficial effects of the ANF analogue A68828 on recovery from ischemic acute renal failure. Ren Fail 14:141–146
142. Neumayer HH, Blossei N, Seherr-Thohs U, Wagner K (1990) Amelioration of postischemic acute renal failure in conscious dogs by human atrial natriuretic peptide. Nephrol Dial Transplant 5:32–38
143. Conger JD, Falk SA, Hammond WS (1991) Atrial natriuretic and dopamine in established acute renal failure in the rat. Kidney Int 40:21–28
144. Margulies KB, McKinley LJ, Cavero PG, Burnett JC (1990) Induction and prevention of radiocontrast-induced nephropathy in dogs with heart failure. Kidney Int 38:1101–1108
145. Pollosk DM, Holst M, Opgenorth TJ (1991) Effect of the ANF analog A68828 in cisplatin-induced acute renal failure. J Pharmacol Exp Ther 257:1179–1183
146. Sands JM, Neylan JF, Olson RA et al. (1991) Atrial natriuretic factor does not improve the outcome of cadaveric renal transplantation. J Am Soc Nephrol 1:1081–1086
147. Smits P, Huysmans F, Hoitsma A et al. (1989) The effect of alpha-human atrial natriuretic peptide on the incidence of acute renal failure in cadaveric kidney transplantation. Transplant Int 2:73–77
148. Mino N, Kobayashi M, Nakajima A et al. (1992) Protective effect of a selective endothelin receptor antagonist, BQ-123, in ischemic acute renal failure in rats. Eur J Pharmacol 221:77–83

Epidemiology of Acute Renal Failure

R.L. Lins, S.L. Chew, and R. Daelemans

Introduction

Acute renal failure (ARF) is a syndrome, not a disease. It has numerous causes and occurs in a wide range of patients, making the evaluation of prognosis very difficult. The most accurate outcome measure is the mortality rate. That of acute renal failure is about 50%. It may be as high as 80% in patients treated in intensive care units (ICU) [1]. This high mortality rate has remained virtually unchanged despite the advent of antibiotics, diuretics, vasoactive drugs, standardization of nutritional measures, and the generalization of nephrology services and ICU so that no patient is denied the possibility of treatment with sophisticated techniques in developed countries.

The main reasons for this paradox are the change in the population susceptible to ARF and the progress of medicine, which succeeds in keeping people alive who would previously have died before developing ARF [2]. In a recent study, however, the mortality of surgical as well as traumatic and medical cases was reduced from 69% in the years 1975–1979 to 48% in the years 1985–1989 [3].

Most studies of prognosis in ARF have analyzed the influence of demographic factors, severity of ARF, nature of diseases causing ARF, coexisting diseases, treatments received, and complications [4–6]. A good prognostic index would allow comparisons to be made between renal centers and between patients enrolled in clinical trials.

Prognosis in ARF has been the subject of some recent reviews, and references to many of the primary sources used for this chapter can be found in these articles [1, 7].

Incidence

Knowledge about the incidence of ARF is necessary because of therapeutic, ethical, and economic implications. However, due to a wide variability in study design, patient populations, definitions of ARF, and renal pathology, data about incidence of ARF must be interpreted carefully. Moreover, a continuous evolution in diagnostic and therapeutic facilities will permanently influence the types and incidence of ARF.

Overall, there is a wide variety in incidence of ARF, ranging from 0.14% for severe ARF in the general population [8] to 33% in critically ill ICU patients [9]. In a recent prospective, community-based study, Feest et al. looked at true population incidence of severe ARF (serum creatinine >5.5 mg/dl). An incidence of 0.14% was found in the total population and in 0.17% of the adults. However, due to study design, the true community incidence was underestimated [8]. Kaufman et al. [10] reported an incidence of community-acquired (i.e., present on admission to the hospital) ARF (serum creatinine >2 mg/dl) of 1% in a prospective study. More than 80% of their patients had a potentially reversible cause for their ARF. In the prospective study of hospital-acquired renal insufficiency by Hou et al. [11], the incidence of ARF (increase of 0.5 mg/dl when serum creatinine was <1.9 mg/dl, 1.0 mg/dl when 2.0–4.9 mg/dl and 1.5 mg/dl when >5.0 mg/dl) was 4.9%. In 20% of the cases, the increase in serum creatinine was more than 3.0 mg/dl. Shusterman et al. [12] showed that in a large teaching hopital (case–control study) ARF (increase in serum creatinine of 0.9 mg/dl or 1.5 mg/dl when baseline serum creatinine was <2.0 mg/dl and >2.0 mg/dl, respectively) occurred in 2% during hospitalization. ARF occurs more frequently in critically ill ICU patients, but here too a wide range in incidence can be found (3%–33%) [9]. In the prospective study by Jochimsen et al. [13], 6.6% of the critically ill patients in a medical ICU developed ARF (rise in serum creatinine >30%). The prevalence found by Groeneveld et al. [9] in a retrospective study in medical ICU patients with ARF (serum creatinine >3.2 mg/dl or a twofold rise in chronic renal failure) was 16%. A change in incidence of the type of ARF has certainly been seen during the last few decades. There has been a significant decline in incidence of obstetric and post-traumatic ARF (2.8%). Surgical ARF has remained constant, except for cardiovascular surgery, where an increase was noted (34%). The increase in medical ARF is significant (60%) [2].

Before relevant therapeutic and economic conclusions can be drawn from all these data, it is obvious that more strict definitions of ARF and better registration are necessary.

Risk Factors – Associated Conditions

In most critically ill and hospital-acquired ARF patients, there is an additive interaction of multiple risk factors, associated conditions, and diagnostic or therapeutic interventions that cause ARF. Therefore, knowledge and recognition of these factors is important to avoid multiple renal injury leading to ARF. A relatively small number of well-known acute events (volume depletion, hypotension, infection, use of vasopressors, and nephrotoxin exposure) are responsible for hospital-acquired ARF. A major role is played by renal hypoperfusion and sepsis [11, 13, 14]. In all, 72% of critically ill ARF patients had sepsis, in 70% occurring before the onset of

ARF [9]. However, multivariate analysis showed that individual prediction is impossible [13]. In critically ill patients, ARF is a part of multiple organ failure (MOF): 73%–87% of ARF patients have failure of other organs before the onset of ARF. The kidneys were the first organ to fail in only 7%–22% of ARF patients [9, 15]. Multivariate analysis showed that prior chronic disease (preexisting chronic renal failure and cardiovascular disease) influenced development of hospital-acquired ARF [9, 15]. Patients with underlying renal disease are also at increased risk for developing community-acquired ARF [10]. Several studies confirm that elderly patients are at a higher risk of developing ARF [8, 16, 17]. Iatrogenic factors often play an important role and occur more in older patients. In a prospective study by Davidman et al. [18], iatrogenic renal disease developed in 1% of all patients admitted to a tertiary care hospital. The most common syndrome was ARF (59%), most often caused by nephrotoxins (46%, medication and contrast media) and volume depletion (45%). In the study by Hou et al. [11], iatrogenic factors accounted for 55% of all ARF episodes.

Cost

Although the cost of financing health care is a big issue in many countries, only few data related to cost-effectiveness can be found in medical literature. The cost of treating critically ill patients with ARF is high. In an American study, the costs of treating ARF increased by 217% between 1967 and 1975 to US$17332 per patient in 1975, despite similar hospitalization times [19]. In a study of dialysis for ARF in an ICU in London lasting 3 years from 1985, the costs were estimated at £65030 per survivor. This is an increase of roughly 623% [20]. In this context, it is important to mention that only 36% of the patients with severe ARF in the community-based study of Feest et al. [8] were referred for nephrological opinion. Jungers et al. [21] recently reported that 30% of chronic renal failure patients were referred at a very late stage for maintenance dialysis with more complications and prolonged hospitalizations as a result. It may be that earlier nephrological advice and referral could influence incidence and cost of ARF as well. Cost of treatment may be a useful and reasonable outcome measure and merits further study and analysis.

Patient Survival

Design of Outcome Studies

There is considerable variability in study design, ranging from large (1347 patients) to small (38 patients) retrospective series, and few studies are prospective; ever fewer use the powerful tool of multivariate analysis or multiple linear or logistic regression [7]. However, even when statistical methodology and patient numbers are similar, inclusion criteria can range from mild rises in creatinine to only dialysis-treated patients. Furthermore, the terms ARF and acute tubular necrosis (ATN) are often used synonymously, and it is clear from exclusion criteria that several series of "ARF" consist predominantly or even exclusively of ATN cases, even if this is not explicitly stated [1].

Rasmussen et al.'s [22] study is an example of the use of multivariate discriminant analysis in this field. They first retrospectively analyzed 23 clinical variables in 148 patients to derive an equation using ten variables, or "discriminant function," giving a discriminant score. At a given level, this discriminant score had a 100%-positive predictive value for death, with a sensitivity of 58%. This was then prospectively evaluated in 113 patients, again with a 100%-positive predictive value, but only 26% sensitivity (in other words, a score above the given level was universally predictive of death, although only 26% of patients who eventually died had a score that reached this level). One group has applied the technique of "receiver operating characteristics" to ARF, which allows the trade-off between specificity and sensitivity at different score values to be calculated [6]. The clinician can then choose score levels which deliver higher sensitivities at the cost of lower specificities. It is essential that details of predictive values, specificities, and sensitivities (and details of the control groups on which these calculations are based) are provided.

Another feature of modern studies is that factors found nonsignificant on univariate analysis can be contributory on multivariate analysis and vice versa [7]. Even the use of two different multivariate regression methods, linear and logistic, can give different results, as showed in the study of Liaño et al. [17]. In this recent study, the outcome of acute tubular necrosis was studied retrospectively (228 patients), prospectively (100 patients) and validated in another center (25 patients). The multiple linear was better than the logistic regression model in terms of many statistical parameters.

Unfortunately, the many, and differing, exclusion criteria limit the use of many scoring systems in ARF in general. For example, postrenal ARF, acute glomerulonephritis (AGN), uric acid nephropathy, acute interstitial nephritis (AIN), and hepatorenal syndrome were excluded by Rasmussen et al. [22]. Also, several equations are probably too cumbersome for everyday use by clinicians. Another problem is the definition of outcome measurements. Most studies have measured hospital survival. Other outcomes, such as length of hospitalization, ought to be evaluated. It is generally longer for hospital survivors (29 days) than those who survive the ICU only to die on outside wards (13.8 days) and those who die in the ICU (13.5 days) [20].

Demographic Factors

There is no consistency in the literature relating age to increased mortality in ARF. The largest series of ARF patients found that prognosis worsened with age. It was, however, in the elderly that outcome had improved over the years, perhaps due to medical advances; potentially adverse factors appear to occur more often in the elderly [2, 23]. Smaller multivariate, but retrospective analyses found age to be an independent predictive factor for death [7]. Sex and race have no predictive value for survival [7].

Causes of Acute Renal Failure

Among medical causes of ARF, toxic causes (contrast, aminoglycosides, and other drugs) have increased and appear to have a good prognosis, with survival rates approaching 80%, while other causes such as sepsis and heart disease have poorer survival rates (approximately 45%) [2, 6].

Many series suggest that medical causes in general have a better prognosis than surgical causes, but there are other studies than find cause of no help in determining prognosis, despite adequate numbers of medical and surgical patients [7].

Series examining surgical patients show survival rates between 19% and 47%, but discriminant analyses have given conflicting results regarding surgery, identifying cardiac and vascular surgery by some and noncardiovascular surgery by other authors as predictive of mortality [24]. The problem appears to lie in the case mix. Others have attempted closer definitions of renal pathologies, using prerenal, postrenal, and the different subtypes of intrinsic renal failure in their classification. In a largely descriptive study of community-acquired ARF, Kaufman et al. [10] found that despite a rapid reversal of ARF in prerenal and postrenal patients, mortality was still high (prerenal 7%, postrenal 24%, intrinsic 55%), possibly reflecting coexisting diseases. The inconsistency in exclusion criteria between the various series makes it difficult to draw conclusions about the usefulness of this sort of classification as far as outcome is concerned.

Coexisting Diseases

In studies using multivariate analysis, hypotension was found to be an independent predictor of mortality [7]. Inotropic drug use for blood pressure support, 1 week after diagnosis, was predictive of death in one multivariate analysis [25]. Chronic heart disease appears less predictive [7], and it was only Rasmussen et al.'s [22] study that found it discriminating (together with acute cardiac disease). Acute respiratory failure or the need for mechanical ventilation are predictors of a bad outcome in most series [7, 9, 24, 26]. In a large study (134 patients) of ARF in an ICU, the need for mechanical ventilation 48 h after admission was a better predictor of mortality than at admission or after 24 h. This study also used multivariate analysis; however, the equations used were not published [27]. An initial requirement for artificial ventilation was also strongly correlated with outcome in a recent study on 250 ICU patients with ARF: 65 of 77 (84%) nonventilated patients and 67 of 173 (39%) ventilated patients survived ($p < 0.001$) [28]. In the study by Bellomo et al. [29], 72.7% of his patients received artificial ventilation and 40.9% had more than four failing organs. The mean APACHE II score was 27.7. ALL patients were treated with continuous haemofiltration. Despite the degree of illness severity, 32.2% survived to discharge from hospital.

Studies of adult respiratory distress syndrome (ARDS) have also found this to be predictive of death [22]. Coma or acute neurological dysfunction have been frequently predictive of death, with a few dissenting studies [7]. In 126 patients needing dialysis, Lohr et al. [30] found that death in coma patients was not independent of the need for mechanical ventilation. Convulsions have not been found to be predictive of mortality [7]. Suspected or proven sepsis were predictive of mortality in many univariate series, with a higher mortality for gram-positive sepsis, compared to gram-negative sepsis and ARF [7]. In contrast, multivariate analyses have failed to find an independent link between sepsis and mortality in surgical patients, ICU patients, a general hospital population, or patients needing dialysis [7].

Malignancy carried a poor prognosis in the largest series of ARF [2, 22]. Vascular surgery was related to death in a multivariate study [31], while another such study found the presence of peripheral vascular disease to be predictive on univariate, but not on multivariate, analysis [17].

Other coexisting diseases studied not predictive of mortality were diabetes mellitus, hypertension, immune deficiencies, urological abnormalities, dehydration, liver failure or disease (except in two series), and alcoholism [7]. Nevertheless, coexisting diseases do play a large role in determining mortality and in generating the variability between studies. Overall, the important predictive factors for mortality in most series appear to be hypotension, acute or chronic heart failure, acute cardiac infarction, mechanical ventilation, acute respiratory failure, ARDS, coma, sepsis, and malignancy. Several of these factors may not be independent predictors of death, especially coma with mechanical ventilation, and sepsis with malignancy [7].

Severity of Renal Injury

Of all the parameters of renal injury, oliguria appears to be the most important and carried major weight in multivariate analyses [7,17, 22].

ARF does not seem to have a worse prognosis in patients already suffering from chronic renal failure [7]. However, Rasmussen et al.'s study is an important exception, finding that chronic renal failure carried intermediate weight in determining a poor prognosis [22]. In another study of 38 patients needing dialysis for more than 4 weeks, chronic renal failure was a predictor of mortality [14].

Serum creatinine at the time of admission or diagnosis of ARF lacks predictive value [7]. Of the laboratory parameters reputed to reflect the severity of renal injury, only the peak creatinine level has been found to relate to outcome in more than one univariate study [7]. One multivariate analysis found the peak creatinine unrelated to outcome [27]. Urea levels (either on admission, at time of diagnosis, rate of rise or peak levels) appear to be unhelpful [7].

Complications

Multivariate analysis in studies of ICU patients show that only cardiovascular failure as a complication of ARF was predictive of death and failed to show a relationship between other organ failures developing after the onset of ARF and mortality [9]. Nevertheless, the mortality of ARF in the setting of the ICU, where it usually occurs as part of the wider syndrome of MOF, remains high (62%–87.5%) [32]. Since the majority of MOF patients die with ARF, and not from it, it is unrealistic to expect to find that different modalities of renal support affect outcome, unless a technique is developed which directly influences the course of MOF, perhaps by the removal of significant amounts of cytokines. Concentrating upon the underlying causes and processes of MOF is far more likely to lead to an improvement in patient survival.

Bleeding diathesis and gastrointestinal bleeding have not been found to worsen prognosis [6, 7, 27]. The role of complications in outcome after ARF has been inadequately studied, but factors occurring before ARF appear to be more closely associated with death than factors developing after ARF onset [7]. In the recent study by Liaño et al. [17], the number of complications during ATN development was higher in nonsurvivors than in survivors (2.2 ± 1.2 versus 0.6 ± 1.1, $p < 0.001$).

Treatment

Central to the treatment of severe ARF is dialysis. Several groups have tried to study the effect of the intensity of dialysis on outcome using control populations and have found no difference [7]. Others reported the need for dialysis to carry a poorer prognosis on univariate analysis; however, this factor did not retain independent predictive value on discriminant analysis [17]. Several series have found no influence of dialysis type or duration on outcome [1, 7].

Inotropic support in ARF patients has been studied in ICU populations, but data are inconclusive [20, 24, 26, 27].

Several groups have tried to examine parenteral nutrition and enteral nutrition, more as markers of the severity of illness rather than as trials of therapy. Methodological flaws make meaningful interpretation of these findings difficult [7].

Other Laboratory Parameters

Potassium and sodium levels, acidosis, blood count, thyroid function, bacteremia, and the renal failure index have not been found to be good predictors of outcome [7]. Other factors that are predictive for mortality on univariate analysis, but failed to be independent factors on multivariate analysis, are raised lipase and amylase levels, albumin and bilirubin levels, and renal biopsy findings [7].

Organ Survival

ARF appears to be something of an "all or nothing" phenomena, and it is usually considered that those leaving hospital should have enough renal function to be able to lead a normal life. However, this is not always the case: about 1% of ARF patients needing dialysis will enter a chronic dialysis program, increasing to a rate of 6% in ARF following aortic aneurysm surgery. Some patients retain functional derangements long after the ARF episode, more frequently in older patients [1, 7]. Despite multiple renal insults and prolonged dialysis support of more than 1 month, 23 (88%) of 26 survivors recovered sufficient renal function to discontinue dialysis [14]. Irreversible renal failure was seen more frequently in patients with preexisting renal insufficiency in this series. Few studies have been done on long-term prognosis. The results of Bonomini et al. [33] show that 5 years after the acute episode, chronic renal failure may be expected to occur in about 50% of patients with ARF due to glomerular and vascular injuries.

Epidemiological Information

A review of the literature on factors influencing outcome in ARF reveals uncertainty about the predictive value of almost every parameter (Table 1). The current situation appears as confused as when Butkus [34] identified the difficulties in this field almost 10 years ago in a seminal editorial. This is due

Table 1. Important prognostic factors in acute renal failure (ARF)

Factor	Number of studies predictive of adverse prognosis	Number of studies not predictive
Age	9	13
Cause[a]	7	4
Hypotension	12	2
Ventilation	12	0
Coma	6	6
Sepsis	8	5
CRF	2	6
Oliguria	9	4
Creatinine[b]	4	8

For more details and complete references, see reference [7].
CRF, chronic renal failure
[a] Surgical causes (poor prognosis) compared to medical causes.
[b] Peak levels (definitions vary depending on authors).

to the lack of large prospective studies using appropriate statistical methods and the differing selection criteria between studies. Multicenter studies are rare, although recently a very interesting prospective multicenter study has been completed in Spain [17]. Thus the factors that should be collected in future studies include age, setting of ARF (obstetric, medical-toxic, medical-others, surgical), hypotension, acute or chronic heart failure, cardiac infarction, mechanical ventilation, ARDS, coma, jaundice, suspected or proven sepsis, neoplasia, pancreatitis, chronic renal failure, oliguria, creatinine, clotting times, glucose, and albumin [7].

Severity Scoring

Although scoring systems may predict with some accuracy the prognosis of a group of patients in the presence of a concrete circumstance and are useful for research, they are unlikely to be useful in the assessment of prognosis in a given individual [1]. In the intensive care literature, diverse methods of establishing prognosis, varying according to the patient's clinical condition, have appeared. Among them, the most noteworthy are: TISS (therapeutic intervention scoring system), APACHE (acute physiology and chronic health evaluation), SAPS (simplified acute physiology score), MPM (mortality prediction model), APACHE II, and APACHE III [1]. Of these, APACHE II, a scoring system based on simple laboratory and clinical parameters, has had the most impact. However, its use in the case of ARF patients has been rare and although it was found promising in retrospective analyses, prospective evaluations failed to confirm this [1, 7].

The characteristics that an ideal system of prognosis evaluation should have, are efficiency, earliness, simplicity, reproducibility, universality, and high discriminative power [1]. High sensitivity and specificity are required for the system to be efficient.

Recently, Liaño et al. [17] proposed the following scoring system for patients with ATN only: the patient's probability of death (ATN individual severity score) = 0.032 (age decades) − 0.086 (sex) − 0.109 (nephrotoxic) + 0.109 (oliguria) + 0.116 (hypotension) + 0.122 (jaundice) + 0.150 (coma) − 0.154 (consciousness) + 0.182 (assisted respiration) + 0.21.

Each clinical variable takes the value of 1 or 0, depending on its presence or absence, with exception of the age, which takes the value of the patient's decade. Hypotension was defined as a systolic blood pressure below 100 mmHg; jaundice was defined as a bilirubinemia of more than 2 mg/dl; and nephrotoxicity was based on a clinical assessment of the etiology of ATN. The parameters mentioned are obtained at referral to the nephrologist or in the first 24 h of hospitalization if it is caused by ATN. This equation allows the use of a discriminative cutoff point of 0.9, above which no patient has survived.

In another recent study [28], logistic regression analysis was also used prospectively in 250 consecutive ARF patients treated with continuous hemofiltration to identify important prognostic factors, and the regression coefficients were used to weight an illness severity scoring system. Outcome was related to age, need for artificial ventilation, use of inotropes, urine volume, serum bilirubin, arterial base deficit, and serum creatinine. With a cutoff point chosen to give approximately equal sensitivity and specificity, this "full model" had a sensitivity of predicting mortality of 81% and a specificity of 80%. In order to produce a manageable scoring system, a simplified model based on the first five of these variables and rounding the coefficients to a whole number had a specificity of predicting death of 67% and a sensitivity of 76%. These authors conclude that the possibility of identifying groups of patients with different risks clearly provides a useful aid to self-audit.

Although it is important for ICU physicians and nephrologists to predict mortality in the first 24 h after hospitalization, relying on one score only can be misleading. One interesting report by Wendon et al. [35] shows that in ARF patients treated with continuous high-volume venous–venous haemofiltration, there was a decrease in the APACHE II score at the first and second day of treatment in those who survived, whereas this was not so in patients who died. Some authors have pointed out that in the case of mechanical ventilation, heart failure and hypotension, evaluation at 48 h may be more useful than at the time of diagnosis [27]. Also, the time between the insult causing ARF and admission to the hospital varies between patients and between the different causes of ARF, which can lead to important differences in progress during the first days of admission. Supportive care, or lack of it, can influence prognosis in the first days. Therefore, a score usable in different centres and for different causes of ARF should be repeated after, say, 48 h. It is obviously important that a poor score does not become a "self-fullfilling" prophecy and lead to therapecutic nihilism [1]. The ideal prognostic index would allow us to predict mortality in an individual patient, to estimate the prognosis of a group of patients, to compare patients enrolled in clinical trials of specific treatments, to compare clinical centres, and to estimate the correct allocation of resources devoted to the treatment of these patients.

Conclusion

A review of the literature on factors influencing outcome in ARF reveals uncertainty about the predictive value of almost every parameter. Future studies should be prospective, multicenter studies, involving a large, heterogeneous population, and results should be analyzed using multivariate analyses. Any scoring system derived from these discriminant functions should be clinician-friendly and should incorporate a system where the components parts of the score can be broken down and read. It is essential that any scoring system be calculable at diagnosis of ARF. However, it may be of value to reassess the parameters after 48 h to determine the predictive value of the response of the patient to appropriate treatment.

It is important not to forget that the mortality of ARF in the setting of the ICU, where it often occurs as part of the wider syndrome of MOF, remains very high. Concentrating upon the underlying causes and pathogenesis of MOF is most likely to lead to an improvement in patient survival in the ICU.

References

1. Liaño F (1993) Severity of acute renal failure: the need of measurement. In: Papadimitriou M, Alexopoulos E (eds) Proceedings of the 3rd international symposium on acute renal failure. University Studio Press, Thessaloniki, pp 181–192
2. Turney JH, Marshall DH, Brownjohn AM, Ellis CM, Parsons FM (1990) The evolution of acute renal failure, 1956–1988. Q J Med 74:83–104
3. Biesenbach G, Zazgornik J, Kaiser W, Grafunger P, Study U, Necek S (1992) Improvement in prognosis of patients with acute renal failure over a period of 15 years: an analysis of 710 cases in a dialysis center. Am J Nephrol 12:319–323
4. Cameron JS (1990) Acute renal failure thirty years on. Q J Med 74:1–2
5. Smithies MN, Cameron JS (1989) Can we predict outcome in acute renal failure? Nephron 51:297–300
6. Corwin HL, Bonventre JV (1989) Factors influencing survival in acute renal failure. Semin Dial 2:220–225

7. Chew SL, Lins RL, Daelemans R, De Broe ME (1993) Outcome in acute renal failure. Nephrol Dial Transplant 8:101–107
8. Feest TG, Round A, Hamad S (1993) Incidence of severe acute renal failure in adults: results of a community based study. Br Med J 306:481–483
9. Groeneveld ABJ, Tran DD, van der Meulen J, Nauta JJP, Thijs JG (1991) Acute renal failure in the medical intensive care unit: predisposing, complicating factors and outcome. Nephron 59:602–610
10. Kaufman J, Dhakai M, Patel B, Hamburger R (1991) Community-acquired acute renal failure. Am J Kidney Dis 17:191–198
11. Hou SH, Bushinsky DA, Wish JB, Cohen JJ, Harrington JT (1983) Hospital-acquired renal insufficiency: a prospective study. Am J Med 74:243–248
12. Shusterman M, Strom BL, Murray TG, Morrison G, West SL, Maislin G (1987) Risk factors and outcome of hospital-acquired acute renal failure. Am J Med 83:65–71
13. Jochimsen F, Schäfer JH, Maurer A, Distler A (1990) Impairment of renal function in medical intensive care: predictability of acute renal failure. Crit Care Med 18:480–485
14. Spurney RF, Fulkerson WJ, Schwab SJ (1991) Acute renal failure in critically ill patients: prognosis for recovery of kidney function after prolonged dialysis support. Crit Care Med 19:8–11
15. Tran DD, Oe PL, de Fijter CWH, van der Meulen J, Cuesta MA (1993) Acute renal failure in patients with acute pancreatitis: prevalence, risk factors and outcome. Nephrol Dial Transplant 8:1079–1084
16. Pascual J, Orofino L, Liaño F et al. (1990) Incidence and prognosis of acute renal failure in older patients. J Am Geriatr Soc 38:25–30
17. Liaño F, Gallego A, Pascual J et al. (1993) Prognosis of acute tubular necrosis: an extended prospectively contrasted study. Nephron 63:21–31
18. Davidman M, Oslon P, Kohen J, Leithert T, Kjellstrand C (1991) Iatrogenic renal disease. Arch Intern Med 151:1809–1812
19. McMurray SD, Luft FC, Maxwell DR et al. (1978) Prevailing patterns and predictor variables in patients with acute tubular necrosis. Arch Intern Med 138:950–955
20. Maher ER, Robinson KN, Scoble JE et al. (1989) Prognosis of critically ill patients with acute renal failure: Apache II score and other predictive factors. Q J Med 72:857–866
21. Jungers P, Zingraff J, Albouze G et al. (1993) Late referral to maintenance dialysis: detrimental consequences. Nephrol Dial Transplant 8:1089–1093
22. Rasmussen HH, Pitt EA, Ibels LS, McNeil DR (1985) Prediction of outcome in acute renal failure by discriminant analysis of clinical variables. Arch Intern Med 145:2015–2018
23. Lameire N, Matthys E, Vanholder R et al. (1987) Causes and prognosis of acute renal failure in elderly patients. Nephrol Dial Transplant 2:316–322
24. Berisa F, Beaman M, Adu D et al. (1990) Prognostic factors in acute renal failure following aortic aneurysm surgery. Q J Med 76:689–698
25. Lien J, Chan V (1985) Risk factors influencing survival in acute renal failure treated by hemodialysis. Arch Intern Med 145:2067–2069
26. Spiegel DM, Ullian ME, Zerbe GO, Berl T (1991) Determinants of survival and recovery in acute renal failure patients dialysed in intensive care units. Am J Nephrol 11:44–47
27. Schaefer JH, Jochimsen F, Keller F, Wegscheider K, Distler A (1991) Outcome prediction of acute renal failure in medical intensive care. Intensive Care Med 17:19–24
28. Barton IK, Hilton PJ, Taub NA et al. (1993) Acute renal failure treated by hemofiltration: factors affecting outcome. Q J Med 86:81–90
29. Bellomo R, Boyce N (1993) Acute continuous hemodiafiltration: a prospective study of 110 patients and a review of the literature. Am J Kidney Dis 21:508–518
30. Lohr JW, McFarlane MJ, Grantham JJ (1988) A clinical index to predict survival in acute renal failure patients requiring dialysis. Am J Kidney Dis 11:254–259
31. Cioffi WG, Ashikaga T, Gamelli RL (1984) Probability of surviving postoperative acute renal failure. Ann Surg 200:205–211

32. Beale R (1993) Outcome of acute renal failure in the intensive care unit, related to the mode of renal replacement. In: Papadimitriou M, Alexopoulos E (eds) Proceedings of the 3rd international symposium on acute renal failure. University Studio Press, Thessaloniki, pp 194–195
33. Bonomini V, Stefoni S, Vangelista A (1984) Long-term patient and renal prognosis in acute renal failure. Nephron 36:169–172
34. Butkus DE (1983) Persistent high mortality in acute renal failure. Are we asking the right questions? Arch Intern Med 143:209–212
35. Wendon J, Smithies M, Sheppard M et al. (1989) Continuous arteriovenous high volume venous-venous hemofiltration in acute renal failure. Intensive Care Med 15:358–363

Measurement of Glomerular Filtration Rate in the Acutely Ill Patient: The Challenge to the Nephrologist in the Intensive Care Unit

J.P. Bosch

Improvements in morbidity and mortality of patients acutely ill admitted to the intensive care unit (ICU) will depend on the ability of the staff to provide, when required, specific organ support.

Organ support in the ICU implies the ability to maintain or replace a given bodily function by providing the necessary intervention. Nutritional support requires the ability to provide amino acids, calories, and other nutrients to maintain metabolic needs. Cardiac support may call for the administration of cardiotonic drugs or vasodilator agents to decrease pre- or afterload; in extreme cases an aortic balloon pump may be required to maintain cardiac output. Respiratory support may need the use of mechanical ventilation to maintain vital gas exchange. Renal support may require the administration of drugs that induce renal vasodilatation and preserve renal blood flow when systemic pressure is reduced. In the absence of significant renal function, this may be replaced by the use of dialysis or continuous therapies.

In order to provide the necessary support, it is fundamental to be able to monitor the specific organ function. The need for nutritional support may be assessed by changes in albumin concentration or by analysis of the protein and caloric requirements of the patient. The necessity for cardiac support may be inferred from hemodynamic and pressure measurements such as cardiac output and pulmonary and arterial pressure. Measurement of arterial blood gases and airway pressure are a fundamental step in assessing lung function. Renal function is evaluated by time changes in plasma concentration of blood urea nitrogen (BUN) and creatinine. Urine flow and creatinine clearance measured over a period of time are also used to assess kidney function.

Once the function of a particular organ has been assessed as inadequate, support can be initiated if available. Depending on the sensitivity and accuracy of the parameter used to assess the function of the organ, the support can be effective in restoring the physiologic function and no further intervention will be required. On the other hand, further and more intense support may sometimes be required (Fig. 1).

If we consider the modern ICU it is clear that those organ systems for which there is an adequate methodology to assess the physiologic function simply, sensitively, accurately, and inexpensively are the ones for which

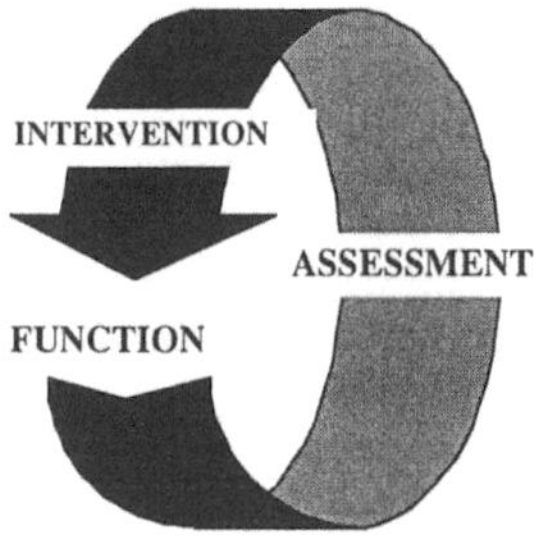

Fig. 1. Organ support in the intensive care unit (ICU). In order to maintain organ function, assessment by an easy, sensitive, accurate, and inexpensive method is essential to plan and time clinical interventions

more sophisticated and effective methods of support have been developed. For example, the ease of determining blood gases has spurred on the development of respiratory support systems with multiple variations. Gas exchange can now be maintained from minimal impairment to a very serious one. In contrast, in nephrology support of renal function is usually given to replace renal function by dialysis or another form of continuous therapy. This "all or nothing" approach to renal support is a consequence of the lack of an easy, sensitive, and accurate method in nephrology to assess changes in the glomerular filtration rate (GFR).

The traditional paramenters used to assess the need for renal support are changes over time of plasma values, urine flow rate, and creatinine clearance.

The use of plasma BUN changes over time to assess acute renal impairment is limited. In patients with decreased urea excretion due to volume depletion or with variable generation of urea over time, a change in concentration from 40 to 60 mg/dl may not indicate a worsening of renal function, but rather reflect increased catabolism or gastrointestinal bleeding. A decrease in BUN from 100 to 80 ml/dl may indicate an improvement of renal function, but also a decrease in catabolism due to the initiation of parenteral nutrition. In the presence of no significant renal function, plasma BUN concentration should increase by about 10–30 mg/dl per day depending on the metabolic status of the patient.

Plasma creatinine changes over time are more reliable indicators of changes in renal function. It must be remembered that an initial plasma creatinine concentration will double when GFR decreases by 50%. A creatinine concentration over 2.0 mg/dl represents a relatively small increase in concentration, but a major abnormality in glomerular filtration. An elevated creatinine concentration is an accurate indicator of renal impairment, but the rate of increase is an insensitive parameter of the seriousness of the derangement of GFR. A rise in creatine from 1.0 to 2.0 mg/dl in 24 h may represent a decrease of 60 ml/min of GFR (120 to 60 ml/min), while in the similar period an increase from 2.0 to 4.0 mg/dl only represents a 30 ml/min decrease (60 to 30 ml/min). In the presence of no significant renal function, plasma creatinine concentration should increase about 1.5 mg/dl or more per day.

The urine flow rate is helpful only when there is anuria, in which obstruction or cortical necrosis must be ruled out. A decrease in urine flow rate may occur in assocration with changes in the GFR, but in general patients may experience a considerable reduction in GFR without increases or decreases in glomerular filtration. In my experience the use of osmolarity, sodium concentration, or fractional excretion of sodium is not practical in the ICU to indicate changes in the severity of parenchymal damage.

The use of creatinine clearance to measure GFR in patients in the ICU is laden with problems. On a meat-free diet, urinary creatinine is derived entirely from endogenous breakdown of muscle creatine and phospocreatine [1]. Creatinine is more concentrated in the urine than any other easily measured, endogenous substance. The creatinine to inulin clearance ratio fluctuates widely in humans, indicating that creatinine clearance may both underestimate and overestimate GFR in some situations. Many potential errors may help explain this variability [1].

1. The accuracy of the endogenous creatinine clearance as a clinical index of GFR depends on a constant rate of creatinine production and excretion. However, 24-h creatinine excretion rates vary widely from day to day in some individuals. Perhaps this is due to changes in intake of meat, an important source of creatinine. Creatinine excretion rates may vary widely even in subjects on a constant protein intake.
2. The presence of significant amounts of nonspecific chromogens in plasma makes the precise measurement of plasma creatinine difficult.
3. Creatinine is not an ideal marker of GFR in humans, because there is significant tubular secretion and there may be reabsorption under conditions of very low urinary flow rate. The rate of secretion may be influenced by drugs. In normal humans, despite unequivocal evidence of creatinine secretion, the creatinine to inulin clearance ratio is close to unity. This may be a fortuitous result of balancing errors. Overestimation of plasma creatinine by standard methods that measure noncreatinine chromogens approximately balances the effect of tubular secretion endogenous creatinine clearance. In renal disease the creatinine to inulin ratio varies widely. In chronic renal failure it progressively increases as GFR falls, because tubular secretion of creatinine increases in absolute magnitude or in relation to the filtered creatinine. When GFR is 15–20 ml/min, endogenous creatinine clearance may overestimate inulin clearance by 50%–100%. When GFR falls below 15 ml/min, the creatinine to inulin ratio again approaches unity, suggesting that creatinine secretion is inhibited or creatinine reabsorption occurs in severely diseased kidneys. Tubular secretion of creatinine may be especially high

when renal failure is due to glomerular disease associated with heavy proteinuria.

In conclusion, at best endogenous creatinine clearance is a poor index of GFR; in the ICU and in patients with any degree of renal failure, it is not only a poor index but impossible to measure over a short period [2].

The use of other markers for the measurement of GFR, e.g., inulin, is also impractical in the ICU. The collection of timed samples and the delay in chemical measurements mean that they are not useful in the introduction of preventive therapeutic maneuvers.

It is evident that at the present time there are no adequate parameters to assess GFR in patients in the ICU. We must rely on indicators that only signal severe renal damage that has occurred in the past. This inability to predict renal dysfunction as it is occurring severely limits our therapeutic interventions (see Fig. 2). We are limited to providing total organ replacement, i.e., dialysis or continuous renal replacement therapies.

Recently, studies by Rabito et al. [2] have reintroduced [3], with modern technology, the use of rate constant for the clearance of an ideal filterable agent to provide a sensitive and accurate estimation of GFR. The basic principle behind this methodology is that an agent is administered to the patient and the disappearance rate of the marker is determined over time by a noninvasive method. From this, the rate constant for the clearance is calculated and it is possible to determine whether GFR increases, decreases, or remains stable during the observation period. The absolute value of GFR can also be determined. Rabito et al. [4] have developed the equipment necessary to determine the rate constant at short intervals. Therefore, using the concept of disappearance rate of a radioactive compound (99 Tc-DTPA, diethylene triamine penta-acetic acid) and an extracorporeal system to monitor the changes in concentration of the compound, these authors are able to monitor GFR continuously in the ICU.

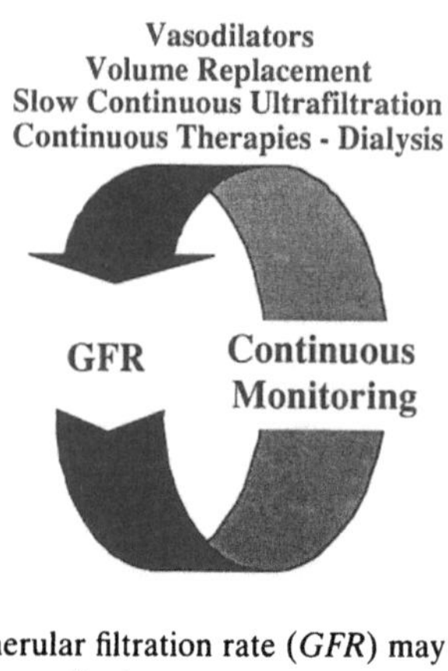

Fig. 2. Ideal renal support. Continuous monitoring of the glomerular filtration rate (*GFR*) may permit the timing of the appropriate clinical intervention to ensure the best outcome

The application of this principle and this technology may permit us, for the first time, to study acute renal failure under actual clinical conditions. Moreover, we may be able to assess the true value of preventive measures that are now commonly used. The utilization of noninvasive real time monitoring of renal function is a fundamental and essential method that has taken too long to arrive.

References

1. Levinsky NG, Lieberthal W (1992) Clearance techniques. In: Windhager EE (ed) Renal physiology. Oxford University Press, New York (Handbook of Physiology, Sect 8)
2. Rabito CA, Panico F, Rubin R, Tolkoff-Rubin N, Teplick R (1994) Noninvasive, real-time monitoring of renal function during critical care. J Am Soc Nephrol 4:1421–1428
3. Cohen LM, Patel JK, Baxter DL (1971) External monitoring of plasma disappearance for the determination of renal function: comparison of effective renal plasma flow and glomerular filtration rate. Pediatrics 48:377–391
4. Rabito CA, Moore RH, Bougas C, Dragotakes SC (1993) Noninvasive, real-time monitoring of the renal function: the ambulatory renal monitor. J Nucl Med 34:199–207

Rhabdomyolysis and Acute Renal Failure

A.G. Fabris and G. Fabris

Introduction

The term rhabdomyolysis defines an injury of skeletal muscle of such severity to cause a disruption of cell integrity and a release of its content into the circulation [1]. The lesion may be confirmed by serum elevation of creatine phosphokinase (CPK), aldolase, and myoglobin. The latter is a iron-containing protein, closely resembling hemoglobin, with a molecular weight of about 17.8 kDa. In healthy subjects its content is about 4 mg/g skeletal muscle [2].

Myoglobin, normally present in very small amounts in the plasma [2], has a renal threshold of 0.5–1.5 mg/dl; thus myoglobin plasma levels must exceed 1.5 mg/dl before entering the urine [2]. At low plasma levels, 50% of myoglobin is bound to α_2-globulin. Once the renal threshold has been exceeded, the possibility of seeing gross myoglobinuria depends on the amount of myoglobin released by the injured muscles, glomerular filtration rate (GFR), extent of the plasma protein binding of myoglobin, and the urine flow rate [3]. Therefore if a patient with normal renal function eliminates highly concentrated urine, visible myoglobinuria can be demonstrated with relatively small quantities of necrotic muscles. In contrast, if GFR is low and the patient is excreting large quantities of dilute urine, visible myoglobinuria may not be seen even if much larger quantities of necrotic muscles are involved [3]. Therefore, owing to the above considerations the term rhabdomyolysis is preferable to myoglobinuria [3].

Since the classic description of the syndrome during the bombing of London in the Second World War [4], many cases have been reported in the international literature [5–15].

Etiological Factors

Table 1 shows the causes of rhabdomyolysis from an etiological point of view. A more rational classification is, however, that in which the causes of rhabdomyolysis are divided into several categories, i.e., an imbalance between muscle energy consumption and production (the latter congenital

Table 1. Factors implicated in rhabdomyolysis

1. Direct muscle injury
   - a) Traumatic
     - Trauma
     - Crush injury
     - Burns
   - b) Immunologic
     - Polymyositis
     - Dermatomyositis
2. Excessive muscular activity
   - Physical exercise
   - Delirium tremens
   - Seizures
   - Status asmathicus
   - Prolonged labor
   - Acut psychosis
3. Drugs
   - Heroin
   - Methadone
   - Phencyclidine
   - LSD (lysergic acid diethylamide)
   - Fibrates
   - Barbiturates
   - Amphetamines
   - epsilon-aminocaproic acid
   - Codeine
   - Glutethimide
4. Infections
   - a) Bacterial
     - Tetanus
     - Legionnaire's disease
     - Leptospirosis
     - *Escherichia coli*
     - *Staphylococcus aureus*
   - b) Viral
     - Influenza
     - Mononucleosis
     - Coxsackievirus
     - Echovirus and adenovirus
5. Toxins
   - Ethanol
   - Carbon monoxide
   - Ethylene glycol
   - Toluene
   - Mercuric chloride
   - Wasp bite
   - Brown spider bite
   - Snake bite
6. Ischemia
   - Compression
   - Vascular occlusion (thrombosis and/or embolism)
   - Sickle cell trait
7. Metabolic disorders
   - a) Diabetes mellitus
     - Hyperosmolar nonketotic coma
     - Ketoacidosis
   - b) Hypokalemia
     - Diuretics
     - Hyperaldosteronism (primary or secondary)
     - Renal tubular acidosis
     - Parenteral nutrition
   - c) Hypophosphatemia
   - d) Hyponatremia
8. Genetic disorders
   - a) Altered carbohydrate metabolism
     - Myophosphorylase deficiency (McArdle syndrome)
     - α-glucosidase deficiency
     - Amylo-1-6-glucosidase deficiency
     - Phosphohexomerase deficiency
     - Phosphofructokinase deficiency
   - b) Altered lipid metabolism
     - Carnitine deficiency
     - Carnitine-palmityl-transferase deficiency
9. Others
   - a) Idiopathic, recurrent
   - b) High-voltage shock
   - c) Hyperthermia
     - Malignant hyperthermia
     - Heat stroke
     - Malignant neuroleptic syndrome
   - d) Hypothermia

or acquired), primary muscle injury, decreased muscle oxygenation, infections, and toxins [16].

According to this classification, rhabdomyolysis and myoglobinuria may be caused not only by a direct muscle injury, but also by a nontraumatic event such as that associated with increased muscle oxygen consumption (severe exercise. delirium tremens, seizures, heat stroke, cramps, hypertermia, and malignant neuroleptic syndrome), decreased muscle energy production (hypokalemia, hyphosphatemia, hypotermia, diabetic ketoacidosis, and genetic enzymatic deficiences), decreased muscle oxygenation (arterial thrombosis or embolism, compressive vascular occlusion, shock, carbon monoxide poisoning), infections, and direct toxins [3]. It is important to note that multiple factors capable of damaging muscles by different mechanisms may be present in the same category [5].

According to Gabow et al. [5], alcoholism and drug abuse appear to be responsible for the majority of cases of rhabdomyolysis. Another common cause is intense exercise, particularly when carried out by untrained subjects in hot, humid climates, although normal trained subjects cannot be considered free of rhabdomyolysis if they perform extremely exhausting exercises [1].

Pathophysiology of Rhabdomyolysis

The release of muscular constituents may be secondary to cell destruction or to alteration in cell membrane integrity, resulting in leakage of intracellular contents. One of the crucial points in the pathophysiology of rhabdomyolysis is the impairment in injured muscles of sarcolemmic sodium–potassium–adenosine–triphosphatase activity [1]. In most forms of rhabdomyolysis, and especially exertional rhabdomyolysis, red muscle fibers (type 2, oxidative) are predominantly affected [1]. In these fibers, damage is closely related to an inadequate resynthesis of adenosine triphosphate (ATP), which depends on local hypoxia [1]. Interference with the production of ATP, the source of energy that acts on active sodium–potassium exchange as well as on sarcolemmic calcium efflux, is followed by a reduction in the extrusion of sodium and calcium from the cells and by an intracellular increase of these ions [17] along with water and chloride [18].

The high levels of cytosolic free calcium activate neutral proteases that in turn cause disruption of myofibrils and Z-bands [19, 20], triggering muscle damage in exertional, ischemic, traumatic, metabolic, and toxic rhabdomyolysis [21]. Such ultrastructural lesions are the early visible alterations in rhabdomyolysis [17].

Intramuscular pressure plays an important role. Some authors have demonstrated that in a simulated limb-compression position, the increase in intramuscular pressure (in some instances up to 240 mmHg) is sufficient to cause ischemia and necrosis by local obstruction to the circultation [22].

Ischemic interference with the regulation of muscular cell volume causes cell swelling, which depends on intracellular solute accumulation and osmotic water influx, an increase in membrane leakiness, and a reduction of ion extrusion [18]. In muscle groups anatomically characterized by a low compliance, edema rapidly elevates the compartment pressure, producing compartment tamponade, and a self-perpetuating edema–ischemia cycle may develop [22]. Other factors such as hypoxia, hypotension, or vascular damage may be important, but compression seems to be the primary factor [22].

Adjunctive factors such as hypokalemia and hypophosphatemia are also important in the pathophysiology of rhabdomyolysis.

In skeletal muscle, blood flow, low at rest, increases rapidly during muscular work in order to deliver fuel for biochemical processes. This increase is important in removing metabolic products and transporting heat to the body surface where it is dissipated in the environment [23]. Although many products of muscle metabolism may play a role as possible mediators of exercise hyperemia, one of the most important is potassium. It is suggested that the increase in potassium concentration in the interstitial fluid of contracting muscle directly dilates muscle arterioles [23]. Therefore, it is possible that potassium deficits can interfere with arterial dilatation so that muscle blood flow during exercise does not rise appropriately, leading to relative ischemia and consequent muscle necrosis [24].

Phosphate deficiency interferes with ATP production, because the formation ATP from adenosine diphosphate (ADP) needs a sufficient quantity of phosphate [17]. Phosphate deficiency is also associated with a decline of 2,3-diphosphoglycerate in red blood cells; this may limit oxygen release at the cellular level [25]. Finally, ATP deficiency can morphologically alter red blood cells, which become spheric and stiff, a condition that increases the possibility of hypoxia [25].

Clinical and Laboratory Features

The usual clinical features of a patient with rhabdomyolysis are muscle pain, stiffness, weakness, tenderness, and swelling. It has been demonstrated both in humans [7] and in animals [26] that a large quantity of fluids, appearing as edema, may be sequestrated in the damaged muscles within hours or days. On the other hand, muscle swelling caused by sequestration of fluids may appear only after intravenous fluid therapy. Therefore, limb swelling after parenteral therapy used for resuscitation may be an important clue to recent rhabdomyolysis [5]. Adjunctive symptoms may be the presence of sweating and signs of circulatory insufficiency such as tachycardia and hypotension, most often secondary to dehydration, as manifested by reduced skin turgor and dryness of mucous membranes, nausea, and vomiting [6]. Sometimes muscle swelling may be extensive and may lead to signs of compression of peripheral nerves and vessels [6, 18]. A certain number of patients, however, complain of minimal symptoms or may be asymptomatic [5]. In these situations an anamnestic recall may help: age, sex (women are rarely affected by exertional rhabdomyolysis [1]), drug and alcohol abuse, physical activity, family history of chronic weakness, or muscle cramps associated with minimal exercise are important indicative elements. The definitive confirmation to the suspicion, however, comes from the laboratory.

Myoglobin

In normal man, the half-life of myoglobin is between 1 and 3 h; myoglobin completely disappears from the circulation in approximately 6 h [3]. Concentrations of about 100 mg/dl are necessary to cause visible staining in plasma [3]. However, to produce a plasma concentration of 100 mg/dl an enormous muscle destruction should be necessary. Taking into account that myoglobin content is 4 mg/g muscle and the distribution space of myoglobin is about 28.5 l [27], the staining of this volume would require elaboration of 28 500 mg myoglobin derived from the destruction of 7.1 kg muscle [3]. The same quantity of muscle contains an enormous quantity of potassium, the release of which would cause a sudden death before plasma myoglobin concentrations reach visible levels [3]. This possibility, together with the high renal clearance of myoglobin, probably explains why in rhabdomyolysis, unless GFR is markedly depressed or myonecrosis is very severe, plasma is usually clear, while urine stains red, red–brown, or brown. Myoglobinuria is confirmed by the positivity of orthotolidine dipstich in the absence of red blood cells at microscopic examination of urine, although some authors demonstrated that myoglobinuria was detected by orthotolidine dipstick in only 50% of patients and hematuria was present in a high percentage of individuals [5].

Enzymatic Syndrome

The most sensitive index of musle involvement is the elevation of CPK, particularly its isoenzyme MM [1]; the values of this enzyme are often greater than 100 000 IU/l. Without further muscle injury, CPK should decline by 50% in about 48 h [3]. A second rise, the so-called second wave phenomenon, may occur if necrosis has involved a muscle in a tight fascial compartment, in which edema produces ischemia and a second bout of necrosis [3].

Other enzymes involved are transaminases, aldolase-1, and lactic acid dehydrogenase (LDH)-4 and particularly LDH-5. Recently an increase in isoenzyme 1 of LDH and an inversion of the LDH-1 to LDH-2 ratio has been reported as characteristic of rhabdomyolysis [28, 29].

Electrolyte and Waste Products

Hyperkalemia, sometimes life-threatening, is often present during muscular destruction. Muscle cell potassium content is about 100 mmol/kg [3]; necrosis of about 150 g muscle will release more than 15 mmol, sufficient to elevate plasma and extracellular fluid potassium concentration by 1.0 mmol/l [5].

Renal function is the most important determinant of potassium levels in rhabdomyolysis. In one study, the average serum potassium concentrations were 4.4, 4.5, and 6.3 mmol/l in patients with rhabdomyolysis without renal failure, with nonoliguric ARF, and with oliguric ARF, respectively [30]. Therefore, the absence of hyperkalemia does not exclude the diagnosis of rhabdomyolysis, particularly when renal function is normal [5].

The phosphorus content of skeletal muscle is about 2.25 g/kg [3]. Massive muscle destruction, therefore, causes an important elevation of serum phosphorus concentration, in some instances up to about 20 mg/dl [6]. In the study by Gabow, however, serum phosphate was not a sensitive marker of rhabdomyolysis, because it was normal in patients without renal failure and elevated in azotemic patients. In the same study phosphate concentration was directly correlated with serum anion gap and inversely with bicarbonate concentration [5].

The serum anion gap in patients with rhabdomyolysis-related ARF was significantly higher than that in patients with non-rhabdomyolysis-related ARF [5]. The mean anion gap was also significantly higher in patients with rhabdomyolysis without renal failure than in other patients randomly selected on a single day from the wards of the hospital [5]. This suggests that unidentified organic acids are of some importance in rhabdomyolysis. Hypocalcemia occurs frequently and early in rhabdomyolysis. Because hypocalcemia varies directly with hyperphosphatemia [31], it has been attributed to the precipitation of calcum phosphate salts in injured muscles [32]. Low plasma levels of 1,25-dihydroxycholecalciferol (1,25-(OH)2 D), depressed by hyperphosphatemia, could also be responsible for the hypocalcemia of rhabdomyolysis [33]. Hyperphosphatemia, however, also stimulates the production of parathyroid hormone (PTH). Despite elevated levels of PTH, the hypocalcemia of rhabdomyolysis is not corrected, suggesting bone resistance to the calcemic action of the hormone [34]. During the diuretic phase of rhabdomyolysis-induced ARF, initially hypocalcemic patients may become hypercalcemic [6]. Possible explanations take into account healing of injured muscles and fall of phosphorus levels. Both of these factors may allow remobilization of calcium previously deposited in muscles [6]. Others factors include high levels of 1,25-(OH)2 D and PTH, suggesting that a rise in vitamin D levels restores the calcemic action of PTH [33].

Marked elevations of uric acid, often greater than 20 mg/dl, are frequent in rhabdomyolysis. It has been suggested that the source of uric acid is the purine released from injured muscles, which is rapidly converted to uric acid in the liver [3]. Comparing a group of patients with alcoholic rhabdomyolysis and a group of patients with exertional rhabdomyolysis, Knochel noted that in the latter group, serum urate was much higher. In fact, in exertional rhabdomyolysis, trained people have a greater muscle mass that releases more precursors which, in turn, are converted into uric acid by the liver. Alcoholics, with similar muscle destruction, but liver disease, cannot convert purine precursors to uric acid at the same rate [3].

Patients with exertional rhabdomyolysis have a disproportionate elevation of uric acid to urea nitrogen [3].

Finally, a disproportionate elevation of serum creatinine concentration with respect to the blood urea nitrogen (BUN) has been described [3]. This phenomenon is the result of the release of massive amounts of creatine from injured muscles, which is then converted to creatinine.

The most frequent major complication of rhabdomyolysis is acute renal failure (ARF), which may develop, as in the study by Gabow, in about one third of patients [5]. However, rhabdomyolysis has been implicated as the cause of overall episodes of ARF in approximately 5%–9% [6, 9, 13].

Pathophysiology of Myoglobinuric Acute Renal Failure

The commonly utilized model for studying ARF in rhabdomyolysis is the induction of myoglobinuria in the rat by intramuscular injection of glycerol [35, 36]. Although this form of injury is not completely comparable to that seen in humans, this model has been extensively used for elucidating the pathogenesis of renal failure. This has been attributed to a direct toxic effect of myoglobin or its breakdown products such as ferrihemate, renal ischemia, tubular obstruction, and backleak of filtrate [12, 37]. Because in experimental pigment nephropathy, tubular transport is depressed without a decrease in O_2 utilization [38], tubular anoxia resulting from an imbalance between O_2 supply (limited by renal ischemia) and continued O_2 demand should be considered as a further factor in the pathogenesis of ARF [3].

Nephrotoxicity of Myoglobin

It has been demonstrated that myoglobin per se is not nephrotoxic [37–40]. However, it becomes highly nephrotoxic when dehydration, acidemia, or both are present [39–41]. Aciduria sems to be an important requisite for myoglobin nephrotoxicity. At pH values less than 5.6, both hemoglobin and myoglobin produce ferrihemate [42]; the release of free iron from the heme portion of the molecule catalyzes the formation of toxic free radicals such as hydroxyl ions and lipid peroxidation [43] and perhaps inhibits the vasodilating effect of endothelial relaxing factors [44]. Dehydration and a concentrated urine potentiate the nephrotoxic effect of myoglobin in the presence of an acidic urine [41]. An otherwise benign level of myoglobinuria also increases its toxic effect when combined with an ischemia produced by temporary renal arterial occlusion [45].

Mechanism of Renal Failure

It has been suggested that increased renal vascular resistances and reduction of cortical blood flow are important factors, at least in the early stages, in the reduction of GFR and development of ARF [46–48]. It is important, however, to note that these functional changes appear to be due, in part, to the decreased circulating blood volume produced in experimental models [49] by the sequestration of fluids in the area of glycerol injection or at the level of damaged muscle in clinical situations [37].

The factors proposed as mediators in the initial vasoconstrition in myoglobinuric ARF are increased sympathetic nerve activity [50], activation of the renin–angiotensin system [51–54], suppressed renal prostaglandin synthesis [55], elevated plasma levels of vasopressin [56, 57], and the presence of glomerular microthrombi in cases of disseminated intravascular coagulation [58]. Finally, another possible mechanism responsible for the decrease in GFR might be a reduction of glomerular permeability [59–61].

The classical histologic picture in myoglobinuric ARF is tubular obstruction by cellular debris and pigmented casts. Some authors demonstrated cast precipitates of myoglobin and Tamm-Horsfall glycoprotein in medullary collecting ducts; however, the cast formation was considered important not in the initial fall in GFR, but in the maintenance of ARF [41].

Finally, it has been suggested that filtrate backleak accounts for only a small portion of the reduction in GFR in the myoglobinuric model of ARF [37].

Because ARF is such a serious complication, some authors have devoted their attention to what factors may be predictive of renal dysfunction.

In a retrospective study, Ward noted that renal failure could be predicted by a higher degree of serum CPK, potassium, and phosphorus [12]. Mean serum calcium and albumin were lower in the renal failure group. These patients also tended to be more acidemic, older, and more likely to have a history of hypertension. Patients presenting with dehydration and hypotension, sepsis, burns, and drug ingestion were most likely to develop renal failure [12].

Gabow introduced the following formula to help predict the risk of developing ARF:

$$R = 0.7(K) + 1.1(\text{creat}) + 0.6(\text{Alb}) - 6.6$$

where K is serum potassium concentration in mmol/l, creat is serum creatinine concentration in mg/dl, and Alb is serum albumin concentration in g/dl.

R values equal to or higher than 0.1 and R values lower than 0.1 represent high and low risk conditions for ARF, respectively [5].

Prevention and Therapy

Prevention and treatment of rhabdomyolysis are directed at the recognition of individuals at high risk. Most of these subjects are starved, volume-depleted, potassium-depleted, phosphate-depleted alcoholics [3].

One of the cornerstones of the prevention of rhabdomyolysis is the rapid and adequate correction of fluid deficits. In the crush syndrome, isotonic saline should initially be infused at a rate of 1.5 l/h, beginning as soon as the patient can be treated [18]. Once the systemic circulation has been stabilized and urine is present, forced mannitol and alkaline diuresis therapy should be started [7]. Using this aggressive and early therapy, none of seven subjects trapped under a collapsed building developed azotemia and renal failure [7]. After initial infusion (carried out before the whole body had been released from compression), patients were treated with an infusion of hypotonic sodium chloride and sodium bicarbonate in 5% glucose solution, to which about 10 g mannitol/l was added in a 20% solution. Once a diuresis of more 300 ml/h was achieved, fluids excreted in the urine were replaced with a solution of 5% dextrose containing sodium and potassium. Sodium bicarbonate was adjusted to maintain urinary pH above 6.5 [7]. This aggressive and abundant fluid replacement, however, was accompanied by a great retention of liquids in the injured muscles. Despite muscle swelling, pulse remained palpable and no new neurologic symptoms developed. Therefore, the positive fluid balance was well tolerated (at least in previously healthy young adults) [7].

The protective role of an alkaline urine against the development of ARF has been demonstrated in animals injected with myoglobin [39]. Animals with a urinary pH of less than 6 developed ARF, while ARF did not appear when pH was higher than 6 [39].

The utility of sodium bicarbonate has been questioned by Knochel, who claimed that a massive solute diuresis by itself results in an urinary pH of sufficient alkalinity to protect against pigment precipitation [3].

The use of loop diuretics is questioned for the prevention of rhabdomyolysis–ARF, because these agents have the theoretical disadvantage of acidifying the urine [18].

The correction of hypovolemia and acidosis, along with diuresis, is sometimes sufficient to control hyperkalemia. Alternatively, the administration of an ion-exchange resin (Kayexalate; sodium polystyrene sulfonate) is prudent, because the administation of glucose and insulin is not as effective as expected [37].

The infusion of calcium salts is not indicated, unless there is danger of hyperkalemic arrhythmia [18]. On the other hand, unless continuously infused, calcium administration corrects hypokalcemia only temporarily, because it is deposited in necrotic muscles. This may aggravate rhabdomyolysis and cause metastatic calcifications [32].

Aggressive use of phosphate-binding antiacids may be needed to control elevated phosphatemia [37].

With regard to fasciotomy, the introduction of intracompartmental manometry and the study of involved muscle with Doppler techniques has improved the management of the compartmental syndrome [18]. Some authors reserve early fasciotomy for patients whose compartmental syndrome is due primarily to interruption of arterial circulation [18]. On the other hand, it has been demonstrated that the use of hypertonic mannitol lowers intracompartmental pressure in the canine model, thus suggesting a possible conservative approach to the management of compartmental syndrome in humans [18].

Finally, in case of need, early dialysis may be required for the treatment of ARF, because patients tend to be severely hypercatabolic. Considering the molecular weight of myoglobin, however, convective techniques such as CAVH that utilize more permeable membranes should be considered as the dialytic technique of choice [62]. It has been demonstrated that with continuous arterovenous hemofiltration–dialysis (CAVH-D, with an average hourly value of ultradiafiltrate of 1500 ml), it is possible to remove 700 mg myoglobin/h from the serum [63]; Thus CAVH-D, by removing largely myoglobin, might have a protective or therapeutic role in the management of rhabdomyolysis even before the development of ARF [63].

In conclusion, rhabdomyolysis is a serious disease frequently observed in the intensive care unit, often complicated by ARF and sometimes by disseminated intravascular coagulation.

It has also been reported that hypophosphatemic rhabdomyolysis occurring in alcoholics or in patients with protein-calorie malnutrition during refeeding without adequate phosphate replacement is often accompanied by respiratory muscle weakness, hypoventilation, severe hypoxia, and hypercapnia [64].

All these complications mean that rhabdomyolysis must be treated vigorously and without delay. The early treatment of water, electrolyte, acid-base, and metabolic derangements is then mandatory to reduce morbidity and mortality.

References

1. Knochel JP (1990) Catastrophic medical events with exhaustive exercise: "white collar rhabdomyolysis". Kidney Int 38:709–719
2. Kagen LJ (1971) Myoglobinemia and myoglobinuria in patients with myositis. Arthritis Rheum 14:457–464
3. Knochel JP (1981) Rhabdomyolysis and myoglobinuria. Semin Nephrol 1:75–86

4. Bywaters EGL, Beall D (1941) Crush injuries with impairment of renal function. Br Med J 1:427–432
5. Gabow PA, Kaehny WD, Kelleher S (1982) The spectrum of rhabdomyolysis. Medicine (Baltimore) 61:141–152
6. Koffler A, Friedler RM, Massry SG (1976) Acute renal failure due to non-traumatic rhabdomyolysis. Ann Intern Med 85:23–28
7. Ron D, Taitelman U, Michaelson M et al. (1984) Prevention of acute renal failure in traumatic rhabdomyolysis. Arch Intern Med 144:277–280
8. Demos MA, Gitin E, Kagen JL (1974) Exercise myoglobinemia and acute exertional rhabdomyolysis. Arch Intern Med 134:669–673
9. Thomas MAB, Ibels LS (1985) Rhabdomyolysis and acute renal failure. Aust N Z J Med 15:623–628
10. Singhall P, Horowitz B, Quinones M et al. (1989) Acute renal failure following cocaine abuse. Nephron 52:76–78
11. Malik GH, Sirwal IA, Reshi AR et al. (1993) Acute renal failure following physical torture. Nephron 63:434–437
12. Ward MM (1988) Factors predictive of acute renal failure in rhabdomyolysis. Arch Intern Med 148:1553–1557
13. Grossman RA, Hamilton RN, Morse BM et al. (1974) Non-traumatic rhabdomyolysis and acute renal failure. N Engl J Med 291:807–811
14. Eneas JF, Schonfeld PY, Humphreys MH (1979) The efect of infusion of mannitol-sodium bicarbonate on the clinical course of myoglobinuria. Arch Intern Med 139:801–805
15. Richter RW, Challenor RA, Hayes PJ, Tedesco FJ (1977) Myoglobinuria and renal failure associated with thyphoid fever. JAMA 238:341–345
16. Glassock RJ (1990) Hematuria and pigmenturia. In: Massry SG, Glassock RJ (eds) Textbook of nephrology, 2nd edn. Williams and Wilkins, Baltimore, pp 491–500
17. Knochel JP (1981) Serum calcium derangements in rhabdomyolysis. N Engl J Med 305:161–163
18. Better OS, Stein JH (1990) Early management of shock and prophylaxis of acute renal failure in traumatic rhabdomyolysis. N Engl J Med 322:825–829
19. Reddy MK, Etlinger JD, Rbinowitz M et al. (1975) Removal of Z-lines and α-actinin from isolated myofibrils by a calcium-activated neutral protease. J Biol Chem 250:4278–4284
20. Blachley JD, Ferguson ER, Carter NW, Knochel JP (1980) Chronic alcohol ingestion induces phosphorus deficiency and myopathy on the dog. Trans Assoc Am Physicians 93:110–122
21. Cheung JY, Bonventre JV, Malis CD, Leaf A (1982) Calcium and ischemic injury. N Engl J Med 314:1670–1676
22. Owen CA, Mubarak SJ, Hargens AR et al. (1979) Intramuscular pressures with limb compression. N Engl J Med 300:1169–1172
23. Knochel JP (1972) Exertional rhabdomyolysis. N Engl J Med 287:927–929
24. Knochel JP, Schlein EM (1972) On the mechanism of rhabdomyolysis in potassium depletion. J Clin Invest 51:1750–1758
25. Knochel JP (1977) The pathophysiology and clinical characteristics of severe hypophosphatemia. Arch Intern Med 137:203–220
26. Bywaters EGL, Popjak G (1942) Experimental crushing injury: peripheral circulatory collapse and other effects of muscle necrosis in the rabbit. Surg Gynecol Obstet 75:612–627
27. Koskelo P, Kekki M, Wager O (1967) Kinetic behaviour of I-labelled myoglobin in human being. Clin Chim Acta 17:339–347
28. Fabris A, Pellanda MV, Gardin C et al. (1989) Rabdomiolisi da bezafibrato. Acta Med 2:907–909
29. Nanji AA, Pudek MR (1983) Unusual lactate dehydrogenase isoenzyme pattern in rhabdomyolysis. Clin Chem 29:1562–1566

30. Cadnaphornchai P, Taher S, McDonald FD (1980) Acute drug-associated rhabdomyolysis: an examination of its diverse renal manifestations and complications. Am J Med Sci 280:66–70
31. Meroney WH, Herndon RF (1954) The management of acute renal insufficiency. JAMA 155:877–883
32. Meroney WH, Arney GK, Segar WE, Balch HH (1957) The acute calcification of traumatized muscle with particular reference to acute post-traumatic renal insufficiency. J Clin Invest 36:825–832
33. Llach F, Felsenfeld AJ, Haussler MR (1981) The pathophysiology of altered calcium metabolism in rhabdomyolysis-induced acute renal failure: interactions of parathyroid hormone, 25-hydroxycholecalciferol, and 1,25-dihydroxycholecalciferol. N Engl J Med 305:117–123
34. Massry SG, Arieff AI, Coburn JW et al. (1974) Divalent ion metabolism in patients with acute renal failure. Studies on the mechanism of hypocalcemia. Kidney Int 5:437–445
35. Ayer G, Grandchamp A, Wyler T et al. (1971) Intrarenal hemodynamics in glycerol-induced myohemoglobinuric acute renal failure in the rat. Circ Res 29:128–135
36. Hsu CH, Kurtz TW, Waldinger TP (1977) Cardiac output and renal blood flow in glycerol-induced acute renal failure in the rat. Circ Res 40:178–182
37. Honda N (1983) Acute renal failure and rhabdomyolysis. Kidney Int 23:888–898
38. Braun SR, Weiss FR, Keller AI et al. (1970) Evaluation of the renal toxicity of heme proteins and their derivatives: a role in the genesis of acute tubular necrosis. J Exp Med 131:443–460
39. Perri GC, Gorini P (1952) Uraemia in the rabbit after injection of crystalline myoglobin. Br J Exp Pathol 33:440–444
40. Lalich JJ (1955) The role of oxyhemoglobin and its derivatives in the pathogenesis of experimental hemoglobinuric nephrosis. Am J Pathol 31:153–160
41. Garcia G, Snider T, Feldman M, Clyne DH (1981) Nephrotoxicity of myoglobin in the rat: relative importance of urine pH and prior dehydration (Abstr). Kidney Int 19:200
42. Bunn HF, Jandl JH (1966) Exchange of heme among hemoglobin molecules. Proc Natl Acad Sci USA 56:974–978
43. Paller MS, Hedlund BE (1988) Role of iron in post-ischemic renal injury in the rat. Kidney Int 34:474–480
44. Martin W, Villani GM, Jothianandan D, Furchgott RF (1985) Selective blockade of endothelium-dependent and glycerol trinitrate-induced relaxation by hemoglobin and by methylene blue in the rabbit aorta. J Pharmacol Exp Ther 232:708–716
45. Mandal AK, Davis JB, Bell RD, Miller JM (1989) Myoglobinuria exacerbates ischemic renal damage in the dog. Nephron 53:261–267
46. Oken DE, Arce ML, Wilson DR (1966) Glycerol-induced hemoglobinuric acute renal failure in the rat. I. Micropuncture study of the development of oliguria. J Clin Invest 45:724–735
47. Flamenbaum W, McNeil JS, Kotchen TA, Saladino AJ (1972) Experimental acute renal failure induced by uranyl nitrate in the dog. Circ Res 31:682–698
48. Chedru MF, Baethke R, Oken BE (1972) Renal cortical blood flow and glomerular filtration in myohemoglobinuric acute renal failure. Kidney Int 1:232–239
49. Reineck HJ, O'Connor GJ, Lifschitz MD et al. (1980) Sequential studies on the pathophysiology of glycerol-induced acute renal failure. J Lab Clin Med 96:356–362
50. McLean D, Thomson AE (1970) Effect of phenoxybenzamine on glycerol-induced acute renal failure in the rat (Abstr). Fed Proc 29:478
51. Di Bona GF, Sawin LL (1971) The renin-angiotensin system in acute renal failure in the rat. Lab Invest 25:528–532
52. Kokot F, Kuska J (1969) Plasma renin activity in acute renal insufficiency. Nephron 6:115–127
53. Tu WH (1965) Plasma renin activity in acute tubular necrosis and other renal diseases associated with hypertension. Circulation 31:686–695

54. McDonald FD, Thiell G, Wilson DR et al. (1969) The prevention of acute renal failure in the rat by long-term saline loading: a possible role for the renin-angiotensin axis. Proc Soc Exp Biol Med 131:610–614
55. Torres VE, Strong CG, Romero JC, Wilson DM (1975) Indomethacin enhancement of glycerol-induced acute renal failure in rabbits. Kidney Int 7:170
56. Hofbauer KG, Konrads A, Bauereiss K et al. (1977) Vasopressin and renin in glycerol-induced acute renal failure. Circ Res 41:424–435
57. Iaina A, Orndorff M, Gavendo S, Solomon S (1980) ADH effects on development of ischemic acute renal failure. Proc Soc Exp Biol Med 163:206–211
58. Blachar Y, Fong JSC, De Chadarevian JP, Drummond KN (1981) Muscle extract infusion in rabbits: a new experimental model of the crush syndrome. Circ Res 49:114–124
59. Cox JW, Baehler RW, Sharm H et al. (1974) Studies on the mechanisms of oliguria in a model of unilateral acute renal failure. J Clin Invest 53:1546–1558
60. Blantz RC (1975) The mechanisms of acute renal failure after uranyl nitrate. J Clin Invest 55:621–635
61. Schor N, Ichikawa I, Renke HR et al. (1981) Pathophysiology of altered glomerular function in amynoglycoside-treated rats. Kidney Int 19:288–296
62. Ronco C, Brendolan A, Bragantini L et al. (1985) Continuous arterio-venous haemofiltration. Contrib Nephrol 48:70–88
63. Berns JS, Cohen RM, Rudnick MR (1991) Removal of myoglobin by CAVH-D in traumatic rhabdomyolysis (Letter). Am J Nephrol 11:73
64. MacKlem PT (1986) Muscular weakness and respiratory function. N Engl J Med 314: 775–779

Drug-Induced Acute Renal Failure

G.J. Kaloyanides

Introduction

Acute renal failure (ARF) is a syndrome characterized by the rapid decline of renal excretory function manifested by depression of glomerular filtration and the accumulation in serum of nitrogenous waste products such as urea and creatinine. Among the leading causes of ARF in hospitalized patients ranks nephrotoxic reactions to drugs. In three prospective studies, drugs were implicated as a major factor in approximately 20% of cases of ARF observed in a hospital setting (Rasmussen and Ibels 1982; Hou et al. 1983; Kleinknecht et al. 1985). In this chapter the pathogenesis of drug-induced ARF commonly encountered in hospitalized patients will be reviewed and strategies for obviating this frequently fatal complication will be discussed.

Major Mechanisms of Drug-Induced Acute Renal Failure

Drug-induced ARF may result from one of four major mechanisms listed in Table 1. Renal hypoperfusion is the fundamental mechanism underlying the well-described syndrome of prerenal azotemia. Absolute or relative extracellular volume depletion secondary to diuretic therapy is probably the most common cause of this syndrome. Prerenal azotemia may be precipitated also by afterload-reducing agents. Because many elderly patients have elevated baseline renal vascular resistance due to fibrointimal hyperplasia accompanying hypertension or atherosclerosis, even modest reductions in mean arterial pressure may exceed their renal autoregulatory capacity and precipitate renal hypoperfusion and a pattern of prerenal azotemia. Patients with renal artery stenosis treated with angiotensin-converting enzyme inhibitors are at particular risk for this complication. Another common cause of this syndome is the use of nonsteroidal anti-inflammatory drugs (NSAID) in patients whose renal function is dependent on an adaptive increase in the synthesis of vasodilator prostaglandins. The diagnosis of prerenal azotemia is supported by a urine sodium of less than 20 mmol/l, a fractional sodium excretion (FE_{Na}) of less than 1.0%, a urine/plasma (U/P) creatinine ratio of more than 40, and a U/P osmolality of more than 1.4.

A second major mechanism of drug-induced ARF is acute tubular necrosis (ATN), which can be caused by a number of nephrotoxic agents (Table 1).

Table 1. Major mechanisms of drug-induced acute renal failure (ARF)

Mechanism	Examples
Renal hypoperfusion	Diuretics, vasodilating agents, converting enzyme inhibitors
Low systemic blood pressure	
Direct renal vasoconstriction	NSAID, amphotericin B, radiocontrast agents
Acute tubular necrosis (ATN)	Aminoglycosides, beta-lactams, amphotericin B, cisplatin
Intratubular obstruction	Sulfadiazine, acyclovir, methotrexate
Allergic interstitial nephritis	Beta-lactam antibiotics, NSAID

NSAID, nonsteroidal anti-inflammatory drug.

The diagnosis of ATN is supported by a urine sodium concentration greater than 40 mmol/l, an FE_{Na} greater than 1.5%, a U/P creatinine ratio less than 20, a U/P osmolality less than 1.2, and findings on examination of the urine sediment of muddy brown casts and tubular epithelial cells.

A third major mechanism of drug-induced ARF is intratubular obstruction caused by the intratubular precipitation of drug in the form of crystals or possibly in combination with protein. The diagnosis is supported by the presence of drug crystals often accompanied by microscopic hematuria in the urine sediment of a patient at risk for this complication. The urinary indices resemble those associated with ATN.

The fourth major mechanism of drug-induced ARF is allergic interstitial nephritis (AIN). The fully developed syndrome of AIN includes systemic manifestations of hypersensitivity often accompanied by skin rash, arthralgias, fever, and eosinophilia in a patient with ARF, hematuria that may be macroscopic, and pyuria that includes eosinophils. Unfortunately, the fully developed syndome is the exception rather than the rule. The urinary indices usually are indistinguishable from those of ATN, which is often the initial diagnosis until a renal biopsy establishes the correct diagnosis. The number of drugs reported to cause this syndome is enormous and continues to expand; however, often the evidence implicating a particular drug is not very compelling, especially when only a single case has been reported.

Determinants of Drug Cytotoxicity

The toxic as well as the therapeutic activity of a drug is critically dependent on the concentration of the active moiety reaching sensitive target sites and the duration of exposure of the target to the offending agent (Kaloyanides 1991). Because the kidney is the major route of excretion of a large number of drugs and their metabolites, this organ is frequently exposed to high concentrations of potentially toxic compounds. Depending on the mechanisms by which a drug is handled by the kidney, e.g., glomerular filtration, active or passive tubular absorption or secretion, metabolic transformation etc., specific cells within the kidney may be exposed to toxic concentrations of an agent. For example certain nephrotoxic drugs are eliminated primarily by secretion via the organic anion transport system of proximal tubular cells, and when the intracellular concentration of drug reaches a critical threshold, toxic injury occurs. In other cases active tubular absorption of drug is responsible for generating toxic concentrations of drug intracellularly. Whenever the fractional tubular absorption of water exceeds the fractional tubular absorption of drug, the intraluminal concentration of drug will rise. Thus, under conditions of antidiuresis, cells lining the distal nephron may be bathed in tubular fluid containing markedly elevated concentrations of potentially toxic drugs or their metabolites. In some cases the resulting rise in intraluminal concentration of drug may exceed the drug's solubility and lead to precipitation of drug in the form of crystals that may cause intratubular obstruction.

The capacity of a drug to interact with specific target sites on the cell membrane or within the cell is another important determinant of cytotoxicity. Some agents are inherently reactive, while in other cases the parent drug during the process of renal excretion undergoes metabolic activation via oxidative, reductive, or hydrolytic reactions to a more reactive species that may induce oxidative stress such as lipid peroxidation or may bind covalently to and inactivate critical macromolecules. Typically, these reactive species are converted via glucuronidation, sulfation, acylation, methylation, and glutathionation reactions to biologically inactive compounds that are water soluble and readily excreted in the urine. Increased accumulation of toxic intermediates may result from a primary increase in their generation or from impaired function of detoxification pathways.

Risk Factors for Nephrotoxic Acute Renal Failure

Hospital-acquired ARF typically results from one or more insults to a patient who, because of comorbidities, is predisposed to develop this complication. This is particularly true in the case of nephrotoxic ARF that develops in an ICU setting. In recent years, clinical investigators have attempted to identify and quantitate risk factors that contribute to ARF in general (Rasmussen and Ibels 1982; Wilkins and Faragher 1983; Shusterman et al. 1987; Groeneveld et al. 1991) and to specific forms of nephrotoxic ARF (Moore et al. 1984, 1992; Smith et al. 1986; Fisher et al. 1989). Clearly much work remains to be done in this area. Nevertheless, from such studies several factors have emerged, that either singly or in combination heighten the risk of a patient to develop ARF after exposure to a nephrotoxic drug:

1. Renal hypoperfusion
   a) Volume depletion

   b) Low cardiac output states
   c) Systemic vasodilatation
   d) Sepsis
2. Advanced age
3. Chronic disease
   a) Cardiac disease
   b) Renal insufficiency
   c) Liver disease
   d) Hypertension
   e) Peripheral vascular disease
   f) Diabetes mellitus
4. Exposure to multiple, potentially nephrotoxic agents

Paramount among these predisposing factors is renal hypoperfusion irrespective of cause. One consequence of depressed renal function is that renal excretion of drugs is impaired, and this may result in the exposure of the kidney to toxic quantities of a drug or metabolite. Prolonged renal hypoperfusion carries the additional risk of causing ischemic injury to tubular cells, and even mild or subclinical degrees of ischemic injury magnify the nephrotoxic potential of drugs even at doses that are considered below the toxicity threshold. Advanced age is another major risk factor for nephrotoxic ARF and may be related to the fact that the elderly patient is more likely to experience hemodynamic instability with renal hypoperfusion and ischemia. The age-related decline of renal function, estimated to be about 10% per decade after age 40, and the resulting loss of renal reserve and reduced capacity for renal tubular cell regeneration and repair also contribute to this risk. Moreover, failure to appreciate the fact that renal function in the elderly patient is often substantially lower than that suggested by the prevailing blood urea nitrogen (BUN) and serum creatinine may lead to inappropriate dosing of potentially nephrotoxic drugs. Similar mechanisms contribute to the increased risk associated with chronic renal insufficiency. Finally, it is common for patients in an ICU to receive multiple potentially nephrotoxic drugs. Often such drugs individually carry a low risk of causing renal injury; however, when administered in combination, they interact synergistically to cause severe nephrotoxicity. Details concerning specific drug interactions and related risk factors will be discussed in subsequent sections.

Outcome of Acute Renal Failure in the Intensive Care Unit

Hospital-acquired ARF has been shown to greatly increase the risk of death (Shusterman et al. 1987). During the past 20 years, mortality rates associated with ARF have ranged from 40% to more than 70% in various series depending on the case mix (Finn 1993; Wilkins and Faragher 1983; Cioffi et al. 1984; Bullock et al. 1985; Lohr et al. 1988; Turney et al. 1990; Groeneveld et al. 1991). Furthermore, renal replacement therapies have had a limited impact on lowering mortality rates in ARF (Finn 1993; Cameron 1986; Turney et al. 1990). It is well recognized that isolated ARF in the absence of serious systemic disease carries a relatively low mortality risk (Finn 1993). However, when ARF occurs as a complication of multiple organ failure, as commonly occurs in an ICU setting, the mortality rate may approach 100% (Wilkins and Faragher 1983; Cioffi et al. 1984; Cameron 1986; Lohr et al. 1988; Maher et al. 1989; Groeneveld et al. 1991). A number of studies have been undertaken to develop models that predict the outcome of ICU patients with ARF (Wilkins and Faragher 1983; Cioffi et al. 1984; Bullock et al. 1985; Rasmussen et al. 1985; Lohr et al. 1988; Maher et al. 1989; Schaefer et al. 1991; Groeneveld et al. 1991; Halstenberg et al. 1994). Factors identified as adversely influencing the prognosis for survival include advanced age, the type (especially cardiac and respiratory) and number of organ system failures, sepsis, and the severity of renal failure.

Given this dismal picture concerning outcome of ARF in ICU patients, the most effective strategy for dealing with this complication is primary prevention. In the case of nephrotoxic ARF, the physician by virtue of his/her decisions concerning diagnostic and therapeutic interventions plays the critical role in trying to obviate this complication. The first step is to be aware of the nephrotoxic potential of an agent or combination of agents especially when administered in a particular clinical setting. The second step is to conduct a risk/benefit analysis. Can another drug be substituted to achieve the same therapeutic goal with lower risk? If no alternative agents are available, then it behooves the physician to carefully assess what steps can be taken to minimize the risk of causing a nephrotoxic insult. Careful attention must be given to optimizing volume status, to improving renal perfusion, to correcting metabolic derangements and nutritional deficiencies, and to eliminating other agents that may potentiate the nephrotoxicity of the proposed drug. The dose of drug and the frequency and duration of its administration must be tailored to the individual patient in light of information about kidney function, cardiac function, liver function, and the influence of organ dysfunction on the pharmacokinetics and toxicity of all drugs. The patient must be closely monitored for signs of nephrotoxicity as well as for changes in the function of other organ systems and in metabolic status that may alter the nephrotoxicity potential of drugs being administered. Only by a process of systematically and thoroughly reassessing on at least a daily basis all the variables known to influence the risk of nephrotoxicity can meaningful progress be made in reducing the frequency of this all too often fatal complication.

Acute Renal Failure Caused by Specific Drugs

Antibiotics

Aminoglycoside Antibiotics

In various studies the incidence of aminoglycoside-induced nephrotoxicity as defined by strict criteria has ranged between 7% and 36% (Kaloyanides 1993). This variability reflects differences with respect to the nephrotoxicity potentials of aminoglycoside antibiotics currently in clinical use as well as differences among the patient populations receiving the drugs. A survey of clinical studies published between 1975 and 1982 reveals that the average incidence of nephrotoxicity caused by specific aminoglycoside antibiotics was: gentamicin, 14%; tobramycin, 12.9%; amikacin, 9.4%; netilmicin, 8.9% (Kahlmeter and Dahlager 1984). In critically ill patients, the incidence of nephrotoxicity was approximately double these figures (Plaut et al. 1979; Schentag et al. 1982).

Aminoglycoside antibiotics are organic polycations with a net cationic charge that at pH 7.4 ranges from +4.47 in the case of neomycin to +2.39 in the case of amikacin (Kaloyanides 1984). Because these compounds are highly hydrophilic, they are poorly absorbed across the intestinal tract and, therefore, must be administered parenterally. They are distributed in a volume that is slightly greater than extracellular fluid and eliminated from the body without metabolic transformation. The route of elimination is almost exclusively by the kidneys, and the mechanism of elimination is glomerular filtration. Of toxicological significance is the fact that a small fraction of filtered drug is transported into proximal tubular cells, primarily by adsorptive endocytosis, and accumulates within the lysosomal compartment, where it resides with a half-life measured in days. When the concentration of drug in renal proximal tubular cells reaches a critical threshold, clinical signs of nephrotoxicity become evident.

The clinical expression of aminoglycoside nephrotoxicity and its pathogenesis have been reviewed recently (Kaloyanides 1993; Humes 1988). Increased urinary excretion of low-molecular-weight proteins and lysosomal and brush-border enzymes are the earliest signs of toxicity and may appear within 24 h of initiating therapy. These changes are followed by increased urinary excretion of tubular epithelial cells, white blood cells, and casts, the magnitude of which correlate with proximal tubular cell injury. The frequency and severity of these changes rise as a function of the dose and duration of therapy. Typically, after 7 or more days of drug therapy, elevations of the BUN and serum creatinine become evident and signify the onset of depression of the glomerular rate (GFR). Nonoliguric ARF is characteristic of aminoglycoside toxicity, and maintenance of urine output at nonoliguric levels commonly persists even as GFR falls to profoundly low levels. If oliguria is observed, it usually signifies the presence of one or more complicating factors, e.g., ischemia or sepsis, especially if oliguria occurs early in the course of aminoglycoside administration. Even after stopping the drug, the BUN and serum creatinine often continue to rise slowly but progressively over a number of days. This implies that the full expression of tubular cell injury caused by these drugs may be delayed for several days. Other manifestations of aminoglycoside toxicity include hypokalemia and hypomagnesemia secondary to renal wasting of these cations. In rare cases a Fanconi-like syndrome may be seen.

Light and electron microscopy studies in animal models (Houghton et al. 1976) and in human kidney tissue (De Broe et al. 1984) implicate the proximal tubule as the principal site of injury. The characteristic ultrastructural lesion of aminoglycoside nephrotoxicity is the lysosomal myeloid body, a multilamellar structure composed of membranes rich in phospholipid that can be seen within 24 h of drug administration. Both the number and size of lysosomal myeloid bodies increase as a function of the dose and duration of drug therapy, which reflects the fact that the formation of myeloid bodies is causally related to the accumulation of aminoglycoside within the lysosomal compartment, where it inhibits the activity of lysosomal phospholipases and blocks the degradation of membrane phospholipid (Laurent et al. 1982; Mingeot-Leclercq et al. 1990). When the concentration of drug and/or the amount of lysosomal phospholipid in the form of myeloid bodies reaches a critical level, an injury cascade is activated that eventuates in proximal tubular cell necrosis. The precise mechanism by which aminoglycosides trigger the injury cascade remains unknown. One theory states that the injury cascade is triggered by the rupture of engorged lysosomes. The resultant release of high concentrations of drug into the cytoplasm leads to the adverse interaction between these organic polycations and a number of critical intracellular processes. Inhibition of mitochondrial respiration, inhibition of microsomal protein synthesis, disruption of the phosphatidylinositol cascade, and generation of hydroxyl radicals have been implicated in the injury cascade of aminoglycoside toxicity in animal studies (Kaloyanides 1993).

Aminoglycoside nephrotoxicity in animal models can be prevented or significantly modified by the administration of polyaspartic acid (Gilbert et al. 1989; Ramsammy et al. 1989; Kishore et al. 1992). This polyanionic compound has been shown to form electrostatic complexes with the cationic aminoglycoside antibiotics and, thereby, prevents these drugs from interacting with critical anionic targets on cell membranes (Ramsammy et al. 1990). The efficacy of polyaspartic acid in obviating aminoglycoside nephrotoxicity in humans has yet to be tested. Therefore, for the present time the primary focus of prevention of aminoglycoside nephrotoxicity in humans is understanding and modifying when possible the risk factors for this complication (Moore et al. 1984; Smith et al. 1986; Bertino et al. 1993).

Risk factors for the development of aminoglycoside nephrotoxicity not readily modifiable clinically include: age, female sex, obesity, preexisting liver disease, preexisting kidney disease, renal hypoperfusion, and sepsis. Factors potentially modifiable clinically include: daily aminoglycoside dose, interval, and duration, specific aminoglycoside, volume depletion, hypokalemia, hypomagnesemia, metabolic acidosis, and concurrent drug therapy (amphotericin B, cephalosporin, vancomycin, cisplatin, furosemide, radiocontrast agents).

Advanced age has been identified as a significant risk factor by Moore et al. (1984). The reason that female sex confers an increased risk remains obscure (Moore et al. 1984). Obesity also carries an increased risk for toxicity that is unexplained by differences in the volume of distribution or renal clearance of drug (Corcoran et al. 1988). Preexisting chronic renal insufficiency is associated with increased risk, primarily due to failure to adjust appropriately the dose of aminoglycoside for the level of impaired kidney function (Moench and Smith 1982). The increased risk associated with chronic liver disease (Moore et al. 1984) may be related to the alterations in extracellular volume, hemodynamics, and electrolyte balance commonly observed in this disorder and all of which are known to promote renal cortical accumulation of drug. Renal hypoperfusion from any cause carries an increased risk for aminoglycoside nephrotoxicity. This can be seen when the renal ischemic insult occurs before (Molitoris et al. 1993), during (Zager 1988), or after the period of drug administration (Zager et al. 1983). The latter observation is especially worthy of note because it implies that the increased risk of nephrotoxicity persists even after the drug has been discontinued. The prolonged half-life of aminoglycosides in renal cortex may contribute to this risk. Three components of the septic state – renal hypoperfusion, endotoxemia, and hyperthermia – have been identified as contributing to the heightened risk of ARF during aminoglycoside therapy (Zager 1992). Renal hypoperfusion and endotoxemia are associated with increased accumulation of drug in renal cortex; however, this factor alone does not explain the increased risk.

Of the risk factors that are potentially modifiable by the physician, the most important are daily drug dose, interval of dosing, and duration of therapy. A direct relationship between total drug dose over time and the incidence and severity of nephrotoxicity has been consistently observed (Kaloyanides 1993). In animal studies, increased nephrotoxicity was observed when the same daily dose of drug was given as a continuous infusion or in divided doses compared to once per day dosing (Gilbert 1991). These observations have stimulated additional studies to assess the antimicrobial efficiacy of once per day dosing with an aminoglycoside administered either alone or in combination with a beta-lactam antibiotic (Levison 1992; Prins et al. 1993; Rozdzinski et al. 1993; EORTC International Antimicrobial Therapy Project Group 1993). All of these studies have demonstrated that once per day dosing was as effective as standard dosing in the treatment of bacterial infection, and in one study (Prins et al. 1993) the incidence of nephrotoxicity was reduced. Additional studies are needed to better define under what clinical circumstances once per day dosing is appropriate. These observations, however, do provide a compelling rationale for prolonging the dosing interval rather than reducing the dose per interval in patients with chronic renal insufficiency.

Comparative studies in humans suggest that the rank order for clinical nephrotoxicity potential is: gentamicin > tobramycin > amikacin > netilmicin (Kahlmeter and Dahlager 1984). This knowledge should be considered when prescribing an aminoglycoside in a patient at increased risk for nephrotoxicity. Volume depletion, hypokalemia, hypomagnesemia, and metabolic acidosis confer increased risk for aminoglycoside nephrotoxicity (Kaloyanides 1993). In the case of volume depletion and hypokalemia, the increased risk appears to be related to increased accumulation of drug in the renal cortex. Importantly, these are risk factors that can be modified by appropriate interventions. Similarly, a number of pharmaceutical agents have been demonstrated to augment aminoglycoside nephrotoxicity in animals and/or in humans. This is particularly true for amphotericin B (EORTC International Antimicrobial Therapy Project Group 1993). Potentiation of aminoglycoside nephrotoxicity in humans has been demonstrated for cephalothin, but not for the third-generation cephalosporins (Rankin and Sutherland 1989).

The prevention of aminoglycoside nephrotoxicity requires that these drugs be used for well-defined indications and that they be prescribed in the appropriate dose and for the appropriate duration to achieve the therapeutic goal. Dosing based on drug pharmacokinetics derived from monitoring serum drug levels is a rational approach for achieving optimum therapy. Unfortunately, prospective studies have failed to demonstrate that dosing based on pharmacokinetics reduces the incidence of nephrotoxicity (Leehey et al. 1993). Nevertheless, frequent monitoring of serum drug concentration is still indicated in high-risk patients to ensure that therapeutic levels are being achieved and that toxic concentrations are being avoided. Even when all appropriate steps have been taken to eliminate or minimize risk factors and the peak and trough drug concentrations are within established guidelines, a certain number of patients will still develop nephrotoxic ARF. Some of these patients exhibit an abnormally high rate of drug accumulation in the renal cortex; in other cases increased sensitivity to a given load of drug appears to be responsible (Schentag et al. 1978). In any event, monitoring for nephrotoxicity is indicated in all patients receiving aminoglycoside antibiotics, with the intensity of monitoring dictated by the relative risk factors. In high-risk patients such as are commonly found in the ICU, daily monitoring of renal function and blood levels may be warranted. The objective is to detect signs of toxicity as early as possible so that appropriate action, e.g., stopping the drug, reducing the dose, lengthening the interval, can be taken to minimize furhter injury. Even when nephrotoxicity is recognized early and the drug is discontinued, nonoliguric renal failure may progress over a number of days with the serum creatinine and BUN rising to disturbingly high levels, and it may remain there for more than several days before renal function begins to slowly improve. No specific therapies have been shown to hasten recovery. The prognosis for recovery of renal function is dictated by the number and severity of associated risk factors.

Beta-Lactam Antibiotics

The penicillins, cephalosporins, and carbapenems comprise the beta-lactam antibiotics. This class of drugs may cause ARF secondary to acute proximal tubular cell necrosis or AIN. The rank order of nephrotoxicity potential as defined in animal studies is: cephaloglycin > cephaloridine >> cefaclor > cefazolin > cephalothin >>> cephalexin, ceftazidime, and penicillins which are not nephrotoxic (Tune 1986, 1993). The potential of these drugs to cause nephrotoxic ARF is determined by two factors. The first is the extent to which these drugs undergo concentrative uptake by the organic anion transport system of proximal tubular cells. The second factor is the intrinsic reactivity of these drugs towards intracellular target proteins. Current evidence implicates inhibition of mitochondrial respiration as the dominant mechanism of toxicity (Tune 1993). In the case of cephaloridine, lipid peroxidation also may play a role in the injury cascade (Goldstein et al. 1986).

The therapeutic to nephrotoxic ratio of these agents is much more favorable than that of aminoglycoside antibiotics. The incidence of serum creatinine elevations observed with the third-generation cephalasporins is difficult to state with certainty, but severe nephrotoxic ARF appears to be distinctly uncommon (Norrby 1987; Winston et al. 1991). Similar to other antibiotics, high doses and prolonged therapy elevate the risk for nephrotoxicity. Animal studies have demonstrated that the incidence and severity of nephrotoxicity assosicated with beta-lactam antibiotics are potentiated by aminoglycoside antibiotics, by renal ischemia, and by endotoxemia (Tune 1993). In three prospective studies in human subjects, the combination of an aminoglycoside antibiotic with cephalothin was associated with a dramatically higher incidence of nephrotoxicity, as manifested by elevation of the serum creatinine concentration, which was significantly higher than that predicted from the incidence of nephrotoxicity observed in subjects treated with either agent alone or in combination with another antibiotic (Klastersky et al. 1975; Wade et al. 1978; EORTC International Antimicrobial Therapy Project Group 1978). Whether other cephalosporins potentiate the nephrotoxicity of aminoglycosides in man is even less clear than the data implicating a synergistic effect of cephalothin. Early reports suggested an interaction between several second-generation cephalosporins and aminoglycoside antibiotics (Rankin and Sutherland 1989); however, in a recent report no interaction was evident between third-generation cephalosporins and aminoglycosides (EORTC International Antimicrobial Therapy Project Group

1993). The clinical experience with carbapenems in humans is relatively limited. Nevertheless, the available data indicate that these agents have the potential to cause toxic injury to renal proximal tubular cells by the same mechanism established for cephalosporin antibiotics (Tune et al. 1990).

The diagnosis of nephrotoxic ARF is suggested by the appropriate clinical setting in combination with a urine sediment and urinary indices typical of ATN. It should be kept in mind that beta-lactam antibiotics can also cause ARF secondary to AIN (Grunfeld et al. 1993). The pattern of rise in the BUN and serum creatinine as well as the urinary indices may be indistinguishable from that seen with ATN. The finding of large numbers of red and white blood cells in the urine sediment, especially if associated with eosinophiluria and eosinophilia, strongly suggests the diagnosis of AIN. However, in many patients these clues are absent or equivocal, and it may be necessary to perform a kidney biopsy to establish the correct diagnosis, especially in patients who exhibit delayed recovery of renal function after stopping the drug.

Vancomycin

The rise in the incidence of methicillin-resistant staphylococcal infection in recent years has stimulated increased clinical use of vancomycin. This drug is poorly absorbed from the gastrointestinal tract; therefore, it usually is administered intravenously for the treatment of systemic infactions. Vancomycin is not metabolized to any appreciable extent and it is eliminated almost completely in the urine, primarily by glomerular filtration, as there is no evidence that the drug undergoes tubular secretion or absorption (Moellering et al. 1981). Therefore, drug dosing must be modified in patients with renal failure. Animal studies demonstrated that vancomycin caused nephrotoxicity and ototoxicity (Wold and Turnipseed 1981). Early clinical experience in humans revealed a significant incidence of nephrotoxicity, which in retrospect may have been related to impurities generated during the initial manufacturing process (Cook and Farrar 1978). More recent reports indicate that the incidence of nephrotoxicity associated with vancomycin when given as sole therapy ranges between 0% and 7% (Appel et al. 1986). Animal studies suggested that vancomycin and aminoglycosides interacted synergistically to cause ARF (Wood et al. 1986). A recent study supports the conclusion that a similar interaction occurs in humans (Goetz and Sayers 1993). A prudent approach dictates that patients at increased risk of nephrotoxic injury be monitored closely for this complication while receiving vancomycin either as sole therapy or in combination with other potentially nephrotoxic antibiotics. The blood level of vancomycin should be measured in such patients to ensure that therapeutic concentrations are achieved and toxic levels are avoided.

Vancomycin has been implicated as a cause of AIN (Eisenberg et al. 1981), but this appears to be an uncommon complication.

Antiviral Agents

Acyclovir

Acyclovir is a potent antiviral agent effective in the treatment of infections caused by herpes simplex virus and herpes zoster virus (Dorsky and Crumpacker 1987). The major route of elimination is by renal excretion, which accounts for approximately 80% of total body clearance of drug (de Miranda and Blum 1983). As the renal clearance of acyclovir exceeds the creatinine clearance several fold, a substantial fraction of excreted drug must be eliminated by tubular secretion, which would favor the attainment of drug concentrations in excess of the drug's solubility estimated to be 1.3 mg/l. Approximately 85% of the drug recovered in the urine is unchanged; the remainder is recovered as the principal metabolite, 9-carboxy-methoxy-methyl-guanine.

Acyclovir has been reported to cause elevation of the BUN and serum creatinine in 10%–15% of cases in several large series (Keeney et al. 1982; Brigden et al. 1982). However, in one series of 23 patients, the incidence of acute renal insufficiency was 48% (Bean and Aeppli 1985). The clinical expression of nephrotoxicity ranges from asymptomatic azotemia to renal colic with nausea and vomiting. Examination of the urine sediment may reveal microscopic hematuria, pyuria, and birefringent crystals. The pathogenesis of acyclovir-induced ARF has been attributed to intratubular obstruction based on the observation in rats that crystals precipitated in the collecting duct (Brigden et al. 1982). In a recent study, acyclovir administration to rats was shown to alter the function of the proximal tubule and thick ascending limb of Henle's loop and to inhibit the response of the inner medullary collecting duct to vasopressin (Campos et al. 1992). These observations suggest that a direct toxic effect may participate in the pathogenesis of acyclovir-induced ARF. A recent case report provides support for this conclusion (Becker et al. 1993).

High drug dose, rapid infusion of drug, and low urine volume predispose to the development of ARF. The onset of azotemia occurs during the first few days of therapy in about half of the cases; it is usually transient and frequently resolves in response to increased fluid intake even while drug therapy is continued. However, severe renal failure has been reported even in patients who were prehydrated (Sawyer et al. 1988). Fortunately, renal function usually recovers even in these cases.

Foscarnet

Foscarnet is an antiviral agent that is being used with increasing frequency for the treatment of cytomegalovirus infections and acyclovir-resistant herpesvirus infections, especially in immunocompromised individuals

(Fanning 1990; Safrin et al. 1991; Dieterich et al. 1993). This agent is excreted unchanged in the urine by glomerular filtration and tubular secretion (Sjovall et al. 1989). ARF, often severe, is the major complication of therapy with this agent (Jacobson et al. 1993; Deray et al. 1989); however, the mechanism of the presumed nephrotoxic insult remains to be established. The incidence and severity of ARF can be greatly reduced by infusing normal saline at 1.5–2.5 l per day (Deray et al. 1989). In addition, foscarnet therapy has been accompanied by electrolyte abnormalities including hypo- and hypercalcemia, hypophosphatemia, hypokalemia, and hypomagnesemia (Gearhart and Sorg 1993; Berns et al. 1991).

Antifungal Agents

Amphotericin B

Amphotericin B continues to be the drug of choice for the treatment of many deep-seated fungal infections, especially in immunocompromised patients (Como and Dismukes 1994; Rowe et al. 1994). Unfortunately, the clinical application of this agent is associated with a number of toxic side effects, the most serious of which is ARF (Maddux and Barriere 1980; Medoff et al. 1983). Amphotericin B is a polyene that consists of a large lactone ring with seven conjugated double bonds, seven hydroxyl groups, and a sugar moiety. The toxicity of this drug has been attributed to its ability to increase membrane permeability to univalent ions and small electrolytes by creating membrane pores estimated to be composed of eight molecules of drug alternating with eight molecules of cholesterol (Bolard 1986). Amphotericin B binds preferentially to ergosterol, the major sterol of fungi, which is presumed to be the explanation of the selective toxicity of this and similar drugs for fungi (Brajtburg et al. 1990).

The reason amphotericin B preferentially causes nephrotoxicity in man and in animals is obscure. Studies of pharmacokinetics do not reveal the answer (Janknegt et al. 1992; Christianson et al. 1985; Atkinson and Bennett 1978). Because amphotericin B is poorly absorbed from the gastrointestinal tract, it is given by i.v. infusion. The volume of distribution is about 4 l/kg. Up to 95% of drug in serum is bound to protein, primarily beta-lipoprotein. The liver is the major depot site for amphotericin B, where up to 41% of administered drug can be recovered, whereas only 6% is found in the lung and 2% in the kidney. No metabolites have been identified. The elimination of amphotericin B from serum is described by a triexponential curve with a half-life of 24 h, 48 h, and 15 days, respectively. Less than 10% of administered drug is recovered in the urine.

Although the kidney is not a major route of elimination, it is the major site of toxicity. The incidence of amphotericin B-induced nephrotoxicity is influenced by a number of factors, including daily drug dose, duration of therapy, and the presence of potentiating risk factors (Fisher et al. 1989; Branch 1988). The clinical expression of amphotericin B nephrotoxicity is dominated by the appearance of azotemia and creatininemia, which may develop early in the course of drug administration (Butler et al. 1964; Medoff and Kobayashi 1980; Branch 1988) and reflects at least initially a reversible depression of renal blood flow (RBF) and GFR due to increased renal vascular resistance. With prolonged therapy, however, depression of renal function may persist due to the development of frank tubular cell injury (Wertlake et al. 1963) and possibly injury to the renal vasculature (Bhathena et al. 1978). Various abnormalities of tubular function may be seen as well including incomplete distal renal tubular acidosis (Patterson and Ackerman 1971), hypokalemia and hypomagnesemia secondary to renal tubular wasting of these cations (Burgess and Birchall 1972; Barton et al. 1984), and loss of urine-concentrating capacity (Barbour et al. 1979). Examination of the urine sediment frequently reveals microscopic hematuria, pyuria, celluria, and cylinduria. Most of these abnormalities are reversible after the drug is discontinued, but full recovery may be delayed for a number of months. Chronic renal insufficiency may occur with prolonged or repeated courses of drug therapy.

Studies in animals have provided insight into the pathogenesis of amphotericin B nephrotoxicity. Administration of amphotericin B causes an acute depression of RBF and GFR in association with an increase in renal vascular resistance by a mechanism that is not mediated by the renal nerves, angiotensin II, endothelium-dependent factors, or tubuloglomerular feedback (Cheng et al. 1982; Tolins and Raij 1988; Sabra et al. 1990; Sawaya et al. 1991). These alterations can be ameliorated by calcium channel blockers (Tolins and Raij 1991), by a selective dopamine A_1 receptor agonist (Brooks et al. 1991), by saline loading (Ohnishi et al. 1989), and by atrial natriuretic peptide or theophylline (Sawaya et al. 1991). Depolarization of vascular smooth muscle secondary to pore formation was postulated to be the basic mechanism by which amphotericin B augmented renal vascular resistance (Sawaya et al. 1991). Amphotericin B also induces tubular dysfunction in the rat that mimics abnormalities observed in humans (Gouge and Andriole 1971). The dominant site of tubular injury in the rat as assessed by light and electron microscopy is the inner stripe of the outer medulla (Heyman et al. 1993b), which is a zone that even under physiological conditions functions on the verge of hypoxia. Investigators have postulated that hypoxic injury to this zone results from the demand for increased oxygen to support increased sodium transport stimulated by the heightened influx of sodium across the apical membrane made permeable by amphotericin B at a time when the supply of oxygen is reduced because amphotericin B depresses RBF (Brezis et al. 1984; Heyman et al. 1993b).

Deoxycholate, the vehicle in which amphotericin B is suspended, has been implicated as a contributory factor in the cytotoxicity associated with amphotericin B (Zager et al. 1992). Of particular interest is the observation that amphotericin B complexed to cholesteryl sulfate was not cytotoxic to renal tubular cells in vitro. This observation reinforces the findings of a growing number of studies that the administration of amphotericin B in liposomes (Janknegt et al. 1992) or with lipid preparations (Caillot et al. 1993) greatly reduces the nephrotoxicity of this agent without compromising its efficacy as an antifungal agent. Further clinical trials are needed to establish the latter point.

In the meantime, the physician is obligated to try to minimize those factors known to potentiate the risk of this complication:

1. Daily drug dose
2. Duration of therapy
3. Chronic renal insufficiency
4. Sodium depletion
5. Renal hypoperfusion
6. Concomitant drug therapy/exposure
   a) Diuretics
   b) Aminoglycosides
   c) Cisplatin
   d) Radiocontrast agents
   e) Cyclosporine

Fisher et al. (1989) observed a 1.8-fold increase in the risk of nephrotoxicity for each 0.1 mg/kg increment in the daily dose of amphotericin B. The risk of nephrotoxicity was increased 15.4-fold in patients who had an elevated serum creatinine prior to the start of amphotericin B therapy and 12.5-fold in patients who received diuretics during the course of amphotericin B therapy. The latter observation presumably reflects the powerful potentiating influence of sodium depletion on this complication. Importantly, sodium loading has been shown to minimize this complication. Thus, every effort should be expended to ensure that the patient is optimally volume repleted prior to the initiation of therapy with this agent. Parenteral flucytosine administered in combination with amphotericin B has been reported to reduce the incidence of nephrotoxicity (Stamm et al. 1987). The renoprotective effect of this combination may be explained by the lower dose of amphotericin B required for successful therapy as well as the fact that flucytosine is often given as an infusion of 0.9% NaCl.

Antiprotozoal Agents

Pentamidine

Pentamidine has been used since the 1950s to treat *Pneumocystis carinii* pneumonia (PCP). In the pre-AIDS (acquired immunodeficiency sydrome) era, pentamidine therapy was complicated by ARF in about 25% of cases

(Walzer et al. 1974). The incidence of this complication in patients with AIDS, however, appears to be substantially higher than this figure, and it is unexplained by greater drug dose, longer duration of therapy, or by concomitant therapy with other potentially nephrotoxic drugs (Lachaal and Venuto 1989). The mechanism of ARF is not known. Initial pharmacokinetic studies that utilized a fluorometric assay indicated that up to 20% of the daily dose of pentamidine was excreted unchanged in the urine and that following cessation of therapy drug was detected in the urine for up to 8 weeks (Waalkes et al. 1970), which implied that pentamidine was being released from tissues stores. More recent pharmacokinetic studies that utilized a high-performance liquid chromatography (HPLC) assay indicate that less than 5% of the daily dose of pentamidine is excreted in the urine each day (Conte et al. 1987; Navin et al. 1987). The mechanism of renal elimination of drug is not known. Of relevance to the nephrotoxicity of pentamidine is the observation that pentamidine is concentrated in the kidney (Waalkes et al. 1970; Waldman et al. 1973; Navin et al. 1987; Farr et al. 1993).

Pentamidine nephrotoxicity presents as nonoliguric ARF begining 7–10 days after the initiation of therapy. Urinalysis reveals mild proteinuria, microscopic hematuria, pyuria, and cylinduria. Most patients experience mild to moderate ARF, but occasionally severe renal failure necessitating dialysis therapy is seen. In one series the azotemia was accompanied by hyperkalemia in association with a picture consistent with hyperchloremic metabolic acidosis (Lachaal and Venuto 1989). Renal magnesium wasting has been observed in several cases (Mani 1992). Recovery of renal function usually begins within a week after discontinuation of drug and in most cases returns to baseline within several weeks.

Chronic renal insufficiency and volume depletion are thought to increase the risk of pentamidine nephrotoxicity in man (Berns et al. 1991). In the rat, pentamidine nephrotoxicity was potentiated by amphotericin B, by tobramycin, and by cyclosporin A, whereas it was ameliorated by fosfomycin, by D-glucaro-1,5-lactam, by verapamil, and by enalapril (Feddersen and Sack 1991).

Sulfadiazine

The sulfonamide antibiotics and their metabolites are excreted primarily via the kidneys by a process that involves glomerular filtration, tubular secretion, and tubular absorption (Weinstein et al. 1960). The high incidence of nephrotoxicity observed with the first generation of sulfonamides was due to their limited solubility, which resulted in intratubular obstruction secondary to the deposition of drug in the form of crystals (Dowling and Lepper 1943). Sulfadiazine, a poorly soluble sulfonamide, continues to be used today in combination with pyrimethamine for the treatment of toxoplasma encephalitis, and nephrotoxicity expressed by hematuria, crystalluria, renal colic, and renal insufficiency may complicate therapy in 5% of cases (Molina et al. 1991; Berns et al. 1991). These abnormalities usually subside with hydration and alkalinization of the urine.

Trimethoprim-Sulfmethoxazole

Trimethoprim-sulfmethoxazole (TMP-SMX) is used as an alternative to pentamidine for the treatment of PCP. An increase in serum creatinine concentration is commonly observed with this agent due to the inhibition of tubular secretion of creatinine by trimethoprim (Berglund et al. 1975; Kainer and Rosenberg 1981). The magnitude of this effect is more pronounced in patients who have chronic renal insufficiency with an elevated baseline serum creatinine. The failure of the BUN to rise in proportion to the rise in serum creatinine should alert the physician to the correct diagnosis. The incidence of ARF secondary to intratubular crystal precipitation declined sharply after the introduction of the more soluble sulfonamides, such as sulfamethoxazole. However, the intravenous administration of TMP-SMX in high concentration for the therapy of PCP carries a finite risk for ARF secondary to crystal deposition of the parent drug or a relatively insoluble metabolite (Siegel 1978; Buchanan 1978). Sulfonamides including sulfamethozazole have been implicated as a cause of hypersensitivity reactions and AIN (Grunfeld et al. 1993). Patients with AIDS experience a high incidence of adverse drug reactions during TMP-SMX therapy (Schneider et al. 1992); however, thus far no increased incidence of AIN has been reported.

Radiocontrast Agents

The radiocontrast agents in clinical use today are water-soluble compounds that are eliminated from the body via the kidneys by glomerular filtration. The expanding use of radiologic diagnostic and therapeutic procedures involving radiocontrast agents has been accompanied by an increase in the frequency of radiocontrast-induced nephropathy (RCIN). The reported incidence of RCIN has varied depending on the criteria used to define this complication as well as the characteristics of the patient population studied. In various prospective studies, the incidence of RCIN has ranged from 0% to 70%; however, a survey of 12 prospective studies revealed an aggregate incidence of 10.2% (Berns 1989).

The clinical expression and course of RCIN has been well described (Berns 1989; Mission and Cutler 1985; Berkseth and Kjellstrand 1984; Byrd and Sherman 1979). The first sign of RCIN may be the appearance of oliguria shortly after the procedure. In many cases, however, the patient remains nonoliguric and the first clue of RCIN is an elevation of the serum creatinine evident 24–48 h after the injection of dye. In most cases the rise in serum creatinine peaks in 3–5 days and returns to baseline in 7–10 days. In more severe cases, however, the serum creatinine may not peak until 7–10 days and may not return to baseline until 14–21 days after the procedure. Such patients may require dialysis support. The urinalysis is usually nonspecific and it is not uncommon to observe an FE_{Na} of less than 1% in oliguric patients. Persistence of a nephrogram 24–48 h after dye study is a characteristic, but not a diagnostic feature of RCIN, as this finding was noted in a number of false-positive cases (D'Elia et al. 1982). Vacuolization and patchy necrosis of proximal tubular cells have been observed in human renal biopsy material (Moreau et al. 1975). In an animal model of RCIN (Heyman et al. 1988), necrosis of the medullary thick ascending limb of Henle's loop was observed, which suggested that hypoxia contributed to the tubular cell injury.

The pathogenesis of renal failure in RCIN has not been unequivocally established. However, the abrupt onset of oliguria, the low FE_{Na}, the persistence of the nephrogram, and the rapid resolution of the ARF are consistent with a reversible renal vasoconstrictor mechanism. It is well established that injection of radiocontrast dye in animals elicits a biphasic response characterized initially by renal vasodilatation followed by prolonged renal vasoconstriction with depression of RBF and GFR (Porter 1993). The magnitude of these hemodynamic changes is influenced by the osmolality, dose, and injection site of the dye. Norepinephrine, the renin–angiotensin system, and renal prostaglandins do not appear to mediate the renal vasoconstriction. Calcium channel blockers (Bakris and Burnett 1985) and adenosine antagonists (Arend et al. 1987; Deray et al. 1990) have been shown to inhibit the depression of RBF and GFR induced by the administration radiocontrast agents to experimental animals. These observations have led to the hypothesis that activation of tubuloglomerular feedback secondary to increased delivery of solute to the macula densa mediates the increase in renal vascular resistance (Porter 1993). Recent studies implicate a role for endothelin in the vasoconstrictor response to radiocontrast agents (Heyman et al. 1992). The fact that radiocontrast agents stimulate increased urinary excretion of enzymes derived from renal proximal tubular cells (Hartmann et al. 1985; Jevnikar et al. 1988; Parvez et al. 1990) suggests that these agents may exert a direct toxic effect on renal tubular cells. This possibility is supported by experiments that demonstrated injury of proximal tubular cells exposed in vitro to radiocontrast media (Humes et al. 1987; Messana et al. 1988). It is likely that intense renal vasoconstriction and the attendant hypoxia related thereto magnifies any direct tubular toxic effect of these agents. The observations that radiocontrast agents stimulate increased urinary excretion of uric acid (Mudge 1980), oxalate (Gelman et al. 1978), and Tamm-Horsfall protein (Hoyer and Seiler 1987) and precipitate Tamm-Horsfall protein in vitro (Schwartz et al. 1970) has fueled speculation about the possibility that intratubular obstruction participates in the pathogenesis of RCIN. Finally, radiocontrast agents have been shown to alter red blood cell (RBC) shape, decrease RBC deformability, increase blood viscosity, and increase platelet aggregation (Berns 1989), the net effect of which would be to depress flow through the microcirculation.

Established, probable, and possible risk factors for RCIN are listed below:

1. Definite
   a) Chronic renal insufficiency
   b) Diabetes mellitus
2. Probable
   a) Renal hypoperfusion
   b) Volume depletion
   c) Dehydration
   d) Concomitant exposure to other nephrotoxic drugs
   e) Age >60 years
   f) Volume of contrast dye injected
   g) Multiple exposures to contrast dye
   h) Congestive heart failure (class III and IV)
   i) Atherosclerotic vascular disease
   j Hypertension
   k) Liver disease
   l) Multiple myeloma
3. Possible
   a) Proteinuria
   b) Hyperuricemia
   c) Anemia

Preexisiting chronic renal insufficiency is the single most important risk factor for RCIN (D'Elia et al. 1982; Berkseth and Kjellstrand 1984; Berns 1989), and the more severe the renal insufficiency, the greater the risk (Tereul et al. 1981; D'Elia et al. 1982; Davidson et al. 1989; Moore et al. 1992). Diabetes mellitus has been the focus of much discussion concerning the risk of RCIN. In the absence of azotemia, the incidence of RCIN in individuals with diabetes mellitus is similar to that of nonazotemic, nondiabetic individuals (Van Zee et al. 1978; Harkonen and Kjellstrand 1979; Parfrey et al. 1989). Diabetic patients with azotemia, however, appear to be at greater risk for RCIN than nondiabetic patients with a similar degree of azotemia (Weinrauch et al. 1977; Harkonen and Kjellstrand 1977; Van Zee et al. 1978; Parfrey et al. 1989; Goldfarb et al. 1993). The evidence linking the remaining factors to increased risk for RCIN is often circumstantial, such as a high prevalence of these abnormalities among patients who experience RCIN (Berns 1989). In studies where multivariate analysis has been performed, an association between a particular factor or group of factors and RCIN has not been consistently identified (Spinler and Goldfarb 1992). Nevertheless, parallels drawn from other studies of nephrotoxicity suggest that the risk of RCIN is likely to be magnified in the presence of an ischemic insult related to renal hypoperfusion, by concurrent therapy with other potentially nephrotoxic drugs, by large doses of dye or multiple contrast studies over a brief period, by advanced age, and by comorbidities, especially if they are associated with depressed renal function. That patients with multiple myeloma are at exceptionally high risk for RCIN has been promoted as dogma for years; however, close scrutiny of the evidence indicates that the risk is not greater than one would predict based on the presence of other identified risk factors such as renal insufficiency and dehydration (Berkseth and Kjellstrand 1984).

The prevention of RCIN begins with an assessment of the risk/benefit ratio. In patients with advanced chronic renal failure (serum creatinine >4 mg/dl), the risk of precipitating an irreversible decline of renal function and initiating permanent dialysis therapy must be weighed against the information to be gained by the radiographic procedure. In such cases careful consideration should be given to substituting an alternate imaging technique. Medications should be systematically reviewed to determine whether it is possible to eliminate or adjust the dose of drugs, e.g., NSAID, diuretics, hypotensive agents, that might potentiate RCIN. Careful attention must be paid to repairing extracellular volume deficits, optimizing renal function prior to the procedure, limiting the dose of dye, and spacing multiple contrast procedures whenever possible. It has become standard practice among nephrologists to "prehydrate" high-risk patients prior to the procedure (Berns 1989), even though controlled studies that document the benefit of this maneuver are lacking. R.L. Eisenberg et al. (1981) reported that infusing saline at high rates (550 ml/h) during the angiographic procedure provided complete protection against RCIN. Other investigators (Anto et al. 1981) have reported that infusing 1500 ml 0.45% saline beginning about 12 h prior to the procedure followed by an infusion of 250 ml 20% mannitol 60 min after the procedure reduced the incidence of RCIN associated with intravenous urography to 22% compared to an expected incidence of 70% based on a prior study by the same group (Shafi et al. 1978). In a subsequent paper, these authors reported that the combination of mannitol plus furosemide was also protective against RCIN in high-risk patients (Porush et al. 1982). The timing of the mannitol infusion is dictated by the procedure. For angiogrphic procedures, Berkseth and Kjellstrand (1984) have recommended infusing a cocktail of mannitol plus furosemide during the procedure in patients with a serum creatinine level greater than 2.0 mg/dl, but they provided no data concerning the effects and benefits of this protocol. In all protocols utilizing mannitol, with or without furosemide, particular attention should be paid to adequate replacment of the increase in urine volume and electrolytes so as to avoid the complications of volume depletion and electrolyte imbalance. It is the author's practice in high-risk patients to infuse 0.9% NaCl at 100 ml/h for 12–18 h prior to the procedure. One hour prior to the intra-arterial injection of radiocontrast agent, an infusion of 250 ml 20% mannitol is started at 100 ml/h along with an infusion of 0.45% NaCl adjusted to match urine output over the ensuing 12 h. Furosemide is injected intravenously as necessary to maintain urine output at 75 ml/h or more. This protocol is modified in patients with impaired cardiac function.

As noted above, studies in animals (Bakris and Burnett 1985) have raised the possibility that calcium channel blockers might be of value in preventing RCIN in humans. Several prospective studies of the protective effect of these drugs have been reported (Russo et al. 1990; Neumayer et al. 1989). While the data demonstrate a beneficial effect of calcium channel blockers in attenuating the adverse effects of radiocontrast agents on renal hemodynamics, the limited number of subjects studied as well as the type of experimental design used in these studies do not provide a definitive answer as to the effectiveness of these agents in preventing RCIN. Other investigators have examined whether the infusion of vasodilators would provide protection against RCIN. Hall et al. (1992) reported that no RCIN was observed in 11 patients with a baseline serum creatinine level of 2.0 mg/dl or more who were infused with dopamine at 3 μg/kg per min commencing the evening before angiography and continuing to the morning following the procedure, whereas the incidence of RCIN in the control group not given dopamine was 62% (eight out of thirteen cases). Weisberg et al. (1994) reported that no RCIN was observed in nondiabetic patients with chronic renal insufficiency infused for 2 h with dopamine, Atrial naturitis peptide (ANP), or mannitol commencing immediately after completion of full instrumentation for cardiac catheterization, whereas the incidence of RCIN was 38% in the control group infused with 0.45% NaCl at 100 ml/h. In diabetic patients with a similar degree of chronic renal failure, the infusion of dopamine, ANP, or mannitol resulted in an increased incidence of RCIN, although the degree of elevation of the serum creatinine was on average less than 50%. While these studies are of interest, once again the small number of patients enrolled as well as the type of experimental design employed limit the conclusions that can be drawn.

The precise role of the low-osmolar, nonionic radiocontrast agents in strategies to prevent RCIN remains a controversial subject. Barrett and Carlisle (1993) conducted a metaanalysis of 24 trials and concluded that low-osmolar agents cause less RCIN in patients with preexisting renal insufficiency than do high-osmolar agents. A recent multicenter trial (Hill et al. 1993) has confirmed the results of previous reports that patients administered iohexol for cardiac angiography experienced fewer side effects and adverse events than did patients administered diatrizoate. Among patients with preexisting renal insufficiency and no diabetes, the incidence of RCIN, as defined by an increase in serum creatinine of 1.0 mg/dl or more was 7% in the diatrizoate group and 4% in the iohexol group; among patients with diabetes mellitus and preexisting renal insufficiency, the incidence of RCIN was 27% and 12%, respectively (Goldfarb et al. 1993). Thus, in high-risk patients it is reasonable to utilize low-osmolar radiocontrast agents in an attempt to reduce the frequency and severity of RCIN.

Antineoplastic Agents

Cisplatin

Cisplatin (*cis*-diaminedichloroplatinum II) is comprised of an inorganic complex of platinum with two ammonia groups and two chloride ligands. It is an alkylating agent that is widely used for the treatment of a number of solid tumors. When cisplatin was first introduced for clinical use, nephrotoxic ARF was recognized as the major dose-dependent complication, with an incidence approaching 33% after a single course of therapy and reaching 75% after multiple courses (Lippman et al. 1973; Madias and Harrington 1978). With the introduction of hydration protocols (vide infra), the incidence of ARF has been reduced significantly but not eliminated. In a recent report of high-dose cisplatin therapy, the incidence of acute nephrotoxicity was 56%; in 30% the renal dysfunction was mild, in 18% it was moderate, and in 8% it was severe (Cooper et al. 1993).

The renal toxicity of cisplatin is causally linked to the mechanism by which this agent is processed by the kidney. When cisplatin is infused intravenously over 6h, plasma platinum levels decline in a biphasic manner with a half-life of less than 60min for the rapid phase and a half-life of 42.2h for the slow component (Loehrer and Einhorn 1984). After intravenous bolus injection, cisplatin shows a triphasic decay pattern with a half-life of 0.3, 1.0, and 24h. In plasma up to 90% of cisplatin is bound to plasma proteins or erythrocytes; the remainder is unbound drug. Binding to tissue proteins also occurs, as evidenced by the rapid redistribution of drug to selected organs, especially the kidney. From 23% to 70% of cisplatin is recovered unchanged in the urine at 24h, but this amount can be augumented by volume expanding with saline or mannitol. The remainder of the drug is recovered in the urine over a variable period of time and presumably reflects the release of drug from tissue stores. The unbound moiety of cisplatin is rapidly excreted in the urine by a process of glomerular filtration and tubular secretion (Jacobs 1986). Microinjection experiments argue against an appreciable absorptive flux (Safirstein et al. 1986). Cisplatin is known to be concentrated within the inner cortex and outer medulla of the kidney in humans and experimental animals. The available evidence indicates that the renal cortical accumulation of cisplatin is mediated by transport of the drug across the basolateral membrne of cells lining the pars recta. Both the organic cation (Bird et al. 1984) and organic anion (Jacobs et al. 1984) transport systems have been implicated in this process. The pars recta is also the tubule segment that manifests cell necrosis following cisplatin administration in the rat (Dobyan et al. 1980; Laurent et al. 1988). In human kidneys lesions have been observed in the distal nephron as well as the proximal tubule (Gonzales-Vitale et al. 1977; Dentino et al. 1978).

The mechanism(s) by which cisplatin causes injury to cells of the pars recta has not been established. Speculation has focused on a metabolite of cisplatin thought to be generated intracellularly, but its identity has remained elusive (Safirstein et al. 1986). Binding to macromoleules causing inactivation of function (Robins 1982), inhibition of protein synthesis (Tay et al. 1988), and oxidative stress (Hannemann and Baumann 1988; Bull et al. 1988) have been implicated in the pathogenesis of cisplatin's cytotoxicity. In addition, cisplatin also perturbs distal tubular function; however, it is not known whether similar or different mechanisms mediate these functional alterations.

In experimental animals, cisplatin causes a dose-dependent polyuric ARF accompanied by derangements of proximal and distal tubular functions (Safirstein et al. 1986; Litterst and Weiss 1987; Daugard 1990; Ammer et al. 1993) that mimic those observed in humans. Despite altered distal tubular function that includes magnesium wasting and vasopressin-resistant polyuria, histopathologic lesions are confined almost exclusively to the pars recta of the proximal tubule. Also of interest is the observation that tubular dysfunction precedes the depression of RBF and GFR, which typically does not occur until 72 h after cisplatin administration. Recovery of renal function begins in 6–8 days, but it usually is incomplete and correlates with chronic histopathologic changes consisting of dilated tubules, cyst formation, and interstitial fibrosis (Dobyan 1985).

In humans cisplatin-induced nonoliguric ARF most commonly occurs after "high"-dose, e.g., 200 mg/m^2, therapy and often in association with other nephrotoxic drugs (Cooper et al. 1993). In patients treated with standard doses of drug after proper hydration, the incidence of ARF as manifested by an acute rise in the BUN and serum creatinine is low. Nevertheless, signs of nephrotoxic injury that initially may be subclinical can be detected in these individuals if sought. These include abnormalities of tubular function such as depression of iodohippurate transport (Groth et al. 1986), increased urinary excretion of β_2-microglobulin and enzymes derived from proximal tubule cells (Jones et al. 1980), increased urinary excretion of amino acids, magnesium, potassium, and calcium (Bitran et al. 1982), sodium wasting (Hutchison 1988), and defective urine concentrating and acidifying capacity (Swainson et al. 1985). The frequency and severity of these abnormalities increase as a function of the dose and the number of cycles of cisplatin therapy, which implies that the nephrotoxic insult is cumulative. It is not uncommon for the clinical picture to be dominated by electrolyte abnormalities of hypomagnesemia, hypokalemia, and hypocalcemia, which are linked to the renal tubular wasting of magnesium (Bell et al. 1985). This tubular defect may persist for a prolonged period of time and require chronic oral supplementation (Schilsky et al. 1982). Elevation of the BUN and serum creatinine does occur in patients treated with standard therapy; however, typically these changes are mild and transient, which was taken as evidence that the nephrotoxic injury was reversible. This conclusion is no longer justified, as several studies have documented that significant depression of GFR may develop at varying intervals after completion of cisplatin therapy even in the absence of an observed rise in serum creatinine (Meijer et al. 1983; Groth et al. 1986). With repeated cycles of therapy, frank and persisting elevations of the BUN and serum creatinine may develop and these changes typically signify the development of chronic interstitial nephritis, which may progess insidiously (Guinee et al. 1993).

The first step in the prevention of cisplatin-induced nephrotoxicity is to ensure optimal expansion of extracellular volume with saline prior to, during, and following drug administration (Finley et al. 1985). This can be accomplished by infusing 3–5 l of normal saline per day beginning the day before the start of drug therapy and continuing for a day after administering the last dose. When high-dose therapy is used, the drug commonly is infused in 3% NaCl in divided doses. Some protocols call for the infusion of mannitol with or without furosemide immediately after completion of cisplatin infusion with the goal of promoting increased urine volume. The mechanism by which volume expansion protects the kidney against cisplatin-induced toxicity has not been established. Increased renal excretion of drug, decreased intratubular concentration of drug, decreased contact time between drug and tubular cells, and decreased formation of a toxic metabolite have been suggested as possibilities.

Because the degree of protection provided by the various hydration protocols is incomplete, especially when high-dose therapy is given, attention has focused on the possibility of modulating the nephrotoxicity of cisplatin using nucleophilic sulfur-containing compounds (Borch 1993). One such chemical modulator is sodium thiosulfate, which forms highly stable platinum (II) adducts. When sodium this sulfate is infused immediately before or simultaneously with cisplatin, it is highly effective in protecting the kidney against cisplatin-associated toxicity. The mechanism is thought to involve the uptake of sodium thiosulfate by renal tubular cells followed by the intracellular binding of toxic cisplatin metabolites. Unfortunately, this agent also reduces the cytotoxicty of cisplatin for neoplastic cells. Therefore, its use is restricted to those cases where cisplatin is administered intraperitoneally to treat intraabdominal disease, which permits sodium thiosulfate to be infused intravenously to provide nephroprotection without blunting cisplatin's therapeutic efficacy. Sodium diethyldithiocarbamate (DDTC) has also been shown to provide nephroprotection in animals and in humans. Unfortunately, its clinical application may be limited due to its profile of side effects. WR2271 is a prodrug that in normal tissue is hydrolyzed by membrane alkaline phosphatase of endothelial cells to WR1065, a diaminothiol which then readily diffuses intracellularly, where it inactivates cisplatin or a toxic metabolite. In tumor tissue, the rate of hydrolysis of WR2271 to WR1065 is often limited because of poor vascularity, which explains the selective protection afforded normal tissue by this agent. Studies in animal models have demonstrated that WR2271 is effective in providing protection against nephro-, myelo-, neuro-, and ototoxicity related to cisplatin therapy (Treskes and van der Vijgh 1993). Clinical trials are in progress. Other pharmacological strategies have focused on blocking the renal tubular uptake of cisplatin using probenecid (Jacobs et al. 1991). Glycine infusion has been shown to protect rats against cisplatin-induced ARF, presumably by blocking the uptake of drug by cells of the pars recta (Heyman et al. 1993a).

Methotrexate

Methotrexate is an antimetabolite whose cytotoxic action is related to inhibition of dihydrofolate reductase. The drug is eliminated from the body primarily via the kidneys by the combined mechanism of glomerular filtration and tubular secretion. Most of the drug appearing in the urine is unchanged; a small fraction is excreted as the 7-hydroxy metabolite. Of toxicological significance is the fact that the solubility of methotrexate is reduced by more than tenfold in acid urine. Moreover, the solubility of 7-hydroxy methotrexate is approximately 25% of that of the parent drug. At conventional doses, the nephrotoxic potential of methotrexate is very low. However, with the introduction of high-dose therapy of $1-7\,g/m^2$ with leucovorin rescue, the incidence of nephrotoxicity increased dramatically – up to 60% in one series (Pitman et al. 1975). The observation that vigorous hydration combined with alkalinization of the urine greatly reduced the frequency of this complication (Pitman and Frei 1977) gave credence to the hypothesis that obstruction secondary to intratubular precipitation of drug was the principal cause of the ARF observed with high-dose methotrexate therapy. Other data, however, suggest that this may not be the only mechanism of nephrotoxicity. For example, significant depression of GFR (range, 17%–77%) was observed 20–40 h after high-dose methotrexate administration in eight of nine hydrated subjects (Abelson et al. 1983). In only three of nine subjects was the depression of GFR accompanied by clinically significant nephrotoxicity, defined as a rise in serum creatinine of 50% or more above baseline. These data imply that high-dose methotrexate usually provokes a transient depression of GFR in most patients. Other investigators (Goren et al. 1986) have reported that high-dose methotrexate therapy in patients subjected to vigorous hydration and urine alkalinization was accompanied by reversible increases in the urinary excretion of enzymes and protein derived from proximal tubular cells. Maximal excretion rates were detected on the second day post-treatment and generally returned to or toward baseline by day 8. These observations suggest that methotrexate may be directly toxic to renal proximal tubular cells and that this toxic effect may be linked to the depression of GFR observed by Abelson et al. (1983). The typical clinical expression of methotrexate-induced nephrotoxicity is nonoliguric ARF, which usually resolves in 10–14 days. Because renal failure results in prolonged elevation of methotrexate in plasma due to impaired renal excretion of drug, the risk of systemic toxicity is greatly magnified, but can be obviated by infusing leucovorin and thymidine until plasma methotrexate levels decline to nontoxic levels (Abelson et al. 1983).

Nonsteroidal Anti-inflammatory Drugs

The therapeutic efficacy of NSAID is linked to their potency as inhibitors of cyclo-oxygenase activity, the first enzymatic step in the metabolism of arachidonic acid to prostaglandins (PG). NSAID are known to cause a number of renal complications (Heinrich 1993; Schlondorff 1993; Murray and Brater 1993), which, with the exception of AIN, are predictable consequences of the pharmacologic action of these drugs as inhibitors of PG synthesis; these complications include:

1. Acute renal failure
   a) Reversible acute renal vasocontriction
   b) Ischemic acute tubular necrosis
   c) Allergic interstitial nephritis (with and without nephrotic syndrome)
2. Fluid and electrolyte abnormalities
   a) Sodium and water retention
   b) Hyponatremia
   c) Hyporeninemic hyponaldosteronism
      α) Hyperkalemia
3. Chronic renal failure
   a) Analgesic nephropathy (papillary necrosis)

Renal PG have been shown to modulate various aspects of kidney function. At the level of the afferent and efferent arterioles, the vasodilating effects of PGI_2 and PGE_2 serve to modulate the vasoconstricting actions of a variety of stimuli including angiotensin II, norepinephrine, endothelin, and arginine vasopressin. PGI_2 modulates renin secretion by the juxtaglomerular cells. PGE_2 inhibits sodium transport along the thick ascending limb of Henle's loop and antagonizes vasopressin's action on water transport along the collecting duct. PG also play a role in the adaptive hyperfiltration of residual nephrons that accompanies virtually all forms of chronic renal failure. In healthy individuals with normal renal function, inhibition of PG synthesis by NSAID has little discernible impact clinically on renal function and fluid and electrolyte metabolism (Sedor et al. 1986). The same is not the case for individuals who suffer from an absolute or relative decline in effective circulating volume, and require heightened activity of the renin–angiotensin system, the sympathetic nervous system, and other vasoconstrictor mechanisms to support systemic hemodynamics (Heinrich 1993; Blackshear et al. 1983). Under these clinical circumstances, the vasodilator PG synthesized at the level of the afferent and efferent arterioles play a critical role in moderating the renal vasoconstricting actions of these stimuli and preserving renal perfusion and glomerular filtration. Inhibition of PG synthesis by NSAID in this setting will provoke an abrupt decline of RBF and GFR and sodium and water excretion that can be detected within 60 min of drug administration (Murray and Brater 1993). The magnitude of the decline in renal function is related to the intensity of activation of the vasoconstrictor mechanisms, which is a function of the degree to which systemic hemodynamics have been compromised.

The typical clinical picture is that of prerenal azotemia manifested by a variable elevation of the BUN (usually greater than the rise in serum creatinine) and a low FE_{Na}. In high-risk individuals (advanced age with underlying heart, liver, or kidney disease), the BUN and serum creatinine may rise rapidly over several days to alarmingly high levels, which may reflect the development of ischemic ATN secondary to intense renal vasoconstriction. In most cases, however, the ARF reverses rapidly with discontinuation of the drug. In some patients the clinical picture is dominated by abnormalities in fluid and electrolyte metabolism. Sodium retention with edema formation, hyponatremia, and escape from control of antihypertensive medication are common complications of NSAID. As a result of their inhibitory effect on renin secretion, NSAID may provoke hyperkalemia, especially in patients with chronic renal insufficiency, in patients with diabetes mellitus, and in patients taking potassium-sparing diuretics.

All NSAID have the potential to cause functional or reversible ARF and to perturb fluid and electrolyte metabolism. Although sulindac has been promoted as a NSAID that protects the kidney from these complications because of its unique renal metabolism (Ciabattoni et al. 1984), in fact this drug has been shown to cause the same alterations in renal function and in fluid and electrolyte metabolism in susceptible individuals (Brater et al. 1986). Of particular relevance to the ICU setting is ketorolac, a NSAID that is being increasingly used for pain control in order to avoid problems of respiratory depression, sedation, and addiction associated with narcotics. This agent has the same potential to cause renal dysfunction as the other NSAID (Pearce et al. 1993). ICU patients, who typically are under great stress from an acute illness that is often accompanied by multiorgan dysfunction including renal insufficiency, are especially prone to develop renal complications from ketorolac (Hayek et al. 1993). This drug, like most NSAID, is metabolized in the liver to an inactive metabolite (Day et al. 1987). In the case of ketorolac, however, the metabolite is an unstable acylglucuronide conjugate that is excreted predominantly in the urine. In patients with chronic renal insufficiency, the metabolite accumulates in plasma and, being unstable, undergoes hydrolysis to reform the active parent drug, thereby magnifying the risk of renal complications. Close monitoring of renal function in such patients is essential.

ARF in patients on NSAID may also result from AIN (Porile et al. 1990), although this complication is far less common than ischemic ARF. Among NSAID fenoprofen has been associated most commonly with this syndrome, but virtually all drugs in this class have been reported to cause AIN. In rare cases the onset of AIN has been observed as early as 1 week after starting therapy. More commonly it develops after more than several months of therapy. The clinical expression of AIN secondary to NSAID is typically devoid of signs of hypersensitivity such as fever, rash, eosinophilia, and eosiniphiluria. Renal insufficiency in association with nephrotic-range proteinuria with or without nephrotic syndrome is highly suggestive of AIN, but the diagnosis can only be established by renal biopsy which typically reveals interstitial inflammation composed predominantly of lymphocytes along with variable numbers of neutrophils and eosiniphils. The dominant finding in the glomerulus is fusion of epithelial cell foot processes. Discontinuation of drug is usually followed by recovery of function over several weeks to several months. The effectiveness of steroid therapy in promoting recovery has not been established.

References

Abelson HT, Fosburg MT, Beardsley P, Goorin AM, Gorka C, Link M, Link D (1983) Methrotrexate-induced renal impairment: clinical studies and rescue from systemic toxicity with high-dose leucovorin and thymidine. J Clin Oncol 1:208–216

Ammer U, Natochin Y, David C, Rumrich G, Ullrich KJ (1993) Cisplatin nephrotoxicity: site of functional disturbance and correlation to loss of body weight. Renal Physiol Biochem 16:131–145

Anot HR, Chou-S-Y, Porush J, Shapiro W (1981) Infusion intravenous pyelography and renal function: effects of hypertonic mannitol in patients with chronic renal insufficiency. Arch Intern Med 141:1652–1656

Appel GB, Given DB, Levin LR, Cooper GL (1986) Vancomycin and the kidney. Am J Kidney Dis 8:75–80

Arend LJ, Bakris GL, Burnett JC Jr, Megerian C, Spielmann WS (1987) Role of intrarenal adenosine in the renal hemodynamic response to radiocontrast media. J Lab Clin Med 110:406–411

Atkinson AJ Jr, Bennett JE (1978) Amphotericin B pharmacokinetics in humans. Antimicrob Agents Chemother 13:271–276

Bakris GL, Bunett JC Jr (1985) A role for calcium in radiocontrast-induced reduction in renal hemodynamics. Kidney Int 27:465–468

Barbour GL, Straub KD, O'Neal BL, Leatherman JW (1979) Vasopressin-resistant nephrogenic diabetes insipidus – a result of amphotericin B therapy. Arch Intern Med 139:86–88

Barrett BJ, Carlisle EJ (1993) Metaanalysis of the relative nephrotoxicity of high- and low-osmolality iodinated contrast media. Radiology 188:171–178

Barton CH, Pahl M, Vaziri ND, Cesario T (1984) Renal magnesium wasting associated with amphotericin B therapy. Am J Med 77:471–474

Bean B, Aeppli D (1985) Adverse effects of high-dose intravenous acyclovir in ambulatory patients with acute herpes zoster. J Infect Dis 151:362–365

Bhathena DB, Bullock WE, Nuttall CE, Luke RG (1978) The effects of amphotericin B therapy on the intrarenal vasculature and renal tubules in man. A study of renal biopsies by light, electron, and immunofluorescence microscopy. Clin Nephrol 9:103–110

Becker BN, Fall P, Hall C, Milan D, Leonard J, Glick A, Schulman G (1993) Rapidy progressive acute renal failure due to acyclovir: case report and review of the literature. Am J Kidney Dis 22:611–615

Bell DR, Woods RL, Levi AJ (1985) Cis-diamminedichloroplatinum-induced hypomagnesemia and renal magnesium wasting. Eur J Cancer Clin Oncol 21:287–290

Berglund F, Killander J, Pompeius R (1975) Effect of trimethoprim-sulfamethoxazole on the renal excretion of creatinine in man. J Urol 114:802–808

Berkseth RO, Kjellstrand CM (1984) Radiologic contrast-induced nephropathy. Med Clin North Am 68:351–370

Berns AS (1989) Nephrotoxicity of contrast media. Kidney Int 36:730–740

Berns JS, Cohen RM, Rudnick MR, Stumacher RJ (1991) Renal aspects of therapy for human immunodeficiency virus and associated opportunistic infections. J Am Soc Nephrol 1:1061–1080

Bertino JS, Booker LA, Franck PA, Jenkins PL, Franck KR, Nafziger AN (1993) Incidence of and significant risk factors for aminoglycoside-associated nephrotoxicity in patients dosed using individualized pharmackinetic modelling. J Infect Dis 167:173–179

Bird JE, Walser MM, Quebbemann AJ (1984) Protective effects of organic cation transport inhibitors on cis-diamminedichloroplatinum-induced nephrotoxicity. J Pharmacol Exp Ther 231:752–758

Bitran JD, Desser RK, Billings AA, Kozloff MF, Shapiro CM (1982) Acute nephrotoxicity following cis-dichlorodiamine-platinum. Cancer 49:1784–1788

Blackshear JL, Davidman M, Stillman T (1983) Identification of risk for renal insufficiency from nonsteroidal anti-inflammatory drugs. Arch Intern Med 143:1130–1134

Bolard J (1986) How do the polyene macrolide antibiotics affect the cellular membrane properties? Biochim Biophys Acta 864:257–304

Borch RE (1993) The nephrotoxicity of antineoplastic drugs. In: Hook JB, Goldstein RS (eds) Toxicology of the kidney, 2nd edn. Raven, New York, pp 283–301

Brajtburg J, Powderly WG, Kobayashi GS, Medoff G (1990) Amphotericin B: current understanding of mechanisms of action. Antimicrob Agents Chemother 34:183–188

Branch RA (1988) Prevention of amphotericin B-induced renal impairment: a review of the use of sodium supplementation. Arch Intern Med 148:2389–2394

Brater DC, Anderson SA, Brown-Cartwright D, Toto RD (1986) Effects of nonsteroidal anti-inflammatory drugs in patients with renal insufficiency and cirrhosis. Am J Kidney Dis 8:351–355

Brezis M, Rosen S, Silva P, Spokes K, Epstein FH (1984) Polene toxicity in renal medulla: injury mediated by transport activity. Science 224:66–68

Brigden D, Rosling AE, Woods NC (1982) Renal function after acyclovir intravenous injection. Am J Med 73 Suppl 1A:182–185

Brooks DP, Mitchell MP, Short BG, Ruffolo RB Jr, Nichols AJ (1991) Attenuation of amphotericin B nephrotoxicity in the dog by fenoldapam prodrug, SKF R-105058. J Pharmacol Exp Ther 257:1243–1247

Buchanan N (1978) Sulfamethoxazole, hypoalbuminemia, crystalluria and renal failure. Br Med J 2:172

Bull JMC, Strebel FR, Sunderland BA, Bulger RE, Edwards M, Siddik Z, Newman RA (1988) O-(β-Hydroxyethyl)-rutoside-mediated protection of renal injury associated with cis-diamminedichloroplatinum (II)/hyperthermia treatment. Cancer Res 48:2239–2244

Bullock ML, Ulman AJ, Finkelstein M, Keene WF (1985) The assessment of risk factors in 462 patients with acute renal failure. Am J Kidney Dis 5:97–103

Burgess JL, Birchall R (1972) Nephrotoxicity of amphotericin B with emphasis on tubular function. Am J Med 53:77–84

Butler WT, Bennett JE, Alling DW, Wertlake PT, Utz JP, Hill GJ (1964) Nephrotoxicity of amphotericin B: early and late effects in 81 patients. Am J Med 61:175–187

Byrd L, Sherman RL (1979) Radiocontrast-induced acute renal failure. A clinical and pathophysiologic review. Medicine (Baltimore) 58:270–279

Caillot D, Casanovas O, Solarz E, Chavenet P, Bonnotte B, Reny G, Entezam F, Lopez J, Bonnin A, Guy H (1993) Efficacy and tolerance of an amphotericin B lipid (intralipid) emulsion in the treatment of candidaemia in neutropenic patients. J Antimicrob Chemother 31:161–169

Cameron JS (1986) Acute renal failure in the intensive care unit today. Intensive Care Med 12:64–70

Campos SB, Seguro AC, Cesar KR, Rocha AS (1992) Effects of acyclovir on renal function. Nephron 62:74–79
Cheng J-T, Witty RT, Robinson RR, Yarger WE (1982) Amphotericin B nephrotoxicity: increased resistance and tubule permeability. Kidney Int 22:626–633
Christiansen KJ, Bernard EM, Gold JWM, Armstrong D (1985) Distribution and activity of amphotericin B in humans. J Infect Dis 152:1037–1043
Ciabattoni G, Cinotti GA, Pierucci A, Simonetti BM, Manzi M, Pugliese F, Barsotti P, Pecci G, Taggi F, Patrono C (1984) Effects of sulindac and ibuprofen in patients with chronic glomerular disease. N Engl J Med 310:279–283
Cioffi WG, Ashikaga T, Gamelli RL (1984) Probability of surviving postoperative acute renal failure: development of a prognostic index. Ann Surg 200:205–211
Como JA, Dismukes WE (1994) Oral azole drugs as systemic antifungal therapy. N Engl J Med 330:263–272
Conte JE, Upton RP, Lin ET (1987) Pentamidine pharmacokinetics in patients with AIDS with impaired renal function. J Infect Dis 156:885–890
Cook FV, Farrar WE (1978) Vancomycin revisited. Ann Intern Med 88:813–818
Cooper WB, Creger RJ, Soegiarso W, Mackay WL, Lazarus HM (1993) Renal dysfunction during high-dose cisplatin therapy and autologous hematopoietic stem cell transplantation: effect of aminoglycoside therapy. Am J Med 94:497–504
Corcoran GB, Salazar DE, Schentag JJ (1988) Excessive aminoglycoside nephrotoxicity in obese patients. Am J Med 85:279–284
Daugard G (1990) Cisplatin nephrotoxicity: experimental and clinical studies. Dan Med Bull 37:1–12
Davidson CJ, Hlatky M, Morris KG, Pieper K, Skelton TN, Schwab SJ, Bashore TM (1989) Cardiovascular and renal toxicity of a nonionic radiocontrast agent after cardiac catheterization. A prospective trial. Ann Intern Med 110:119–124
Day RO, Grahm GG, Williams KM, Champion GD, De Jager J (1987) Clinical pharmacology of nonsteroidal anti-inflammatory drugs. Pharmacol Ther 33:383–433
De Broe ME, Paulus GJ, Verpooten GA, Roels F, Buyssens N, Wedeen R, Van Hoof F, Tulkens PM (1984) Early effects of gentamicin, tobramycin and amikacin on the human kidney. Kidney Int 25:643–652
D'Elia JA, Gleason RE, Arday M, Malarick C, Godfrey K, Warran J, Kladany A, Weinrauch LA (1982) Nephrotoxicity from angiographic contrast material. A prospective study. Am J Med 72:719–725
De Miranda P, Blum MR (1983) Pharmacokinetics of acyclovir after intravenous and oral administration. J Antimicrob Chemother 12 Suppl B:29–37
Dentino M, Luft FC, Yum MN, Williams SD, Einhorn LH (1978) Long term effect of cis-diamminedichloride platinum (CDDP) on renal function and structure in man. Cancer 41:1274–1281
Deray G, Martinez F, Katlama C, Levaltier B, Beaufiles H, Danis M, Rozenheim M, Baumelou A, Dohin E, Gentilini M, Jacobs C (1989) Foscarnet nephrotoxicity: mechanism, incidence and prevention. Am J Nephrol 9:316–321
Deray G, Martinez F, Cacoub P, Baumelou B, Baumelou A, Jacobs C (1990) A role for adenosine, calcium and ischemia in radiocontrast-induced intrarenal vasoconstriction. Am J Nephrol 10:316–322
Dieterich D, Poles MA, Dicker M, Tepper R, Lew E (1993) Foscarnet treatment of cytomegalovirus gastrointestinal infections in acquired immunodeficiency syndrome patients who have failed ganciclovir induction. Am J Gastroenterol 88:542–548
Dobyan DC (1985) Long-term consequences of cisplatin-induced renal injury: a structural and functional study. Anat Rec 212:239–249
Dobyan DC, Levi J, Jacobs C, Kosek J, Weiner MW (1980) Mechanism of cis-platinum nephrotoxicity. II. Morphologic observations. J Pharmacol Exp Ther 213:551–556
Dorski DI, Crumpacker CS (1987) Drugs five years later: acyclovir. Ann Intern Med 107:859–874

Dowling HF, Lepper MH (1943) Toxic reactions following therapy with sulfapyridine, sulfathiazole and sulfadiazine. JAMA 121:1190–1194

Eisenberg ES, Robbins N, Lenci M (1981) Vancomycin and interstitial nephritis. Ann Intern Med 95:658

Eisenberg RL, Bank WO, Hedgcock MW (1981) Renal failure after major angiography can be avoided with hydration. AJR 136:859–861

EORTC International Antimicrobial Therapy Project Group (1978) Three antibiotic regimens in the treatment of infection in febrile granulocytic patients with cancer. J Infect Dis 137:14–29

EORTC International Antimicrobial Therapy Project Group (1993) Efficacy and toxicity of single daily doses of amikacin and ceftriaxone versus multiple doses of amikacin and ceftazidime for infection in patients with cancer and granulocytopenia. Ann Intern Med 119:584–593

Fanning MM (1990) Foscarnet therapy of cytomegalovirus retinitis in AIDS. J AIDS 3:472–479

Farr SJ, Jones HE, Blundell GK, Richards RJ (1993) Dose-dependent distribution of ^{3}H-pentamidine following intra-tracheal administration to rats. Xenobiotica 23:53–60

Feddersen A, Sack K (1991) Experimental studies on the nephrotoxicity of pentamidine in rats. J Antimicrob Chemother 28:437–446

Finley RS, Fortner CL, Grove WR (1985) Cisplatin nephrotoxicity: a summary of preventive interventions. Drug Intell Clin Pharmacol 19:362–367

Finn WF (1993) Recovery from acute renal failure. In: Lazarus JM, Brenner BM (eds) Acute renal failure. Churchill Livingstone, New York, pp 553–596

Fisher MA, Talbot GH, Maislin G, McKeon BP, Tynan KP, Strom BL (1989) Risk factors for amphotericin B-assocoiated nephrotoxicity. Am J Med 87:547–552

Gearhart MO, Sorg TB (1993) Foscarnet-induced severe hypomagnesemia and other electrolyte disorders. Ann Pharmacother 27:285–289

Gelman LM, Rowe JW, Coggins CH (1978) Effects of an angiographic contrast agent on renal function. Cardiovasc Med 4:313–318

Gilbert DN (1991) Once-daily aminoglycoside therapy. Antimicrob Agents Chemother 35:399–405

Gilbert DN, Wood CA, Kohlhepps SJ, Kohnen PW, Houghton DC, Finkbeiner HC, Lindsley J, Bennett WM (1989) Polyaspartic acid prevents experimental aminoglycoside nephrotoxicity. J Infect Dis 159:945–953

Goetz MB, Sayers J (1993) Nephrotoxicity of vancomycin and aminoglycoside therapy separately and in combination. J Antimicrob Chemother 32:325–334

Goldfarb S, Spinler S, Berns JS, Rudnick MR (1993) Low-osmolality contrast media and the risk of contrast-associated nephrotoxicity. Invest Radiol 28:S7–S10

Goldstein RS, Pasino DA, Hewitt WR, Hook JB (1986) Biochemical mechanism of cephaloridine nephrotoxicity: time and concentration dependence of peroxidative injury. Toxicol Appl Pharmacol 87:297–305

Gonzales-Vitale JC, Hayes DM, Cvitkovic E, Sternberg SS (1977) The renal pathology in clinical trial of cis-platinum. II. Diamminedichloride. Cancer 39:1362–1371

Goren MP, Wright RK, Horowitz ME, Meyer WH (1986) Enhancement of methotrexate nephrotoxicity after cisplatin therapy. Cancer 58:2617–2621

Gouge TH, Andriole VT (1971) An experimental model of amphotericin B nephrotoxicity with renal tubular acidosis. J Lab Clin Med 78:713–724

Groeneveld AB, Tran DD, van der Meulen J, Nauta JJP, Thijs LG (1991) Acute renal failure in the medical intensive care unit: predisposing, complicating factors and outcome. Nephron 59:602–610

Groth S, Nielson H, Sorensen JB, Christensen AB, Pedersen AG, Rorth M (1986) Acute and long-term nephrotoxicity of cis-platinum in man. Cancer Chemother Pharmacol 17:191–196

Grunfeld J-P, Kleinknecht D, Droz D (1993) Acute interstitial nephritis. In: Schrier RW, Gottschalk CW (eds) Diseases of the kidney, 5th edn. Little, Brown, Boston, pp 1331–1353

Guinee DG, Van Zee B, Houghton DC (1993) Clinically silent progressive tubulointerstitial disease during cisplatin chemotherapy. Cancer 71:4050–4054
Hall KA, Wong RW, Hunter GC, Camazine BM, Rappaport WA, Smyth SH, Bull DA, McIntyre KE, Bernhard VM, Misiorowski RL (1992) Contrast-induced nephrotoxicity: the effects of vasodilator therapy. J Surg Res 53:317–320
Halstenberg WK, Goormastic M, Paganini EP (1994) Utility of risk models for renal failure and critically ill patients. Semin Nephrol 14:23–32
Hannemann J, Baumann K (1988) Cisplatin-induced lipid peroxidation and decrease of gluconeogenesis in rat kidney cortex: different effects of antioxidants and radical scavengers. Toxicology 15:119–132
Harkonen S, Kjellstrand CM (1977) Exacerbations of diabetic renal failure following intravenous pyelography. Am J Med 63:939–946
Harkonen S, Kjellstrand CM (1979) Intravenous pyelography in nonuremic diabetic patients. Nephron 24:268–270
Hartmann HG, Braedel HE, Jutzler GA (1985) Detection of renal tubular lesions after abdominal aortography and selective arteriography by quantitative measurements of brush-border enzymes in the urine. Nephron 39:95–101
Hayek M, Vitting K, Castely P, Comer C, Yoganathan T, Stark B (1993) Effects of ketorolac on renal function after coronary bypass graft surgery. J Am Soc Nephrol 4:317A
Heinrich WL (1993) Nephrotoxicity of nonsteroidal anti-inflammatory agents. In: Schrier RW, Gottschalk CW (eds) Diseases of the kidney, 5th edn. Little, Bromn, Boston, pp 1203–1217
Heyman SN, Brezis M, Reubinoff CA, Greenfield C, Lechene FH, Epstein FH, Rosen S (1988) Acute renal failure with selective medullary injury in the rat.J Clin Invest 82:401–412
Heyman SN, Clark BA, Kaiser N, Spokes K, Rosen S, Brezis M, Epstein FH (1992) Radiocontrast agents induce endothelial release in vivo and in vitro. J Am Soc Nehprol 3:58–65
Heyman SN, Spokes K, Egorin MJ, Epstein FH (1993a) Glycine reduces early renal parenchymal uptake of cisplatin. Kidney Int 43:1226–1228
Heyman SN, Stillman IE, Brezis M, Epstein FH, Spokes K, Rosen S (1993b) Chronic amphotericin B nephropathy: morphometric, electron microscopic and functional studies. J Am Soc Nephrol 4:69–80
Hill JA, Winneford M, Cohen MB, Van Fossen DB, Murphy MJ, Halpern EF, Ludbrook PA, Wexler L, Rudnick MR, Goldfarb S (1993) Multicenter trial of ionic versus nonionic contrast media for cardiac angiography. Am J Cardiol 72:770–775
Hou SH, Bushinsky DA, Wish JB, Cohen JJ, Harrington JT (1983) Hospital acquired renal insufficiency; a prospective study. Am J Med 74:243–248
Houghton DC, Hartnett M, Campbell-Boswell M, Porter G, Bennett WM (1976) A light and electron microscopic analysis of gentamicin nephrotoxicity in rats. Am J Pathol 82:589–612
Hoyer JR, Seiler MW (1987) Pathophysiology of Tamm-Horsfall protein. Kidney Int 16:279–289
Humes HD (1988) Aminoglycoside nephrotoxicity. Kidney Int 33:900–911
Humes HD, Hunt DA, White MD (1987) Direct toxic effect of the radiocontrast agent diatrizoate on renal proximal tubule cells. Am J Physiol 252:F246–F255
Hutchison FN, Perez EA, Gandara DR, Lawrence HJ, Kaysen GA (1988) Renal salt wasting in patients with cisplatin. Ann Intern Med 108:21–25
Jacobs C (1986) The handling of platinum by the human kidney. In: McBrien DCD (ed) Biomedical mechanisms of platinum antitumor drugs. IRL Oxford, pp 147–170
Jacobs C, Coleman CN, Rich L, Hirst K, Weiner MW (1984) Inhibition of cis-diamminedichloroplatinum secretion by the human kidney with probenecid. Cancer Res 44:3632–3635
Jacobs C, Kaubisch S, Halsey J, Lum BL, Gosland M, Coleman CN, Sikic B (1991) The use of probenecid as a chemoprotector against cisplatin nephrotoxicity. Cancer 67:1518–1524
Jacobson MA, Causey C, Polsky B, Hardy D, Choun M, Davis R, O'Donnell JJ, Kuppermann BD, Heinemann M-H, Holland GN, Mills J, Feinberg JE (1993) A dose-ranging study of

daily maintenance intravenous foscarnet therapy for cytomegalovirus retinitis in AIDS. J Infect Dis 168:444–448
Janknegt R, de Marie S, Bakker-Woudenberg IAJM, Crommelin DJA (1992) Liposomal and lipid formulations of amphotericin B. Clin Pharmacokinet 23:279–291
Jevnikar AM, Finnie KJC, Dennis B, Plummer DT, Avila A, Linton AL (1988) Nephrotoxicity of high- and low-osmolality contrast media. Nephron 48:300–305
Jones BR, Gralla RA, Mladek J (1980) Comparison of methods of evaluating nephrotoxicity of cis-platinum. Clin Pharmacol Ther 27:557–562
Kahlmeter G, Dahlager J (1984) Aminoglycoside toxicity – a review of clinical studies between 1975 and 1982. J Antimicrob Chemther 13 Suppl A:9–22
Kainer G, Rosenberg AR (1981) Effect of co-trimoxazole on the glomerular filtration of healthy adults. Chemotherapy 27:229–232
Kaloyanides GJ (1984) Renal pharmacology of aminoglycoside antibiotics. Contrib Nephrol 42:148–167
Kaloyanides GJ (1991) Metablic interactions between drugs and tubulo-interstitial cells: role in nephrotoxicity. Kidney Int 39:531–540
Kaloyanides GJ (1993) Aminoglycoside nephrotoxicity. In: Schrier RW, Gottschalk CW (eds) Diseases of the kidney, 5th edn. Little, Brown, Boston, pp 1131–1164
Keeney RE, Kirk LE, Brigden D (1982) Acyclovir tolerance in humans. Am J Med 73 Suppl 1A:176–181
Kishore BK, Ibrahim S, Lambricht P, Laurent G, Maldague P, Tulkens PM (1992) Comparative assessment of poly-l-aspartic and poly-l-glutamic acids as protectants against gentamic-induced renal lysosomal phospholipidosis and phospholipiduria and cell proliferation in rats. J Pharmacol Exp Ther 262:424–432
Klastersky J, Hensgens G, Debusscher L (1975) Empiric therapy for cancer patients: comparative study of ticarcillin-tobramycin, ticarcillin-cephalothin and cephalothin-tobramycin. Antimicrob Agents Chemother 7:640–645
Kleinknecht D, Laudais P, Goldfarb B (1985) Drug associated acute renal failure. A prospective multicenter report. Proc Eur Dial Tromsplant Assoc 22:1002–1007
Lachaal M, Venuto R (1989) Nephrotoxicity and hyperkalemia in patients with AIDS treated with pentamidine. Am J Med 87:260–263
Laurent G, Carlier MB, Rollman B, Van Hoof F, Tulkens P (1982) Mechanism of aminoglycoside-induced lysosomal phospholipidosis: in vitro and in vivo studies with gentamicin and amikacin. Biochem Pharmacol 31:3861–3870
Laurent G, Yernaux V, Nonclercq D, Toubeau G, Maldague P, Tulkens PM, Heusen-Stiennon JA (1988) Tissue injury and proliferative response induced in rat kidney by cis-diammine dichloroplatinum. II. Virchows Archiv [B] 55:129–145
Leehey DL, Braun BI, Tholl DA, Chung LS, Gross CA, Roback JA, Lentino JR (1993) Can pharmacokinetic dosing decrease nephrotoxicity with aminoglycoside therapy? J Am Soc Nephrol 4:81–90
Levinson ME (1992) New dosing regimens for aminoglycoside antibiotics. Ann Intern Med 117:693–694
Lippman AJ, Helson C, Helson L, Krakoff IH (1973) Clinical trials of cis-diamminedichloroplatinum. Cancer Chemother Rep 57:191–200
Litterst CL, Weiss RB (1987) Clinical and experimental nephrotoxicity of chemotherapeutic agents. In: Bach PH, Lock EA (eds) Nephrotoxicity in the experimental and clinical situation. Nijhoff, Dordrecht, pp 771–816
Loehrer PJ, Einhorn EH (1984) Cisplatin. Ann Intern Med 100:704–713
Lohr JW, McFarlane MJ, Grantham JJ (1988) A clinical index to predict survival in acute renal failure patients requiring dialysis. Am J Kidney Dis 11:254–259
Maddux MS, Barriere SL (1980) A review of complications of amphotericin B therapy: recommendations for prevention and management. Drug Intell Clin Pharmacol 14:177–181
Madias NE, Harrington JT (1978) Platinum nephrotoxicity. Am J Med 65:307–314

Maher ER, Robinson KN, Scoble JE, Farrimond JG, Browne DRG, Moorhead JF (1989) Prognosis of critically ill patients with acute renal failure: APACHE II score and other predictive factors. Q J Med 72:857–866

Mani S (1992) Pentamidine-induced renal magnesium wasting. AIDS 6:594–595

Medoff G, Kobayashi GS (1980) Strategies in the treatment of systemic fungal infections. N Engl J Med 302:145–155

Medoff G, Brajtburg J, Kobayashi GS, Bolard J (1983) Antifungal agents useful in therapy of systemic fungal infections. Annu Rev Pharmacol Toxicol 23:303–330

Meijer S, Sleifjer DT, Mulder NH, Sluiter WJ, Marrink J, Koops HS, Browers TM, Oldhoff J, van der Hem GK, Mandema E (1983) Some effects of combination therapy with cis-platinum on renal function in patients with nonseminomatous testicular carcinoma. Cancer 51:2035–2040

Messana JM, Gieslinski DA, Nguyen VD, Humes HD (1988) Comparison of the toxicity of the radiocontrast agents iopamidol and diatrizoate to rabbit renal proximal tubule cells in vitro. J Pharmacol Exp Ther 244:1139–1144

Mingeot-Leclercq MP, Piret J, Brasseur R, Tulkens PM (1990) Effect of acidic phospholipids on the activity of lysosomal phospholipases and on their inhibition by aminoglycoside antibiotics. I. Biochemical analysis. Biochem Pharmacol 40:489–497

Mission RT, Cutler RE (1985) Radiocontrast-induced renal failure. West J Med 142:657–664

Moellering RC, Krogstad DJ, Greenblatt DJ (1981) Pharmacokinetics of vancomycin in normal subjects and in patients with reduced renal function. Rev Infect Dis 3 Suppl:S230–S235

Moench TR, Smith CR (1982) Risk factors for aminoglycoside nephrotoxicity. In: Whelton A, Neu HC (eds) The aminoglycosides: microbiology, clinical use and toxicology. Dekker, New York, pp 401–415

Molina J-M, Belenfant X, Doco-Lecompte T, Idatte J-M, Modai J (1991) Sulfadiazine-induced crystalluria in AIDS patients with toxoplasma encephalitis. AIDS 5:587–589

Molitoris BA, Meyer, C, Dahl R, Geerdes A (1993) Mechanism of ischemia-enhanced aminoglycoside binding and uptake by proximal tubule cells. Am J Physiol 264:F907–F916

Moore RD, Smith CR, Lipsky JL, Mellits ED, Lietman PS (1984) Risk factors for nephrotoxicity in patients treated with aminoglycosides. Ann Intern Med 100:352–357

Moore RD, Steinberg EP, Powe NR, Brinker JA, Fishman EK, Graziano S, Gopalan R (1992) Nephrotoxicity of high-osmolality versus low-osmolality contrast media: randomized clinical trial. Radiology 182:649–655

Moreau JF, Droz D, Sabto J, Jungers P, Kleinknecht D, Hinglais N, Michel JR (1975) Osmotic nephrosis induced by water-soluble triiodinated contrast media in man. Radiology 115:329–336

Mudge GH (1980) Nephrotoxicity of urographic drugs. Kidney Int 18:540–552

Murray MD, Brater DC (1993) Renal toxicity of nonsteroidal anti-inflammatory drugs. Annu Rev Pharmacol Toxicol 32:435–465

Navin TR, Dickinson CM, Adam SR, Mayersohn M, Juranek DD (1987) Effect of azotemia in dogs on the pharmacokinetics of pentamidine. J Infect Dis 155:1021–1026

Neumayer HH, Junge W, Kufner A, Wenning A (1989) Prevention of radiocontrast-media induced nephrotoxicity by the calcium channel blocker nitrendipine: a prospective randomized clinical trial. Nephrol Dial Transplant 4:1030–1036

Norrby SR (1987) Side effects of cephalosporins. Drugs 34 Suppl 2:105–120

Ohnishi A, Ohnishi T, Stevenhead W, Robinson RD, O'Day DH, Jackson EK, Branch RA (1989) Sodium status influences amphotericin B nephrotoxicity in the rat. Antimicrob Agents Chemother 3:1222–1227

Parfrey PS, Griffiths SM, Barrett BJ, Paul DM, Genge M, Withers J, Farid N, McManomon P (1989) Contrast material-induced renal failure in patients with diabetes mellitus, renal insufficiency or both. N Engl J Med 320:143–149

Parvez Z, Ramamurstby S, Patel NB, Moncada R (1990) Enzyme markers of contrast media-induced renal failure. Invest Radiol 25:5133–5134

Patterson RM, Ackerman GL (1971) Renal tubular acidosis due to amphotericin B nephrotoxicity. Arch Intern Med 127:241–244
Pearce CJ, Gonzalez FM, Wallin JD (1993) Renal failure and hyperkalemia associated with ketorolac tromethamine. Arch Intern Med 153:1000–1002
Pitman SW, Frei E III (1977) Weekly methotrexate-calcium leucovorin rescue: effect of alkalinization on nephrotoxicity; pharmacokinetics in the CNS; and use in CNS non-Hodgkin's lymphoma. Cancer Treat Rep 61:695–701
Pitman SW, Parker LW, Tattersall MHN, Jaffe N, Frei E III (1975) Clinical trial of high-dose methotrexate (NSC-740) with citrovorum factor (NSC-3590): toxicologic and therapeutic observations. Cancer Chemother Rep 6(3):43–49
Plaut ME, Schentag JJ, Jusko WJ (1979) Aminoglycoside nephrotoxicity: comparative assessment in critically ill patients. J Med 10:257–266
Porile JL, Bakris GL, Garella S (1990) Acute interstitial nephritis with glomerulopathy due to nonsteroidal anti-inflammatory agents: a review of its clinical spectrum and effects of steroid therapy. J Clin Pharmacol 30:468–475
Porter GA (1993) Effects of contrast agents on renal function. Invest Radiol 28:S1–S5
Porush JG, Chou S-Y, Anto HR, Oguagha C, Shapiro WB, Faubert PF (1982) Infusion pyelography and renal function: effects of hypertonic mannitol and furosemide in patients with chronic renal insufficiency. In: Eliahou HE (ed) Acute renal failure. Libbey, London, pp 161–167
Prins JM, Buller HR, Kuijper EJ, Tange RA, Speelman P (1993) Once versus thrice daily gentamicin in patients with serious infections. Lancet 341:335–339
Ramsammy LS, Josepovitz C, Lane BP, Kaloyanides GJ (1989) Polyaspartic acid protects against gentamicin nephrotoxicity in the rat. J Pharmacol Exp Ther 250:149–153
Ramsammy LS, Josepovitz C, Lane B, Kaloyanides Gj (1990) Polyaspartic acid inhibits gentamicin-induced perturbations of phospholipid metabolism. Am J Physiol 258:C1141–1149
Rankin GO, Sutherland CH (1989) Nephrotoxicity of aminoglycosides and cephalosporins in combination. Adverse Drug React Acute Poisoning Rev 8:73–88
Rasmussen HH, Ibels LS (1982) Acute renal failure: multivariate analysis of causes and risk factors. Am J Med 73:211–218
Rasmussen HH, Pitt EA, Ibels LS (1985) Prediction of outcome in acute renal failure by discriminant analysis of clinical variables. Arch Intern Med 145:2015–2018
Robins AB (1982) The binding of platinum ethylendiammine dichloride to proteins in vitro and in vivo. Chem Biol Interact 38:349–356
Rowe JM, Ciobanu N, Ascensao J, Stadtmauer EA, Weiner RS, Schenkein DP, McGlave P, Lazarus HM (1994) Recommended guidelines for the management of autologous bone marrow transplantation: a report from the Eastern Cooperative Oncology Group. Ann Intern Med 120:143–158
Rozdzinski E, Kern WV, Reichle A, Moritz T, Schmeiser T, Gaus W, Kurle E (1993) Once-daily versus thrice-daily dosing of netilmicin in combination with β-lactam antibiotics as empirical therapy for febrile neutropenic patients. J Antimicrob Chemother 31:585–598
Russo D, Testa A, Della Volpe L, Sansone G (1990) Randomized prospective study on renal effects of two different contrast media in humans: protective role of a calcium channel blocker. Nephron 55:254–257
Sabra R, Takahashi K, Branch RA, Badr KF (1990) Mechanisms of amphotericin B-induced reduction of the glomerular filtration rate: a micropuncture study. J Pharmacol Exp Ther 253:34–37
Safirstein R, Winston J, Goldstein M, Moel D, Dikman S, Guttenplan J (1986) Cisplatin nephrotoxicity. Am J Kidney Dis 8:356–367
Safrin S, Crumpacker C, Chatis P (1991) A controlled trial comparing foscarnet with vidarabine for acyclovir-resistant mucocutaneous herpes simplex in the acquired immunodeficiency syndrome. N Engl J Med 325:551–555

Sawaya BP, Weihprecht H, Campbell WR, Lorenz JN, Webb RC, Briggs JP, Schnermann J (1991) Direct vasoconstriction as a possible cause for amphotericin B-induced nephrotoxicity in rats. J Clin Invest 87:2097–2107
Sawyer MH, Webb DF, Balow JE, Strauss SE (1988) Acyclovir induced renal failure: clinical course and histology. Am J Med 84:1067–1071
Schaefer JH, Jochimsen F, Keller F (1991) Outcome prediction of acute renal failure in medical intensive care. Intensive Care Med 17:19–24
Schentag JJ, Cumbo TJ, Jusko WJ, Plaut ME (1978) Gentamicin tissue accumulation and nephrotoxic reactions. JAMA 240:2067–2069
Schentag JJ, Cerra FB, Plaut ME (1982) Clinical and pharmacokinetic characteristics of aminoglycoside nephrotoxicity in 201 critically ill patients. Antimicrob Agents Chemother 21:721–726
Schilsky RL, Barlock A, Ozols RF (1982) Persistent hypomagnesemia following cisplatin chemotherapy for testicular cancer. Cancer Treat Rep 66:1767–1769
Schlondorff D (1993) Renal complications of nonsteroidal anti-inflammatory drugs. Kidney Int 44:643–653
Schneider MME, Hopelman AIM, Schattenkerk JKME, Nielsen TL, van der Graaf Y, Frissen JPH, van der Ende IME, Kolsters AFP, Borleffs JCC (1992) A controlled trial of aerosolized pentamidine or trimethoprim-sulfamethoxazole as primary prophylaxis against Pheumocystis cariini pneumonia in patients with human immunodeficiency virus infection. N Engl J Med 327:1836–1841
Schwartz RH, Berdon WE, Wagner HE, Becker J, Baker DH (1970) Tamm-Horsfall urinary mucoprotein precipitation of urographic contrast agents. AJR 108:698–701
Sedor JR, Davidson EW, Dunn MJ (1986) Effects of nonsteroidal anti-inflammatory drugs in healthy subjects. Am J Med 81 Suppl 2B:58–70
Shafi T, Chou S-Y, Porush J, Shapiro W (1978) Infusion intravenous pyelography and renal function: effects in patients with chronic renal insufficiency. Arch Intern Med 138:1218–1221
Shusterman N, Strom BL, Murray TG, Morrison G, West SL, Maisten G (1987) Risk factors and outcome of hospital-acquired acute renal failure. Am J Med 83:65–71
Siegel WH (1978) Unusual complication of therapy with sulfamethoxazole-trimethoprim. J Urol 117:397
Sjovall J, Bergdahl S, Gunille M (1989) Pharmacokinetics of foscarnet and distribution to cerebrospinal fluid after intravenous infusion in patients with human immunodeficiency virus infection. Antimicrob Agents Chemother 33:1023–1031
Smith CR, Moore RD, Lietman PS (1986) Studies of risk factors for aminoglycoside nephrotoxicity. Am J Kidney Dis 8:308–313
Spinler SA, Goldfarb S (1992) Nephrotoxicity of contrast media following cardiac angiography: pathogenesis, clinical course, and preventive measures including the role of low-osmlality contrast media. Ann Pharmacother 26:56–72
Stamm AM, Diasio RB, Dismukes WE, Shadomy S, Cloud GA, Bowles CA, Karam GH, Espilel-Ingroff A (1987) Toxicity of amphotericin B plus flucytosine in 194 patients with cryptococcal meningitis. Am J Med 83:236–242
Swainson CP, Colls BM, Fitzharris BM (1985) Cis-platinum and distal tubule toxicity. N Z Med J 98:375–378
Tay LK, Bregman CL, Masters BA, Williams PD (1988) Effects of cis-diaminedichloroplatinum (II) on rabbit kidney in vivo and on rabbit proximal tubule cells in culture. Cancer Res 48:2538–2543
Tereul JL, Marcer R, Onaindia JM, Serano A, Quereda C, Ortuno J (1981) Renal function impairment caused by intravenous urography. Arch Intern Med 141:1271–1274
Tolins JP, Raij L (1988) Adverse effect of amphotericin B administration on renal hemodynamics in the rat. Neurohumoral mechanisms and influence of calcium channel blockade. J Pharmacol Exp Ther 245:594–599

Tolins JP, Raij L (1991) Chronic amphotericin B nephrotoxicity in the rat: protective effect of calcium channel blockade. J Am Soc Nephrol 2:98–102
Treskes M, van der Vijgh WJF (1993) WR2721 as a modulator of cisplatin- and carboplatin-induced side effects in comparison with other chemoprotective agents: a molecular approach. Cancer Chemother Pharmacol 33:93–106
Tune BM (1986) The nephrotoxicity of cephalosporin antibiotics: structure-activity relationships. Commun Toxicol 1:145–170
Tune BM (1993) The nephrotoxicity of beta-lactam antibiotics. In: Hook JB, Goldstein RS (eds) Toxicology of the kidney, 2nd edn. Raven, New York, pp 257–287
Tune BM, Fravert D, Hsu C-Y (1990) Thienamycin nephrotoxicity: mitochondrial injury and oxidative effects of imipenem in the rabbit kidney. Biochem Pharmacol 38:3779–3783
Turney JH, Marshall DH, Brownjohn AM, Ellis CM, Parson FM (1990) The evolution of acute renal failure, 1956–1988. Q J Med 74:83–104
Van Zee BE, Hoy WE, Talley TE, Jaenike JR (1978) Renal injury associated with intravenous pyelography in nondiabetic and diabetic patients. Ann Intern Med 89:51–54
Waalkes TM, Denhem C, De Vita VT (1970) Pentamidine: clinical pharmacologic correlations in man and mice. Clin Pharmacol Ther 11:505–512
Wade JC, Petty BG, Conrad G, Smith CR, Lipsky JJ, Ellner J, Lietman PS (1978) Cephalothin plus an aminoglycoside is more nephrotoxic than methicillin plus an aminoglycoside. Lancet 2:604–606
Waldman R, Pearce D, Martin R (1973) Pentamidine isothionate levels in lungs, liver and kidneys of rats after aerosol or intravenous administration. Am Rev Respir Dis 108:1004–1006
Walzer PD, Perl DP, Krogstad DJ, Rawson PG, Schultz MG (1974) Pneumoncystis cariini pneumonia in the United States. Epidemiologic, diagnostic and clinical features. Ann Intern Med 80:83–93
Weinrauch LA, Healy RW, Leland OS, Goldstein HH, Kassissieh SD, Libertino JA, Takacs FJ, D'Elia JA (1977) Coronary angiography and acute renal failure in azotemic diabetic nephropathy. Ann Intern Med 86:56–59
Weinstein L, Madoff MA, Samet CM (1960) The sulfonamides. N Engl J Med 263:793–800
Weisberg LS, Kurnik PB, Kurnik BRC (1994) Risk of radiocontrast nephropathy in patients with and without diabetes mellitus. Kidney Int 45:259–265
Wertlake PT, Butler WT, Hill GJ II, Utz JP (1963) Nephrotoxic tubular damage and calcium deposition following amphotericin B therapy. Am J Pathol 43:449–457
Wilkins RG, Faragher EB (1983) Acute renal failure in an intensive care unit: incidence, prediction and outcome. Anesthesia 38:628–634
Winston DJ, Winston GH, Bruckner DA, Champlin RE (1991) Beta-lactam antibiotic therapy in febrile granulocytopenic patients: a randomized trial comparing cefoperazone plus piperacillin, ceftazidime plus piperacillin and imipenem alone. Ann Intern Med 115:849–859
Wold JS, Turnipseed SA (1981) Toxicology of vancomycin in laboratory animals. Rev Infect Dis 3 Suppl:S224–S229
Wood CA, Kohlhepp SJ, Kohnen PW, Houghton DC, Gilbert DN (1986) Vancomycin enhancement of experimental tobramycin nephrotoxicity. Antimicrob Agents Chemother 30:20–24
Zager RA (1988) Gentamicin nephrotoxicity in the setting of acute renal hypoperfusion. Am J Physiol 254:F574–F581
Zager RA (1992) Endotoxemia, renal hypoperfusion and fever: interactive risk factors for aminoglycoside and sepsis-associated acute renal failure. Am J Kidney Dis 20:223–230
Zager RA, Sharma HM, Johannes GA (1983) Gentamicin increases renal susceptibility to an acute ischemic insult. J Lab Clin Med 101:670–678
Zager RA, Bredl CR, Schimpf BA (1992) Direct amphotericin B-mediated tubular toxicity: assessment of selected cytoprotective agents. Kidney Int 41:337–345

Hepatorenal Syndrome – Current Concepts of Pathophysiology and Therapy

M. Epstein

Introduction

The hepatorenal syndrome (HRS) is a unique form of acute renal failure occurring in patients with liver disease for which a specific cause cannot be elucidated. Despite the intense clinical and investigative interest that this syndrome has stimulated, until recently relatively little progress has been made in the understanding and management of this syndrome. The past several years have witnessed newer insights in both the pathophysiology and therapeutics of this syndrome. The application of newer methodology such as tracer kinetics have more rigorously delineated the role of a number of pathogenic mechanisms including activation of the sympathetic nervous system. The characterization of endothelin and the nitric oxide–arginine pathway and their roles in biology and medicine has provided additional new insights with regard to the pathogenesis of hepatorenal syndrome. Finally, recently initiated therapeutic approaches lend a note of optimism to the future management of a syndrome that is so often incompatible with recovery.

It is not my intent to compile an exhaustive survey of the pathophysiology and therapeutics of the hepatorenal syndrome. Because there are major derrangements of renal function, volume homeostasis, and cardiac performance in this syndrome, these patients are often seen and treated in an intensive care setting. Rather, emphasis will be on selective issues that I believe are timely and have recently attracted increased attention and investigative interest.

Clinical Features

Progressive oliguric renal failure commonly complicates the course of advanced hepatic disease [1–4]. Although this condition has been designated by many names, including "functional renal failure," "hemodynamic renal failure," "hepatic nephropathy," "renal failure of cirrhosis," and others, the more appealing, albeit less specific, term HRS is the most commonly used. For the purpose of this discussion, HRS is defined as unexplained renal failure occurring in patients with liver disease in the absence of clinical, laboratory, or anatomic evidence of other known causes of renal failure.

The clinical features of HRS have been detailed in several recent reviews [1–4]. In brief, HRS usually occurs in cirrhotic patients who are alcoholic, although cirrhosis is not a sine qua non for development of HRS. HRS may complicate other liver diseases, including acute hepatitis, fulminant hepatic failure, and hepatic malignancy [5–7]. Although renal failure may develop in patients in whom normal serum creatinine levels have been previously documented within a few days of onset of HRS, this does not imply that these patients had a normal glomerular filtration rate (GFR). The serum creatinine has been shown to be a poor index of renal function in patients with chronic liver disease, often masking markedly reduced GFR [7]. Implicit in such a formulation is the concept that HRS patients may have a low GFR for weeks to months prior to coming to medical attention. We are therefore dealing with kidneys that are almost certainly susceptible to further insult by hemodynamic or other stimuli.

The development of renal failure in the course of Laennec's cirrhosis is of grave prognostic significance [1, 4, 8]. The majority of patients die within 3 weeks of onset of azotemia. Despite the bleak prognosis, it is difficult to attribute the poor outcome directly to renal failure in patients in whom azotemia is moderate. Such observations suggest that the renal failure may be more of a reflection of a broader lethal event and that in most instances it is not in itself the major determinant of survival. A truly uremic death is a rarity.

Pathogenesis

A substantial body of evidence lends strong support to the concept that the renal failure in HRS is functional in nature. Despite the severe derangement of renal function, pathological abnormalities are minimal and inconsistent [1, 4, 9]. Furthermore, tubular functional integrity is maintained during the renal failure, as manifested by a relatively unimpaired sodium reabsorptive capacity and concentrating ability. Finally, more direct evidence is derived (a) from the demonstration that kidneys transplanted from patients with HRS are capable of resuming normal function in the recipient [10] and (b) by the return of renal function when the patient with HRS successfully receives a liver transplant [11].

Despite extensive study, the precise pathogenesis of HRS has not been delineated. Many studies utilizing diverse hemodynamic techniques have documented a significant reduction in renal perfusion [12–14]. Since a similar decrement of renal perfusion is compatible with urine volumes exceeding 1 l in many patients with chronic renal failure, it is unlikely that a decrease in mean blood flow per se is responsible for the encountered oliguria [15].

Our laboratory applied the ^{133}Xe washout technique and selective renal arteriography to the study of HRS and demonstrated a significant reduction in calculated mean blood flow as well as a preferential reduction in cortical perfusion [13]. In addition, cirrhotic patients manifested marked vasomotor instability that was characterized not only by variability between serial xenon washout studies, but also by instability within a single curve [13]. This phenomenon has not been encountered in renal failure of other etiologies. In addition, Epstein and coworkers [13] performed simultaneous renal arteriography to delineate further the nature of the hemodynamic abnormalities. Selective renal arteriograms disclosed marked beading and tortuosity of the interlobar and proximal arcuate arteries and an absence of distinct cortical nephrograms and vascular filling of the cortical vessels (Fig. 1A). Postmortem angiography performed on the kidneys of five patients studied during life disclosed a striking normalization of the vascular abnormalities with reversal of all the vascular abnormalities in the kidneys (Fig. 1B). The peripheral vasculature filled completely, and the previously irregular vessels became smooth and regular. These findings provide additional evidence for the functional basis of the renal failure, operating through active renal vasoconstriction [13].

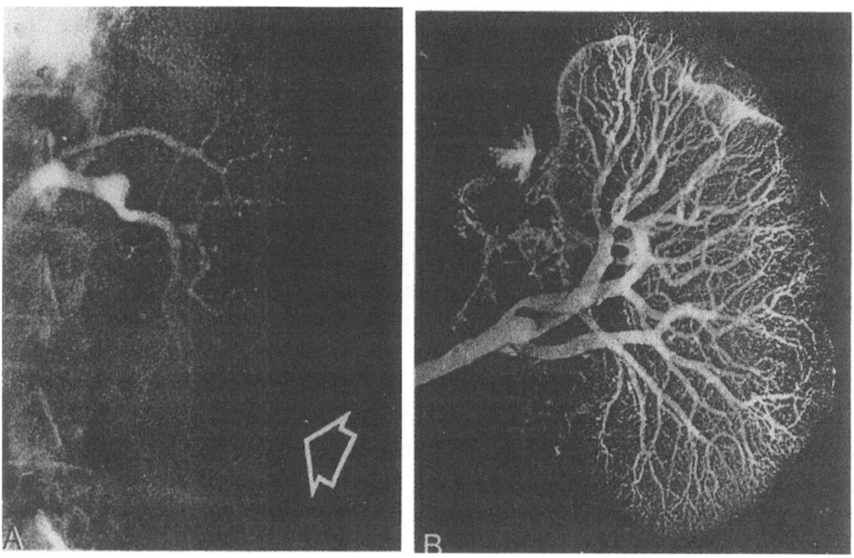

Fig. 1. A Selective renal arteriogram carried out in a patient with oliguric renal failure and cirrhosis. Note the extreme abnormality of the intrarenal vessels, including the primary branches off the main renal artery and the interlobar arteries. The arcuate and cortical arterial system is not recognizable, nor is a distinct cortical nephrogram present. The *arrow* indicates the edge of the kidney. **B** Angiogram carried out postmortem of the same kidney with the intra-arterial injection of micropaque in gelatin as the contrast agent. Note filling of the renal arterial system throughout the vascular bed to the periphery of the cortex. The peripheral arterial tree that did not opacify in vivo now fills completely. The vascular attenuation and tortuosity is no longer present. The vessels were also histologically normal. (From [13], with permission)

Although renal hypoperfusion with preferential renal cortical ischemia has been shown to underlie the renal failure of HRS [13, 16], the factors responsible for sustaining reduction in cortical perfusion and suppression of filtration in HRS have not been fully elucidated. A consideration of the pathogenetic events leading to the intrarenal hemodynamic derangement and the decrease in GFR is simplified by a consideration of the afferent and efferent events that lead to this derangement. The discussion of afferent events will include a consideration of the extracellular fluid translocations or sequestration into serous spaces or interstitial fluid compartments characterizing advanced liver disease. The section considering efferent events will encompass a survey of the hormonal and neural mechanisms proposed or implicated in the pathogenesis of the renal failure. Emphasis will be placed on recent studies characterizing the sympathetic nervous system, renal thromboxanes, nitric oxide–arginine pathway, and the possible contribution of endothelin.

Afferent Events

Traditionally, it has been proposed that a contraction of the effective blood volume constitutes a pivotal event in predisposing to HRS [1–4, 17–19]. In this context, it is important to note that the term "effective plasma volume" refers to that part of the total circulating volume that is effective in stimulating volume receptors. The concept is somewhat elusive, since the actual volume receptors remain incompletely defined. A diminished effective volume may reflect subtle alterations in systemic hemodynamic factors such as decreased filling of the arterial tree, a diminished central blood volume, or both. Despite massive retention of salt and water, effective blood volume remains functionally contracted because of a disturbance in the Starling forces that govern the distribution of fluid within the extracellular fluid (ECF) compartment.

The mechanisms contributing to the appearance of a diminished effective volume are multiple. Traditionally, it has been proposed that ascites formation in cirrhotic patients begins when a critical imbalance of Starling forces in the hepatic sinusoids and splanchnic capillaries causes an excessive amount of lymph formation, exceeding the capacity of the thoracic duct to return this excessive lymph to the circulation [1, 17–19]. Consequently, excess lymph accumulates in the peritoneal space as ascites, with a subsequent contraction of circulating plasma volume. Thus, as ascites develops, there is a progressive redistribution of plasma volume.

Although an imbalance of Starling forces in the hepatosplanchnic microcirculation is thought to contribute importantly to the relative decrease in effective blood volume, it should be emphasized that this is not the sole mechanism. An additional determinant is the significant diminution of total peripheral resistance in most patients with cirrhosis who are retaining sodium and water [20, 21]. This decrease in peripheral vascular resistance is no doubt partially related to anatomical arteriovenous shunts and possibly to some undefined vasodilator (either produced by or not inactivated by the diseased liver). Thus, despite an increase in total plasma volume, the relative "fullness" of the arteriovenous tree is diminished. In summary, several hemodynamic events act in concert to diminish effective volume, thereby activating the mechanisms promoting a decrease in renal perfusion and GFR. Regardless of cause, the resultant diminution of effective volume is thought to constitute an afferent signal to the renal tubule to augment salt and water reabsorption and to decrease GFR. Thus, the traditional underfill formulation suggests that the renal retention of sodium is a *secondary* rather than primary event.

Peripheral Arterial Vasodilation Theory (Revised Underfill Theory)

The principal distinguishing feature of a newly proposed revision of the underfill theory is that the decrease in effective blood volume is attributable primarily to an early occurring increase in vascular capacitance [21]. Thus, peripheral vasodilation is the initial determinant of intravascular underfilling, and an imbalance between the expanded capacitance and available volume constitutes a diminished effective volume. This concept brings the hypothesis into accord with some experimental observations that were not consistent with the original postulate. For example, recent careful balance studies in animals with experimental cirrhosis have clearly shown that sodium retention precedes ascite formation [22].

Primary systemic hemodynamic changes characterized by peripheral vasodilation occur very early in experimental cirrhosis and in humans with compensated cirrhosis [20, 22, 23]. The decrease in effective volume induced by these hemodynamic alterations is compounded further by an impaired pressor response to vasoactive agents including exogenous angiotensin II and noradrenaline [4, 21]. Even in those patients who eventually develop an increase in total plasma volume, the relative fullness of the arteriovenous tree is decreased.

According to the peripheral arterial vasodilation hypothesis, the hepatorenal syndrome constitutes an extreme extension of underfilling of the arterial circulation, with the most extreme elevations of vasoactive hormones including plasma renin activity (PRA), norepinephrine, and vasopressin and the most extreme degree of renal vasoconstriction [21].

Overflow Theory

An alternative hypothesis to the two underfill theories is the overflow theory of ascites formation [22, 24]. In contrast to the underfill formulation, the overflow theory postulates that the initial *primary* event is the inappropriate retention of excessive amounts of sodium by the kidneys, unrelated to defense of the plasma volume (and thought to be due to intrahepatic hypertension). In the setting of abnormal Starling forces in the portal venous bed and hepatic sinusoids (both portal venous hypertension and a reduction in plasma colloid osmotic pressure), the expanded plasma volume is sequestered preferentially in the peritoneal space, with ascite formation. Thus, renal sodium retention and plasma volume expansion *precede rather than follow* the formation of ascites.

In summary, both underfill theories provide a possible explanation of why fluid retention often fails to attenuate the stimulus for neurohormonal activation and continuing sodium and water retention. Despite a progressive increase in total ECF volume, fluid is sequestered into one or more of the other fluid compartments without succeeding in normalizing effective blood volume. Since the interstitial fluid (ISF) and its associated spaces, for example the peritoneum, are largely limitless in capacity, the kidneys encounter great difficulty in filling such a space and the sodium retention becomes relentless. Only correction of the disturbance in the forces governing fluid distribution and reversing the peripheral arterial vasodilatation will permit a reexpansion of effective blood volume to normal. Importantly, the peripheral arterial vasodilation theory highlights the florid systemic hemodynamic disturbances and the importance of attempting to correct not only the renal hemodynamic disturbances, but the concomitant systemic hemodynamic derangements as well.

An alternate formulation has emphasized that the renal vasoconstriction is attributable to unique events independent of a contracted volume, i.e., a primary cause. According to this theory advanced liver damage, in conjunction with some other unknown abnormality, induces a primary disorder in one or more of the modifiers regulating renal vascular tone. The renal ischemia, it is argued, is not an expression of the normal neural and hormonal response to liver damage, but represents either an alteration in the synthesis, degradation, or potency of a vasoactive substance or a malfunction of the normal feedback regulation of its release. Such abnormalities might result from impaired hepatic degradative or excretory capacity, portosystemic shunting of blood, or altered neural connections between liver and kidney.

Although many investigators have focused on a contraction of effective arterial blood volume (EABV) as a major etiological factor in the pathogenesis of HRS, there is lack of unanimity on this point. Some authors have proposed that because a diminished EABV causes the typical syndrome of prerenal failure (easily reversible with volume replacement) sometimes leading to acute tubular necrosis (ATN), it cannot be considered as the prepotent etiological factor for HRS. Although I agree that HRS is primarily a syndrome induced by a unique cause for renal ischemia not necessitating a contracted EABV, a contributory role for a contracted EABV need not be excluded. Rather, it is tempting to postulate that a contracted EABV and/or the concomitant activation of neurohormonal mediators that attend such hypovolemia amplify the renal vasoconstrictive effects of the putative, as yet undefined, mediators. Indeed, because the majority of studies have reported that a reduction of EABV is a typical feature of patients with HRS, this alteration in volume status may be a necessary but not sufficient factor predisposing to HRS.

An alternate formulation to reconcile the presence of contracted EABV in both prerenal azotemia and HRS posits that they represent differences in degree, occupying disparate points on a continuum [21]. Conceivably, patients with moderate contraction of EABV develop prerenal azotemia which is reversible by volume depletion. With advancing liver disease, the magnitude of the contraction becomes greater and at some point is no longer reversible by volume-expansive maneuvers. Presumably at this point we are facing the transition from prerenal azotemia to HRS.

Efferent Events

The effectors that promote renal ischemia and a decrease in GFR remain incompletely defined. Several major hypotheses have been implicated or suggested, including the following:

1. Hormonal
   a) Activation of the renin–angiotensin system
   b) Alterations in renal eicosanoids
      α) Diminished vasodilatory prostaglandins
      β) Increased vasoconstrictor thromboxanes
   c) Enhanced nitric oxide production
   d) Elevated plasma endothelin levels
   e) Endotoxemia
   f) Relative impairment of renal kallikrein production
   g) Diminished atrial natriuretic peptides
   h) Vasoactive intestinal peptide
   i) Glomerulopressin deficiency
2. Neural and hemodynamic
   a) An increase in sympathetic nervous system activity
   b) Alterations in intratenal blood flow distribution

Renin–Angiotensin System

Several lines of evidence suggest a role for the renin–angiotensin axis in sustaining the vasoconstriction in HRS [25]. Patients with decompensated cirrhosis frequently manifest marked elevations of plasma renin levels

[25–29]. An examination of the relationship between renal function and plasma renin levels has disclosed that cirrhotic patients with impaired renal function manifested the most profound elevations in plasma renin levels. Although the elevation of plasma renin is attributable in part to decreased hepatic inactivation of renin, it is evident that the major determinant is increased renin secretion by the kidney. It is noteworthy that the elevation of plasma renin often occurs despite diminished hepatic synthesis of the α_2-globulin, renin substrate [25].

The activation of the renin–angiotensin system has profound implications for renal function. In light of compelling experimental evidence that angiotensin plays an important role in the control of the renal circulation [30], it is tempting to speculate that enhanced angiotensin levels contribute to renal vasoconstriction and reduction in filtration rate of renal failure in cirrhosis. Observations by Cade et al. [31] have underscored the role of angiotensin II in mediating the reduction in renal perfusion and GFR in patients with HRS. The infusion of angiotensin II caused a marked reduction of renal plasma flow in GFR, with a marked increase in filtration fraction.

The availability of pharmacological agents that interrupt the renin–angiotensin axis has suggested a possible approach for defining further the role of angiotensin as a determinant of the state of the renal vasculature [32]. Unfortunately, attempts to block the renin–angiotensin system in cirrhotic humans have been complicated by a striking fall in blood pressure and by the intrinsic activity of the partial agonists in use, which may have blunted the influence on GFR. Synthesis of more specific angiotensin antagonists that may act preferentially at the level of the renal vascular bed without inducing concomitant hypotension may contribute to the further characterization of the pathogenesis of HRS [32].

Role of Renal Prostaglandins

Alterations of renal prostaglandin also participate in mediating the renal failure of cirrhosis. Attempts to investigate the role of renal prostaglandins in modulating renal hemodynamics and mediating the sodium retention in cirrhosis have encompassed two manipulations: (1) administration of exogenous prostaglandins and (2) alteration of the endogenous production of prostaglandins by inhibition of prostaglandin synthesis. Initially, the problem was approached by examining the renal hemodynamic response to the administration of exogenous prostaglandins [33]. Unfortunately, the relevance of such studies in cirrhotic humans is tenuous, since any action of prostaglandins on the kidney must be as a local tissue hormone [34]. Thus, any evaluation of the physiological role of prostaglandins in renal function necessitates an experimental design in which the endogenous production of the lipids is altered.

Several investigators have demonstrated that the administration of inhibitors of prostaglandin synthetase (both indomethacin and ibuprofen) resulted in significant decrements in GFR and effective renal plasma flow (ERPF) in patients with alcoholic liver disease and ascites [35, 36]. Of interest, the decrement in renal hemodynamics varied directly with the degree of sodium retention, i.e., the patients with the most avid sodium retention manifested the largest decrements in GFR [36–38].

Since the above-cited studies have examined the effect of inhibiting endogenous production of renal prostaglandins, it was of great interest to assess an opposite experimental manipulation, i.e., assessing the effects on renal function of augmentation of endogenous prostaglandins. Epstein et al. [39] have utilized water immersion to the neck, an experimental maneuver that redistributes blood volume with concomitant central hypervolemia and enhances prostaglandin E (PGE) excretion in normal humans. They demonstrated that decompensated cirrhotic patients manifested an increase in mean PGE excretion that was threefold greater than that observed in normal subjects studied under identical conditions [40]. This was attended by a marked natriuresis and an increase in creatinine clearance. When interpreted in concert with the earlier studies utilizing prostaglandin synthetase inhibitors, these findings suggest that derangements in renal PGE production contribute to the renal dysfunction of cirrhosis. Specifically, it is tempting to postulate that in the setting of cirrhosis of the liver, the ability to enhance prostaglandin synthesis constitutes a compensatory or adaptive response to incipient renal ischemia. The corollary of this formulation is that the administration of agents that impair such an adaptation can induce a clinically important deterioration of renal function.

Additional studies have suggested that alterations of thromboxanes may contribute to the renal dysfunction. Thromboxane A_2 (TxA_2), a potent proaggregatory and vasoconstrictor substance, is synthesized by platelets and a large number of other cell types and tissues, including the kidney [41, 42]. Renal TxA_2 production is thought to be involved in the regulation of glomerular hemodynamics because of its action on glomerular capillary filtration surface area [41, 42] and by modulating the tone of afferent and efferent arterioles [42]. It has been proposed that the ratio of the vasodilator PGE_2 to the vasoconstrictor prostaglandin thromboxane A_2 (TxA_2) i.e., E_2/TxA_2, rather than absolute levels of PGE_2, may determine the degree of renal vasoconstriction of HRS. Zipser et al. [43] determined urinary excretion of PGE_2 and TxB_2 (the nonenzymatic metabolite of TxA_2) in 14 patients with HRS. They observed that whereas PGE_2 levels were decreased in comparison with those of healthy controls as well as those of patients with acute renal failure, TxB_2 levels were markedly elevated. The authors interpreted their data to suggest that an imbalance of vasodilator and vasoconstrictor metabolites of arachidonic acid contribute to the pathogenesis of HRS.

It should be noted, however, that the findings of others of an increase in TxB_2 are somewhat different. Rimola et al. [44] reported that patients with HRS failed to manifest increases in urinary PGE_2, 6-keto-$PGF_{1\alpha}$, and TxB_2, in contrast to the findings of Zipser et al. [43]. Additional studies will be required to assess alterations in the differing eicosanoids with progressive renal functional impairment.

In light of the above findings suggesting that thromboxanes may contribute to the development of HRS, there have been attempts to modify the course of HRS by administration of selective inhibitors of thromboxane synthesis and thromboxane receptor antagonists [45–47]. As detailed below, such interventions have either been negative or have failed to substantively augment GFR. Additional studies with thromboxane receptor antagonists in patients with widely varying degrees of acute renal insufficiency will be required to further define the role of TxA_2 as a major determinant of the renal vasoconstriction in HRS.

Increase in Sympathetic Nervous System Activity

An increase in sympathetic nervous system activity also contributes to the renal failure of cirrhosis. It is now well established that alterations in the input of cardiopulmonary receptors induce changes in renal sympathetic activity [48–51]. Thus, a decrease in effective blood volume is sensed as a decrease in left atrial pressure (the sensor of the low pressure vascular system). This "unloads" the left atrial mechanoreceptors, which in turn discharge into afferent vagal fibers that have appropriate central nervous system representation. As a consequence, efferent renal sympathetic nerve activity (ERSNA) is augmented [49, 50, 52]. Such an increase in sympathetic tone would tend to produce renal vasoconstriction and a decrease in GFR.

Although these theoretical considerations suggest a role for the sympathetic nervous system in the renal vasoconstriction and sodium retention of cirrhosis, only recently have studies been conducted to test this possibility. Studies to assess the activity of the sympathetic nervous system in cirrhotic humans have measured plasma catecholamine levels during basal conditions and following postural manipulations [50, 52–57]. Most observers agree that mean peripheral norepinephrine levels are elevated in cirrhotic patients [54–57], Ring-Larsen et al. [54] have determined plasma norepinephrine and epinephrine concentrations in differing vascular beds of cirrhotic patients at the time of hepatic venous catheterization. Based on differences in regional norepinephrine levels, they concluded that the elevated norepinephrine levels in patients with cirrhosis were attributable to enhanced sympathetic nervous system activity rather than decreased metabolism.

As detailed in several recent reviews [58–60], however, the plasma concentrations of norepinephrine are an inadequate guide to either total or regional sympathetic activity. Global measures of sympathetic activity, such as plasma norepinephrine measurements, fail to identify sources of norepinephrine release and cannot delineate regional patterns of sympathetic nervous activation. Recently, Esler et al. [60] conducted a physiologic and neurochemical evaluation of patients with cirrhosis, applying tracer kinetic techniques using radiolabeled norepinephrine, thereby allowing more precise description of regional pattern of the sympathetic nervous derangement in cirrhosis. They demonstrated that the elevated plasma norepinephrine concentration in patients with cirrhosis is attributable to higher overall rates of spillover of the neurotransmitter to plasma and not to reduced plasma clearance caused by liver disease. Administration of clonidine reduced previously elevated norepinephrine overflow rates for the whole body, kidneys, and hepatomesenteric circulation. This sympathetic inhibition was accompanied by several potentially clinically beneficial effects: the lowering of renal vascular resistance, an augmentation of GFR, and the reduction of portal venous pressure [60].

In summary, the available data indicates that the sympathetic nervous system is activated in cirrhosis, both in the kidney and in other regional vascular beds, consequently contributing to the renal vasoconstriction and sodium retention of cirrhosis [52, 60].

Endotoxins

Systemic endotoxemia may participate in the pathogenesis of the renal failure of cirrhosis. Endotoxins, the lipopolysaccharide constituents of the cell wall of certain bacteria, are potent renal vasoconstrictors [61]. It has been hypothesized that enteric endotoxin is liberated into the systemic circulation through naturally or surgically created portosystemic shunts, thus bypassing the hepatic Kupffer cells, the major site of endotoxin removal. Several investigators have measured endotoxin by the limulus lysate technique and reported that endotoxin is present in the portal and systemic circulation of many cirrhotic patients, particularly those with ascites. Since several investigators have demonstrated a high frequency of positive limulus assays in cirrhotic patients with renal failure but not in the absence of renal failure, endotoxins may contribute to the pathogenesis of the renal failure. Endotoxemia is appealing as a possible humoral agent not only because it may cause renal vasoconstriction, but also because it may produce vasodilatation in other circulatory beds and may be a treatable condition [61, 62]. Indeed, Vallance and Moncada have proposed that endotoxemia induces nitric oxide synthase in peripheral blood vessels with resultant vasodilation (vide infra).

Nitric Oxide

A more recent approach to investigation of the pathogenesis of the hepatorenal syndrome has focused on the florid systemic hemodynamic disturbances that invariably accompany the syndrome. These include a hyperdynamic circulation, increased heart rate and cardiac output, and decreased blood pressure and systemic vascular resistance [4, 20–22]. These observations have suggested the likelihood of excess production of a vasodilator [63]. A number of vasodilators have been postulated including prostacyclin, bradykinin, substance P, and atrial natriuretic peptide (ANP), but clear evidence of involvement of any of them is lacking [4, 63].

Recently, attention has focused on the role of nitric oxide as a mediator of both the hyperdynamic circulation and renal failure [64]. Nitric oxide, a vasodilator synthesized from L-arginine, accounts for the biological activity of endothelium-derived relaxing factor [65, 66]. In animals, agonist-induced release of nitric oxide from vascular endothelium leads to peripheral vasodilation, a fall in blood pressure, and tachycardia [67, 68]. These effects are short-lived, however, and vascular tone returns to normal once the agonist infusion is stopped. On the other hand, there is second, distinct, inducible nitric oxide synthase that occurs in response to bacterial lipopolysaccharide endotoxin. Once induced, this enzyme releases nitric oxide for many hours without the need for further stimulation.

Based on these considerations, Vallance and Moncada [64] have postulated that endotoxemia induces a nitric oxide synthase in peripheral blood vessels and that this increased nitric oxide synthesis and release accounts for the associated hyperdynamic circulation.

If this hypothesis is correct, inhibition of nitric oxide synthesis should restore sensitivity to vasoconstrictors and reverse these hemodynamic abnormalities. Specific inhibitors of either the constitutive or the inducible nitric oxide synthase theoretically should facilitate a more precise manipulation of nitric oxide synthesis and help to establish the pathophysiological importance of nitric oxide in endotoxemia and cirrhosis.

In a recent preliminary communication, these investigators reported that serum nitrite and nitrate levels, an index of nitric oxide production, were elevated in a group of cirrhotic patients [69]. The patients with ascites manifested higher nitrite and nitrate levels than cirrhotic patients without ascites. Furthermore, there was a direct correlation between serum nitrite and nitrate levels and endotoxemia. Additional studies will be required to substantiate this hypothesis.

Endothelin

Endothelin, a recently characterized peptide elaborated by endothelial cells grown in culture, is reported to be the most potent mammalian vasoconstrictor peptide described to date [70–73]. We and others have characterized the renal microvascular and hemodynamic actions of endothelin. We have demonstrated that endothelin is a potent vasoconstrictor that acts predominantly on the afferent arteriole with a modest efferent arteriolar effect. As a consequence of this microvascular action, endothelin decreases GFR in normal isolated perfused kidneys. Furthermore, endothelin provokes prominent renal microvascular vasomotion. Finally, we have demonstrated that both nifedipine [72] and isradipine [73] reverse the afferent arteriolar actions of endothelin, suggesting that this peptide elicits renal vasoconstriction, at least in part, by a mechanism involving dihydropyridine-sensitive channels.

Recently, Moore et al. [74] and Moller et al. [75] have suggested the possibility that alterations in endothelin may play a pathogenetic role in the renal failure of the hepatorenal syndrome. They reported that patients with hepatorenal syndrome had markedly elevated plasma endothelin-1 and endothelin-3 concentrations compared with normal subjects, patients having acute or chronic renal failure, and patients with liver disease without renal dysfunction. These investigators interpreted their results to support the hypothesis that these substances play a role in the pathogenesis of the hepatorenal syndrome. As I have noted in a recent editorial, it is equally possible, if not probable, that the results merely represent pari passu events [76]. Thus, elevated plasma endothelin concentrations might be attributable to decreased renal disposal of endothelin. Additional studies are required to assess further the pathogenetic role of endothelin concentrations in this syndrome.

Role of Biologically Active Atrial Peptides

Another hormone that should be included in any consideration of pathogenetic mechanisms of HRS is ANF or atriopeptin. Since the demonstration by DeBold et al. [77] in 1981 that saline extracts of rat heart atria, but not ventricles, caused a marked natriuresis and diuresis when injected into normal rats, there has been much interest in the role of ANF as a mediator of volume homeostasis. Micropuncture studies in rats have shown that ANF, given by either bolus injection or continuous infusion, causes a significant increase in GFR [78] as well as natriuresis and diuresis [79, 80].

Because ANF has thus been shown to be of importance in volume homeostasis and because volume homeostasis is of critical importance in patients with cirrhosis and portal hypertension, a number of investigators have sought a role for ANF in severe hepatic disease [80].

Despite proposals that ANF deficiency may contribute to the renal dysfunction of liver disease, the available data fail to support this formulation. Most investigators have found ANF levels in plasma either normal [81, 82] or increased [83, 84] in cirrhotics with ascites. Morgan et al. [85] compared circulating ANF levels in seven patients with hepatorenal syndrome and seven patients with advanced alcoholic liver disease and ascites but normal serum creatinine levels. They demonstrated that ANF levels were twofold higher in the patients with HRS, indicating that a deficiency of ANF does not contribute to the renal failure.

Acute Renal Failure

Although much attention has been directed to HRS, it should be borne in mind that cirrhotic patients are as vulnerable as noncirrhotic patients to the development of ATN. Among liver disease patients in whom renal failure developed, the etiology of renal failure is more commonly ATN than HRS [1–4]. The increased frequency of ATN may relate to the hypotension, bleeding dyscrasias, infection, and multiple metabolic disorders that complicate the clinical course of these patients. There have been several attempts to develop diagnostic tests to reliably discriminate between acute renal failure and HRS [86–90]. To date these tests that rely on enzymuria or electrolyte excretory patterns are often suggestive but lack sufficient selectivity to be relied on.

Differential Diagnosis

It must be emphasized that the abrupt onset of oliguria in a cirrhotic patient does not necessarily imply the presence of HRS. Prerenal causes are important to differentiate, particularly since they constitute reversible conditions if recognized and treated in the incipient phase. Volume contraction or cardiac pump failure may present as a "pseudohepatorenal" syndrome. Furthermore, as already emphasized, it is not uncommon for patients with alcoholic cirrhosis to develop classic ATN. In many instances, the differentiation from HRS can be made readily by recognition of the

Table 1. Differential diagnosis of acute azotemia in patients with liver disease: important differential urinary findings

	Prerenal azotemia	Hepatorenal syndrome	Acute renal failure (ATN)
Urinary sodium concentration (mEq/1)	<10	<10	>30[a]
Urine to plasma creatinine ratio	>30:1	>30:1	<20:1
Urine osmolality	At least 200 mOsm > plasma osmolality	At least 200 mOsm > plasma osmolality	Relatively similar to plasma osmolality
Urine sediment	Normal	Unremarkable	Casts, cellular debris

The numbers cited in the table are arbitrary and are meant to highlight the salient differences in these three diagnostic categories. However, the values vary. As an example urinary sodium concentration occasionally may exceed 10 mEq/l.

[a] Radiocontrast agents and sepsis may lower urinary sodium concentration in patients with ATN. When urinary output is very low, the concentration of sodium may rise. Urinary sodium levels may also rise when vasoconstriction is so severe that acute tubular necrosis sets in.

precipitating event and by characteristic laboratory findings. Table 1 lists laboratory features helpful in differentiating the three principal causes of acute azotemia in patients with liver disease. The most uniform urinary finding of HRS patients is a strikingly low sodium concentration, usually less than 10 mEq/l and occasionally as low as 2–5 mEq/l. Unfortunately, prerenal azotemia is associated with similarly low urinary sodium concentrations. In contrast, patients with oliguric ATN frequently have urinary sodium concentrations exceeding 30 mEq/l and usually even higher.

Although avid renal sodium retention is evident in the majority of patients with HRS, occasional patients with HRS have been recognized in whom the urinary sodium concentration is consistently greater than 10 mEq/l. In some of these patients, the urinary sodium concentration is initially low but increases to levels of approximately 40 mEq/l as renal impairment progresses, and it has been suggested that this late increase in urinary sodium concentration may represent the possible transition to ATN. Other patients have been recognized in whom HRS has developed and progressed in the presence of a urinary sodium concentration persistently in the range of 20–30 mEq/l [1, 4].

Both HRS and prerenal azotemia manifest well-maintained urinary-concentrating ability characterized by a urine to plasma osmolality ratio (U/P_{osm}) exceeding 1.0, whereas ATN patients excrete a relatively isoosmotic urine (i.e., urine that is neither concentrated nor dilute). The urine to plasma creatinine ratio (U/P creatinine) is greater than 30:1 (and at times 40:1) in both prerenal failure and HRS, whereas U/P creatinine is 20:1 or less in ATN. Proteinuria is absent or minimal in HRS.

In summary, the finding of a low urinary sodium concentration in the presence of oliguric acute renal failure usually precludes the diagnosis of ATN. Only when prerenal failure and ATN are excluded can one establish the diagnosis of HRS.

Treatment

General Considerations

The management of HRS has been discouraging in view of the absence of any reproducible effective treatment modality. Since knowledge about the pathogenesis of HRS is inferential and incomplete, therapy to the present time has been supportive. Because iatrogenic events often precipitate this syndrome and therapy is difficult once the syndrome is established, prevention constitutes the linchpin of management.

The initial step in the management of a cirrhotic patient with acutely reduced renal function is to not equate decreased renal function with HRS, but rather to search diligently for and treat correctable causes of azotemia such as volume contraction, cardiac decompensation, and urinary tract obstruction. The diagnosis of ATN (acute intrinsic renal failure) should clearly be considered, since ATN occurs commonly in cirrhotic patients and they may be expected to recover if supported with dialytic therapy.

Although we commonly invoke the caveat of primum non nocere, it now takes on greater meaning in the HRS patient. As noted previously, it is well established that nonsteroidal anti-inflammatory drugs, which inhibit prostaglandin synthetase activity, often adversely influence renal function in the patient with liver disease and ascites [35, 36, 38]. Similarly, the broad-spectrum antibiotic demeclocycline may induce acute azotemia in the patient with cirrhosis and ascites [91, 92]. Finally, we should be cognizant of the fact that drugs that may be indicated for the management of complications of liver disease (i.e., lactulose for the treatment of hepatic encephalopathy) are capable of inducing profound hypovolemia (secondary to diarrhea) with resultant azotemia.

In excluding reversible prerenal azotemia, there are several management considerations. Since HRS and prerenal azotemia have similar urinary diagnostic indices, one must often use a functional maneuver, i.e., administration of volume expanders to differentiate between these two entities. In this regard, it should be underscored that our frame of reference for the cirrhotic patient may be quite different from that pertaining to other disease states. The degree of volume expansion necessary to replete the cirrhotic patient may at times be marked, occasionally requiring the infusion of massive amounts of colloid.

There is no defined regimen that allows one to predict the amount of volume expanders necessary to replete the cirrhotic patient suspected of being hypovolemic. I recommend that the expanders should be infused in a setting in which alteration of clinical status (blood pressure, urine flow rate, creatinine clearance) as well as central hemodynamics (central venous pressure, CVP; data derived from Swan-Ganz catheter) are monitored. Furthermore, it should be stressed that it is usually the change in CVP that often is important rather than the absolute level, i.e., although a CVP reading may not be extremely low, it may not change (increase) until large amounts of expanders are administered. Such guidelines do not presuppose that there is a correlation between central hemodynamics and the volume deficit. Rather, we utilize manometric determinations as a guideline to assist in determining when to discontinue volume expansion so as to avoid overt fluid overload. Of note, volume expansion carries with it the risk of opening up fragile esophageal varices with secondary bleeding, although in my experience this is a infrequent occurrence.

Basic Management

Once correctable causes of renal functional impairment are excluded, the mainstay of the therapy of HRS to prevent clinical deterioration is careful restriction of sodium and fluid intake. A number of specific therapeutic measures have been attempted, but only a few have proved to be of practical value. Attempts at volume expansion with different agents have resulted in only transient improvement in renal hemodynamics without significant alteration of the outcome. Similarly, attempts at reinfusion of concentrated ascitic fluid have not provided any lasting improvement. Major new approaches that have attracted investigative attention and may possibly warrant future considerations will be enumerated.

Paracentesis

A role of paracentesis in the treatment of HRS, with or without simultaneous plasma volume expansion, has not been established. The potential renal benefit of a reduction of ascitic fluid volume includes diminished intra-abdominal pressure with possible relief of inferior vena caval obstruction and augmentation of cardiac output. Improvement in renal function, when it occurs, is transient, because the abnormal hydraulic pressures that sustain ascites formation are not altered by paracentesis. Continued fluid removal is necessary and may result in progressive depletion of intravascular volume with subsequent deterioration in cardiac function and renal perfusion. Nevertheless, over the past several years the Barcelona group has marshalled evidence that paracentesis may induce a more favorable renal excretory and hormonal response than previously thought [93–96].

Dialysis

Dialysis was previously reported to be ineffective in the management of HRS [97, 98]. Our own recent experience, however, suggests that such a sweeping condemnation should be qualified [99]. Although most of the published literature indeed suggests a dismal prognosis for patients who are dialyzed, such early reports have dealt with patients with chronic end-stage liver disease. In a few instances we have undertaken dialysis in HRS patients with acute hepatic disease and have been gratified by the ultimate favorable outcome. Our experience suggests that in selected patients, i.e., those with acute hepatic dysfunction in whom there is reason to believe that the renal failure may reverse coincident with resolution of the acute hepatic insult, dialytic therapy is indicated.

With the recent maturation and refinement of orthotopic liver transplantation and its acceptance as the treatment of choice for end-stage liver disease, dialysis has assumed an extremely important ancillary role. Dialysis is now widely used as a supportive measure in the management of many patients awaiting liver transplantation.

Continous Hemofiltration

In addition to stabilizing renal function, it is often necessary to remove fluid, either to prevent life-threatening emergencies such as acute pulmonary edema or to permit administration of requisite fluids such as bicarbonate solutions or hyperalimentation. Intermittent hemodialysis has been used for the treatment of fluid overload and ascites. This procedure, however, may be attended by hemodynamic instability and bleeding, and fluid removal is difficult. To circumvent this problem, slow continuous ultrafiltration (SCUF), continuous arteriovenous or venovenous hemofiltration (CAVH or CVVH), and continuous arteriovenous or venovenous hemodialysis (CAVHD or CVVHD) have been introduced for the removal of fluids and solutes in critically ill patients with liver disease [100, 101]. These procedures use small filters with a membrane highly permeable to water and low-molecular-weight solutes. With SCUF, CAVH, and CAVHD, the patient's own blood pressure is usually sufficient to maintain filtration, and high rates of fluid removal (0.4–12 l/h) can be achieved.

We believe that continuous hemofiltration may prove to have a valuable role in the management of some patients with massive ascites. Because information concerning the above-mentioned emerging modalities is not yet readily available to clinicians, we provide herein considerable detail, albeit prior to confirmation of the efficacy and safety of these techniques in this setting.

CAVH requires the use of either temporary access to the circulation (via femoral catheters) or a semipermanent Scribner shunt. Blood propelled by the patient's own arterial pressure flows through a low-resistance hemofilter and returns to the patient through the venous limb (Fig. 2). Heparinization of the device is necessary to prevent clotting; however, continuous therapy has been successfully performed in patients with liver failure without anticoagulation of the extracorporeal circuit [102]. Pump-assisted CAVH can be utilized to achieve higher blood flows. In addition, CVVH, using a blood pump, has been introduced to eliminate the need of arterial cannulation in CAVH. Close patient monitoring is necessary when blood pumps are utilized.

The ultrafiltrate is collected into a plastic bag. According to the need for fluid removal, part of the ultrafiltrate is replaced by intravenous administration of a solution such as isotonic NaCl or Ringer's lactate. Replacement fluid can be infused together with heparin through a port that is either proximal to the hemofilter (predilution mode) or distal to it in the venous limb (postdilution mode).

Treatment is continuous (24 h a day) until ultrafiltration is no longer needed. It is not unusual for a patient to be treated for several days. Using the postdilution technique with CAVH, urea clearance approximates the amount of filtrate that is replaced. Thus, with a fluid removal rate of 500 ml/h, clearance would be about 12 l/day.

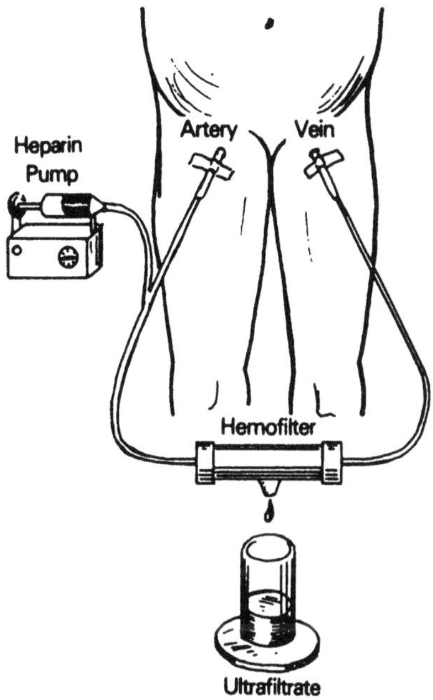

Fig. 2. Procedure employed for continuous arteriovenous hemofiltration (CAVH). Access to the patient's vascular system in this case consists of femoral arterial and venous catheters. The hemofiltration cartridge acts as an ultrafilter, retaining cellular components and proteins in the circulation and allowing water and crystalloids to pass through the pores of hollow fiber membranes. Heparinization of the device is necessary. (From [99], with permission)

Since their initial introduction in the early 1980s, hemofilters have undergone design modifications that have enhanced their applicability to an increasing patient population. As an example, the Diafilter-30 hemofilter (Amicon Scientific Systems Division, Danvers, USA) has had a second port added to its housing. This permits the option of circulating a dialysis solution around its hollow fibers and combining diffusive transport with ultrafiltration for a net gain in blood clearance (CAVHD). The Amicon Diafilter-10 device, having a larger number of capillary fibers but a shorter length than the original Amicon Diafilter-20 hemofilter, has a similar membrane area but produces less resistance to blood flow. This design is particularly advantageous with patients having low blood flow due to very low blood pressure or limited vascular access. Alternatively, dialyzers such as the Fresenius F-40 polysulfone dialyzer can be used at a lesser cost.

We have used CAVH for the treatment of refractory ascites in a patient with advanced liver cirrhosis [100, 103]. The procedure safely induced a negative fluid balance of 4 l and restored the sensitivity to diuretics without causing hypotension, bleeding, or decreases in renal function. Similarly, in a preliminary communication, Kaplan [101] reported on the successful application of CAVH in the management of two patients with hepatic insufficiency and concomitant renal failure.

In conclusion, the optimal interventional treatment of truly intractable ascites and renal insufficiency in the patient with advanced liver disease has not been established. Large-volume paracentesis is effective in the treatment of resistant ascites [93, 94]. The dialytic techniques discussed above are more difficult to institute but may be used in patients requiring frequent paracentesis and may occasionally result in a return of responsiveness to diuretics. Finally, the peritoneovenous (PV) shunt may provide a more permanent solution but entails more risk and expense (see below). Additional experience and controlled studies will be necessary in order to establish the role of continuous hemofiltration in these patients.

Peritoneovenous (LeVeen) Shunt

An advance that has engendered major controversy in the management of HRS is the development of PV shunting [104–107]. The past 20 years have witnessed a flurry of enthusiasm for the use of PV (LeVeen) shunting in the management of HRS. Since the underlying abnormality is thought to be a maldistribution of ECF with a resultant diminished effective blood volume, attention has focused on developing procedures to redistribute body fluids between compartments, so that the central compartment is replenished despite decreasing ascites. Unfortunately, although there have been a few well-documented successes [105, 107], the majority of reports have been anecdotal with insufficient details to allow critical assessment. Even where sufficient data were available, we must conclude that the majority of putative successes occurred in patients who were not clearly documented to have HRS; rather, many patients probably had reversible azotemia secondary to a diminished effective blood volume [106, 107].

Only two prospective randomized studies of the role of the PV shunt in the treatment of HRS have been performed [108, 109]. Linas et al. [108] prospectively compared the effects of the PV shunt ($n = 10$) or medical therapy ($n = 10$) on renal function and mortality in 20 patients with the HRS associated with alcoholic liver disease. After 48–72 h, body weight and serum creatinine were increased with medical therapy and decreased (from 3.6 ± 0.4 to 3.0 ± 0.5; $p < 0.05$) in patients with the shunt. Despite improvement of renal function, only one patient with the PV shunt had a prolonged survival (210 days). In the remainder, survival was 13.8 ± 2.2 days compared to 4.1 ± 0.6 days with medical therapy. The investigators concluded that whereas PV shunting often stabilizes renal function, it does not prolong life in patients with HRS. Additional studies are currently underway in HRS patients with less advanced disease.

In the VA Cooperative study [109], although there were seven long-term survivals in a group of 14 patients treated with PV shunting the results were not statistically significant when compared with those of a group of 19 patients undergoing medical therapy. The mean survival of patients treated with the shunt did not differ significantly from that of controls. Of note, the group of patients with HRS was carefully selected, and patients with severe complications of chronic liver disease were excluded.

Based on the available data, it is apparent that a beneficial role for the PV shunt in the treatment of HRS has not been established. Although some patients exhibit an improvement in renal function, further controlled studies with larger number of patients are necessary to delineate the effect of the PV shunt on long-term survival, quality of life, and the incidence of complications.

Orthotopic Liver Transplantation

Orthotopic liver transplantation (OLTX) has recently become the accepted treatment for end-stage liver disease [110]. Of interest, many of these patients present with varying degrees of concomitant renal dysfunction, including HRS. OLTX has been reported to reverse HRS acutely [11, 111, 112]. Gonwa et al. [110] reviewed the extensive experience of the Baylor University transplant group and have reported a good long-term survival with return of acceptable renal function for prolonged periods. They retrospectively reviewed the first 308 patients undergoing OLTX. The incidence of HRS was 10.5%. HRS patients manifested an increase in GFR from a baseline of 20 ± 4 ml/min to a mean of 33 ± 3 ml/min at 6 weeks, with a further increase to 46 ± 6 ml/min at 1 year. GFR remained stable at 2 years postoperatively (38 ± 6 ml/min). There was no difference in perioperative (90-day) mortality between HRS and non-HRS patients, despite a worse preoperative status and a rockier postoperative course. The actuarial 1- and 2-year survival rate for the HRS patients was 77%, not different from non-HRS patients. These investigators concluded that with aggressive pre- and post-transplant management, one can anticipate excellent results following OLTX in patients with HRS.

Newer Experimental Modalities

As noted previously, nonsteroidal anti-inflammatory drugs have been shown to induce reversible decrements in renal perfusion and renal function in patients with decompensated cirrhosis [35–38]. Conversely, we have shown that augmentation of renal prostaglandins induced by water immersion is associated with marked increments in creatinine clearance [39, 40].

Attempts to extend these observations by investigating the effects of administration of a prostaglandin E_1 analogue (misoprostol) on renal function initially suggested that this approach may be beneficial [113]. Unfortunately, these investigators, or other groups, have failed to confirm these initial observations.

Other Treatment Modalities

In view of the prominent role assigned to renal cortical ischemia in the pathogenesis of HRS, it is not altogether surprising that there have been numerous attempts to treat HRS with vasodilators. Intrarenal infusion of nonspecific vasodilators such as acetylcholine and papaverine improve renal blood flow, but do not augment GFR [114]. Similarly, blockade of vasoconstrictor α-adrenergic nerves by intrarenal infusion of phentolamine or phenoxybenzamine or stimulation of vasodilator β-adrenergic nerves with isoproterenol has no significant effect on GFR [13].

Direct stimulation of renal dopaminergic receptors by infusion of nonpressor doses of dopamine produces renal vasodilation, but again GFR and urine flow are virtually unaffected, despite infusions for as long as 24 h [29, 115, 116].

Finally, a variety of other treatment modalities have been proposed, including prednisone, exchange transfusion, charcoal hemoperfusion, xenobiotic cross-circulation, and ex vivo baboon liver perfusion [4, 117]. None are of demonstrated benefit, and the actual and potential complications are of sufficient magnitude to dictate great hesitation in their clinical use.

Considerations for Future Therapeutic Approaches

An additional investigative approach that has not been undertaken but merits consideration is the possible role of calcium antagonists. Studies from several laboratories, including our own, have demonstrated profound effects of these calcium antagonists on renal vascular smooth muscle and concomitant alterations in renal function [118–120]. Specifically, calcium antagonists have been shown to augment and restore GFR in diverse experimental settings characterized by renal vasoconstriction. This effect is due, in part, to the selective reduction of afferent arteriolar resistance. In essence, calcium antagonists may constitute selective renal vasodilators reversing or attenuating renal ischemia [121]. Indeed, studies from several laboratories have recently demonstrated that calcium antagonists are effective in the prophylaxis of acute renal insufficiency in diverse clinical settings including cadaveric kidney transplantation and radiocontrast-induced renal dysfunction [121]. Because patients with hepatorenal syndrome manifest a more extreme degree of preferential renal cortical ischemia, it appears reasonable to anticipate that calcium antagonists can induce a similar salutary effect on renal hemodynamics. If it can be demonstrated that calcium antagonists can be safely administered to patients with decompensated cirrhosis without inducing concomitant hypotension, they may constitute an additional therapeutic approach to the management of HRS.

Vasoconstrictor Therapy

A final therapeutic approach that warrants consideration is the administration of vasoactive agents that preferentially reverse the decreased systemic vascular resistance without increasing renal vascular resistance. As discussed previously [21, 122], there has been a resurgence of interest in the role of peripheral vasodilation as the primary determinant of intravascular underfilling. The resultant imbalance between the expanded capacitance and the available volume eventuates in a diminished effective volume. Such a formulation dictates that therapy should be directed toward a correction of the diminished systemic vascular resistance in HRS patients. Such an approach is not novel. Thirty years ago, Gornel et al. [123] demonstrated that the administration of the pressor amine metaraminol in cirrhotic patients is often followed by increased GFR, an increase in urine flow, and the elaboration of a more dilute urine. Although the use of metaraminol was fraught with problems, it would appear that the general approach of administering pressor agents might be valid.

Twenty-six years ago, Cohn et al. [124] demonstrated that a synthetic analogue of lysine vasopressin (Octapressin; PLV-2) had the unique property of producing renal vasodilation combined with systemic vasoconstriction, thereby producing a redistribution of blood flow to the kidney. These investigators studied the systemic and renal hemodynamic effects of PLV-2 in patients with decompensated cirrhosis of the liver and observed that PLV-2 in small doses produced renal vasodilatation and in larger doses preferential extrarenal vasoconstriction resulting in redistribution of blood flow to the kidney. Based on these findings, Cohn et al. [124] proposed a possible role for PLV-2 in the management of HRS. Unfortunately, additional studies were not undertaken.

Recently, there has been renewed interest in the hemodynamic derangements and attempts to improve renal function by countervailing this hyperdynamic state. Lenz et al. [125] investigated the effects of infusion of ornipressin on renal and circulatory function. In a preliminary report, they observed that ornipressin reversed the hyperdynamic state. Concomitantly there was improvement in renal function as assessed by a more than 70% increase in creatinine clearance and a doubling in urine flow. These preliminary observations lend support to the concept that the peripheral vasodilation of liver disease contributes importantly to the renal dysfunction. Consequently, maneuvers which counter the vasodilatation may possibly prove of benefit in improving renal function. In this regard, clinical trials attempting to reverse HRS should be undertaken with additional vasoactive agents that selectively increase systemic vascular resistance. Such studies would be ideally suited for conduct in the intensive care setting.

Summary of Therapeutic Options

Figure 3 summarizes my recommended approach to the management of acute renal failure in cirrhosis. As discussed above, the three important diagnostic considerations are prerenal azotemia, ATN, and HRS. The FE_{Na} or the urinary sodium concentration in a spot urine and the pulmonary capillary wedge pressure (PCWP) or the CVP may help to distinguish among these diagnostic possibilities. There is, however, considerable overlap between the three categories, and more than one diagnosis may be applicable to a given patient. For example, patients with HRS often exhibit ATN, and HRS and prerenal failure often coexist. In fact, the response to colloid infusion is the only feature that helps differentiate the latter two conditions. Of note, because of the low peripheral resistance associated with cirrhosis, volume expansion frequently does not result in a marked increase in CVP or PCWP. Intensive hemodialysis and/or hemoperfusion is indicated for the management of HRS complicating acute (reversible) liver injury. In patients with chronic cirrhosis, dialysis may maintain the patient until a suitable liver donor is found.

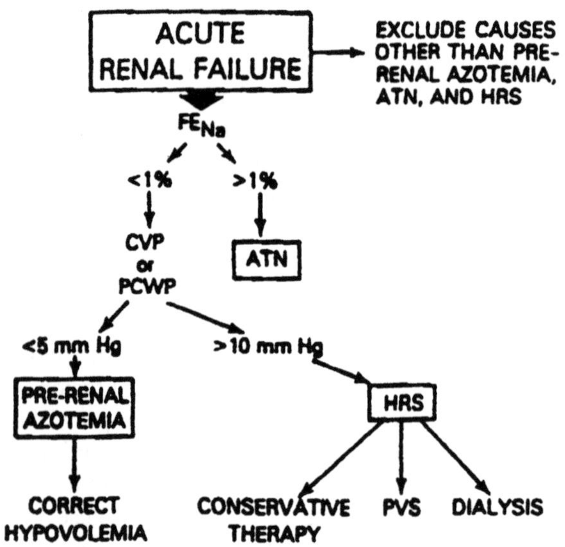

Fig. 3. Algorithm for the evaluation and management of a cirrhotic patient with acute renal failure. *ATN*, acute tubular necrosis; *HRS*, hepatorenal syndrome; *CVP*, central venous pressure; *PCWP*, pulmonary capillary wedge pressure; *PVS*, peritoneovenous shunting. (From [4], with permission)

Summary

In summary, despite considerable progress in the past three decades, we still lack a comprehensive understanding of the pathogenetic cascade that produces HRS. Although there has been some progress in characterizing the pathogenesis of this condition, therapy is largely empirical. The past two decades have witnessed much progress in the delineation of the intrarenal hemodynamic alterations that underlie HRS. The numerous attempts at treating HRS empirically with vasodilators have not resulted in important therapeutic innovations. The failure of many HRS patients to survive despite partial correction of their renal hemodynamic abnormality is a reflection of the precarious state of the patient with liver failure. Hemorrhage, infection, and hepatic coma are the usual causes of demise in these patients.

It is apparent that any future breakthroughs providing definitive treatment of HRS must be predicated on greater clarification of mechanisms and delineation of mediators. The role of hemodialysis has recently undergone reappraisal, and it is apparent that dialysis clearly has a role in supporting patients awaiting hepatic transplantation. Dialysis also may be warranted as a supportive measure in some patients with apparently reversible hepatic dysfunction. Hepatic transplantation has evolved over the past decade to the point where it constitutes definitive therapy for patients with hepatic dysfunction and concomitant renal failure. Although anecdotal information suggests that PV shunting has a role in the management of selected patients with HRS, the results of available prospective studies have failed to confirm such an approach. Finally, the advent of the peripheral vasodilation theory and its focus on the generalized hemodynamic perturbations in the patient with HRS have refocused attention on the florid extrarenal hemodynamic derangements. This suggests that pharmacological interventions that counter the peripheral vasodilatation may afford benefit with regard to both systemic hemodynamics and renal function. Hopefully, future clinical trials will establish the precise contribution of each of these treatment modalities and their respective roles in the therapeutic armamentarium.

Acknowledgments. We thank Elsa V. Reina for her expert secretarial help. Portions of this review have been adapted with permission from earlier reviews by the author: Epstein M (1988) The hepatorenal syndrome. In: Epstein M (ed) The kidney in liver disease, 3rd edn. Williams and Wilkins, Baltimore, pp 89–118 and Epstein M (1994) Hepatorenal syndrome: Emerging perspective of pathophysiology and therapy. J Am Soc Nephrol 4: 1735–1753.

References

1. Papper S (1983) Hepatorenal syndrome. In: Epstein M (ed) The kidney in liver disease, 2nd edn. Elsevier, New York, pp 87–106
2. Epstein M (1990) Functional renal abnormalities in cirrhosis: pathophysiology and management. In: Zakim D, Boyer TD (eds) Hepatology. A textbood of liver disease, 2nd edn. Saundes, Philadelphia, pp 493–512
3. Epstein M (1990) Liver disease. In: Massry SG, Glassock RJ (eds) Textbook of nephrology. Williams and Wilkins, Baltimore, pp 6.304–6.313
4. Epstein M (1988) Hepatorenal syndrome. In: Epstein M (ed) The kidney in liver disease, 3rd edn. Williams and Wilkins, Baltimore, pp 89–118
5. Ritt DJ, Whelan G, Werner DJ, Eigenbrodt EH, Schenker S, Combes B (1969) Acute hepatic necrosis with stupor or coma. Medicine (Baltimore) 48:151–172
6. Epstein M, Oster JR, DeVelasco RE (1976) Hepatorenal syndrome following hemihepatectomy. Clin Nephrol 5:128–133
7. Papadakis MA, Arieff AJ (1987) Unreliability of clinical evaluation of renal function in cirrhosis: a prospective study. Am J Med 82:945–952
8. Goldstein H, Boyle JD (1965) Spontaneous recovery from the hepatorenal syndrome. Report of four cases. N Eng J Med 272:895–898
9. Shear L, Kleinerman J, Gabuzda GJ (1965) Renal failure in patients with cirrhosis of the liver. I. Clinical and pathologic characteristics. Am J Med 39:184–198
10. Koppel MH, Coburn JW, Mims MM, Goldstein H, Boyle JD, Rubini ME (1969) Transplantation of cadaveric kidneys from patients with hepatorenal syndrome. Evidence for the functional nature of renal failure in advanced liver disease. N Engl J Med 280: 1367–1371
11. Iwatsuki S, Popovtzer MM, Corman JL, Ishikawa M, Putnam CW, Katz FH, Starzl TE (1973) Recovery from hepatorenal syndrome after orthotopic liver transplantation. N Engl J Med 289:1155–1159
12. Schroeder ET, Shear L, Sanceta SM, Gabuzda GJ (1967) Renal failure in patients with cirrhosis of the liver. III. Evaluation of intrarenal blood flow by para amino-hippurate extraction and response to angiotensin. Am J Med 43:887–896
13. Epstein M, Berk DP, Hollenberg NK, Adams DF, Chalmers TC, Abrams HL, Merrill JP (1970) Renal failure in the patient with cirrhosis: the role of active vasoconstriction. Am J Med 49:175–185
14. Epstein M, Schneider N, Befeler B (1977) Relationship of systemic and intrarenal hemodynamics in cirrhosis. J Lab Clin Med 89:1175–1187
15. Hollenberg NK, Epstein M, Basch RI, Oken DE, Merrill JP (1968) Acute oliguric renal failure im man: evidence for perferential renal cortical ischemia. Medicine (Baltimore) 47:455–474
16. Kew MC, Varma RR, Williams HS, Brunt PW, Hourigan KJ, Sherlock S (1971) Renal and intrarenal blood flow in cirrhosis of the liver. Lancet 2:504–510
17. Epstein M (1980) Determinants of abnormal renal sodium handling in cirrhosis: a reappraisal. Scand J Clin Lab Invest 40:689–694
18. Witte CL, Witte MH, Dumont AE (1980) Lymph imbalance in the genesis and perpetuation of the ascites syndrome in hepatic cirrhosis. Gastroenterology 78:1059–1066
19. Better OS, Schrier RW (1983) Disturbed volume homeostasis in patients with cirrhosis of the liver. Kidney Int 23:303–311
20. Cohn JN (1981) Renal hemodynamic alterations in liver disease. In: Suki WN, Eknoyan G (eds) The kidney in systemic disease, 2nd edn. Wiley, New York, pp 509–519
21. Schrier RW, Arroyo V, Bernardi M, Epstein M, Henriksen JH, Rodés J (1988) Peripheral arterial vasodilation hypothesis: a proposal for the initiation of renal sodium and water retention in cirrhosis. Hepatology 8:1151–1157
22. Levy M (1988) Pathophysiology of ascites formation. In: Epstein M (ed) The kidney in liver disease, 3rd edn. Williams and Wilkins, Baltimore, pp 209–243

23. Tristani FE, Cohn JN (1967) Systemic and renal hemodynamics in oliguric hepatic failure: effect of volume expansion. J Clin Invest 46:1894–1906
24. Lieberman FL, Denison EK, Reynolds TB (1970) The relationship of plasma volume, portal hypertension, ascites and renal sodium retention in cirrhosis: the overflow theory of ascites formation. Ann NY Acad Sci 170:202–212
25. Epstein M, Norsk P (1988) Renin-angiotensin system in liver disease. In: Epstein M (ed) The kidney in liver disease, 3rd edn. Williams and Wilkins, Baltimore, pp 331–355
26. Schroeder ET, Eich RH, Smulyan H, Gould AB, Gabuzda GJ (1970) Plasma renin level in hepatic cirrhosis. Am J Med 49:186–191
27. Epstein M, Levinson R, Sancho J, Haber E, Re R (1977) Characterization of the renin-aldosterone system in decompensated cirrhosis. Circ Res 41:818–829
28. Barnardo DE, Summerskill WHJ, Strong CB, Baldus WP (1970) Renal function, renin activity and endogenous vasoactive substances in cirrhosis. Am J Dig Dis 15:419–425
29. Barnardo DE, Baldus WP, Maher FT (1970) Effects of dopamine on renal function in patients with cirrhosis. Gastroenterology 58:524–531
30. Levens NR, Peach MJ, Carey RM (1981) Role of the intrarenal renin-angiotensin system in the control of the renal function. Circ Res 48:157–167
31. Cade R, Wagemaker H, Vogel S, Mars D, Hood-Lewis D, Privette M, Peterson J, Schlein E, Hawkins R, Raulerson D, Campbell K (1987) Hepatorenal syndrome: studies of the effect of vascular volume and intraperitoneal pressure on renal and hepatic function. Am J Med 82:427–438
32. Hollenberg NK (1988) Renin, angiotensin, and the kidney: assessment by pharmacological interruption of the renin-angiotensin system. In: Epstein M (ed) The kidney in liver disease, 3rd edn. Williams and Wilkins, Baltimore, pp 375–389
33. Arieff AI, Chidsey CA (1974) Renal function in cirrhosis and the effects of prostaglandin A_1. Am J Med 56:695–703
34. McGiff JC, Miller MJS (1986) Renal functional aspects of eicosanoid-dependent mechanisms. In: Fisher JW (ed) Kidney hormones. Academic, New York, pp 363–395
35. Boyer TD, Zia P, Reynolds TB (1979) Effect of indomethacin and prostaglandin A_1 on renal function and plasma renin activity in alcoholic liver disease. Gastroenterology 77: 215–222
36. Zipser RD, Hoefs JC, Speckart PF, Zia PK, Horton R (1979) Prostaglandins. Modulators of renal function and pressor resistance in chronic liver disease. J Clin Endocrinol Metab 48:895–900
37. Epstein M, Lifschitz MD (1980) Volume status as a determinant of the influence of renal PGE on renal function. Nephron 25:157–159
38. Epstein M (1986) Renal prostaglandins and the control of renal function in liver disease. Am J Med 80 Suppl 1A:46–55
39. Epstein M, Lifschitz M, Hoffman DS, Stein JH (1979) Relationship between renal prostaglandin E and renal sodium handling during water immersion in normal man. Circ Res 45:71–80
40. Epstein M, Lifschitz M, Ramachandran M, Rappaport K (1982) Characterization of renal PGE responsiveness in decompensated cirrhosis: implications for renal sodium handling. Clin Sci 63:555–563
41. Mené P, Dunn MJ (1986) Contractile effects to TxA_2 and endoperoxide analogues on cultured rat glomerular mesangial cells. Am J Physiol 251:F1029–F1035
42. Loutzenhiser R, Epstein M, Horton C, Sonke P (1986) Reversal of renal and smooth muscle actions of the thromboxane mimetic U-44069 by diltiazem. Am J Physiol 250: F619–F626
43. Zipser RD, Radvan GH, Kronborg KJ, Duke R, Little TE (1983) Urinary thromboxane B_2 and prostaglandin E_2 in the hepatorenal syndrome: evidence for increased vasoconstrictor and decreased vasoconstrictor and decreased vasodilator factors. Gastroenterology 84:697–705

44. Rimola A, Ginés P, Arroyo V, Camps J, Pérez-Ayuso RM, Quintero E, Gaya J, Rivera F, Rodés J (1986) Urinary excretion of 6-keto-prostaglandin F1 alpha, thromboxane B_2 an prostaglandin E_2 in cirrhosis with ascites. Relationship to functional renal failure (hepatorenal syndrome). J Hepatol 3:111–117
45. Zipser RD, Kronborg I, Rector W, Reynolds T, Daskalopoulos G (1984) Therapeutic trial of thromboxane synthesis inhibition in the hepatorenal syndrome. Gastroenterology 87:1228–1232
46. Gentilini P, Laffi G, Meacci E, La Villa G, Cominelli F, Pinzani M, Buzzelli G (1988) Effects of OKY 046, a thromboxane-synthase inhibitor, on renal function in non-azotemic cirrhotic patients with ascites. Gastroenterology 94:1470–1477
47. Laffi G, Marra F, Carloni V, Azzena G, De Feo ML, Pinzani M, Tosti-Guerra C, Gentilini P (1992) Thromboxane-receptor blockade increases water diuresis in cirrhotic patients with ascites. Gastroenterology 103:1017–1021
48. Thames MD (1977) Neural control of renal function: contribution of cardiopulmonary baroreceptors to the control of the kidney. Fed Proc 37:1209–1213
49. DiBona GF (1982) The functions of the renal nerves. Rev Physiol Biochem Pharmacol 94:75–181
50. DiBona GF (1984) Renal neural activity in hepatorenal syndrome. Kidney Int 25:841–853
51. Epstein M (1992) Renal effects of head-out water immersion in humans: a 15 year update. Physiol Rev 72:563–621
52. Zambraski EJ, DiBona GF (1988) Sympathetic nervous system in hepatic cirrhosis. In: Epstein M (ed) The kidney in liver disease, 3rd edn. Williams and Wilkins, Baltimore, pp 469–485
53. Bichet DG, VanPutten VJ, Schrier RW (1982) Potential role of increased sympathetic activity in impaired sodium and water excretion in cirrhosis. N Engl J Med 307:1552–1557
54. Ring-Larsen H, Hesse B, Henriksen JH, Christensen NJ (1982) Sympathetic nervous activity and renal and systemic hemodynamics in cirrhosis: plasma norepinephrine concentration, hepatic extraction and renal release. Hepatology 2:304–310
55. Henriksen JH, Ring-Larsen H, Christensen NJ (1984) Sympathetic nervous activity in cirrhosis: a survey of plasma catecholamine studies. J Hepatol 1:55–65
56. Epstein M, Larios O, Johnson G (1985) Effects of water immersion on plasma catecholamines in decompensated cirrhosis. Implications for deranged sodium and water homeostasis. Miner Electrolyte Metab 11:25–34
57. Bichet DG, Groves BM, Schrier RW (1983) Mechanisms of improvement of water and sodium excretion by immersion in decompensated cirrhotic patients. Kidney Int 24: 788–794
58. Kopp UC, Dibona GF (1992) The neural control of renal function. In: Seldin DW, Giebisch G (eds) The kidney: physiology and pathophysiology, 2nd edn. Raven, New York, pp 1157–1204
59. Folkow B, DiBona G, Hjemdahl P, Thoren P, Wallin BG (1983) Measurements of plasma norepinephrine concentration in human primary hypertension – a word of caution concerning their applicability for assessing neurogenic contribution. Hypertension 5:399–403
60. Esler M, Dudley F, Jennings G et al. (1992) Increased sympathetic nervous activity and the effects of its inhibition with clonidine in alcoholic cirrhosis. Ann Intern Med 116: 446–455
61. Liehr H, Jacob AI (1983) Endotoxin and renal failure in liver disease. In: Epstein M (ed) The kidney in liver disease, 2nd edn. Elsevier, New York, pp 535–551
62. Bourgoignie JJ, Valle GA (1988) Endotoxin and renal dysfynction in liver disease. In: Epstein M (ed) The kidney in liver disease, 3rd edn. Williams and Wilkins, Baltimore, pp 486–507
63. Bosch J, Ginés P, Arroyo V, Navasa M, Rodés J (1988) Hepatic and systemic hemodynamics and the neurohumoral systems in cirrhosis. In: Epstein M (ed) The kidney in liver disease, 3rd edn. Williams and Wilkins, Baltimore, pp 286–305

64. Vallance P, Moncada S (1991) Hyperdynamic circulation in cirrhosis: a role for nitric oxide? Lancet 337:776–778
65. Palmer RMJ, Ferrige AG, Moncada S (1987) Nitric oxide release accounts for the biological acitivity of endothelium-derived relaxing factor. Nature 327:524–526
66. Palmer RMJ, Ashton DS, Moncada S (1988) Vascular endothelial cells synthesize nitric oxide from L-arginine. Nature 333:664–666
67. Rees DD, Palmer RMJ, Moncada S (1989) The role of endothelium-derived nitric oxide in the regulation of blood pressure. Proc Natl Acad Sci USA 86:3375–3378
68. Aisaka K, Gross SG, Griffith OW, Levi R (1989) L-arginine availability determines the duration of acetylcholine-induced systemic vasodilation in vivo. Biochem Biophys Res Commun 163:710–717
69. Tomás A, Soriano G, Guarner C et al. (1992) Increased serum nitrite and nitrate in cirrhosis: relationship to endotoxemia (Abstr). J Hepatol 16 Suppl 1:4
70. Yanagisawa M, Kurihara H, Kimura S, Tomobe Y, Kobayashi M, Mitsui Y, Yazaki Y, Goto K, Masaki T (1988) A novel potent vasoconstrictor peptide produced by vascular endothelial cells. Nature 332:411–415
71. Goetz KL, Madwed JB, Zhu JL, Leadley RJ (1988) Cardiovascular, renal and endocrine responses to intravenous endothelin in conscious dogs. Am J Physiol 255:R1064–R1068
72. Loutzenhiser R, Epstein M, Hayashi K, Horton C (1990) Direct visualization of the effects of endothelin on the renal microvasculature. Am J Physiol 258:F61–F68
73. Takenaka T, Forster H, Epstein M (1993) Protein kinase C and calcium channel activation as determinants of renal vasoconstriction by angiotensin II and endothelin. Circ Res 73:743–750
74. Moore K, Wendon J, Frazer M, Karani J, Williams R, Badr K (1992) Plasma endothelin immunoreactivity in liver disease and the hepatorenal syndrome. N Engl J Med 327: 1774–1778
75. Moller S, Emmeluth C, Henriksen JH (1993) Elevated circulating plasma endothelin-1 concentrations in cirrhosis. J Hepatol 19:285–290
76. Epstein M (1992) The hepatorenal syndrome: newer perspectives (editorial). N Engl J Med 327:1810–1811
77. DeBold AJ, Borestein HR, Veress AT, Sonnenberg H (1981) A rapid and potent natriuretic response to intravenous injection of atrial myocardial extracts in rats. Life Sci 28:89–94
78. Cantin M, Genest J (1985) The heart and the atrial natriuretic factor. Endocr Rev 6: 107–127
79. Needleman P, Adams SP, Cole BR, Currie MG, Geller DM, Michener ML, Saper CB, Schwartz D, Standaert DG (1985) Atriopeptins as cardiac hormones. Hypertension (NY) 7:469–482
80. Atlas SA, Epstein M (1988) Atrial natriuretic factor: implications in cirrhosis and other edematous disorders. In: Epstein M (ed) The kidney in liver disease, 3rd edn. Williams and Wilkins, Baltimore, pp 429–455
81. Fyhrquist F, Totterman KJ, Tikkanen I (1985) Infusion of atrial natriuretic peptide in liver cirrhosis with ascites. Lancet 2:1439
82. Epstein M, Loutzenhiser R, Norsk P, Atlas S (1989) Relationship between plasma ANF responsiveness and renal sodium handling in cirrhotic humans. Am J Nephrol 9:133–143
83. Epstein M (1989) Atrial natriuretic factor in patients with liver disease. Am J Nephrol 9:89–100
84. Gerbes AL, Arendt RM, Ritter D, Jungst D, Zahringer J, Paumgartner G (1985) Plasma atrial natriuretic factor in patients with cirrhosis. N Engl J Med 313:1609–1610
85. Morgan TR, Imada T, Hollister AS, Inagami T (1988) Plasma human atrial natriuretic factor in cirrhosis and ascites with and without functional renal failure. Gastroenterology 95:1641–1647
86. Dudley FJ, Kanel GC, Wood LJ, Reynolds TB (1986) Hepatorenal syndrome without avid sodium retention. Hepatology 6:248–251

87. Zarich S, Fang LS, Diamond JR (1985) Fractional excretion of sodium. Exceptions to its diagnostic value. Arch Intern Med 145:108–112
88. Sherman RA, Eisinger RP (1983) Urinary sodium and chloride during renal salt retention. Am J Kidney Dis 3:121–123
89. Cabrera J, Arroyo V, Ballesta AM, Rimola A, Gual J, Elena M, Rodés J (1982) Aminoglycoside nephrotoxicity in cirrhosis. Value of urinary β_2-micoglobulin to discriminate functional renal failure from acute tubular damage. Gastroenterology 82:97–105
90. Rector WG Jr, Kanel GC, Rakela J, Reynolds TB (1985) Tubular dysfunction in the deeply jaundiced patient with hepatorenal syndrome. Hepatology 5:321–326
91. Oster JR, Epstein M, Ulano HB (1976) Deterioration of renal function with demeclocycline administration. Curr Ther Res 20:794–801
92. Carrilho F, Bosch J, Arroyo V, Mas A, Viver J, Rodés J (1977) Renal failure associated with demeclocycline in cirrhosis. Ann Intern Med 87:195–197
93. Arroyo V, Ginés P, Planas R, Panés J, Rodés J (1988) Paracentesis in the management of cirrhotics with ascites. In: Epstein M (ed) The kidney in liver disease, 3rd edn. Williams and Wilkins, Baltimore, pp 578–592
94. Ginés P, Arroyo V, Vargas V et al. (1991) Paracentesis with intravenous infusion of albumin as compared with peritoneovenous shunting in cirrhosis with refractory ascites. N Engl J Med 325:829–835
95. Planas R, Ginés P, Arroyo V et al. (1990) Dextran-70 versus albumin as plasma expanders in cirrhotic patients with tense ascites treated with total paracentesis. Results of a randomized study. Gastroenterology 99:1736–1744
96. Ginés P, Arroyo V, Quintero E et al. (1987) Comparison of paracentesis and diuretics in the treatment of cirrhotics with tense ascites. Results of a randomized study. Gastroenterology 93:234–241
97. Pérez GO, Oster JR (1978) A critical review of the role of dialysis in the treatment of liver disease. In: Epstein M (ed) The kidney in liver disease. Elsevier, New York, pp 325–336
98. Wilkinson SP, Weston MJ, Parsons V, Williams R (1977) Dialysis in the treatment of renal failure in patients with liver disease. Clin Nephrol 8:287–292
99. Pérez GO, Epstein M, Oster JR (1988) Role of dialysis and ultrafiltration in the treatment of the renal complications of liver disease. In: Epstein M (ed) The kidney in liver disease, 3rd edn. Williams and Wilkins, Baltimore, pp 613–624
100. Epstein M, Perez GO, Bedoya LA, Molina R (1986) Continuous arteriovenous ultrafiltration in cirrhotic patients with ascites or renal failure. Int J Artif Organs 9:253–256
101. Kaplan AA (1986) Clinical trials with predilution and vacuum suction enchancing the efficiency of the CAVH treatment. Trans Am Soc Artif Intern Organs 32:49–51
102. Smith D, Paganini EP, Suhoza K, Eisele G, Swann S, Nakamoto S (1986) Non heparin continuous renal replacement therapy is possible. In: Nose Y, Kjellstrand C, Ivanovich P (eds) Progress in artificial organs. ISAO, Cleveland, pp 226–230
103. Epstein M, Pérez GO (1986) Continuous arterio-venous ultrafiltration in the management of the renal complications of liver disease. Int J Artif Organs 9:217–218
104. Epstein M (1982) The peritoneovenous shunt in the management of ascites and the hepatorenal syndrome. Gastroenterology 82:790–799
105. Pladson TR, Parrish RM (1977) Hepatorenal syndrome: recovery after peritoneovenous shunt. Arch Intern Med 157:1248–1249
106. Epstein M (1980) The LeVeen shunt for ascites and hepatorenal syndrome. N Engl J Med 302:628–630
107. Epstein M (1988) Role of the peritoneovenous shunt in the managment of ascites and the hepatorenal syndrome. In: Epstein M (ed) The kidney in liver disease, 3rd edn. Williams and Wilkins, Baltimore, pp 593–612
108. Linas SL, Schaffer JW, Moore EE, Good JT Jr, Giansiracusa R (1986) Peritoneovenous shunt in the management of the hepatorenal syndrome. Kidney Int 30:736–740
109. Stanley MM, Ochi S, Lee KK et al. (1989) Peritoneovenous shunting as compared with medical treatment in patients with alcoholic cirrhosis and massive ascites. N Engl J Med 321:1632–1638

110. Gonwa TA, Morris CA, Goldstein RM et al. (1991) Long-term survival and renal function following liver transplantation in patients with and without hepatorenal syndrome – experience in 300 patients. Transplantation 51:428–430
111. Wood RP, Ellis D, Starzl TE (1987) The reversal of the hepatorenal syndrome in four pediatric patients following successful orthotopic liver transplantation. Ann Surg 205: 415–419
112. Gunning TC, Brown MR, Swygert TH et al. (1991) Perioperative renal function in patients undergoing orthotopic liver transplantation. Transplantation 51:422–427
113. Fevery J, Van Cutsem E, Nevens F et al. (1990) Reversal of hepatorenal syndrome in four patients by peroral misoprostol (prostaglandin E1 analogue) and albumin administration. J Hepatol 11:153–158
114. Cohn JN, Tristani FE, Khatri M (1970) Renal vasodilator therapy in the hepatorenal syndrome. Med Ann DC 39:1–7
115. Bennett WM, Keeffe E, Melnyk C et al. (1975) Response to dopamine hydrochloride in the hepatorenal syndrome. Arch Intern Med 135:964–971
116. Wilson JR (1977) Dopamine in the hepatorenal syndrome. JAMA 238:2719–2720
117. Horisawa M, Reynolds TB (1976) Exchange transfusion in hepatorenal syndrome with liver disease. Arch Intern Med 136:1135–1137
118. Loutzenhiser RD, Epstein M (1985) The effects of calcium antagonists on renal hemodynamics (Editorial). Am J Physiol 249:F619–F629
119. Loutzenhiser RD, Epstein M, Horton C, Sonke P (1986) Reversal of renal and smooth muscle actions of the thromboxane mimetic U-44069 by diltiazem. Am J Physiol 250: F619–F626
120. Loutzenhiser R, Epstein M (1990) Renal hemodynamic effects of calcium antagonists. In: Epstein M, Loutzenhiser R (eds) Calcium antagonists and the kidney. Hanley and Belfus, Philadelphia, pp 33–75
121. Epstein M (1992) Calcium antagonists and renal protection: current status and future perspectives. Arch Intern Med 152:1573–1584
122. Epstein M (1988) Renal sodium handling in liver disease. In: Epstein M (ed) The kidney in liver disease, 3rd edn. Williams and Wilkins, Baltimore, pp 3–30
123. Gornel DL, Lancestremere RG, Papper S, Lowenstein LM (1962) Acute changes in renal excretion of water and solute in patients with Laennec's cirrhosis induced by the administration of the pressor amine, metaraminol. J Clin Invest 41:594–605
124. Cohn JN, Tristani FE, Khatri IM (1968) Systemic vasoconstrictor and renal vasodilator effects of PLV-2 (Octapressin) in man. Circulation 38:151–157
125. Lenz K, Hortnagl H, Druml W et al. (1989) Beneficial effect of 8-ornithin vasopressin on renal dysfunction in decompensated cirrhosis. Gut 30:90–96

Acute Renal Failure in the Neonate: Treatment by Continuous Renal Replacement Therapy

C. Ronco

Introduction

Acute renal failure (ARF) in infancy may result from a variety of pathologic events. The syndrome is generally defined by a decrease in urine output ($\leq$1 ml/kg per h in the newborn) and a parallel increase of urea nitrogen and creatinine serum levels [1–3].

The main cause of ARF in the neonate is renal hypoperfusion due to volume depletion, perinatal aphyxia, and severe hypotension. Conditions such as renal vein thrombosis, urinary tract infections, congenital uropathies, hemolytic uremic syndrome, and cardiac failure may also cause ARF.

Fluid and electrolyte imbalances, metabolic acidosis, and severe catabolic state are frequently seen in these patients.

Conservative treatment with drugs and diet may prevent further deterioration, but sometimes the degree of fluid overload and solute intoxication requires substitutive therapy.

Recent advances in technology have made hemodialysis possible even in small patients. This technique, however, is difficult and is not routinely applied [4]. Peritoneal dialysis has been used with satisfactory results [5]. This technique is simpler than hemodialysis, can be safely used in a large number of pediatric departments, and does not require specialized equipment. Neonatal ARF, however, is generally associated with severe cardiovascular instability, respiratory problems and other medical complications. Under these conditions, hemodialysis may be technically and clinically contraindicated [6]. Recent abdominal surgery, skin infections, and other technical problems may contraindicate the use of peritoneal dialysis. For instance, peritoneal dialysis cannot always effectively treat severe fluid overload because of its low ultrafiltration efficiency. This is secondary to low blood flow in the peritoneal capillary network and high lymphatic reabsorption [7–10]. Finally, due to immunological immaturity and a very thin subcutaneous tissue plane, the risk of peritonitis may be higher than in adults [7–10].

An alternative treatment is needed to maintain adequate metabolic control and avoid dangerous derangement in the body fluid balance and composition [11].

Continuous arteriovenous hemofiltration (CAVH) is a simple method for blood purification and fluid control that was originally described by Kramer et al. in 1977 [12]. A small hemofilter is connected to an artery and a vein, and the arteriovenous pressure gradient generated by the heart moves the blood through the circuit, producing slow continuous ultrafiltration. Blood purification is mainly achieved by convection. Replacement of ultrafiltrate by substitution solutions contributes to lower solute levels in the blood. No pumps are used in the method originally described, and the system operates with low blood flow and low transmembrane pressure [11–14].

In recent years CAVH has been widely used in adults as an alternative treatment for critically ill patients [12, 13, 15]. Simplicity, easy institution, and good clinical tolerance represent the typical advantages of the technique. CAVH is also a reliable treatment for infants and children [16–19]. In these patients the technique presents some special advantages: low priming volume of the extracorporeal circuit, low rate of heparinization [15, 16], low blood flow, and slow continuous removal of isotonic fluid. The historical course and new developments in hemofilters, supplies, and procedures of continuous renal replacement therapy will also be reviewed in detail in the following.

Vascular Access

Vascular access in CAVH is the source of blood for the extracorporeal circuit and generates the hydrostatic gradient that moves blood through it [16, 20, 21]. Vascular access should achieve the highest arteriovenous hydrostatic pressure gradient. Short cannulas with a large diameter are critical for the achievement of adequate blood flow and the avoidance of unnecessary pressure loss. Flexibility without reduction of the inner lumen of the cannula and good clinical tolerance are other important features of vascular access [19].

Several vascular access routes can be utilized in infants: the choice should be made according to the patient's clinical condition and ease of insertion. In the small infant, the umbilical vessels are still open and can be safely used for both arterial and venous access. In the neonate, however, this type of access cannot be used for a long time. It cannot be used at all in patients more than 4–5 days old [15–17, 21–26]. Brachial or femoral artery cannulation may represent a reliable arterial access route. Surgical preparation of the vessels is strongly advised to avoid hematomas, hemorrage, or accidental disconnection of the cannula from the artery. For this purpose small, flexible, 18- to 20- gauge Teflon cannulas (20–25 mm long) can be employed. Cannulas should also be fixed to the skin to avoid disconnection and maintain adequate blood flow despite changes in patient position. In some cases, percutaneous cannulation of the above-mentioned vessels can be performed with the standard Seldinger technique. Peripheral artery cannulation can reduce distal blood flow, producing ischemic lesions or even causing complete thrombosis of the vessel. For this reason, periodic inspection of the cannulation site and of the regional perfusion is strongly recommended.

The jugular or subclavian veins are the most common routes for venous return. Standard connections for venous infusion (such as those for parenteral nutrition and central venous pressure measurement), however, are extremely thin and too long to be used for CAVH. Short lines with a large inner diameter are useful to reduce undesired resistance in the extracorporeal circuit. If venous access is used for a prolonged period of time, peripheral vein cannulation should be avoided because of the high risk of thrombosis. Furthermore, hyperosmotic substitution fluids should be infused centrally.

Blood flow during CAVH ranges from 15 to 50 ml/min and depends on the mean arterial pressure (MAP) of the patient; in the newborn, MAP ranges between 35 and 50 mmHg [17–19].

Higher and stable blood flows can be obtained with the use of a blood pump. In this case, the treatment is named continuous venovenous hemofiltration (CVVH), and two veins or a single vein with a double lumen catheter are cannulated. This approach may reduce the risk of bleeding, but it introduces the risk of air embolism. Furthermore, the priming volume of the extracorporeal circuit becomes clinically important, and it is advisable to start the procedure with a prefilled circuit. When the patient is older and the body weight exceeds 5 kg, a procedure for blood access similar to that for adults can be used [23, 25–27].

Extracorporeal Circuit

Different circuits for continuous therapies are shown in Fig. 1 with all their possible modifications. Standard pediatric hemodialysis lines (inner diameter, 0.3 cm) can be modified in order to obtain arterial and venous lines adequate for CAVH. There are now commercially available blood tubings especially created for CAVH in infants. The arterial line should be as short as possible in order to avoid unnecessary pressure drops along the length of the circuit. Since CAVH operates at low pressures, a loss of 5–10 mmHg may seriously affect the ultrafiltration rate and consequently treatment efficiency. For the same reason, a hemofilter with very low end-to-end pressure drop is required and short connections with an adequate diameter should be employed between the venous line and the jugular cannula. The arterial line should have a port for continuous heparin infusion and another port for arterial blood sampling. The sampling port could also be used for pressure measurements or for the use of the filter in a predilutional mode [18, 19, 21, 22, 27–33].

The venous line must have a port for the infusion of replacement solutions and a venous blood sampling port, which can also be used for pressure

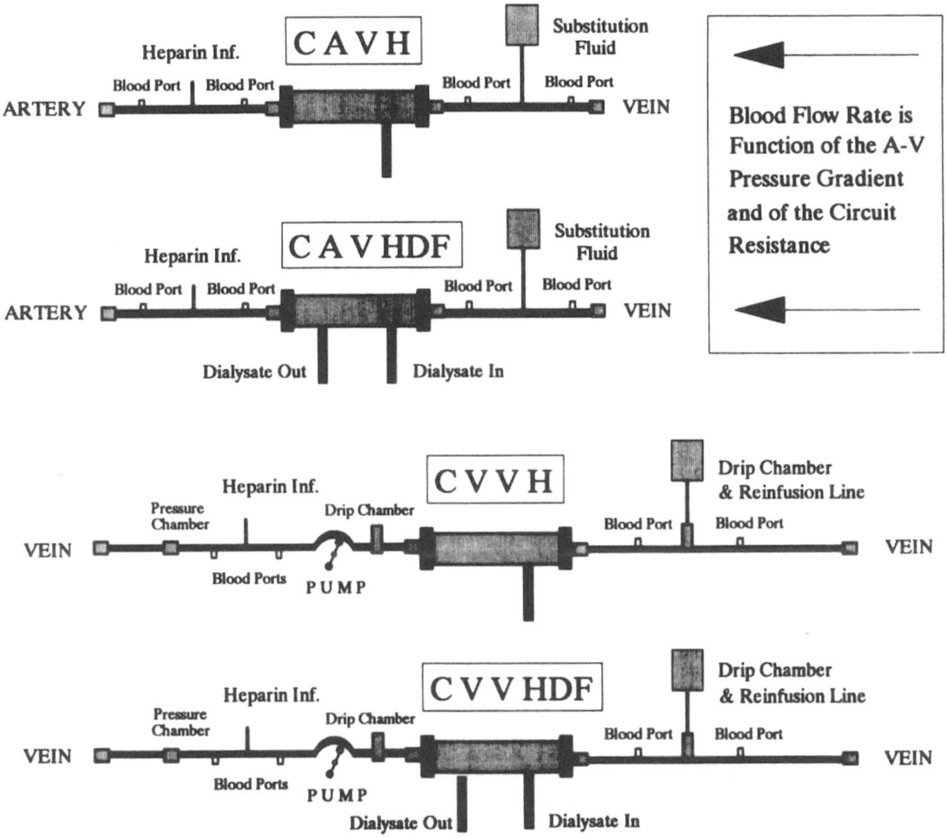

Fig. 1. Circuits utilized for continuous therapies. *CAVH*, continuous arteriovenous hemofiltration; *CAVHDF/CAVHD*, continuous arteriovenous hemodiafiltration/hemodialysis; *CVVH* continuous venovenous hemofiltration; *CVVHDF/CVVHD*, continuous venovenous hemofiltration/hemodialysis

measurements. At the inlet and outlet of the circuit, wide-bore, three-way taps should be placed in order to exclude the patient's circulation during lavage of the filter with heparinized saline solution. Folding of the arterial and venous lines should be carefully avoided during treatment [19, 27–34].

The ultrafiltrate line should be maintained as long as possible in order to maximize the negative pressure exerted on the membrane by the ultrafiltration column. This pressure definitely contributes to increase ultrafiltration. The low priming volume (less than 15 ml with the standard minifiter and 21 ml with the minifilter plus) further increases the clinical tolerance to the treatment. When a blood pump is used in venovenous mode (CVVH), two veins are cannulated and all these aspects lose importance since a constant blood flow is provided by the pump. At blood flows between 20 and 80 ml/

min, pressure-sensitive blood modules are strongly recommended to avoid any damage to the vessels. Nevertheless, access and tubings with low resistance permit operations at low-pressure regimens in the circuit.

Recently, a blood module specifically designed for CVVH in neonates has been made available (HP150; Medica, Medolla, Italy). This pump presents a very low priming volume of the circuit and a continuous monitoring of the pre- and postfilter pressures, thus making it possible to evaluate the patency of the blood compartment in the filter [35].

Acute renal failure is observed in approximately one tenth of neonates treated by extracorporeal membrane oxygenation (ECMO) or extracorporeal CO_2 removal ($ECCO_2R$). The hemofilter can be incorporated into these circuits, thus permitting an adequate fluid balance during treatment [26, 36, 37]. The hemofilter can also be used as a hemoconcentration device after open heart surgery.

Filters

The availability of adequate filters is the key point in performing CAVH in infants. The small filters for standard hemodialysis used at the beginning were inadequate. In CAVH, low priming volumes must be coupled with a very low resistance in the blood compartment of the filter. These conflicting objectives could not be achieved with standard fibers and designs, and a definite improvement came from the development of a new polysulfone hollow fiber with a larger inner diameter (1100 μm).

Hemofilters especially made for CAVH in infants and children are now commercially available. Our initial clinical experience was in 1982 with a polysulfone hollow fiber hemofilter (0.005 m^2 surface area) made by Amicon (Danvers, Mass., USA). A few years later, this prototype was improved (0.015 m^2) with optimized flowdynamic design, and was called the "minifilter." This minifilter, however, was, in some instances, still insufficient to guarantee an adequate amount of ultrafiltrate per day, even though remarkable clinical results were achieved in several pediatric departments. To meet all possible requirements of efficiency and performance, a newer series of minifilters has recently been developed and two models are available today; the specifications are summarized in Table 1.

These filters are designed to operate with minimal end-to-end pressure drop during CAVH in infants. Figure 2 shows the hydraulic properties of the filters tested in vitro. Panel a shows the blood flows achieved through the two filters at different perfusion pressures obtained by gravity. The low resistance is the main feature of these two filters, since high flows are obtained even at very low perfusion pressures. Panel b depicts the inlet pressure at various blood flow rates and the end-to-end pressure drop inside the two filters. The resistance of the blood path appears very low and adequate to operate in conditions of arteriovenous circulation. In panel c,

Table 1. Characteristics of the minifilter series

	First prototype	Minifilter (old version)	Minifilter (present version)	Minifilter plus
Overall length (cm)	13	11.5	17	17
Effective length (cm)	7	8	12.7	12.7
Diameter (cm)	1.5	1.7	1.7	2.5
Membrane type	Asymmetric PSF	Asymmetric PSF	Asymmetric PSF	Asymmetric PSF
Membrane area (cm^2)	50	150	210	800
Fiber internal diameter (μm)	1100	1100	1100	570
Priming volume (ml)	2.8	6	7.6	15
Maximal TMP (mmHg)	500	500	500	500
Maximal blood flow (ml/min)	500	500	500	500
Pressure drop (50 ml/min; mmHg)	2.5	3.1	3.5	5
Range of ultrafiltration (ml/min)	0.2–0.5	0.5–1.5	1–2.5	1–8
Number of fibers	25	60	60	450

TMP, transmembrane pressure; PSF, polysulfone.

the spontaneous ultrafiltration rate (Qf) is plotted against blood flow (Qb). In such conditions, ultrafiltration ranges between 0.5 and 2 ml/min, respectively, at the blood flows generally achieved in CAVH. In this graph, however, the rate of ultrafiltration is measured in the absence of additional pressure. When the filters are utilized in clinical conditions, additional factors, such as the negative pressure exerted by the ultrafiltrate column, help to increase the rate of ultrafiltration. The standard minifilter may in fact reach ultrafiltration rates between 0.5 and 1.5 ml/min for transmembrane pressure (TMP) values between 20 and 70 mmHg with a plateau value at 2.0–2.5 ml/min. At similar pressures, the minifilter plus displays ultrafiltration rates significantly higher and the plateau is reached above 8 ml/min (panel d).

As the blood moves through the filter, water is removed and the protein concentration increases, with a parallel increase in oncotic pressure. In adults treated with CAVH and standard hemofilters, this pressure may even equal the hydrostatic pressure and arrest the filtration process, creating the condition of filtration pressure equilibrium (18-29-39) [22, 29, 38].

In newborns treated with minifilters, filtration pressure equilibrium (hydrostatic = oncotic) does not occur, because of the low resistance of the filters, and low filtration fractions are obtained. This permits an extended filter life span and lower heparin requirements compared to those observed in hemofilters for adults [19, 28, 32].

The new minifilters have two ports in the ultrafiltrate compartment and this permits the use of a countercurrent flow of dialysate. In this case the treatment is named CAVHDF-CVVHDF (continuous arteriovenous or

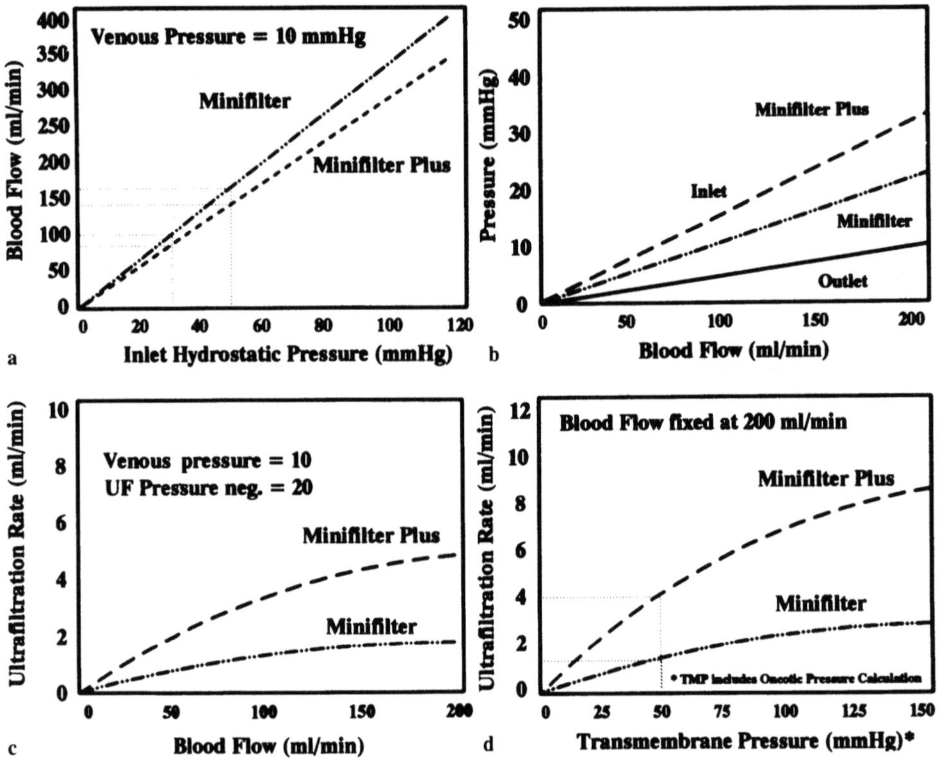

Fig. 2a–d. Hydraulic properties of the two filters used for continuous arteriovenous hemofiltration (CAVH) in the neonate (minifilter and minifilter plus). **a** Blood flows obtained at various perfusion pressures (created by gravity) are reported. **b** Resistance of the filters at various blood flows demonstrated by the pressure drop in the blood compartment. **c** Spontaneous filtraction obtained as a function of blood flow. **d** Ultrafiltration rates obtained at different transmembrane pressures are reported

Table 2. Population treated with different minifilters

	First prototype	Minifilter (old version)	Minifilter (present version)	Minifilter plus
Patients (*n*)	5	12	4	5
Age (days)	2–12	1–110	2–45	3–94
Tx duration (days)	2–4	2–32	1–14	2–16
Blood flow (ml/min)	15–28	13–35	16–44	25–48
Plasma flow (ml/min)	9–19	7–24	10–25	11–26
UF rate (ml/min)	0.6–1.0	0.7–1.1	0.9–1.4	1.6–2.9
Heparin (IU/h)	25–40	33–50	30–50	35–70
Survivors (*n*)	2	5	3	2

Tx, treatment; UF, ultrafiltration.

venovenous hemodiafiltration), since both diffusive and convective transports are present. In this treatment, dialysate flows of up to 10 ml/min can be used [39–42].

Table 2 lists the operational parameters of the filters recorded in 26 CAVH-treated patients aged 1–110 days.

Recently, other hemofilters for children have been developed (Gambro FH22; Gambro, Sweden), making it possible to choose from a wider spectrum of products [43].

Solute Removal and Membrane Characteristics

Asymmetric synthetic polysulfone or polyamide membranes are commonly employed in CAVH-CVVH filters. The process of convective transport is quite similar to the physiological function of the human glomeruli; the clearance of different solutes with molecular weights lower than the membrane's cutoff point presents similar values. In CAVH, this property results in an ultrafiltrate with the same characteristics as plasma water [42, 44, 45].

In our experience, no reduction in membrane permeability has been noted after as long as 86 h of treatment [19]. Periodic lavages of the filter with small quantities of heparinized saline further help to prevent the negative effect of protein "concentration polarization" [22, 25, 33, 34].

CAVH and CVVH take maximum advantage of convective solute removal, i.e., from high filtration rates and high sieving coefficients (35–47). When dialysis fluid is circulated in the filters (CAVHDF-CVVHDF), a mixed diffusive–convective transport takes place with a consequent enhancement of small solute clearance [41, 42, 46].

Anticoagulation

Preparation of the filter for CAVH treatment is extremely important for its function and duration during therapy [19, 28, 42]. After assembly, the filter and circuit should be rinsed with 500–1000 ml heparinized saline solution (5000 IU of heparin/l). During the washing procedure the venous line and the ultrafiltration line should be clamped periodically in order to remove all air bubbles from the system.

Since the population treated with CAVH is often at risk of bleeding, the main goal of anticoagulation is to achieve an adequate local effect without systemic consequences. Whole blood-activated clotting time or partial thromboplastin time must be carefully monitored [19, 28, 47, 48]. After the determination of these parameters under baseline conditions, if they are within normal ranges, a bolus of heparin should be administered (100 IU/kg body weight). The neonate usually metabolizes heparin rapidly, and coagu-

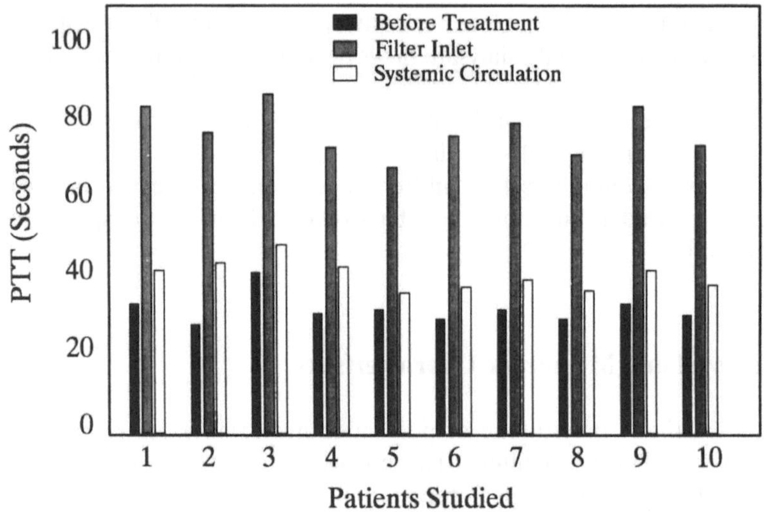

Fig. 3. Effects of heparin infusion at different points of the system in ten patients treated with continuous arteriovenous hemofiltration (CAVH). Maximal anticoagulation is achieved inside the filter while clotting time values close to normal are restored in the systemic circulation. *PTT*, partial thromboplastin time

lation parameters return to normal after less than 1 h. This practice, therefore, ensures a maximal anticoagulant effect during the first few minutes of contact between blood and membrane. This is likely to be critical for subsequent filter function.

After these procedures, a continuous heparin infusion of 5–10 IU/kg body weight per h is generally adequate to maintain effective extracorporeal anticoagulation with minimal systemic effects [34]. However, this amount must be adjusted case by case, since the rate of heparin metabolism may vary significantly in the newborn. Figure 3 shows the effects of heparin infusion in ten patients after 24 h of CAVH treatment. Maximal anticoagulation is achieved in the filter with minimal effects in the systemic circulation. This anticoagulation generally permits a filter to be kept in use for days without clotting of the fibers and the consequent need for replacement of the unit. The dose of heparin required by the minifilters is lower than in adults. This depends on the peculiar geometry of the blood compartment and hollow fiber diameter. The blood travels faster in the fibers, so that lower filtration fractions are achieved with a reduction in secondary layer formation and protein–membrane interactions. All these factors contribute to the longer survival of the filters. Periodic lavages of the circuit with saline help to assess the condition of the filter and to assure the complete absence of clots. To avoid acute fluid overload during this procedure, patients must be excluded from the circuit using the three-ways taps.

Substitution Fluid

The removal of large amounts of ultrafiltrate from the patient (1–2 l/day) requires the administration of substitution fluid. Depending on the patient's requirements, ultrafiltrate can be replaced in part, in whole, or even in excess. The replacement solution can be adeministered by manual, semiautomatic, or completely automatic systems, regulating the rate of replacement on the basis of the ultrafiltration rate during the antecedent 15-min period. Particular care has to be placed in obtaining the scheduled fluid balance because of the high sensitivity of the neonate even to small variations in body fluid balance and composition. In our experience, a simple gravimetric control system (Equaline; Medica, Medolla, Italy) is safe and reliable for precise fluid balance during CAVH over a prolonged period of time [33, 45, 46].

The composition of the replacement solution must be adapted to the metabolic requirements and to the electrolyte imbalances recorded in the patient. In our experience lactate-containing replacement solutions used for chronic hemofiltration may be adequate in the majority of patients. Because of enzyme deficiency in immature babies and consequent lactate intolerance, sometimes bicarbonate-containing replacement solutions must be used. In such cases, calcium and magnesium must be separately administered. The composition of these solutions can be manually modified as far as potassium content is concerned. Finally, such fluids can be safely used also as dialysate in the case of hemodiafiltration treatments [49–51].

Indications and Clinical Management

CAVH is not a substitute for any of the depurative therapies already in use, but it complements them as a further modality of renal replacement therapy. The simplicity of the technique allows rapid application and easy monitoring, even where hemodialysis or peritoneal dialysis cannot be used because of technical or logistic problems.

On the other hand, the clinical tolerance and the peculiar operational characteristics of the technique permit the use of CAVH-CVVH when other types of treatment might be dangerous or contraindicated (severe cardiovascular instability, multiorgan failure, abdominal surgery, septic shock) [14–19, 21–45]. After some years of clinical experience, we consider CAVH-CVVH to be the first-choice treatment in most cases of neonatal ARF. The causes of ARF in our population are reported in Table 3. In all patients urine output at the beginning of the treatment was less than 1 ml/kg per h. In the majority of the patients, ARF developed after abdominal or cardiac surgery and peritoneal dialysis was contraindicated because of the risk of leakage and infections [7–9]. Other patients had severe cardiovascular instability and hemodialysis was contraindicated. Among the medical causes

Table 3. Causes of acute renal failure (ARF) in the treated population

Diagnosis	Patients
Gastrointestinal surgery	6
Urologic surgery	4
Cardiac surgery	4
Septic shock	2
Perinatal asphyxia	2
Abruptio placentae	1
Intravascular coagulation	1
Hemolytic uremic syndrome	2
Multiple organ failure	2
Dehydration-hypotension	2

of ARF, renal hypoperfusion due to hemorrage, volume depletion, and sepsis were the most common. In all patients the treatment was well tolerated and monitoring was easily carried out. The treatment duration varied from 30 h to 32 days with a low rate of complications related to the treatment. Twelve patients recovered renal function and regular diuresis was restored.

In five cases CAVHDF was utilized in conjunction with CAVH to increase treatment efficiency.

Fluid Overload

Fluid overload with pulmonary edema may occur in the newborn. It can be due to renal failure, cardiac failure, or be iatrogenic (excessive fluid intake in the case of oliguria). When oliguria is refractory to diuretic therapy, body fluid balance is difficult to control. Under those conditions CAVH may effectively reduce fluid overload if constantly negative balance between ultrafiltrate and replacement fluid is maintained [52].

The slow and continuous removal of isotonic fluid is generally well tolerated and produces a reduction in preload and a negative sodium balance. The latter may be responsible for the observed decrease in peripheral vascular resistance and the increase in cardiac index with consequent stability of arterial blood pressure [19, 23, 37, 42]. Figure 4 shows the cardiovascular response to CAVH in terms of arterial pressure and heart rate. Removal of fluid is hemodynamically well tolerated in CAVH and CVVH, as demonstrated by the constant arterial pressure and heart rate. Two patients had altered arterial pressure and heart rate from the beginning of the treatment, due to congenital left ventricular hypoplasia.

The removal of isotonic fluid allows continuous plasma refilling due to the oncotic effect of proteins. This promotes the resolution of peripheral and

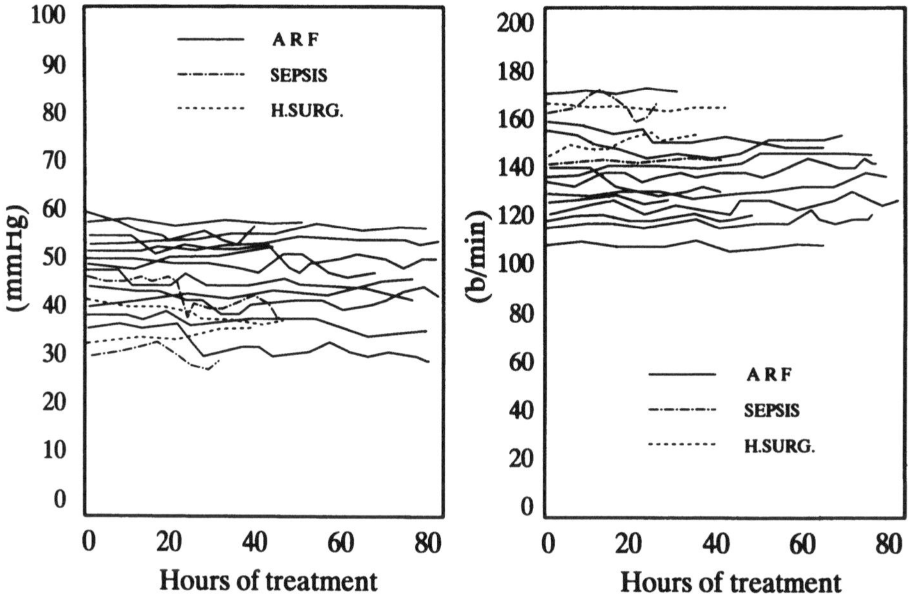

Fig. 4. Behavior of mean arterial pressure (*left*) and heart rate (*right*) in patients treated with continuous arteriovenous hemofiltration (CAVH). The stability in blood pressure is generally obtained thanks to a reduction of peripheral resistance and a parallel increase in cardiac output. *ARF*, acute renal failure; *H. SURG.*, heart surgery

cerebral edema. Finally, cardiovascular stability and intravascular blood volume maintenance may help to restore renal perfusion [28, 30, 48].

Electrolyte and Acid-Base Derangements

The manipulation of extracellular fluid achievable with CAVH permits the treatment of several electrolyte derangements. Hyponatremia, hypernatremia, hypercalcemia, and hyperkalemia can be managed by changing the composition of the replacement solution. The speed of correction depends on the ultrafiltration rate and on the amount and composition of substitution fluid. During a day, CAVH may produce 1–2 l ultrafiltrate (five to ten times the circulating volume in a neonate of 3 kg body weight). Furthermore, if we consider a body water pool of about 2 l, an average ultrafiltration of 2 l in 24 h achieves a daily purification index (liters of clearance/liters of body water) of 1 or more. This relatively high turnover of fluid can be used to vary not only the concentration, but also the absolute body content of some electrolytes. This effect is particularly useful in treating edematogenic states with increased total body sodium.

Recent filters and the use of blood pumps have contributed to increase daily UF volumes with a consequent increase in treatment efficiency. In severe catabolic states; however, a greater degree of blood purification is needed. In these cases CAVHDF may be indicated and the addition of diffusion usually achieves adequate blood urea nitrogen (BUN) control.

Hyperkalemia can also be corrected with CAVH. Potassium removal is directly related to ultrafiltrate production.

CAVH is also reliable in the treatment of hypercalcemia or in acute renal failure associated with alkalosis, where hemodialysis or peritoneal dialysis might worsen the clinical condition of the patient.

In CAVHDF, efficiency depends on the dialysate composition and flow. The kinetics of solute transport is similar to that of hemodialysis, and a final solute balance is sometimes difficult [40, 41, 49–51].

During all these procedures one should consider ultrafiltrate fluid and electrolyte losses, gastrointestinal losses, increased insensible perspiration associated with prematurity, and the use of extracorporeal temperature control systems. Hypocalcemia may occur in the newborn due to immaturity of the parathyroid glands, especially during an exchange transfusion. Seizures may than occur, requiring the urgent administration of calcium. Calcium solutions may induce thrombophebitis. During CAVH, however, calcium supplements can be diluted in the replacement solution, which is then rapidly distributed in the venous circulation. In the absence of seizures, calcium gluconate supplementation can be scheduled as an addition to the replacement solution and a continuous infusion can be provided at the rate of 5 mg/kg per h. Calcium solutions are incompatible with sodium bicarbonate solutions and separate bags must be utilized.

Hypomagnesemia may occur if diphenylhydantoin is given to the mother for the treatment of toxemia in pregnancy. Treatment with 1% magnesium sulfate should not exceed 5–10 ml at the rate of 0.5–1 ml/min. Ultrafiltrate losses should be considered.

In acid-base derangements, different situations should be considered. Bicarbonate loss during CAVH can easily be measured directly in the ultrafiltrate or by using the formula

$$HCO3(f) = UF \times HCO3(s) \times 1.124$$

where HCO3(f) is the bicarbonate concentration in the ultrafiltrate, HCO3(s) is the bicarbonate concentration in the serum, UF is the total amount of ultrafiltrate, and 1.124 is the average sieving coefficient for bicarbonate.

When CAVH is applied without substitution fluid in order to reduce the patient's fluid overload, bicarbonate losses are compensated by the reduction of the body volume distribution for the buffer and the serum concentration does not change significantly.

On the other hand, when replacement solutions are infused to maintain body fluid balance, the amount lost in the ultrafiltrate must be replaced. Finally, when CAVH is used to correct metabolic acidosis, the amount of bicarbonate in the replacement solution must exceed the amount lost in the ultrafiltrate.

In conclusion, when correction of water, electrolyte, or acid-base derangements is required, the rate of ultrafiltration and replacement, the initial plasma concentrations and rate of production, the amount lost in the ultrafiltrate, other losses, and the contents of the replacement solution must be considered for all different solutes in order to achieve the desired physiological targets.

Solute Removal and Metabolic Balance

Despite the remarkable amount of ultrafiltration, treatment may sometimes fail to achieve metabolic balance. Due to the identical composition of ultrafiltrate and plasma water and the purely convective nature of the treatment, CAVH has limited efficiency in small molecule removal. Figure 5 reports the BUN levels recorded in 16 newborns treated with CAVH for ARF. Treatment was effective in removing urea nitrogen in most patients. In three patients BUN levels increased progressively despite therapy. The limited efficiency of CAVH is most evident in severely catabolic patients. Several strategies can then be used when urea nitrogen generation rates exceed 1.2–1.8 g/day. First, ultrafiltration rate should be maximized. Second, protein catabolic rate and urea generation should be reduced. To achieve a positive nitrogen balance and BUN level control, early parenteral nutrition should be instituted.

Hyperalimentation in the newborn must be carried out with special attention to the patient's fluid and electrolyte requirements. Glucose solutions

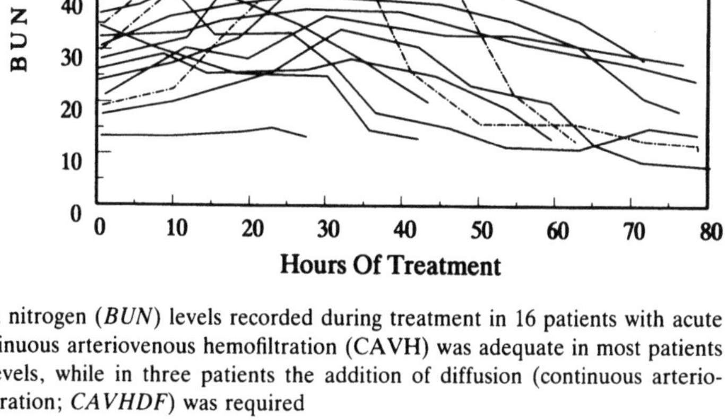

Fig. 5. Blood urea nitrogen (*BUN*) levels recorded during treatment in 16 patients with acute renal failure. Continuous arteriovenous hemofiltration (CAVH) was adequate in most patients to control BUN levels, while in three patients the addition of diffusion (continuous arteriovenous hemodiafiltration; *CAVHDF*) was required

and mixed essential and nonessential amino acid solutions should be provided in order to obtain an energy intake of about 100–150 Cal/kg per day and adequate dietary protein. In some cases, even the above steps are inadequate.

The new filters permit a daily ultrafiltrate increase to up to 4 l with the use of a blood pump. Furthermore, they are provided with a second port in the ultrafiltrate compartment. Dialysate fluid can thus administered at counterflow into the ultrafiltration compartment performing CAVHDF or CVVHDF. This procedure permits improved efficiency of the treatment by adding diffusive transport to convection. If the dialysate circulates at flows of 2–3 ml/min, it is still possible to have a concentration of solutes in the dialysate close to that of plasma (equilibrium dialysis). Under these conditions clearance equals dialysate flow and treatment efficiency can be doubled [40, 41, 49–51].

Monitoring and Complications

Although CAVH is a safe and simple method, technical or clinical complications may occur during the treatment.

The main feature of CAVH is its simplicity. Once the circuit and the filter are assembled and primed, a final check should be performed, paying attention to the following points:

1. CAVH: arterial and venous blood access, connections between lines and filter, heparin infusion system, replacement solution composition and infusion system, ultrafiltrate collecting system
2. CVVH: double venous cannulation or double lumen catheter, connections between lines and filter, blood pump and pressure alarms, venous drip chamber and air trap, heparin infusion system, replacement solution composition and infusion system, ultrafiltrate collecting system
3. CAVHDF-CVVHDF: same as above plus infusion rate and composition of dialysate

Once these checks have been performed, the treatment can be initiated and baseline blood samples should be taken from the arterial line for coagulation parameter measurement. Arterial and venous blood samples for hematocrit and total protein permit the calculation of blood flow and filtration fraction according to the classical formulas [13–26]. An accurate reading of the ultrafiltration rate should be carried out every 15 min. Ultrafiltrate samples from the collecting bag can be used for sieving coefficient calculations. During treatment, ultrafiltrate can be drawn to measure urea, creatinine, electrolyte, and bicarbonate concentration in plasma, avoiding unnecessary blood sampling.

The patient's vital signs (heart rate, arterial pressure, breathing etc.) should be monitored, and body temperature should be controlled to avoid dangerous hypothermia. If necessary, a heating system should be applied to the extracorporeal circuit. Progressive measurements of the blood chemical levels and the ultrafiltration rate should be used to regulate the rate of replacement and the composition of the substitution fluid. Additional check of the body fluid balance can be made with a graduated scale.

Clinical Complications

There has been concern about depletion syndromes (nonspecific loss of vitamins, amino acids, hormones etc.) as well as hypophosphatemia. We have not experienced any of these complications, possibly because specific parenteral nutrition support was provided during treatment. Electrolyte and acid-base imbalances can occur if inappropriate replacement solutions are prescribed. Bleeding episodes can be observed if excessive doses of heparin are given. Hyper- or hypovolemia may also occur with errors in fluid balance. We suggest the use of micromethods for blood chemistry determinations in order to avoid iatrogenic anemia. When necessary, blood transfusions can be provided via the replacement solution infusion port. Finally, drug dosage should be varied according to target plasma concentrations, protein binding, and molecular size of the drug. All of these affect the pharmacodynamics of the molecule during CAVH.

Techinical Complications

Blood loss can occur if a hollow fiber develops a leak. This potential problem is negligible because of the low pressures operating in the system. Should it occur, the high visibility of the red blood cells in the filtrate renders the problem rapidly detectable and a rapid filter exchange can be scheduled. When ultrafiltration rates drop below 0.5 ml/min, a general inspection of the filter, blood access, blood lines, and patient arterial pressure should be carried out. If clotting in the fibers is suspected, lavage can be performed using 50–100 ml heparinized solution via the three-way taps, excluding the patient's circulation. If this is unsuccessful, the filter should be replaced. Finally, air embolism is impossible in this system, as it operates under conditions of positive pressure. Special care must, however, be taken when umbilical vessels are used for blood access or when a blood module is utilized for CVVH. In our experience the use of a pressure-sensitive blood module permitted us to detect increases in the end-to-end pressure drop in the filter due to fiber clotting and to replace the unit before significant reductions in efficiency occurred.

Conclusions

CAVH can be used as an alternative treatment in infants and children as well as in adults. The small size of the patients may present special problems. Clinical experience so far suggests that such technical problems can be overcome. CAVH is simple, safe, and effective in conditions in which hemodialysis or peritoneal dialysis are contraindicated. These features make it a new substitutive therapy in the neonate. The recent development of devices especially designed for CAVH in infants will certainly increase its future use. Deeper knowledge of the mechanisms involved in acute renal failure, septic shock, and multiple organ failure will further encourage the use of continuous therapies in the critically ill patient, not only for blood purification purposes, but also for the removal of possible mediators of tissue and organs injury [53, 54].

References

1. Donkerwolcke RA, Chantler C, Brojer MJC (1983) Paediatric dialysis. In: Drukker W, Parsons FM, Maher JF (eds) Replacement of renal function by dialysis. Nijhoff, Boston, pp 514–535
2. Knochel J (1983) Biochemical, electrolyte and acid-base disturbances in acute renal failure. In: Brenner BM, Lazarus JM (eds) Acute renal failure. Saunders, Philadelphia, pp 568–585
3. Stokke T, Kettler D (1985) Komplikationen der kontinuierlichen arteriovenosen Hemofiltration. Anaesthesist 34:528–533
4. Trachtman H, Hackney P, Tejani A (1986) Pediatric hemodialysis: a decade's (1974–1984) perspective. Kidney Int 30:S15–S22
5. Potter DE, San Luis E, Wippler JE, Portale AA (1986) Comparison of continuous ambulatory peritoneal dialysis and hemodialysis in children. Kidney Int 30:S11–S14
6. Myers BD, Moran SM (1986) Hemodynamically mediated acute renal failure. N Engl J Med 314:97–103
7. Balfe JW (1987) Peritoneal dialysis. In: Holliday MA, Barratt IM, Vernier RC (eds) Pediatric nephrology, 2nd edn. William and Wilkins, Baltimore, pp 814–822
8. Fine RN (1994) Peritoneal dialysis in infants, children and adolescents. Perit Dial Int 14:4–6
9. Zaramella P, Andretta B, Zanon GF, Murer L, Montini G, Cantarutti F, Zacchello G (1994) Continuous peritoneal dialysis in newborns. Perit Dial Int 14:22–25
10. Geary DF, Harvey EA, Balfe JW (1994) Mass transfer area coefficients in children. Perit Dial Int 14:30–33
11. Kramer P, Bohler J, Kehr A, Grone HJ, Schrader J, Matthaei D, Scheler F (1982) Intensive care potential of continuous arteriovenous hemofiltration. Trans Am Soc Artif Intern Organs 28:28–33
12. Kramer P, Wigger W, Rieger J, Matthaei D, Scheler F (1977) Arteriovenous hemofiltration: a new and simple method for treatment of overhydraten patients resistant to diuretics. Klin Wochenschr 55:1121–1125
13. Lauer A, Saccaggi A, Ronco C, Belledonne M, Glabman S, Bosch JP (1983) Continuous artriovenous hemofiltration in the critically ill patient. Ann Intern Med 99:455–461
14. Zobel G, Kuttnig M, Ring E, Grubbauer HM (1990) Clinical scoring systems in children with continuous extracorporeal renal support. Child Nephrol Urol 10:14–17
15. La Creca G, Fabris A, Ronco C (eds) (1986) CAVH. Proceedings of the international symposium on CAVH, Vicenza. Wichtig, Milan
16. Jenkins RD, Harrison HL, Jackson EC, Fink JE (1991) Continuous renal replacement in infants and toddlers. Contrib Nephrol 93:245–249
17. Ronco C, Brendolan A, Bragantini L, La Greca G (1985) Treatment of acute renal failure in newborns by continuous arteriovenous hemofiltration. Trans Am Soc Artif Intern Organs 41:634–638

18. Lieberman KV, Nardi L, Bosch JP (1985) Treatment of acute renal failure in an infant using continuous arterio-venous hemofiltration. J Pediatr 106:646–649
19. Ronco C, Brendolan A, Bragantini L, La Greca G (1986) Treatment of acute renal failure in the newborn by continuous arteriovenous hemofiltration. Kidney Int 29:908–915
20. Olbricht CJ, Schurek HJ, Stolte H, Koch KM (1985) The influence of vascular access modes on the efficiency of CAVH. In: Sieberth HG, Mann H (eds) Continuous arteriovenous hemofiltration. Karger, Basel, pp 14–24
21. Ronco C, Brendolan A, Bragantini L, La Greca G (1986) Studies on blood flow dynamic and ultrafiltration kinetics during continuous arteriovenous hemofiltration. Blood Purif 4:220–226
22. Ronco C, Brendolan A, Bragantini L, La Greca G (1984) Self limited dehydration during CAVH. Blood Purif 2:88–93
23. Ronco C, Brendolan A, Bragantini L, La Greca G (1985) Continuous arterio-venous hemofiltration. Contrib Nephrol 48:70–78
24. Bartlett R, Bosch JP, Paganini EA, Geronemus R, Ronco C (1987) Continuous arterio-venous hemofiltration. Trans Am Soc Artif Intern Organs 38:345–352
25. Paganini EP (1986) Acute continuous renal replacement therapy. Nijhoff, Boston
26. Bartlett RH (1990) Extracorporeal life support for cardiopulmonary failure. Curr Probl Surg 27:621–705
27. Olbricht CJ, Schurek HJ, Tytul S, Muller C, Stolte H (1985) Comparison between Scribner shunt and femoral catheters as vascular access for continuous arteriovenous hemofiltration. In: Kramer P (ed) Arteriovenous hemofiltration. Springer, Berlin Heidelberg New York, pp 57–66
28. Zobel G, Trop M, Muntean W, Ring E, Gleispach H (1988) Anticoagulation for continuous arteriovenous hemofiltration in children. Blood Purif 6:90–95
29. Ronco C, Bosch JP, Lew S (1986) Technical and clinical evaluation of a new hemofilter for CAVH: theoretical concepts and practical applications od a different blood flow geometry. In: La Greca G, Fabris A, Ronco C (eds) CAVH proceedings of the international symposium on CAVH, Vicenza. Wichtig, Milan, pp 55–61
30. Golper TA, Ronco C, Kaplan AA (1988) Continuous arterio-venous hemofiltration: improvements, modifications and future directions. Semin Dial 1:50–54
31. Pallone TL, Peterson J (1987) Continuous arteriovenous hemofiltration, an in vivo simulation. Trans Am Soc Artif Intern Organs 33:304–308
32. Ronco C, Brendolan A, Borin D et al. (1988) Continuous arterio-venous hemofiltration in newborns. In: Sieberth H, Mann H (eds) Proceedings of the international conference on CAVH, Aachen. Karger, Basel, pp 76–79
33. Kramer P (1985) Limitations and pitfalls of continuous arteriovenous hemofiltration. In: Kramer P (ed) Arteriovenous hemofiltration. Springer, Berlin Heidelberg New York, pp 206–211
34. Ronco C (1994) Acute renal failure in infancy: treatment by continuous renal replacement therapy. Intensive Care Med (in press)
35. Ronco C, Fecondini L, Gavioli L, Conz P, Dell'Aquila R, Bragantini L, Chiaramonte S, Brendolan A, Crepaldi C, Feriani M, La Greca G (1994) A new blood module for continuous renal replacement therapies. Int J Artif Organs 17:29–33
36. Stolar CJ, Snedecor SM, Bartlett RH (1991) Extracorporeal membrane oxygenation and neonatal respiratory failure: experience from the extracorporeal life support organization. J Pediatr Surg 26:563–571
37. Zwischenberger JB, Bartlett RH (1990) Extracorporeal circulation for respiratory or cardiac failure. Semin Thorac Cardiovasc Surg 2:320–331
38. Pappenheimer AM Jr (1953) Passage of molecules through capillary walls. Physiol Rev 33:387–423
39. Bosch JP, Ronco C (1989) Continuous arterio venous hemofiltration. In: JF Maher (ed) Replacement of renal function by dialysis, 3rd edn. Kluwer, Dordrecht, pp 347–361

40. Geronemus R, Schnaider N (1987) Continuous arteriovenous hemodialysis. In: Paganini E, Geronemus R (eds) Proceedings of the third international symposium on acute continuous renal replacement therapy. Fort Lauderdale, pp 77–85
41. Ronco C (1985) Arterio-venous hemodiafiltration (AVHDF): a possible way to uncrease urea removal during CAVH. Int J Artif Organs 8:61–62
42. Ronco C, Burchardi H (1993) Management of acute renal failure in the patient critically ill. In: Dhainaut JF, Pinsky M (eds) Pathophysiologic foundations of critical care. Williams and Wilkins, Baltimore, pp 630–676
43. Ronco C (1992) Continuous renal replacement therapies and the polyamide membrane. Contrib Nephrol 96:111–123
44. Ronco C, Brendolan A, Bragantini L, La Greca G (1987) Solute and water transport during continuous arterio-venous hemofiltration. Int J Artif Organs 10:179–184
45. Brendolan A, Ronco C, Crepaldi C, Feriani M, Milan M, Fecondini L, La Greca G (1993) Clinical use of a new fluid balancing system: a useful complement to continuous replacement therapies. J Nephrol 6:149–152
46. Ronco C (1987) Continuous arterio-venous hemofiltration: optimization of technical procedures and new directions. In: Horl WH, Schollmeyer P (eds) New perspectives in hemodialysis, peritoneal dialysis, arteriovenous hemofiltration and plasmapheresis. Plenum, New York, pp 167–181
47. Zobel G, Ring E, Kuttnig M, Grubbauer HM (1991) Continuous arterio-venous hemofiltration versus continuous veno-venous hemofiltration in critically ill pediatric patients. Contrib Nephrol 93:257–260
48. Zobel G, Ring E, Kuttnig M, Grubbauer HM (1991) Five years experience with continuous extracorporeal renal support in pediatric intensive care. Intensive Care Med 17:315–319
49. Ronco C, Brendolan A, Bragantini L, La Greca G (1986) Arteriovenous hemodiafiltration associated with continuous arteriovenous hemofiltration. A combined therapy in the hypercatabolic patient. In: La Greca G, Fabris A, Ronco C (eds) CAVH proceedings of the international symposium on CAVH, Vicenza. Wichtig, Milan, pp 171–183
50. Geronemus R, Schneider N (1984) Continuous arterio-venous hemodialysis: a new modality for treatment of acute renal failure. Trans Am Soc Artif Intern Organs 30:610–613
51. Sigler MH, Teehan BP, Valkenburgh DV (1987) Solute transport in continuous hemodialysis. A new treatment for acute renal failure. Kidney Int 32:562–570
52. Zobel G, Stein JI, Kuttnig M, Beitzke A, Metzler H, Riegler B (1991) Continuous extracorporeal fluid removal in children with low cardiac output after cardiac operations. J Thorac Cardiovasc Surg 101:593–597
53. Bellomo R, Tipping P, Boyce N (1991) Tumor necrosing factor clearances during venovenous hemodiafiltration in the critically ill. Trans Am Soc Artif Intern Organs 37:322–323
54. DeVries I, van Deventer SJH, Debetes J (1990) Endotoxin induced cytokines in human septicemia. Adv Exp Med Biol 256:635–640

Conventional Hemodialysis for Acute Renal Failure

G.M. Chertow, W.F. Owen, Jr., and J.M. Lazarus

Overview and Historical Perspective

Much of the history of acute renal failure and its managment is derived from wartime experience. The phenomenon of acute post-traumatic renal failure was recognized by Bywaters and Beall [1] in military and civilian casualties during World War II; unfortunately, hemodialysis was not yet available at that time. Conventional hemodialysis was first used in clinical practice in 1944, when Kolff [2] successfully dialyzed a 45-year-old woman with drug-induced oliguric acute renal failure and uremic encephalopathy. By the early 1950s, Swan and Merrill [3] were able to achieve a survival rate of 54% in 85 acute renal failure patients, using the Kolff-Brigham coil hemodialyzer [4]. These techniques were later applied successfully during the Korean War.

During the past three decades, the clinical and demographic characteristics of critically ill patients with acute renal failure have changed dramatically. In 1994, acute renal failure can be seen in populations as diverse as bone marrow transplant recipients and octogenarians after coronary artery bypass surgery. However, the goals of dialytic therapy have remained the same: to replace the important functions of volume control and clearance of metabolic byproducts and, with as little disruption as possible, to allow functional recovery of the kidney and other vital organs. This chapter will focus on the use of conventional hemodialysis as opposed to continuous renal replacement therapy for acute renal failure in the critically ill.

Indications for Acute Conventional Hemodialysis

The goals of acute dialytic therapy differ substantially from those which are applied in the care of patients with chronic or end-stage renal disease. In cases of acute renal failure, we are less concerned with many of the important long-term sequelae of impaired or absent kidney function, such as anemia, metabolic bone disease, or β_2-microglobulin amyloidosis. Rather, we are focused on replacing those aspects of kidney function that affect other vital organs, such as the heart, lungs, and central nervous system, as well as in maintaining metabolic balance and appropriate disposition of pharmaceutical agents. The indications for acute dialysis are the same for all forms of renal replacement therapy.

Absolute Indications

Volume Overload

The most common reason for initiating acute hemodialysis in the intensive care unit is volume overload with pulmonary edema. Acute renal failure may result in extravascular (e.g., peripheral edema, ascites, pleural effusions) as well as intravascular (e.g., hypertension, pulmonary congestion) volume expansion. Although the extravascular manifestations of volume overload can be dramatic, they are rarely of sufficient morbidity to warrant dialytic intervention by themselves; however, save the case of isolated right heart failure, intra- and extravascular overload nearly always accompany each other and, when severe, often require dialytic intervention.

Acute renal failure with oliguria has traditionally been defined as less than 400 ml urine output per day. Even among patients with nonoliguric acute renal failure, however, there is often some degree of volume retention, particularly in those individuals with preexisting states of sodium avidity, such as congestive heart failure, hepatic cirrhosis, and sepsis. Volume overload may be iatrogenic in origin. Obligatory fluids are administered, frequently in excess of 4 l per day, to critically ill patients for multiple medications, such as antibiotics and vasoactive drugs, and enteral or parenteral nutrition. In the absence of intravascular monitoring, parenteral fluid challenges are often attempted in patients with acute renal failure to correct suspected hypovolemia or other reductions in renal perfusion. These fluid challenges may ultimately result in pulmonary congestion, especially in patients with concurrent cardiac or pulmonary insufficiency. Sodium salts of various medications (e.g., ticarcillin-clavulanic acid), alkali loads (e.g., sodium bicarbonate), cationic exchange resins (e.g., sodium polystyrene sulfonate), and hyperalimentation may occasionally contribute to volume overload; especially in the setting of oliguric acute renal failure, these otherwise therapeutic measures can lead to pulmonary edema.

Changes in body composition during critical illness can indirectly result in hypervolemia. For example, a patient with sepsis or trauma may be hypercatabolic and may not have his or her nutritional needs met by standard enteral or parenteral nutritional formulations [5]. Such a patient may lose up to 0.5–1.0 kg lean body mass per day. The proportional reduction in body cell mass (visceral and somatic protein plus intracellular water) may be even more dramatic, as body water is typically distributed from the intracellular to the extracellular space during critical illness [6]. Thus, extracellular (intravascular and interstitial) volume may be markedly elevated in the presence of stable or mildly reduced total body weight.

A diuretic challenge should be undertaken in all patients with volume overload before ultrafiltration or dialysis is initiated. A loop diuretic, such as furosemide (200–400 mg) or bumetanide (5–10 mg) can be administered intravenously in combination with a thiazide agent, such as chlorthiazide (250–500 mg) or oral metolazone (5–10 mg), if initial attempts at inducing diuresis with loop agents alone are unsuccessful. Aminophylline (125–250 mg) [7] or low-dose dopamine (1–2 mg/kg per min) [8] may be added to the diuretic regimen to augment renal perfusion and increase natriuresis.

The efficacy of a loop diuretic may be enhanced over time by continuous low-dose intravenous infusion (e.g., 10–40 mg furosemide/h) [9] or administration in combination with salt-poor albumin [10]. Even in the absence of an adequate diuretic effect, the vasodilatory effect of parenteral furosemide may ameliorate the symptoms of pulmonary congestion by increasing venous capacitance [11]. Additionally, the use of topical or intravenous nitrates and parenteral narcotic analgesic agents (e.g., morphine sulfate) should be considered to control dyspnea while dialysis is being arranged.

Ultrafiltration can be accomplished by conventional hemodialysis, hemofiltration or hemodiafiltration, or peritoneal dialysis. In past years, some nephrologists chose to avoid conventional hemodialysis in unstable, critically ill patients with volume overload because of the risk of inducing hypotension by the removal of 3 kg or more per h from the vascular space. In recent years, improvements in conventional hemodialysis techniques (e.g., bicarbonate dialysate, ultrafiltration controllers, sodium modeling, sequential ultrafiltration hemodialysis, see below) have made conventional hemodialysis efficient and safe for the management of symptomatic hypervolemia with acute renal failure in the majority of intensive care unit patients.

Hyperkalemia

Hyperkalemia sufficient to cause disturbances of cardiac conduction may complicate acute renal failure in the critically ill. Typically, individuals with primary disorders associated with hypercatabolism and tissue breakdown are at highest risk; these include patients with concurrent rhabdomyolysis, hemolytic anemia, disseminated intravascular hemolysis, gastrointestinal hemorrhage, or tumor lysis syndrome. Hyperkalemia can be aggravated by certain drugs, including distal diuretics (e.g., spironolactone, amiloride, triamterene), nonsteroidal anti-inflammatory drugs, angiotensin-converting enzyme inhibitors, nonselective β-blockers (e.g., propranolol, nadolol), trimethoprim-sulfamethoxazole [12], and potassium–penicillin preparations. Efforts to direct extracellular potassium excess into the intracellular compartment with insulin and glucose, nebulized or subcutaneous β-agonists (e.g., albuterol) [13], and sodium bicarbonate are effective short-term, but will not reduce total body potassium burden. An enterally administered cation exchange resin is an efficient potassium binder (sodium polystyrene sulfonate, 50–60 g every 1–2 h per os or per rectum) [14], but its use is limited in some critically ill patients who are postoperative or who have ileus or gastrointestinal hemorrhage. It should be noted that the per rectum administration of sodium polystyrene sulfonate with sorbitol has been reported to result in intestinal necrosis; therefore, when used by this route, sodium polystyrene sulfonate should be administered with water alone [15]. Nevertheless, hyperkalemia can be managed quite safely with conservative therapy in the vast majority of patients. The appearance of hyperkalemia along with other manifestations of uremia, however, often requires more prompt rather than delayed dialytic intervention.

The rapid removal of potassium is one of several advantages to conventional hemodialysis compared to peritoneal dialysis or the other continuous renal replacement therapies. The maximal rate of potassium removal by peritoneal dialysis appears to be approximately 12 mEq/h [16], while conventional hemodialysis with maximal blood and dialysate flows is three to four times as efficient. Although the time-averaged small solute clearance achieved with hemodiafiltration can meet or exceed that achieved with conventional hemodialysis, its capacity to remove a large quantity of potassium rapidly is limited. Therefore, conventional hemodialysis should be performed if hyperkalemia is life-threatening and cannot be controlled by conservative means. The risk of ventricular arrhythmia during dialytic treatment of hyperkalemia appears to depend on the absolute potassium level as well as the rate of reduction induced by the technique. Generally, when hyperkalemia is accompanied by electrocardiographic abnormalities, it is advisable to initially utilize a 1–3 mEq/l potassium dialysate and subsequently lower the dialysate potassium, rather than expose the patient to a dialysate which is potassium free, in an effort to limit the risk of ventricular ectopy [17].

Uremia

Unlike pulmonary edema or hyperkalemia, which can be readily diagnosed, the clinical consequences of uremia may be difficult to detect in the intensive care unit. For instance, encephalopathy, a clinical hallmark of uremia, is common among seriously ill patients and may be due to medication-related effects, sleep disturbance, or advanced hepatic failure. Likewise, asterixis, neuromuscular irritability, impaired cognition, somnolence, stupor, and coma can be observed in critically ill patients due to multiple causes. Another complication of uremia, pericarditis, may be seen following cardiac surgery, after myocardial infarction, or as a complication of infectious (e.g., pneumonia), neoplastic (e.g., carcinoma of the breast or lung), or autoimmune (e.g., systemic lupus erythematosus) disease. Pulmonary infiltrates associated with uremia can mimic the adult respiratory distress syndrome, independent of the effects of volume overload. Uremia can also lead to a bleeding diathesis due to platelet malfunction, although underlying coagulopathy (e.g., disseminated intravascular coagulation associated with multiple organ failure), stress gastritis, or anticoagulant and antiplatelet drugs are equally likely culprits. If uremia is contributing to a bleeding diathesis, transfusion of packed red blood cells [18], infusion of cryoprecipitate [19], or administration of deamino-8-D-arginine vasopressin (0.3 mg/kg) [20] can afford some short-term improvement in hemostasis.

Each of the uremic complications alone could probably be safely tolerated without introducing the patients to the risks of complications associated with dialysis (see below). However, these conditions are often manifested together or with volume overload and therefore usually require acute intervention. An important example of this "package deal" phenomenon is the development of acute renal failure in the setting of severe deep tissue ischemia or infection with abscess formation, often in postoperative patients. In the presence of necrotic tissue, the development of azotemia, as well as hyperkalemia and acidemia, is accelerated and may be unremitting unless the underlying condition is surgically repaired. In such a case, frequent and intense conventional hemodialysis treatments may be required.

Of the complications of uremia, those of the central nervous system generally improve most rapidly with dialysis [21], and others usually improve within several days, regardless of the dialytic modality. Conventional hemodialysis is usually preferred in those patients who require increased solute clearance and who are unable to tolerate systemic anticoagulation.

Acidemia

Metabolic acidosis almost invariably accompanies acute renal failure, as endogenously generated organic acids are retained, and the kidney suffers a diminished ability to retain bicarbonate and to maximally acidify the urine. In intensive care unit patients, acidosis can be worsened by hypoventilation, diarrhea, or the composition of intravenous fluids and hyperalimentation.

Metabolic acidosis is usually well tolerated until the systemic pH declines below 7.2. Less severe acidemia may have untoward metabolic effects [22, 23], but can usually be corrected conservatively. The administration of oral alkali (e.g., sodium bicarbonate) at 0.5–1.0 mEq per kg per day is uaually sufficient to match endogenous acid production in the nonhypercatabolic patients. Although sodium citrate is more palatable than sodium bicarbonate, acute aluminum intoxication has been reported in the setting of combined administration of aluminum and citrate [24], so that its use should generally be avoided in intensive care unit patients, particularly those receiving aluminumbased phosphate binders and sucralfate. As both forms of alkali are sodium salts, volume expansion complicating management can result.

More severe acidemia (pH less than 7.2) is frequently associated with cardiovascular dysfunction. Alkali therapy for patients with lactic acidosis due to low cardiac output or hypoxemic states may be contraindicated, as the administration of sodium bicarbonate to this subgroup of critically ill patients may paradoxically worsen acidosis [25]. Therefore, dialysis is usually indicated if severe acidemia is not readily reversed. Hemodynamic instability should be anticipated in these patients, and efforts aimed at reducing hemodialysis-associated hypotension should be entertained (see below).

Both acetate and bicarbonate have been employed as alkali in conventional hemodialysis. Historically, bicarbonate was the first of the pair to be used, but fell into disfavor in the 1960s because of instability at neutral pH, especially in the presence of calcium and magnesium. Acetate acts as a buffer by its metabolism predominantly in liver and muscle to acetyl coenzyme A, a conversion that consumes a proton and therefore liberates a molecule of bicarbonate [26]. At the relatively high acetate flux rates achieved with conventional hemodialysis, metabolic capacity may be exceeded, resulting in the accumulation of acetate itself and the development of hypotension, reduced cardiac output, and worsening of acidemia. Therefore, the use of acetate in acute renal failure has been largely discontinued. Indeed, more than 90% of chronic conventional hemodialysis in the United States is performed with bicarbonate as the base. Bicarbonate and acetate hemodialysis are further compared in a later section.

Relative Indications

Disorders of calcium, magnesium, and uric acid only rarely require dialytic management. Hypocalcemia typically accompanies acute renal failure and can usually be treated effectively with intravenous or oral calcium supplementation and a metabolically active form of vitamin D, such as calcitriol. Hypercalcemia, in contrast, is usually managed with volume expansion and loop diuretics; if refractory, treatment with biphosphanates, corticosteroids, or mithramycin may be required. If hypercalcemia is severe and unresponsive to conservative therapy, a modified dialysate calcium concentration should be formulated (0–1 mEq/l) and conventional hemodialysis initiated. Conventional hemodialysis offers the most rapid and efficient correction of calcium excess among the available dialytic modalities.

When magnesium toxicity results in respiratory depression, as with excessive ingestion of magnesium-containing antacid preparations, conventional hemodialysis can be performed with a magnesium-free dialysate. Similarly, uric acid can be effectively removed by dialysis in the setting of tumor lysis with acute renal failure. Usually, allopurinol, volume expansion, and alkalinization allow for the conservative management of this syndrome.

Conventional hemodialysis and hemoperfusion can be used for toxic ingestions with small water-soluble compounds, such as methanol and ethylene glycol. The extracorporeal treatment of toxic ingestions will not be addressed in this chapter. However, it should be stated that conventional hemodialysis rather than peritoneal dialysis or hemofiltration should be employed in the face of ingestions, as drug removal can be achieved more rapidly with the former technique.

Timing

There is no consensus on the appropriate time to initiate renal replacement therapy for acute renal failure. A single prospective randomized study in patients with post-traumatic renal failure ($n = 18$) compared frequent and early hemodialysis aimed to maintain blood urea nitrogen levels below 70 mg/dl and serum creatinine below 5 mg/dl, with delay until predialysis urea nitrogen and creatinine levels were 150 and 10 mg/dl, respectively. The group who underwent "prophylactic" hemodialysis had improved outcome (36% versus 80% mortality) [27]. A second study ($n = 34$) demonstrated no difference in patient mortality between two groups stratified by treatment intensity (measured by blood urea nitrogen concentration) [28]. These studies were unfortunately limited by reduced statistical power, the absence of blinding, and insufficient control of confounding variables, including comorbid disease and residual renal function.

The potential benefits of early, more intense dialysis for acute renal failure must be weighed carefully against the effects of dialysis on residual renal function and the time course of functional renal recovery (discussed below, see "Biocompatibility"). In view of the questionable benefit of prophylactic dialysis, it is advisable to delay initiation of dialysis in "asymptomatic" patients, especially those who are nonoliguric and tolerating full-scale nutritional therapy, in the hope of maximizing the odds of native renal recovery.

Biophysical Principles of Conventional Hemodialysis

Clearance

The movement of solute between blood and dialysate can be accomplished by diffusive or convective transport. In conventional hemodialysis, most solute clearance is accomplished by diffusion, which can be expressed mathematically by Fick's law:

$$J = -DA(\mathrm{dc}/\mathrm{dx})$$

where J describes the flux of the solute and D the degree of diffusion, A is the area of the diffusion front, and dc the concentration difference over the distance of diffusion, dx. For a model dialyzer, dx is constant, and for an individual solute at fixed temperature, D is constant as well.

The following equation describes the solute transfer from blood to dialysate (e.g., urea nitrogen, potassium):

$$K = Q_{\mathrm{Bi}}(C_{\mathrm{Bi}} - C_{\mathrm{Bo}})/C_{\mathrm{Bi}}$$

where K is the diffusive clearance of a solute from the blood, Q_{Bi} is the blood flow rate, C_{Bi} is the solute concentration of the blood entering the dialyzer, and C_{Bo} is the concentration of the blood as it exits the dialyzer and returns to the patient. This mathematical description assumes that the solute of interest is not present in the dialysate, the dialysate undergoes a single pass through the dialyzer, and the solute is not removed by convection (i.e., ultrafiltration). Thus, the diffusive clearance of a solute during dialysis can be defined as the volumetric removal of solute from the patient's blood.

Likewise, the solute transfer from dialysate to blood (e.g., calcium, bicarbonate) can be described as:

$$K = Q_{\mathrm{Di}}(C_{\mathrm{Do}} - C_{\mathrm{Di}})/C_{\mathrm{Bi}}$$

where Q_{Di} represents the dialysate flow rate, C_{Di} is the concentration of solute in the dialysate entering the dialyzer, and C_{Do} is the concentration of solute leaving the dialyzer [29].

With the above equations, one can determine components of the dialysis prescription that can be altered in order to modify the rate of diffusive solute clearance. These include a change in D, which varies across different model dialyzers. In general, a larger surface area dialyzer would be expected to increase diffusivity, thereby increasing flux J and enhancing solute clearance. Similarly, increases in Q_{Bi} and Q_{Di} augment solute clearance, although the increase is not linear as the above equations might suggest. First, the solute concentration gradient (ΔC) is attenuated along the dialyzer path, resulting in less efficient solute transfer compared to the single-pass model described above. Second, as blood and dialysate flow rates are increased, resistance and turbulence within the dialyzer increase, which also attenuate diffusive solute clearance. Practically, this limitation is observed in conventional ("low flux" usually cellulosic dialyzers at blood flow rates exceeding 300 ml/min and at dialysate flow greater than 500 ml/min. In contrast, the performance limitation in "high-flux" dialyzers is generally not reached until blood flows are in excess of 400 ml/min or dialysate flows are more than 800 ml/min. Therefore, diffusive solute clearance can be increased, albeit nonlinearly, in high-flux dialyzers by increasing blood and dialysate flows.

Patients with acute renal failure, however, are less likely to reach maximal blood flows (400–500 ml/min), by nature of their vascular accesses, invariably double-lumen venous catheters. In addition to an associated reduction in diffusive clearance due to limitations in Q_{Bi}, acute conventional hemodialysis via a double-lumen catheter is prone to recirculation, further limiting dialysis efficiency. In cases in which increased diffusive clearance of small solutes is required, as in a hypercatabolic patient with azotemia and hyperkalemia, it is advisable to empirically extend the duration of dialysis treatment or increase the treatment frequency (e.g., daily) to correct for the above-noted reductions in efficiency and to measure clearance of a marker substance (e.g., urea) to ensure adequate delivery system function.

Low molecular weight substances such as urea and potassium have high diffusive clearance rates that are not markedly effected by the flux of water during dialysis (i.e., convective transport). For solutes evaluated in vitro, molecular weight alone determines the degree of diffusive clearance. However, important biologic mechanisms, such as protein binding, membrane interactions, solute aggregation, and Gibbs-Donnan effects, often result in substantially diminished diffusive clearances in vivo compared with in vitro studies [30].

In contrast, solutes larger than 300 Da (so-called middle molecules), such as β_2-microglobulin, depend largely upon ultrafiltration for optimal clearance. The relationship between diffusive clearance and convective transport can be mathematically expressed as follows:

$$J = (K(1 - Q_F/Q_{Bi}) + Q_F)C_{Bi} = K'C_{Bi}$$

where K, as above, is the diffusive clearance and Q_F is the ultrafiltration rate. If K is large relative to Q_F, as for urea nitrogen, the influence of Q_F is negligible. Alternatively, if K is small, as for vitamin B_{12}, the contribution of clearance due to ultrafiltration is greater and will increase progressively with increasing Q_F. K' is the sum of diffusive and convective clearances [29, 31, 32].

Whereas increased Q_{Bi} and Q_{Di} are critical factors determining the rate of diffusive clearance, these parameters are of less importance with regard to clearance of larger molecules. Therefore, in order to maximize clearance of middle and larger moleculars, such as vitamin B_{12}, insulin, and β_2-microglobulin, Q_F must be increased.

The practical application of solute transport by ultrafiltration is seen with hemofiltration, which can be performed with conventional hemodialysis equipment or by an arteriovenous or venovenous continuous method. Intermittent hemofiltration has been successfully performed long-term, predominantly for patients with recalcitrant hemodialysis-associated hypotension [33, 34]. Unfortunately, diminished small solute clearance and the expense and technical difficulty of administering up to 30 l replacement fluid during 4–5 h make intermittent hemofiltration impractical. Additionally, hemofiltration alone rarely provides sufficient clearance of low molecular weight substances for the patient with acute renal failure. Similar limitations apply to continuous hemofiltration. Therefore, diffusive clearance with countercurrent intrafilter dialysate flow can be applied (continuous arteriovenous hemodiafiltration, CAVHDF, or continuous venovenous hemodiafiltration, CVVHDF [35–37]. Continuous hemofiltration and hemodiafiltration will be addressed elsewhere in the text.

Ultrafiltration

The ultrafiltration coefficient of a dialyzer is defined functionally as the water flux divided by the transmembrane pressure and mathematically as:

$$U = Q_F/(P_B - P_D)$$

where Q_F is the ultrafiltration rate, P_B the mean pressure in the blood compartment, and P_D the mean pressure in the dialysate compartment [29, 31]. The ultrafiltration coefficient defines the volume of ultrafiltrate formed per unit time for a given pressure across the dialysis membrane (transmembrane pressure, TMP). In general, the ultrafiltration coefficient is dependent on the composition of the dialyzer membrane and porosity. Synthetic dialyzers, such as those manufactured from polysulfone, polyacrylonitrile, polyamide, and polymethylmethacrylate, possess a much higher ultrafiltration capacity than those dialyzers comprised of cuprophan or modified cellulose (see below).

In order to achieve a specific volume (l or kg) of ultrafiltration during a single dialysis treatment, an estimate of the ultrafiltration coefficient U and dialysis time T_D are determined, so that TMP can be calculated:

$$\text{TMP} = \text{kg}/(U \times T_D)$$

This equation serves only as an approximation, as U may be under- or overestimated by the manufacturer and affected by biologic and technical factors, such as dialyzer reprocessing.

For example, an intensive care unit patient with acute renal failure and volume overload requires 5 h of conventional hemodialysis on alternate days in order to maintain blood urea nitrogen levels below 100 mg/dl. Employing a dialyzer with an ultrafiltration coefficient of 4.0 ml/mmHg per h, a TMP of 200 mmHg would be required to achieve a 4.0 kg weight loss in a single treatment.

The net pressure exerted across the dialyzer is the difference between the hydraulic pressures in the blood (determined largely by Q_{Bi}) and dialysate (determined largely by Q_{Di}) compartments:

$$P_{net} = (P_{Bi} - P_{Bo})/2 - (P_{Di} - P_{Do})/2$$

It is appropriately assumed that the contribution of blood and dialysate oncotic pressures are negligible. Therefore, returning to the example, if the net pressure across the dialysis membrane is 100 mmHg, an additional 100 mmHg negative pressure would be required in order to achieve the desired volume of ultrafiltrate.

Calculations such as these are of historical and biomechanical importance, since the performance of ultrafiltration during conventional hemodialysis has been simplified (and markedly improved) by the development of ultrafiltration control systems. A typical ultrafiltration control device depends on a flow sensor, which monitors the transfer of dialysate to and from the dialyzer and automatically adjusts the TMP to achieve the desired rate of ultrafiltration. A delivery system with ultrafiltration control can improve the precision of volume removal and offers the advantage of a more uniform weight reduction over dialysis time. Although ultrafiltration control mechanisms differ among dialysis delivery systems, all are typically accurate to whthin 100–200 ml (<5%) of the desired ultrafiltrate volume.

Conventional Hemodialysis Prescription

Dialyzers

Since the 1950s, dialyzers have become progressively smaller and more efficient. Virtually all conventional hemodialyzers available today are of the hollow-fiber variety. The composition and porosity of the membrane-forming fibers are of increasing interest, as more is learned about accumulated products in uremia and the immunologic consequences of the blood–dialyzer contact. These immunologic effects may be particularly important for patients with acute renal failure, in whom the kidney, often ischemic due to surgery, shock, sepsis, or nephrotoxin exposure, is most vulnerable to further, potentially irreversible injury.

Dialyzers are composed of a wide variety of materials, including regenerated cellulose, modified cellulose (e.g., cuprophan, hemophan, cellulose acetate), and newer synthetic materials such as polymethylmethacrylate, polyamide, polysulfone, and polyacrylonitrile. These materials vary widely in their capacity for solute transport (i.e., flux) and ultrafiltration, interaction with cellular and soluble components of the blood (i.e., biocompatibility), and cost.

Flux

Nearly all hollow-fiber dialyzers used in conventional hemodialysis share the capacity to efficiently remove small solutes such as potassium and urea nitrogen. Dialyzers are considered either low flux or high flux according to their hydraulic permeability and the ability to transport compounds with a molecular mass exceeding 10 kDa, the so-called middle or larger molecules. Perhaps the most widely studied of these molecules is β_2-microglobulin, a 50-kDa protein implicated in the development of dialysis-associated amyloidosis and bone cysts [103]. Although of clear importance in end-stage renal disease, the impact of middle molecules such as β_2-microglobulin on the course of acute renal failure is unknown. However, it is known that dialyzers or hemofilters comprised of polymethylmethacrylate, polysulfone, and polyacrylonitrile are capable of removing or binding the anaphylatoxins C3a and

C5a [38] as well as inflammatory cytokines, such as tumor necrosis factor alpha (TNF-α) and interleukin-1 [39], so that increased membrane porosity may affect common mediators of critical illness. Nevertheless, it is difficult to separate the specific effects of membrane flux from the concordant effects of biocompatibility.

A potential disadvantage to high-flux dialyzers is that the larger pore configuration may permit the backfiltration of bacterial cell wall products (e.g., lipopolysaccharide) from unsterile dialysate to the patient. Although rare, dialysate backfiltration may result in an acute febrile illness mimicking sepsis syndrome and may occur more often with reprocessed dialyzers [40, 41].

Biocompatibility

Since the advent of renal replacement therapy, nephrologists have observed that the urine output of a patient with acute renal failure usually drops off after the initiation of hemodialysis. This phenomenon has been attributed to the removal of osmotically active compounds, such as urea nitrogen, which sustained urine output during the predialysis phase, and to repeated bouts of ischemia associated with dialysis-induced hypotension. However, it has become clear that other factors may also be important. Experimental evidence has suggested that the injured kidney lacks the capacity to autoregulate blood flow normally [42, 43]. This has been attributed to neurohumoral disarray and an imbalance between local vasodilatory and vasoconstrictive mediators. In addition, it has been shown that the interaction of blood with an extracorporeal circuit can induce important immunologic sequelae, all of which may be relevant to the management of critically ill patients with acute renal failure [44].

Pulmonary leukosequestration has been demonstrated in animals undergoing hemodialysis, in association with hypoxemia and transient leukopenia [37]. This phenomenon is thought to result from complement elaboration due to the membrane-induced activation of blood monocytes. Similarly, activation of complement has been implicated in the anaphylactoid reactions associated with the use of new cuprophan dialyzers and in the promotion of catabolism in acute and chronic renal failure. Conventional hemodialysis has been associated with enhanced cell surface expression of leukocyte adhesion molecules such as MAC-1 and LAM-1 [45], stimulation of synthesis of reactive oxygen species such as superoxide [46], systemic release of thromboxane [47], and augmented monocyte elaboration of interleukin-1, interleukin-6, and TNF [48, 49] along with other immunologic effects. Many of these molecules are abundant in multiple organ failure, although the effect of their modulation by hemodialysis remains unknown. Cuprophan hemodialyzers appear to initiate these processes more so than synthetic dialyzers [50]. Additionally, experimental evidence suggests that biocompatibility may favorably affect the course of acute renal failure in rats [51] and possibly in humans [52]. Factors relevant to conventional hemodialyzer selection in acute renal failure include the following:

1. Patient-specific factors:
   - Pulmonary reserve
   - Cardiovascular reserve
   - Tolerance of anticoagulant
   - Sepsis
   - Multiple organ failure
   - Catabolism
   - Medication clearance
   - Angiotensin-converting enzyme – inhibition
2. Dialyzer-specific factors:
   - Ultrafiltration coefficient
   - Solute clearance
   - Membrane flux
   - Biocompatibility
   - Blood compartment volume
   - Cost
   - Reprocessing capacity

As far as tolerance of anticoagulant is concerned, membranes comprised of polymethylmethacrylate and polysulfone may be used with less heparin than cellulosic or other synthetic membranes. In patients on angiotensin-converting enzyme inhibitors, polyacrylonitrile (specifically AN-69) membranes have been associated with anaphylactoid reactions, possibly a bradykinin-mediated reaction [99, 100].

Dialysate

One of the major advantages to conventional hemodialysis is the ability to individualize therapy for the patient with acute renal failure, with regard to duration, drugs, dialyzer, delivery system, and dialysate. By manipulation of all five, conventional hemodialysis has become more effective and safe for critically ill patients. Below we review separately each of the dialysate components and their relevance in acute renal failure management.

Sodium

Sodium is the principle determinant of dialysate osmolality, so that modifications of dialysate sodium concentration can effect major changes in the process and results of the procedure. In past years, dialysate sodium concentrations less than 135 mEq/l were employed to limit intradialytic hypertension and thirst. However, the use of hyponatric dialysate can be complicated by headaches, cramps, nausea, and vomiting [53] and may contribute to the development of the dialysis disequilibrium syndrome, presumably associated with cerebral edema due to the osmotic transfer of water into the intracellular space [54, 55]. Most patients with acute renal failure are hypervolemic and generally require 2 l or more ultrafiltration per treatment session. Many are hypotensive, due to cardiovascular disease or multiple organ failure. For these patients, the use of a dialysate serum sodium concentration of 140–145 mEq/l is advisable. During conventional hemodialysis, osmotically active solute (e.g., urea nitrogen) is removed, resulting in a relative reduction in extracellular osmolality. This results in the further loss of extracellular fluid (into the intracellular space), with the potential for hemodynamic instability. Maintaining dialysate sodium concentration at or above the serum sodium concentration attenuates this hemodynamic effect in most patients. Although increased dialysate sodium concentration can result in thirst and polydipsia, resulting in increased interdialytic weight gain, these complications are of less concern in the acute setting.

Newer dialysate delivery systems permit on-line adjustment of dialysate sodium, which may stabilize hemodynamics in critically ill patients. This "sodium modeling" is accomplished by the use of variable dilution proportioning systems rather than the use of a fixed dialysate solute to water ratio. Typically, sodium concentration at the initiation of treatment is 145–150 mEq/l, to allow for more vigorous ultrafiltration without systemic hypotension, with a step, linear, or exponential reduction toward 138–140 mEq/l toward the end of the session. In addition, symptoms associated with increased ultrafiltration (e.g., leg cramps) may be reduced with this technique. Although dialysate sodium concentration has been modeled from 145–150 mEq/l to 130–135 mEq/l in as little as 2–3 h, little is known about the potential central nervous system consequences of such a practice, and marked hemodilution is probably inadvisable to employ in the acute setting. Rather, the dialysate sodium concentration should be maintained at or near 140 mEq/l to reduce the risk of complications (see above). Although sodium modeling reduces the frequency of hypotension during ultrafiltration without a decrease in time committed to diffusive clearance (see "Sequential Ultrafiltration Hemodialysis" below), it is unclear whether this technique is safer than treatment with a fixed dialysate concentration of 140–145 mEq/l [56].

Potassium

As noted above, the rapid and efficient removal of potassium is one of the major advantages to conventional hemodialysis in the acute setting. However, the degree of potassium removal is unpredictable and highly variable among individuals [104]. The major reason for this variability is that only a small fraction of the total body potassium is present in the extracellular space, and the flux of potassium from the intracellular to the extracellular space, the source of the majority of potassium removed [57], is dependent on patient-specific and dialysate-specific factors [58]. As a result of intracellular to extracellular flux after dialysis, a potassium rebound occurs, resulting in an increased serum potassium concentration at 1–2 h after the completion of treatment. It is consequently unwise to monitor the immediate postdialysis potassium concentration as a measure of adequacy of potassium removal, and supplements should not be administered until sufficient time has elapsed to account for rebound.

Another practical implication of the double-pool distribution of potassium is that optimal potassium removal will be achieved with daily treatments rather than protracted treatments every other day, particularly in patients with excess potassium delivery, as with transfusion. The integrity of the vascular access is another important patient-specific component of potassium removal, because of recirculation. As such, patients dialyzed via a temporary venous catheter for acute renal failure may not achieve the degree of removal of potassium otherwise expected.

In addition to these patient-specific variables, the composition of other dialysate elements (e.g., glucose, alkali) may alter the degree of potassium removal. It is probably inadvisable to delivery glucose-free dialysate to a critically ill patient, given the potential risks of hypoglycemia, particularly in individuals with hepatic dysfunction. Nevertheless, the use of glucose-free dialysate can augment potassium clearance by up to 30%, by minimizing insulin release and transcellular potassium uptake [57]. Rapid increases in systemic pH, as may occur in acidemic patients begun on bicarbonate-buffered dialysis, will augment transcellular potassium uptake, resulting in diminished potassium dialysance. Effects of the potassium gradient on base transfer have also been observed. With a 1 mEq increase in the blood to dialysate potassium gradient, the uptake of bicarbonate is reduced by 50 mEq (roughly equivalent to 50 cc 8.4% sodium bicarbonate solution). Therefore, the correction of acidemia in a critically ill patient with acute renal failure may be attenuated if concurrent hyperkalemia necessitates a 0–2 mEq/l dialysate potassium concentration. In such cases, parenteral alkali therapy may be additionally required.

Recognizing that many factors contribute to the efficiency of potassium removal with conventional hemodialysis, the initial dialysate potassium concentration is usually chosen empirically. For those patients with severe hyperkalemia (i.e., more than 8 mEq/l) or ongoing extracellular potassium excess (e.g., trauma, hemolysis etc.), a final dialysate potassium concentration of 0–1 mEq/l will usually be required to maintain intradialytic potassium concentrations below 5–6 mEq/l. However, the patient should be begun on a dialysate potassium concentration of 2–3 mEq/l for 30 min to 1 h to attenuate the rate of reduction. For most intensive care unit patients, a concentration of 2–3 mEq/l throughout the treatment is usually optimal. Rarely, in patients with cardiac arrhythmias or those on digoxin, a dialysate potassium concentration of 4 mEq/l may be prescribed. In addition, one should consider gastrointestinal losses of potassium (e.g., diarrhea, nasogastric suction) even among patients with oliguric acute renal failure, when planning the hemodialysis prescription.

Alkali

The two forms of alkali available for use as buffers in hemodialysate are acetate and bicarbonate. Acetate-based conventional hemodialysis should not be routinely employed in the care of critically ill patients with acute renal failure. Acetate is a direct peripheral vasodilator and myocardial depressant and can be very poorly tolerated in some settings. The acetate flux rates (in excess of 300 mmol/h) which are usually achieved with conventional hemodialysis typically exceed the body's metabolic capacity, particularly in individuals with hepatic dysfunction and/or underperfused skeletal muscle, where acetate is primarily metabolized. With acetate accumulation, hypotension, nausea, vomiting, and transient worsening of metabolic acidosis can occur [59, 60]. This complication appears to be more common among women, the elderly, and patients who are malnourished [61]. Hypoxemia, independent of the membrane-associated effects noted above, can also occur with acetate hemodialysis. This is most likely due to the loss of large amounts of carbon dioxide into the dialysate, resulting in a substantial (approximately 25%) decrease in alveolar and minute ventilation [105].

Most of these complications can be averted or attenuated with the use of a bicarbonate-buffered dialysate; thus, bicarbonate has become the buffer of choice for acute conventional hemodialysis. There are two important disadvantages to the use of bicarbonate-buffered dialysate, although both can be readily managed. First, bicarbonate forms insoluble salts with calcium and magnesium after prolonged exposure in solution. Second, bicarbonate-based solutions support the growth of certain hydrophillic gram-negative rod bacteria, including *Pseudomonas*, *Xanthomonas*, *Acinetobacter*, and *Flavobacterium* species [62]. Therefore, a bicarbonate solution is usually mixed daily from a powdered or liquid concentrate source, avoiding the need for storage, and safely added to other dialysate components by a computerized delivery system.

In order to limit hypoventilation and hypoxemia, hemodialysate comprised of bicarbonate at concentrations of less than 35 mEq/l should be used. The intravenous fluids administered during the intradialytic interval should be scrutinized to avoid excessive chloride administration and to optimize control of the metabolic acidosis that often accompanies critical illness.

Glucose

Historically, the dialysate glucose concentration was altered for patients with diabetes mellitus or as a means to modify the ultrafiltration rate. However, patients with acute renal failure should be dialyzed against a dialysate with glucose at a concentration of 100–250 mg/dl. It is important to recognize that glucose-free dialysate should be avoided in patients with acute renal failure. First, 8–12 g or more amino acids can be lost with each hemodialysis treatment [63, 64], and most nutritionally compromised intensive care unit patients can ill afford the further loss of calories. Second, acute renal failure may predispose a patient to hypoglycemia, because of impaired renal gluconeogenesis as well as diminished clearance of endogenous insulin. Patients with concomitant hepatic failure and those on sulfonylurea-derived hypoglycemic agents are at substantially increased risk for this complication.

Calcium

Hypocalcemia is a common complication of acute and chronic renal failure. As in chronic renal failure, hypocalcemia associated with acute renal failure may be due to phosphate retention with reduced glomerular filtration rate, impaired formation of 1,25-dihydoxycholecalciferol resulting in diminished intestinal calcium absorption, and skeletal resistance to the calcemic effects of parathyroid hormone. Severe hyperphosphatemia, secondary to trauma, rhabdomyolysis, or the tumor-lysis syndrome, may lead to more acute hypocalcemia than other causes of acute renal failure because of calcium-phosphate binding and deposition; similarly, patients with pancreatitis may have more marked hypocalcemia because of calcium–fatty acid soap formation accompanying pancreatic inflammation and dysfunction.

The standard dialysate calcium concentration for chronic hemodialysis has been reduced from 3.5 to 2.5 mEq/l at many institutions, because of more widespread use of calcium-based dietary phosphate binders and more aggressive supplementation with vitamin D analogues to control hyperparathyroidism in patients with end-stage renal failure. Although extremely important in the long-term, the management of metabolic bone disease is less pressing in the acute setting, where the complications of hypocalcemia (e.g., tetany, cardiac arrhythmias, seizures) can be otherwise devastating. Patients with metabolic or respiratory alkalosis (e.g., due to nasogastric suctioning or hyperventilation, respectively) are at increased risk of hypocalemic complications because of a relative reduction in ionized calcium induced by alkalemia.

It is advisable to consider the cause of acute renal failure and concomitant clinical factors prior to choosing the dialysate calcium concentration. It has been determined that to achieve positive calcium balance during hemodialysis, the dialysate calcium concentration must be at least 3.5 mEq/l [65]. For many patients, this higher dialysate calcium concentration would be preferred. In contrast, the rare patient with disseminated carcinoma or myeloma and hypercalcemia may require a reduced dialysate calcium concentration (0–1 mEq/l). Parenteral vitamin D is rarely administered in the acute renal failure setting.

Magnesium

Formerly largely ignored, magnesium has enjoyed closer attention in recent years as a potentially important determinant in critical illness. Hypomagnesemia has been implicated in the pathogenesis of atrial [66] and ventricular arrhythmias [67] and as a regulator of bronchial smooth muscle tone in asthma and chronic obstructive pulmonary disease [68]. Renewed interest in this cation has led to more frequent monitoring of blood levels and more liberal parenteral and enteral supplementation, despite the fact that blood levels are known to be poorly predictive of total body magnesium.

As the kidneys are the predominant site of magnesium excretion, mild to moderate hypermagnesemia is commonly observed in association with acute renal failure. A dialysate magnesium concentration of 1.0 mEq/l is usually employed. Magnesium-free dialysate is manufactured and might be preferred with severe hypermagnesemia and respiratory failure. Rarely, drug-induced renal failure, secondary to aminoglycosides, *cis*-platinum, or amphotericin B may be accompanied by frank hypomagnesemia. In these cases, it is prudent to carefully supplement the patient with oral or intravenous magnesium, rather than increasing the magnesium concentration of dialysate.

Anticoagulation

The interaction between a patient's blood and the hemodialyzer membrane promotes local platelet adherence and thrombus formation. If substantial clotting within the hollow fibers occurs, it can render both clearance and ultrafiltration ineffective. If the entire system clots, 150–250 ml whole blood can be lost;fortunately there appears to be little risk of systemic venous embolization. Therefore, some form of anticoagulation is usually employed in acute conventional hemodialysis. Patient- and equipment-specific factors which influence anticoagulation requirements are outlined below:

1. No heparin or regional anticoagulation with heparin or citrate
   a) Gastrointestinal or other active bleeding
   b) Underlying disorder of hemostasis
   c) Pericarditis
   d) Vascular or abdominal surgery within 7 days

e) Intracranial surgery within 14 days
f) Needle or forceps biopsy of visceral organ or bone within 3 days
g) Anticipated catheter placement or surgical procedure within hours

2. Fractional anticoagulation with heparin
a) Any of above prior to instituting full-dose systemic therapy
b) Minor surgical procedure within 3 days
c) Diabetic retinopathy with acute retinal hemorrhage

Monitoring the intensity of anticoagulation is usually done with the whole-blood activated clotting time (ACT), as intradialytic time constraints typically prevent the use of the more commonly employed partial thromboplastin time (PTT) or international normalized ratio (INR). The ACT is an assay which uses a fixed quantity of an extrinsic clotting cascade activator, such as ground glass, kaolin, or diatomaceous earth, mixed with 0.4 ml whole blood at the bedside. The tube is maintained at 37°C and gently tilted every 5 s to ensure adequate mixing. The normal range is 90–140 s.

In general, there are three methods of anticoagulant administration. The simplest method is systemic administration, in which 2000–5000 units of heparin are administered intravenously at the initiation of treatment, followed by additional boluses of 1000 units/h to keep the target ACT 50% above baseline. A less intensive and more precise means of anticoagulation has been termed "fractional anticoagulation," in which the target ACT is maintained at approximately 15% ("tight fractional") or 25% ("fractional") above baseline. Specifically, 500–3000 units of heparin are administered at dialysis initiation, followed by a continuous intravenous infusion (typically 500–1000 units/h). Lastly, regional or extracorporeal anticoagulation can be performed by experienced personnel, resulting in minimal risk of systemic anticoagulant exposure. With this method, approximately 500 units of heparin are administered at dialysis initiation, and 500–750 units/h are infused into the arterial line. In parallel, 3.75 mg/h protamine, a heparin antagonist, are infused into the venous line. The ACT of the patient is maintained at baseline, while the ACT within the machine components is kept 10 s or more longer. To account for the extended half-life of heparin compared with protamine, an additional 50 mg protamine should be given at the completion of dialysis [69]. In the event of protamine hypersensitivity or an allergy or thrombocytopenic reaction to heparin, regional anticoagulation can be achieved with sodium citrate as the anticoagulant; infused citrate binds with ionized calcium to form a dialyzable salt, which depletes the intrinsic and extrinsic clotting cascade of calcium, an obligatory cofactor [70]. This method proceeds in a similar manner to heparin-protamine regional anticoagulation. A 45% sodium citrate solution is infused into the arterial blood line at 30 ml/h. The serum ionized calcium should be measured at least hourly, and parenteral calcium gluconate administered intravenously if hypocalcemia ensues. In addition to the usual complications associated with acute conventional hemodialysis (see below), hemodialysis with citrate anticoagulation can result in life-threatening hypocalcemia and metabolic alkalosis (from citrate dialysance).

It is not uncommon to encounter critically ill patients who are poor candidates for regional anticoagulation, yet require conventional hemodialysis. In such high-risk situations, acute hemodialysis can be performed heparin free. This method requires frequent flushing (every 15–20 min) of the dialyzer with saline and generally requires brisk blood flows and minimal ultrafiltration. Patients with liver failure, severe thrombocytopenia, or other forms of coagulopathy may tolerate heparin-free dialysis without the need for frequent saline flushes. The following clinical settings require increased anticoagulation intensity:

- Increased hematocrit
- Increased blood viscosity
- Hypercoagulable state (e.g., adenocarcinoma, protein C/S deficiency)
- Increased catheter length and decreased diameter
- Increased tubing length and decreased diameter
- Recirculation
- Increased ultrafiltration
- Reduced blood flow
- Blood transfusions
- Intravenous nitroglycerin therapy
- Cuprophan versus cellulose acetate versus synthetic dialyzer

Clinical settings requiring decreased anticoagulation intensity include:

- Advanced uremia
- Liver disease
- Thrombocytopenia
- Antiplatelet therapy (e.g., aspirin, ticlopidine)
- Malnutrition
- Congestive heart failure
- Broad spectrum parenteral antibiotics
- Oral gut decontamination
- Frequent saline flush of dialyzer

At the present time, heparin and citrate are the only anticoagulants available for use in acute hemodialysis. Dextran cannot be used because of its nephrotoxicity [106]. There has been relatively little experience with low molecular weight heparin in acute renal failure. Although its therapeutic index may be more favorable than standard heparin preparations, it is unlikely to be well-tolerated in individuals with hypersensitivity to heparin or with heparin-induced thrombocytopenia. The development of recombinant analogues of leech-derived anticoagulants, such as hirudin and hirulog, currently under intensive study in cardiovascular disease, may provide safe and effective alternatives to heparin within the next several years.

Dialysis Dose

The nephrology community has addressed in great detail the importance of treatment adequacy in the chronic dialysis setting [71–73]. However, surprisingly little attention has been paid to analogous issues in acute renal failure. Although an elevated blood urea nitrogen level often sparks consultation and intervention in critically ill patients with acute renal failure, alone it is a poor surrogate for uremia and an unacceptable gauge of dialysis adequacy. Furthermore, the gap between dialysis prescribed and dialysis delivered, which may be in excess of 20% or more in end-stage disease [74], may be even more pronounced with acute renal failure, given hemodynamic instability, reduced blood flows, shortened time because of scheduled procedures or diagnostic tests, and suboptimal vascular access, usually a temporary catheter prone to recirculation. Carefully controlled trials of varying levels of dialysis dose with conventional hemodialysis, as well as alternative techniques in acute renal failure, are required to clarify these issues.

Often the major determinant of dialysis dose in critically ill patients is the accompanying need for fluid removal. Assessing adequate ultrafiltration may be even more challenging than for solute clearance, because of the lack of a detectable serum marker. If intravascular monitoring is available, adjusting the state of intravascular hydration to an optimal pulmonary capillary or central venous pressure is advisable. However, in other cases, ultrafiltration often proceeds until mild to moderate hypotension develops. A modest dose of dopamine (e.g., 2–10 µg/kg per min), or salt-poor albumin in individuals with severe hypoproteinemia, may attenuate blood pressure reduction and allow more vigorous ultrafiltration in selected instances.

Despite the current lack of information, we would extrapolate from outcome data in end-stage renal disease and recommend that acute conventional hemodialysis be prescribed to achieve a urea reduction ratio (the change in pre-post dialysis blood urea nitrogen concentration divided by pre-dialysis concentration) of 65% or greater [72]. Conventional hemodialysis should be dosed daily in many cases of hypercatabolic acute renal failure, to allow more liberal administration of intravenous fluids and hyperalimentation. The dangers of using moderate or low blood urea nitrogen or creatinine levels (potentially the result of low dietary protein intake and diminished somatic protein mass, respectively) as measures of treatment adequacy cannot be overemphasized.

Nutritional Support

Acute renal failure, particularly when associated with sepsis, trauma, or multiple organ failure, can be marked by increased energy expenditure and protein catabolism [5, 75]. The optimal means of providing nutrients to such patients, given concerns about urea generation, uremia, and extracellular volume overload, have been elusive. Indeed, the widespread use of parenteral nutrition in the course of acute renal failure has led to the increasingly frequent need to initiate dialysis because of obligate nutrition-related fluid administration.

When possible, enteral nutrition is preferred, as it allows for reduced fluid administration compared with total parenteral nutrition and eliminates the need for a dedicated central venous catheter. More importantly, the potential risks of central venous catheter-associated bacteremia and fungemia are reduced. Likewise, enteral feeding may preserve intestinal mucosal integrity and limit the translocation of gram-negative bacteria and endotoxin, which may result in sepsis syndrome and multiple organ failure [76, 77]. Nevertheless, parenteral nutrition is often required in intensive care unit patients because of abdominal surgery or ischemia, or refractory ileus.

In spite of thorough investigation over the past two decades, the optimal parenteral nutrition formulation for patients with acute renal failure is unknown. An early study compared hypertonic glucose alone with a solution containing essential amino acids and demonstrated increased survival and return of renal function in the latter group [78]. However, no significant differences in survival, renal recovery, or laboratory evidence of nitrogen balance were seen in several subsequent studies which examined modifications of the type (essential versus nonessential or mixed) and quantity of amino acid supplement provided [79–81].

A present, we recommend the administration of at least 1.4 g protein and 35–45 kCal/kg per day for patients with acute renal failure requiring dialysis; substantially more protein and calories may be required for those patients with sepsis or multiple organ failure, who are often markedly hypercatabolic, and somewhat less for obese persons or those ventilated and paralyzed. Efforts to quantify protein needs, by calculation of urea appearance or protein catabolic rate, may help to guide administration of protein or amino acid therapy. Although amino acids are lost during hemodialysis, parenteral nutrition should not be withheld before or during hemodialysis; approximately 90% of infused amino acids are retained even during treatment [63]. For patients with renal and respiratory failure, reductions in carbohydrate content and increased lipids may be necessary to reduce the respiratory quotient toward 0.8. The use of agents to enhance or accelerate anabolism, such as growth hormone [82, 83] or insulin growth factor-1, should be carefully studied in conjunction with nutrient administration. In short, nutrition must be considered an integral part of the conventional hemodialysis prescription.

Drug Disposition

Drug-induced nephrotoxicity is a relatively common contributing cause of acute renal failure in the critically ill [84]. Culprit agents that are frequently employed in the intensive care unit setting include intravenous contrast, antibacterial agents (e.g., aminoglycosides, penicillins, cephalosporins, sulfa drugs), other antimicrobials (e.g., polymixin B, amphotericin B, pentamidine, foscarnet), cancer chemotherapeutic agents and immunosuppressants (e.g., *cis*-platinum, adriamycin, cyclosporin A, FK 506), and nonsteroidal antiinflammatory drugs. The potential adverse renal effects of these and other drugs are well recognized.

In contrast, the important effects of renal function on drug disposition have received less attention and intellectual rigor. The altered disposition of drugs commonly prescribed in critically ill patients with acute renal failure is outlined below (for a detailed review, see Bennett et al. [101, 102]):

1. Drugs to avoid:
   - Dextran
   - Meperidine
   - Pancuronium
   - Succinylcholine
   - Tubocurarine
   - Methotrexate
   - Phenelzine
   - Chlorpropamide
2. Reduced dosage required:
   - Digoxin
   - Procainamide
   - Atenolol
   - Amrinone
   - Sodium nitroprusside (avoid use for longer than 24 h)
   - Fentanyl
   - Morphine
   - Aminoglycosides
   - Vancomycin
   - Trimethoprim-sulfamethoxazole
   - Acyclovir
   - Gancyclovir
   - Pentamidine
   - Selected pencillins (e.g., penicillin G, ampicillin, ureidopenicillins)
   - Selected cephalosporins (e.g., cefazolin, cefotaxime, ceftazadime)
   - Imepenem
   - Histamine-2 receptor antagonists

3. Supplementation after dialysis recommended:
   - Aminoglycosides
   - Most antibiotics
   - Vancomycin (with high-flux dialyzers)

Sequential Ultrafiltration Hemodialysis

Sequential ultrafiltration hemodialysis is a particularly useful and easy-to-implement modification of conventional hemodialysis. This technique is based on the observed improvement of vascular and cardiac hemodynamics during the temporal and physical segregation of ultrafiltration and solute clearance [85]. When performed with diffusive dialysis, ultrafiltration-induced fluid loss is not met by a compensatory increase in peripheral vascular resistance, perhaps related to the concurrent diffusive loss of osmotically active substances and transcellular fluid and electrolyte (e.g., sodium, calcium) shifts. In contrast, when ultrafiltration is performed alone, it is usually accompanied by an increase in peripheral vascular resistance, such that up to 4 l/h can be removed without systemic hypotension [86].

Although some convective clearance is performed during the ultrafiltration phase of sequential ultrafiltration hemodialysis (usually 60–90 min), it is important to maintain a satisfactorily long diffusive phase in order to achieve the desired intensity of small-solute clearance. Therefore, the usual duration of conventional hemodialysis should be prescribed for the clearance phase. As noted above, intermittent hemofiltration alone would not provide adequate solute clearance for a patient with severe acute renal failure.

Vascular Access for Acute Conventional Hemodialysis

Efficient conventional hemodialysis requires access to the circulation at a site large enough to provide blood flow rates in excess of 250 ml/min. In contrast to patients with chronic renal failure, those with acute renal failure typically do not warrant creation of an endogenous arteriovenous fistula or synthetic graft, as most individuals will eventually recover native renal function or unfortunately expire due to the complications of critical illness. Conventional hemodialysis angioaccess requires cannulation of either the femoral, subclavian, or internal jugular vein with a relatively large, double-lumen catheter. In critically ill patients, the site of choice is usually determined by the patients' underlying disease. For example, those patients with coagulopathy are more safely managed with a femoral venous catheter, that site being more amenable to compression in the event of inadvertent arterial puncture. Similarly, patients with severe pulmonary disease may be more safely accessed at the femoral site because of the risk of pneumothorax with internal jugular or subclavian catheter placement. However, a femoral catheter is prone to infection and is less convenient than a subclavian or internal jugular venous catheter. A femoral catheter limits the patient's mobility, as sitting up in bed or ambulating increases the risk of catheter malfunction and local bleeding. As a result, immobility may delay wound healing and physical and nutritional rehabilitation.

Although hemodialysis access at the subclavian site has been commonly performed for the past two decades, recent evidence that prolonged cannulation of the subclavian vein with a percutaneous catheter may markedly increase the risk of venous stenosis has tempered enthusiasm for this technique [87–89]. Percutaneous cannulation of the internal jugular vein has been described and successfully employed by Uldall et al. [90]. More often patients now undergo surgical or fluoroscopic placement of a tunneled internal jugular venous catheter for acute hemodialysis. The right internal jugular vein is preferred because the passage into the superior vena cava is more direct, and less frequently associated with kinking or catheter dysfunction [91]. A Dacron cuff on a semipermanent internal jugular venous catheter may result in fewer catheter-associated bacteremias, by inducing a protective fibrotic reaction along the catheter–vessel interface; however, definitive evidence for this protective effect is lacking. In addition, chronic venous stenosis appears to be less common after prolonged cannulation of the internal jugular vein, compared with the subclavian vein. A single reservation to the use of an internal jugular catheter for acute hemodialysis is the potential risk of bacterial colonization from tracheal secretions in mechanically ventilated intensive care unit patients.

Careful local management is critical to catheter performance. The site should be kept sterile at all times, and dedicated to hemodialysis alone. Heparin (7500 units) is routinely instilled into each catheter lumen after the completion of the dialysis session. If in spite of heparin the catheter becomes occluded with thrombus or fibrin, urokinase (5000 units per port) may be instilled for 20–30 min, achieving thrombolysis with negligible systemic absorption.

If adequate blood flow cannot be achieved with a double-lumen catheter, one should consider cannulation at two separate sites with single-lumen catheters. In addition to the potential for improved blood flow, physical separation of the arterial and venous port to the dialysis delivery system should result in less recirculation of blood and a modest improvement in clearance.

Although of historical importance, the use of an external shunt, such as the Quinton-Scribner shunt, is unwise, given difficulty with sustaining adequate blood flow and an increased risk of clotting and infectious complications.

Unlike the continuous arteriovenous techniques, conventional hemodialysis requires access only to the venous system. Therefore, atherosclerotic disease of the femoral vessels or a history of vascular bypass grafting are not contraindications to the use of conventional hemodialysis. Rarely, all appropriate venous sites have been occupied by intravascular devices (e.g., central venous line for hyperalimentation, pulmonary artery catheter, intraaortic balloon pump), or coagulopathy is so severe that even venous puncture is intolerable. In such cases, acute peritoneal dialysis would clearly be preferred.

Complications of Acute Conventional Hemodialysis

Major complications of acute conventional hemodialysis and their potential remedies are listed in Table 1. The most common complication of acute conventional hemodialysis is systemic hypotension, resulting from both the removal of extracellular fluid with ultrafiltration as well as other factors, less well understood, resulting from vasodilitation due to diffusive solute clearance and blood membrane interactions (see above). Perhaps the most often overlooked and easily prevented cause of hypotension is the injudicious use of vasodilators and other antihypertensive agents proximal to the time of dialysis. Many popular antihypertensive agents have been formulated as long-acting preparations (e.g., calcium antagonists, α- and β-adrenergic antagonists, nitrates) and/or have prolonged elimination with renal dysfunction (e.g., angiotensin-converting enzyme inhibitors, α-methyldopa) and are frequently prescribed to intensive care unit patients with cardiovascular disease. Avoiding administration of these medications during the 4h or more before dialysis (depending on drug half-life) will attenuate the ultrafiltration-associated drop in blood pressure, which may be particularly steep in patients treated with vasodilators who become dependent on preload for maintanence of blood pressure.

Additionally, the patient should be carefully screened for pericardial disease or occult blood loss. The critically ill patient who develops uremic pericarditis may bleed into the pericardium as a result of concurrent coagulopathy or heparinization during dialysis. Although the absence of a rub may indicate resolution of uremia, a pericardial rub may become diminished when fluid (e.g., blood) enters the pericardial sac. Pericardial tamponade can be easily recognized and remedied when discovered. Similarly, the possibility of occult blood loss in critically ill patients (e.g., retroperitoneal bleeding, secondary to hemorrhagic pancreatitis, perforated duodenal ulcer, or hemorrhage from femoral arterial or venous cannulation) should be investigated thoroughly.

More often, hypotension results from the underlying disease process (e.g., sepsis, cardiogenic shock) and is exacerbated by the hemodialysis procedure. The hemodialysis regimen can be modified in several ways to attenuate procedure-related hypotension. The ultrafiltration rate can be reduced to allow for more gradual recruitment of interstitial fiuid into the vascular space, or sequential ultrafiltration hemodialysis should be performed. The dialysate sodium concentration should be maintained at or

Table 1. Complications of acute conventional hemodialysis

Complication	Potential remedies
Hypotension	Hold antihypertensive drugs prior to hemodialysis Reduce ultrafiltration rate if appropriate Increase dialysate sodium concentration Perform sequential ultrafiltration hemodialysis Add inotropic or vasoconstrictive agents Add salt-poor albumin or fresh frozen plasma Reduce dialysate temperature Maintain dialysate calcium concentration at 3.5 mEq/l Screen carefully for pericardial disease (e.g., tamponade) Rule out occult blood loss
Hypoxemia	Add supplemental oxygen during hemodialysis Use biocompatible dialyzer Use dialysate bicarbonate concentration of 35 mEq/l or less Transfuse if anemic
Arrhythmia	Increase dialysate potassium concentration Step reduction in dialysate potassium Limit sympathomimetic agents if tolerated Modify digoxin dose for reduced glomerular filtration rate
Seizure/dialysis disequlibrium	Increase dialysate sodium concentration Limit solute clearance: reduction in membrane surface area, reduction in blood and dialysate flows, cocurrent blood and dialysate flow Mannitol or hypertonic glucose administration Phenytoin
Catheter-associated infection	Parenteral antimicrobial agents Removal of catheter; placement at alternative site
Pyrogen reaction or hemolysis	Parenteral antimicrobial agents Rule out septicemia Supportive care (e.g., inotropic or vasoconstrictive agents) Avoid dialyzer reprocessing Increase ultrafiltration rate to limit backfiltration of dialysate
Hemorrhage	Correct or repair bleeding site Regional or no anticoagulation Deamino-D-argine vasopressin (DDAVP) or alternative agents to improve hemostasis Correction of underlying coagulopathy (e.g., fresh frozen plasma)
Delayed renal functional recovery	Limit ultrafiltration Use biocompatible dialyzer

above 140 mEq/l, and, if tolerated, the dialysate can be cooled to 35–36°C to promote peripheral vasoconstriction [92, 93].

Stopping Therapy

Recovery from acute renal failure usually occurs within 4 weeks, but may take up to 8 weeks or more. It is imperative to periodically examine factors that may be associated with functional recovery, such as an increased urine output, a decrease or decreased rate of rise of serum creatinine during the intradialytic interval, or an improvement in metabolic acidosis. Paradoxically, the blood urea nitrogen may increase during recovery because of improved tubular resorptive capacity. Nephrologic care must be individualized, balancing the risks of holding dialysis against the risks of dialysis-associated complications.

Stopping therapy in the face of declining clinical status can be far more difficult. When acute renal failure affects the critically ill, in-hospital mortality exceeds 50% in most studies [4, 94–98]. In our recent experience, overall in-hospital mortality for patients with acute renal failure who required dialysis was 70%; those with multiple organ system failure and malignancy were at even higher risk (unpublished data).

The decision to withdraw dialysis may be appropriate when further aggressive care is futile, but will almost certainly hasten death. Like most dilemmas faced by intensive care unit staff, the clinical and ethical care of the patient with acute renal failure must be carefully thought out and individualized. The institution of hemodialysis, or any other dialytic modality, should not mandate that treatment be continued indefinitely. As with other invasive procedures, it may be advisable to recommend a trial period of 1–2 weeks, after which the clinical condition of the patient, and appropriateness of dialysis therapy, can be reassessed.

Summary

The critically ill patient with acute renal failure poses many challenges to the intensivist and nephrologist. Recent advances in conventional hemodialysis technology and important modifications in procedural technique have allowed for more efficient, safe, and effective dialytic therapy. As a result of these improvements, conventional hemodialysis can be performed in almost all patients who are candidates for renal replacement therapy.

The mortality rate of critically ill patients with acute renal failure remains distressingly high. Although much of this excess mortality is undoubtedly due to comorbid diseases, it is incumbent upon us to prospectively investigate crucial clinical issues, such as the roles of the dialysis intensity, nutritional support, and cytokine kinetics, in an effort to improve the clinical outcome of acute renal failure patients.

References

1. Bywaters E, Beall O (1941) Crush injuries with impairment of renal function. Br J Med 1:427–436
2. Kolff W (1946) The artificial kidney. Medical dissertation, University of Groningen
3. Swan R, Merrill J (1953) Clinical course of acute renal failure. Medicine (Baltimore) 32:215
4. Murphy W, Swan R, Walter C, Weller J, Merrill J (1952) Use of an artificial kidney. III. Current procedures in clinical hemodialysis. J Lab Clin Med 40:436–444
5. Wilmore D (1991) Catabolic illness: strategies for enhancing recovery. N Engl J Med 325(10):695–702
6. Ziegler T, Young L, Manson J, Wilmore D (1988) Metabolic effects of recombinant human growth hormone in patients receiving parenteral nutrition. Ann Surg 208:6–16
7. Bidani A, Churchill P (1983) Aminophylline ameliorates glycerol-induced acute renal failure in rats. Can J Physiol Pharmacol 61(6):567–571
8. Parker S, Carlon G, Isaacs M, Howland W, Kahn R (1981) Dopamine administration in oliguric and non-oliguric renal failure. Crit Care Med 9:630–632
9. Rudy D, Voelker J, Greene P, Esparza F, Brater D (1991) Loop diuretics for chronic renal failure: a continuous infusion is more efficacious than bolus therapy. Ann Intern Med 115(5):360–366
10. Inoue M, Okajima K, Itoh K et al. (1987) Mechanism of furosemide resistance in analbuminemic rats and hypoalbuminemic patients. Kidney Int 32(2):198–203
11. Anderson C, Shahvari M, Zimmerman J (1979) The treatment of pulmonary edema in the absence of renal function – a role for sorbitol and furosemide. JAMA 241:1008–1110
12. Choi M, Fernandez P, Patnaik A et al. (1993) Brief report: trimethoprim-induced hyperkalemia in a patient with AIDS. N Engl J Med 328(10):703–706
13. Hohnloser S, Verrier R, Lown B (1987) Influence of beta 2-adrenoceptor stimulation and blockade on cardiac electrophysiologic properties and serum potassium concentration in the anesthetized dog. Am Heart J 113(5):1066–1070
14. Flinn R, Merrill J, Wlezant W (1961) Treatment of the oliguric patient with a new sodium exchange resin and sorbitol. N Engl J Med 264:111–114
15. Gerstman B, Kirkman R, Platt R (1992) Intestinal necrosis associated with postoperative orally administered sodium polystyrene sulfonate in sorbitol. Am J Kidney Dis 20:159–161
16. Brown T, Ahern D, Nolph K (1973) Potassium removal with peritoneal dialysis. Kidney Int 4:67–69
17. Hou S, McElroy P, Nootens J, Beach M (1989) Safety and efficacy of low-potassium dialysate. Am J Kidney Dis 13:137–143
18. Remuzzi G, Pusineri F (1988) Coagulation defects in uremia. Kidney Int Suppl 24:S13–S17
19. Janson P, Jubeliere S, Weinstein M, Deykin D (1980) Treatment of the bleeding tendency of uremia with cryoprecipitate. N Engl J Med 303(23):1318–1322
20. Mannucci P, Remuzzi G, Pusineri F et al. (1983) Deamino-8-D-arginine vasopressin shortens the bleeding time in uremia. N Engl J Med 308(1):8–12
21. Locke S, Merrill J, Tyler H (1961) Neurologic complications of acute uremia. Arch Intern Med 108:75–83
22. Mitch W, May R, Maroni B (1989) Mechanisms for abnormal protein metabolism in uremia. J Am Coll Nutr 8(4):305–309
23. Mitch W, May R, Maroni B, Druml W (1989) Protein and amino acid metabolism in uremia: influence of metabolic acidosis. Kidney Int Suppl 27:S205–S207
24. Molitoris B, Froment D, Mackenzie T, Huffer W, Alfrey A (1989) Citrate: a major factor in the toxicity of orally administered aluminum compounds. Kidney Int 36(6):949–953
25. Androgue H, Rashad M, Gorin A, Yacoub J, Madias N (1989) Assessing acid-base status in circulatory failure: differences between arterial and central venous blood. N Engl J Med 320:1312–1315

26. Kveim M, Nesbakken R (1975) Utilization of exogenous acetate during hemodialysis. Trans Am Soc Artif Intern Organs 21:138–143
27. Conger J (1975) A controlled evaluation of prophylactic dialysis in post-traumatic acute renal failure. J Trauma 15:1056–1063
28. Gillum D, Dixon B, Yanover M et al. (1986) The role of intensive dialysis in acute renal failure. Clin Nephrol 25:249–255
29. Sargent J, Gotch F (1989) Principals and biophysics of dialysis. In: Maher J (ed) Replacement of renal function by dialysis. Kluwer, Dordrecht, p 87
30. Babb A, Farrell P, Uvelli D, Scribner B (1972) Hemodialyzer evaluation by examination of solute molecular spectra. Trans Am Soc Artif Intern Organs 18:98–105
31. Henderson L (1989) Biophysics of ultrafiltration and hemofiltration. In: Maher J (ed) Replacement of renal function by dialysis. Kluwer, Dordrecht, p 300
32. Nolph K, Nothum R, Maher J (1974) Ultrafiltration: a mechanism for removal of intermediate molecular weight substances in coil dialyzers. Kidney Int 6:55–60
33. Baldamus C (1983) Clinical value and technical feasibility of long-term hemofiltration. Trans Am Soc Artif Intern Organs 6:192–195
34. Davison A, Roberts T, Mascie-Taylor B, Lewins A (1982) Haemofiltration for profound dialysis-induced hypotension: removal of sodium and water without blood-pressure change. Br Med J 285:87–89
35. Geronemus R, Schneider N (1984) Continuous arteriovenous hemodialysis: a new modality for treatment of acute renal failure. Trans Am Soc Artif Intern Organs 30:610–612
36. Bellomo R, Ernest D, Love J, Parkin G, Boyce N (1990) Continuous arteriovenous haemodiafiltration: an optimal therapy for acute renal failure in the intensive care setting. Aust N Z J Med 20:237–242
37. Bellomo R, Parkin G, Love J, Boyce N (1992) Management of acute renal failure in the critically ill with continuous venovenous hemodiafiltration. Ren Fail 4:183–186
38. Jorstad S (1988) Generation and removal of anaphylatoxins during hemofiltration with 5 different membranes. Blood Purif 6:325–335
39. Bellomo R, Tipping P, Boyce N (1993) Continuous venovenous hemofiltration with dialysis removes cytokines from the circulation of septic patients. Crit Care Med 21: 522–526
40. Flaherty J, Garcia-Houchins S, Chudy R, Arnow P (1993) An outbreak of gram-negative bacteriemia traced to contaminated O-rings in reprocessed dialyzers. Ann Intern Med 119:1072–1078
41. Gordon S, Tipple M, Bland L, Jarvis W (1988) Pyrogenic reactions associated with the reuse of disposable hollow-fiber hemodialyzers. JAMA 260:2077–2081
42. Conger J (1983) The role of blood flow autoregulation in pathophysiology of acute renal failure. Circ Shock 11:235–244
43. Adams P, Adams P, Bell P, Navar L (1980) Impaired renal blood flow autoregulation in ischemic acute renal failure. Kidney Int 18:68–76
44. Schulman G (1993) A review of the concept of biocompatibility. Kidney Int Suppl 41:S209–S212
45. Himmelfarb J, Zaoui P, Hakim R (1992) Modulation of granulocyte LAM-1 and MAC-1 during dialysis – a prospective randomized controlled trial. Kidney Int 41:388–395
46. Himmelfarb J, Lazarus J, Hakim R (1991) Reactive oxygen species production to monocytes and polymorphonuclear leukocytes during dialysis. Am J Kidney Dis 17: 271–276
47. Cheung A, Baranowski R, Wayman A (1987) The role of thromboxane in cuprophan-induced pulmonary hypertension. Kidney Int 31:1072–1079
48. Shaldon S, Lonnemann G, Koch K (1989) Cytokine relevance in biocompatibility. Contrib Nephrol 79:227–236
49. Schindler R, Lonnemann G, Shaldon S, Koch K, Dinarello C (1990) Transcription, not synthesis, of interleukin-1 and tumor necrosis factor by complement. Kidney Int 37:85–93

50. Canivet E, Lavaud S, Wong T, Guenounou M, Willemin J, Potron G (1994) Cuprophane but not synthetic membrane induces increases in serum tumor necrosis factor-alpha levels during hemodialysis. Am J Kidney Dis 23:41–46
51. Schulman G. Fogo A, Gung A, Badr K, Hakim R (1991) Complement activation retards resolution of acute ischemic renal failure in the rat. Kidney Int 40:1069–1074
52. Hakim R, Wingard R, Parker R (1994) Dialysis membranes in the treatment of patients with acute renal failure. N Engl J Med 331:1338–1342
53. Wilkenson R, Barber S, Robson V (1977) Cramps, thirst, and hypertension in hemodialysis patients. Clin Nephrol 7:101–105
54. Port F, Johnson W, Klass D (1973) Prevention of dialysis disequilibrium syndrome by use of high sodium concentration in the dialysate. Kidney Int 3:327–333
55. VanStone J, Bauer J, Carey J (1980) The effect of dialysate sodium concentration on body fluid distribution during hemodialysis. Trans Am Soc Artif Intern Organs 26:383–386
56. Raja R, Kramer M, Barber K, Chin S (1983) Sequential changes in dialysate sodium during dialysis. Trans Am Soc Artif Intern Organs 29:649–651
57. Ward R, Wathen R, Williams T, Harding G (1987) Hemodialysate composition and intradialytic metabolic, acid-base, and potassium changes. Kidney Int 32:129–135
58. Sherman R, Hwang E, Bernhole A, Eisinger R (1986) Variability in potassium removal by hemodialysis. Am J Nephrol 6:284–288
59. Henrich W (1986) Hemodynamic instability during hemodialysis. Kidney Int 30:605–612
60. Wolff J, Pendersen T, Rossen M, Cleeman-Rasmussen K (1986) Effects of acetate and bicarbonate dialysis on cardiac performance, transmural myocardial perfusion and acid-base balance. Int J Artif Organs 9:105–110
61. Vinay P, Prud'homme M, Vinet B et al. (1987) Acetate metabolism and bicarbonate generation during hemodialysis: 10 years of observation. Kidney Int 31:1194–1204
62. Ebben J, Hirsh D, Luchmann D, Collins A, Kehaviah P (1987) Microbiologic contamination of liquid bicarbonate concentrate for hemodialysis. Trans Am Soc Artif Intern Organs 33:269–273
63. Wolfson M, Jones M, Kopple J (1982) Amino acid losses during hemodialysis with infusion of amino acids and glucose. Kidney Int 21:500–506
64. Ikizler A, Flakoll P, Hakim R (1993) Amino acid losses in hemodialysis with different dialysis membranes. J Am Soc Nephrol 4(3):127P
65. Raman A, Chong Y, Sreenevasan G (1976) Effects of varying dialysate calcium concentrations on the plasma calcium fractions in patients on dialysis. Nephron 16:181–187
66. Vliskin S, Belhassen B, Sheps D, Laniado S (1992) Clinical and electrophysiologic effects of magnesium sulfate on paroxysmal supraventricular tachycardia and comparison to adenosine triphosphate. Am J Cardiol 70:870–885
67. Roden D (1989) Magnesium treatment of ventricular arrhythmias. Am J Cardiol 63:43G–46G
68. Skobeloff E, Spivey W, McNamara R, Greenspon L (1989) Intravenous magnesium sulfate in the treatment of acute asthma in the emergency department. JAMA 262: 1210–1213
69. Hampers C, Blaufox M, Merrill J (1966) Anticoagulation rebound after hemodialysis. N Engl J Med 255:1063–1067
70. VonBrecht J, Flanagan M, Freeman R, Lim V (1986) Regional anticoagulation: hemodialysis with hypertonic trisodium citrate. Am J Kidney Dis 8:196–201
71. Harter H (1983) Review of findings from the National Cooperative Dialysis Study and recommendations. Kidney Int 23 Suppl 13:S107–S112
72. Owen W, Lew N, Liu Y, Lowrie E, Lazarus J (1993) The urea reduction ratio and serum albumin concentration as predictors of mortality in patients undergoing hemodialysis. N Engl J Med 329(14):1001–1006
73. Held P, Levin N, Bovberg R, Pauly M, Diamond L (1991) Mortality and duration of hemodialysis treatment. JAMA 257(5):645–650

74. Parker T (1992) Trends and concepts in the prescription and delivery of dialysis in the US. Semin Nephrol 12(3):267–275
75. Bartlett R, Dechert R, Mault J, Ferguson S, Kaiser A, Erlandson E (1982) Measurement of metabolism in multiple organ failure. Surgery 92:771–778
76. Langkamp-Henken B, Glezer J, Kuosk K (1992) Immunologic structure and function of the gastrointestinal tract. Nutr Clin Pract 7(3):100–108
77. Haglund U (1993) Systemic mediators released from the gut in critical illness. Crit Care Med 21 Suppl 2:S15–S18
78. Abel R, Beck C, Abbott W, Ryan J, Barnett G, Fischer J (1973) Improved survival from acute renal failure after treatment with intravenous essential l-amino acids and glucose. N Engl J Med 288(14):695–699
79. Blumenkrantz M, Kopple J, Koffler A et al. (1978) Total parenteral nutrition in the management of acute renal failure. Am J Clin Nutr 31:1831–1840
80. Feinstein E, Blumenkrantz M, Healy M et al. (1981) Clinical and metabolic responses to parenteral nutrition in acute renal failure. Medicine (Baltimore) 60(2):124–137
81. Mirtallo J, Schneider P, Mavko K, Ruberg R, Fabri P (1982) A comparison of essential and general amino acid infusions in the nutritional support of patients with compromised renal function. JPEN J Parenter Enteral Nutr 6(2):109–113
82. Schulman G, Wingard R, Hutchinson R, Lawrence P, Hakim R (1993) The effects of recombinant human growth hormone and intradialytic parenteral nutrition in malnourished hemodialysis patients. Am J Kidney Dis 21(5):527–534
83. Ziegler T, Lazarus J, Young L, Hakim R, Wilmore D (1991) Effects of recombinant human growth hormone in adults receiving maintenance hemodialysis. J Am Soc Nephrol 2(6):1130–1135
84. Hou S, Bushinsky D, Wish J, Cohen J, Harrington J (1983) Hospital-acquired renal insufficiency: a prospective study. Am J Med 74:243–248
85. Shinaberger J, Brautbar N, Miller J, Gardner P (1978) Successful application of sequential hemofiltration followed by diffusion dialysis with standard dialysis equipment. Trans Am Soc Artif Intern Organ 24:677–681
86. Asaba H, Bergstrom J, Furst P et al. (1976) Sequential ultrafiltration and diffusion as alternatives to conventional hemodialysis. Proc Clin Dial Transplant Forum 6:129–135
87. Vanholder R, Lameire N, Verbank J, von Rattinghe R, Kunnen M, Rigoir S (1982) Complications of subclavian catheter hemodialysis: a 5-year prospective study in 257 consecutive patients. Int J Artif Organs 5(5):297–303
88. Cimochowski G, Worley E, Rutherford W, Sartain J, Blondin J, Harter H (1990) Superiority of internal jugular over the subclavian access for temporary dialysis. Nephron 54(2):154–161
89. Uldall P (1994) Subclavian cannulation is no longer necessary or justified in patients with end-stage renal failure. Semin Dial 7:161–164
90. Uldall P, DeBruyne M, Besley M, McMillan J, Simons M, Fraicoer R (1993) A new vascular access catheter for hemodialysis. Am J Kidney Dis 21(3):270–277
91. Moss A, McLaughlin M, Lempert K, Holley J (1988) Use of a silicone catheter with a Dacron cuff for dialysis short-term vascular access. Am J Kidney Dis 12(6):492–498
92. Sherman R, Faustino E, Bernholc A, Eisinger R (1984) Effect of variations in dialysate temperature on blood pressure during hemodialysis. Am J Kidney Dis 4:66–68
93. Jost C, Agarwal R, Khair-el-Din T, Grayburn P, Victor R, Henrich W (1993) Effects of cooler temperature dialysate on hemodynamic stability in problem hemodialysis patients. Kidney Int 44:606–612
94. Stott R, Cameron J, Ogg C, Bewick M (1972) Why the persistently high mortality in acute renal failure? Lancet 2:75–79
95. Lohr J, McFarlane M, Grantham J (1988) A clinical index to predict survival in acute renal failure patients requiring dialysis. Am J Kidney Dis 11:254–259
96. Cioffi W, Ashikaga T, Gamelli R (1984) Probability of surviving postoperative acute renal failure. Ann Surg 200:205–211

97. Spiegel D, Ullian M, Zerbe G, Berl T (1991) Determinants of survival and recovery in acute renal failure patients dialyzed in intensive care units. Am J Nephrol 11:44–47
98. Corwin H, Teplick R, Schreiber M, Fang L, Bonventre J, Coggins C (1987) Prediction of outcome in acute renal failure. Am J Nephrol 7:8–12
99. Tielemans C, Madhoun P, Lenaers M, Schandene L, Goldman M, Vanderweghem J (1990) Anaphylactoid reactions during hemodialysis on AN69 membranes in patients receiving ACE inhibitors. Kidney Int 38:982–984
100. Schulman G, Hakim R, Arias R, Silverberg M, Kaplan A, Arbeit L (1993) Bradykinin generation by dialysis membrane: possible role in anaphylactic reactions. J Am Soc Nephrol 3:1536–1539
101. Bennett W, Muther R, Parker R, Feig P, Morrison G, Golper T (1980) Drug therapy is renal failure: dosing guidelines for adults. Ann Intern Med 93:62–89
102. Bennett W, Aronoff G, Morrison G, Golper T, Pulliam J, Wolfson M (1983) Drug prescribing in renal failure: dosing guidelines for adults. Am J Kidney Dis 3:155–193
103. Campistol JM, Skinner M (1993) β_2-Microglobulin anyloidosis: an overview. Sem Dial 6:117–126
104. Sherman RA, Hwang ER, Bernholc AS, Eisinger RP (1986) Variability in potassium removal by hemodialysis. Am J Nephrol 6:284–288.
105. Nissenson AR, Kraut JA, Shinaberger JH (1984) Dialysis-associated hypoxemia: pathogenesis and prevention. ASAIO J 7:1–12
106. Mailoux L, Schwartz CD, Capizzi R et al. (1967) Acute renal failure after administration of low-molecular weight dextran. N Engl J Med 277:113–118

Continuous Hemofiltration in Acute Renal Failure

H. Kierdorf and H.G. Sieberth

Introduction

In 1977, Kramer et al. [1] published the first report of continuous extracorporeal treatment for patients with acute renal failure (ARF). The arteria femoralis had mistakenly been punctured instead of the femoral vein. Kramer left the arterial catheter in place and was able to demonstrate that the arterial blood pressure was sufficient for a filter to achieve satisfactory filtration capacity without a blood pump. This continuous arteriovenous hemofiltration (CAVH) was the first form of therapy allowing continuous artificial replacement of an organ system. Owing to its surprising simplicity, CAVH quickly gained ground. However, blood pressure-dependent filtration capacity could not control azotemia adequately in hemodynamically unstable patients with acute hypercatabolic renal failure, so the early enthusiasm for this method soon waned. A number of treatment methods aimed at combining the advantages of continuous therapy with a higher effectiveness have been developed since the beginning of the 1980s [2]. The common feature of these new methods, for instance continuous arteriovenous hemodialysis (CAVHD) and pump-assisted venovenous methods such as continuous venovenous hemofiltration (CVVH) or continuous venovenous hemodialysis (CVVHD), is that their greater effectiveness enables them to treat even hemodynamically unstable hypercatabolic patients with ARF and multiorgan failure (MOF) satisfactorily [3].

Advantages and Disadvantages of Continuous Hemofiltration

A number of theoretical benefits are claimed for continuous extracorporeal treatment as opposed to intermittent hemodialysis. These include:

- Slow ultrafiltration, hemodynamic stability
- Avoidance of rapid fluid and electrolyte shift
- Unlimited alimentation
- Elimination of mediators (?)
- Easier drug dosage
- Simple equipment (CAVH)

Greater hemodynamic stability is seen as the main advantage of and the main indicator for using continuous methods, especially with MOF patients. Roughly 10% of all ARF patients cannot be treated by intermittent hemodialysis, but can almost invariably benefit from continuous hemofiltration [4]. A positive long-term effect on the patients' hemodynamic situation, not explained solely by the ultrafiltration level and not encountered in intermittent hemodialysis, is also reported [5]. Continuous methods avoid fluctuations in the electrolyte and fluid balance almost completely [1, 6].

Due to the high fluid turnover rate, no limitation on fluids is necessary; parenteral nutrition can be adapted without restriction to the needs of hypercatabolic patients, even in cases of anuria. With intermittent methods, adequate nutrition must often be sacrificed in order to avoid short-term fluid overloads. MOF patients in particular have benefited from a needs-adapted energy and protein intake, which avoids the impact of malnutrition on mortality in these critically ill patients [6]. The slow continuous correction of electrolyte status and fluid balance significantly reduces cerebral alterations in continuously treated patients, because rapid sodium and fluid shifts in intermittent hemodialysis were demonstrated to be responsible for cerebral side effects.

The dosage of drugs is easier in continuous than in intermittent hemodialysis, preventing under- or overdosing of medication in these severely ill patients. The total clearance calculated from the filtrate volume and the residual renal clearance allows doses and dosing intervals for the filtered medication to be taken from dosing tables for renal insufficiency patients [7]. Continuous hemofiltration may also improve elimination of high-molecular substances. This is especially relevant to mediator substances which play a role in the development and persistence of ARF and MOF, such as tumor necrosis factor and interleukin-1 [8]. By comparison, intermittent hemodialysis cannot effectively eliminate these molecules with a relative molecular mass of 15–50 kDa.

Significant disadvantages cited for continuous treatment methods are the lactate load, the arterial punction (not necessary in pump-assisted venovenous methods), and inadequate elimination of urea, creatinine, and of potassium. The inadequate control of azotemia is caused by low filtrate volumes, and additional dialysis becomes necessary. This disdvantage does not apply to the more effective continuous methods. Filtrate amounts of 20–25 l or more a day or CAVHD with a dialysis amount of 1.5–2 l/h will always lead to a sufficient control of urea.

It is, of course, impossible to mobilize patients on continuous treatment, but the critically ill patients concerned are generally immobilized in any case, due to the primary disease.

The most important and perhaps the only significant disadvantage of the continuous methods is the continuous anticoagulation they require. Here, the advantage of intermittent hemodialysis is that anticoagulation is needed only for a limited period or can even be dispensed with altogether [9]. On the other hand, continuous therapy without any anticoagulation also appears to be possible (see "Anticoagulation" below).

Practical Applications

Different Methods of Treatment

Arteriovenous Treatment

CAVH was the first continuous method used in the clinic. Its undisputed advantage is its simplicity. Apart from arterial and venous access (see access), the sole requirements are a hemofilter and tube systems (Fig. 1). The force required for this form of treatment comes exclusively from the patient's arterial blood pressure. Effective treatment is usually possible with a systolic blood pressure above 80–90 mmHg. Net filtrate performance depends on blood pressure, on venous resistance to the blood flow resulting from arterial pressure and venous counterpressure, on the properties of the hemofilter (type of surface, surface area, and internal resistance), on the patient's hematocrit and protein concentration, on the colloidal osmotic pressure, on the dialysate flow (CAVHD) and on the total resistance of the extracorporeal system. The effective membrane pressure which determines filtrate performance may be calculated from the mean arterial pressure, the venous resistance, the colloid osmotic pressure, and the negative pressure

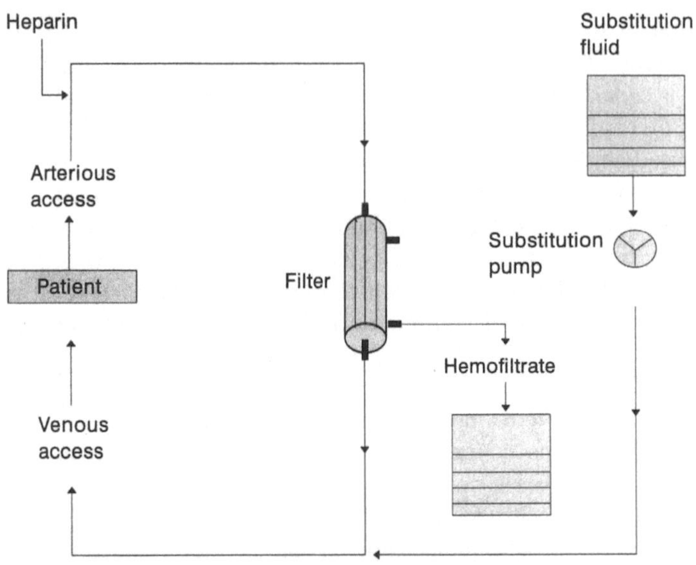

Fig. 1. Continuous arteriovenous hemofiltration (CAVH)

prevailing on the outer side of the membrane. This negative pressure on the outer membrane surface is caused by the enclosed flow of the filtrate to a collecting vessel. The greater the distance between the hemofilter and the collecting vessel, the higher will be the resulting differential pressure.

In order to increase the effectiveness of the method, it is important to avoid a decrease in arterial pressure or an increase in venous resistance. Additional infusion points (three-way taps) should not be integrated in CAVH circulation systems. The length of the blood tube systems must be kept to a minimum to prevent pressure losses within the system. The hemofiltrate must be drawn off in a such a way that volumes can be determined precisely. Substitution is by means of various solutions (see "Substitution solutions") and can be performed manually or with the aid of a balancing unit (see "Balancing").

The ineffectiveness of CAVH with hypercatabolic patients has led to the development of CAVHD [2]. The techniques and apparatus used for this method are comparable with those for CAVH (Fig. 2). Unlike CAVH, however, CAVHD does not replace the ultrafiltrate produced at the filter by a sterile substitution solution, but passes a defined quantity of dialysate on the outer side of the hemodialysator, using the counterflow principle. The dialysate flow is generated by gravity or controlled by volumetric infusion pumps. Substances such as creatinine and urea are therefore exchanged mainly by diffusion, as in hemodialysis. A certain quantity of ultrafiltrate is

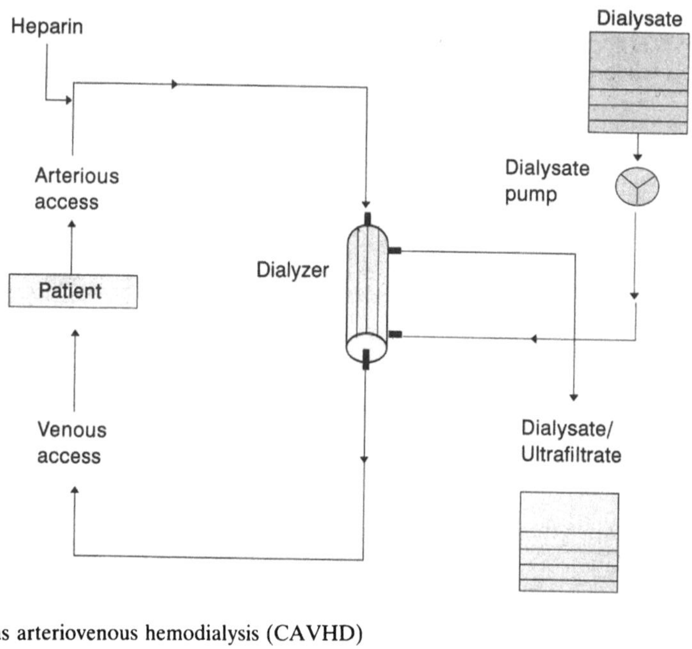

Fig. 2. Continuous arteriovenous hemodialysis (CAVHD)

still produced, so that the therapy represents a combination of dialysis and filtration, i.e., of diffusive and convective transport. The dialysate flow rate is 1–2 l/h. CAVHD is significantly more effective than CAVH. At a blood flow rate of 100 ml/min, the daily hemofiltrate quantity for CAVH is about 15 l, corresponding to a clearance of 10 ml/min for a freely interchangeable substance. At the same blood flow rate, CAVHD with a dialysate flow rate of 1.5 l/h usually achieves a clearance of 15–20 ml/min [3].

Venovenous Treatment Methods

Venovenous treatment methods require the use of a blood pump. The technical effort demanded for this form of therapy is therefore significantly greater than in the case of CAVH. The use of blood pumps in the extracorporeal circulation demands various control and safety devices, e.g., air-free valves, automatically working clamps etc.

Pump-assisted therapy can be performed as an exclusively filtrative treatment (CVVH; Fig. 3). The pressure at the membrane is provided by a blood pump, with the significant advantage that the filtrate volume can be adapted to the patient's needs at any time, even in hemodynamically unstable hypercatabolic patients. Additional intermittent hemodialysis, often needed in CAVH therapy alone, is not necessary with this method. A daily hemofiltrate volume of 30 l can usually be achieved at a blood flow rate of 100–200 ml/min. CVVH has no additional negative impact on circulation, even in

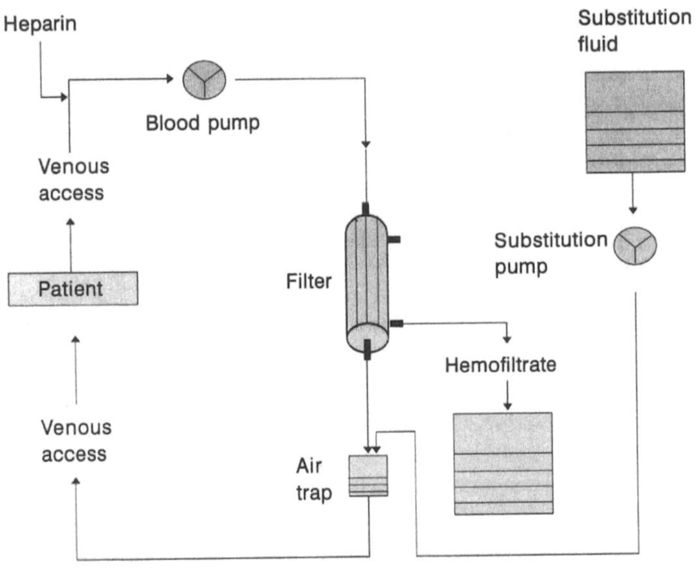

Fig. 3. Continuous venovenous hemofiltration (CVVH)

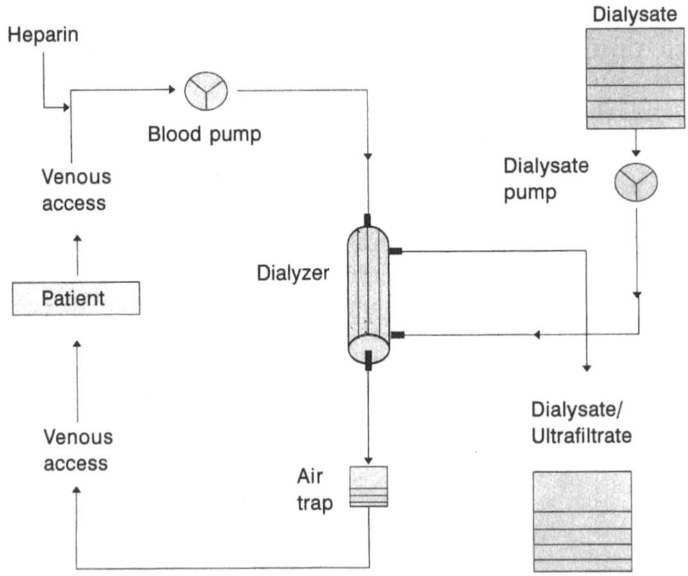

Fig. 4. Continuous venovenous hemodialysis (CVVHD)

critical hemodynamic situations, for example when intra-aortal balloon counterpulsation is used simultaneously in patients with systolic blood pressure values below 70 mmHg. In long-term studies, no clinically relevant hemolysis was observed at blood flow rates of 100–150 ml/min.

An alternative is CVVHD (Fig. 4), where the exchange of substances occurs in the same way as in CAVHD. The technical requirements correspond to those for CVVH, the material exchange to that in CAVD.

Technical requirements for a venovenous treatment are therefore considerably higher than those for CAVH. Using blood pumps involves fitting a variety of control and safety equipment, including air traps, check valves, automatically working clamps, and pressure gauges to monitor the pressure before and behind the filter.

Vascular Access

Arterial Access

In order to perform arteriovenous therapy, it is always necessary to access a large artery and a large vein. Arterial access is almost exclusively via the arteria femoralis. In the Seldinger technique, a short (7–12.5 cm) Shaldon catheter with an external diameter of 2.5–2.7 mm is inserted. Longer catheters tend to increase the incidence of vessel thromboses and have a higher flow resistance. Thicker catheters, which can reduce flow resistance, are ruled out because of higher thrombogenicity and the greater trauma for the vessel. Arterial punctures should be performed with extreme care, since accidental injury to the posterior wall of the artery above the inguinal ligament may cause large retroperitoneal hematomas. Because the patient is generally unconscious or under sedation, this complication is frequently overlooked. Arterial puncture is one of the chief disadvantages of the arteriovenous methods. Local complications in the vicinity of the puncture location (infections, aneurysma, thromboses with embolization in the peripheral extremities) and undetected disconnection bleeding are additional problems for these high-risk patients. An alternative is surgical fitting of a Scribner shunt. In isolated cases, a Cimino-Brescia shunt can be used for continuous treatment, but this method entails a high risk of thrombosis in long-term treatment.

Venous Access

With the arteriovenous methods, venous return flow is via the vena femoralis [1] or the superior vena cava (vena jugularis, vena subclavia). A large Shaldon catheter (external diameter up to 3.0 mm) is installed using the Seldinger technique. A large catheter cross-section should be ensured, especially with arteriovenous methods, since flow resistance increases with decreasing vessel cross-section.

Pump-assisted venovenous methods can be performed using two Shaldon catheters, installed almost exclusively in the superior vena cava. Shaldon catheters with two lumina, allowing venovenous treatment via a single access in a central vein, are increasingly popular. The venous back-pressure of these catheters is tolerable even at a blood flow rate of 300 ml/min. The outside diameter of this two-lumina catheter is 3.2–3.8 mm. The position of a central vein catheter must always be checked radiologically.

Balancing

Fluid balancing is a great problem for all continuous therapy methods. A daily hemofiltrate volume of 25 l or more is usually desirable in CVVH. To avoid endangering the patient, the daily balancing error for this filtrate volume should not exceed 100 ml. Kramer et al. [1] recommend balancing with calibrated filtrate-collecting vessels and subsequent manual regulation of the substitution volume. In clinical practice, such accurate manual measurements are often impractical in intensive care. A further difficulty of manual regulation is that the true content of commercial substitution solutions differs by 5%–10% from their nominal content. Automated balancing devices should therefore always be used where continuous treatment lasts several days or weeks. An essential requirement for such a device is a 1:1 balance of filtrate and substitute and a maximum daily balancing error of 100 ml. The device must also allow preselection of a negative balance. Mechanical and electronic balancing devices [10] exist for this purpose. Our own experience with untolerably high differences indicates that balancing with two identical calibrated pumps cannot be recommended.

Hemofilters

A variety of filters using different membrane materials are available for continuous treatment methods. Different advantages are claimed for each of these synthetic membrane materials. The filters have different sieving coefficients depending on the membrane material used, which is important especially for substances with molecular, masses between 15 and 50 kDa.

The membrane in most widespread use throughout the world is the AN 69, a polyacrylonitrile type manufactured by Hospal, France.

CAVH requires the smallest possible filter with a low inherent resistance. Table 1 reviews different membranes offered for continuous treatment methods.

Substitution Solutions

In continuous hemofiltration, the hemofiltrate is replaced completely by a substitution solution. Physiological solutions developed primarily for intermittent hemofiltration are generally used. Solutions used in peritoneal dialysis are recommended as an alternative, but their high glucose concentration leads to incomplete metabolization by the often critically ill hypermetabolic patients or requires additional insulin intake. Table 2 shows the compositions of commonly used substitution solutions. Commercial

Table 1. Different types of hemofilters/hemodialyzers for continuous forms of extractorporeal treatment

Company	Membrane material	Trade name
Hospal, France	Polyacrylonitrile (AN 69)	Multiflow Cardioflow
Amicon, USA	Polysulfone	D20, D30
Gambro, Sweden	Polyamide	FH 22, FH 66 FH 77, FH 88
Fresenius, Germany	Polysulfone	AV 400, AV 600
Asahi, Japan	Polyacrylonitrile	PAN

Table 2. Different substitution solutions for continuous extracorporeal treatment

	Lactate-buffered solution (mmol/l)	Bicarbonate-buffered sloution (mmol/l)
Sodium	135–144	140
Chloride	100–110	110
Bicarbonate	0	345
Lactate	38–44.5	3.0
Calcium	1.0–2.0	1.75
Magnesium	0.5–1.0	0.5
Glucose	0–17.5	5.6
Osmolarity	286–320	302

solutions usually contain lactate (30–45 mmol/l) as a buffer. However, negative effects on metabolic parameters, e.g., enhanced protein catabolism, and on hemodynamic parameters are ascribed to the lactate. In patients with lactacidosis and liver failure, conversion of lactate into bicarbonate is also disturbed. Bicarbonate-buffered substitution solutions are available as an alternative. The disadvantage of this solution is that owing to its limited period of stability, the bicarbonate must be supplied directly, prior to the application of the substitution solution (Table 2).

The solutions referred to above can be used with identical compositions for continuous hemodialysis. It is also possible to employ any ready-to-use commercial dialysis solution.

None of the solutions contain phosphate; to prevent phosphate impoverishment of the body, phosphate must be replaced by means of an additional dose of 1.0–2.0 mmol/l.

Anticoagulation

Continuous anticoagulation can usually be performed with conventional heparin or with low-molecular heparin. If conventional heparin is used, coagulation can generally be checked directly at the patient's bedside (anticoagulation test, ACT). Heparin doses can also be adapted to the activated thromboplastin time (double the standard value) or on the activated full blood coagulation time, which is easily determined at the bedside in the ACT. If low-molecular heparin is used, the dose must be chosen to achieve a concentration of roughly 0.3–0.6 anti-Xa units. A total of 500 units of conventional or 400 units of low-molecular heparin per hour are generally sufficient to meet these requirements.

Continuous anticoagulation thus requires a daily heparin intake which is administered to most patients as a prophylactic heparin dose. For patients at

Table 3. Anticoagulation in different forms of continuous extracorporeal treatment

Reference	Dosage	Filter running time (h)	Form of treatment
[6]	500 IU heparin/h	30	CAVH
[11]	371 IU heparin/h	32	CAVHD
[12]	500 IU heparin/h	52.5	CAVHD
[13]	500 IU heparin/h	62	CVVH
[11]	–	10	CAVHD
[14]	5–10 mg prostacyclin/kg body weight per min	14	CAVH/CVVH

CAVH, continuous arteriovenous hemofiltration; CAVHD, continuous arteriovenous hemodialysis; CVVH, continuous venovenous hemofiltration.

risk of bleeding, the heparin dose can be reduced significantly by increasing the blood flow rate to values above 150 ml/min. Table 3 shows minimum heparin doses for various continuous treatment methods [6, 11–14]. Alternatives are regional anticoagulation and, especially, the use of prostacyclin at a dosage of 5–10 ng/kg body weight per min [14]. Taking into account the side effects of prostacyclin (reduced blood pressure, tachycardia), this substance appears to be a promising alternative, especially in view of its intervention in endothelial cell- and mediator-controlled processes in MOF.

Patient Monitoring

The following checks are necessary daily, even if electronic balancing aids are used:

1. Clinical parameters
   a) Hydration status
2. Hemodynamic parameters
   a) Pulse rate
   b) Central venous blood pressure
   c) Pulmonary capillary pressure
3. Respiratory function
4. Fluid balance
5. Laboratory checks
   a) Sodium
   b) Potassium
   c) Phosphate
   d) Urea
   e) Creatinine
   f) Blood gases

Preparation of the Extracorporeal Circulation and System Checks

Prior to commencement of the treatment, the entire system is flushed with 1 l sodium solution with 5000 added units of heparin. Flushing is repeated with 1 l heparin-free NaCl solution immediately before the treatment.

During the flushing cycle, the entire system is inspected visually for leaks, especially in CAVH and CAVHD, where no additional safety devices are available. In pump-assisted methods, the automatic clamp devices and the intermediate air traps must be function checked.

A daily hemofiltrate volume of 25 l and more is desirable in CVVH to allow adequate control of azotemia. In CAVHD, a dialysate volume of 1.5–2 l/h is usually enough to ensure adequate control of substances usually eliminated in the urine. Since no other parameters are available at present, continuous extracorporeal therapy should be oriented on the urea concentration (<25 mmol/l) and/or the creatinine concentration (<300 μmol/l). Adequate compensation of renal acidosis (base excess, BE < −5) should also be achieved.

Outcome in Acute Renal Failure and Multiple Organ Failure: Influence of Continuous Treatment?

Prospective studies comparing the outcome in ARF correlated to different forms of treatment are not present. Three relevant retrospective studies compare intermittent hemodialysis with continuous treatment. Barzilay et al. [15] demonstrated a statistically significant increase in the survival rate of MOF patients treated by continuous methods as compared to conventional therapy. Surprisingly, the MOF patients with the highest chance of survival were those treated by a combined method using CAVHD and plasma separation, unfortunately not explained in greater detail. A criticism of this study is that the information on the MOF and on the patient data is very limited. For example, it is not noted whether any of the patients suffered from a renal failure or, if so, to what extent [15].

Mauritz et al. [16] compared hemodialysis, CAVH, and CVVH. This detailed study showed no statistical significance for one of the three groups in terms of their survival rate, but indicated a clear trend in favor of a higher survival rate for patients treated with pump-driven continuous filtration. In addition, the authors described a statistically higher renal recovery rate in the CVVH group.

We carried out a retrospective study comparing 73 patients treated by continuous hemofiltration from 1986 to 1988 with 73 patients treated by intermittent hemodialysis. These 73 intermittently treated patients were randomized retrospectively from a total of 243 patients, so that the group was comparable to the continuous treatment group in terms of age, sex, and number of vital function disturbances. There was a significantly lower mortality in the CVVH group: only 57 of the 73 patients died, as compared to 68 in the group of 73 dialyzed patients. In addition, there was a correlation between mortality and the number of vital function disturbances in both groups [17].

Despite the fact that in retrospective analyses continuous methods appear to reduce mortality in critically ill patients with ARF, randomized prospective studies are necessary to demonstrate clearly the benefit compared to intermittent forms of treatment.

Further Development

A number of attempts have been made to explain the advantages of continuous as opposed to intermittent hemodialysis which are apparent in retrospective analyses. One important and noncontroversial aspect is certainly the ability to provide adequate parenteral nutrition suited to the individual circumstances.

The phenomenon may also be attributable to a greater hemodynamic stability or to an increased elimination of mediator substances such as tumour necrosis factor and interleukins [8] which are involved in the progress of ARF and MOF.

In the coming years, prospective studies should therefore address the following questions:

1. Does the choice of extracorporeal therapy influence the prognosis of ARF and MOF?
2. Do extracorporeal treatment methods succeed in eliminating mediators adequately in ARF and MOF (e.g., in the hemofiltrate and/or through adsorption) and does this improve the prognosis for the patient?
3. Can changes in membrane manufacture through the development of membranes with a higher exclusion limit or enhanced adsorptive properties reduce the high mortality rate for these critically ill patients?

References

1. Kramer P, Wigger W, Rieger J, Matthai D, Scheler F (1977) Arteriovenous hemofiltration: a new and simple method for treatment of overhydrated patients resistant to diuretics. Klin Wochenschr 55:1121–1122
2. Geronemus R, Schneider N (1984) Continuous arteriovenous hemodialysis: a new modality for treatment of acute renal failure. Trans Am Soc Artif Intern Organs 30:610–613
3. Kierdorf H (1991) Continuous versus intermittent treatment: clinical results in acute renal failure. Contrib Nephrol 93:1–12
4. Paganini EP, O'Hara P, Nakamoto S (1984) Slow continous ultrafiltration in hemodialysis resistant oliguric acute renal failure patients. Trans Am Soc Artif Intern Organs 30: 173–178

5. Lauer A, Alvis R, Avram M (1988) Hemodynamic consequences of continuous arteriovenous hemofiltration. Am J Kidney Dis 12:110–115
6. Bartlett RH, Bosch J, Geronemus R, Paganini E, Ronco C, Swartz R (1988) Continuous arteriovenous hemofiltration for acute renal failure. Trans Am Soc Artif Intern Organs 34:67–77
7. Sieberth HG (1987) Dosierung von Pharmaka und Auswahl der Substitutionslösung unter kontinuierlicher Hämofiltration. In: Lawin P, Peter K, Aken HV, Prien T (eds) Intensivmedizin. Thieme, Stuttgart, pp 79–86
8. Bellomo R, Tipping P, Boyce N (1993) Continuous veno-venous hemofiltration with dialysis removes cytokines from the circulation of septic patients. Crit Care Med 21: 522–526
9. Casati S, Moia M, Graziani G, Cantaluppi A, Citterio A, Mannucci PM, Ponticelli C (1984) Hemodialysis without anticoagulants: efficiency and hemostatic aspects. Clin Nephrol 21:102–105.
10. Schultheis R, Brings W, Glöckner WM, Sieberth HG (1985) Device for controlled cylic substitution during spontaneous filtration. In: Sieberth HG, Mann H (eds) Continuous arteriovenous hemofiltration. Karger, Basel, pp 64–66
11. Geronemus RP (1988) Slow continuous hemodialyisis. Trans Am Soc Artif Intern Organs 34:59–60
12. Van Geelen JA, Vincent HH, Schalekamp MADH (1988) Continuous arteriovenous hemofiltration and hemodiafiltration in acute renal failure. Nephrol Dial Transplant 2:181–186
13. Canaud G, Carred LJ, Christol JP, Aubas S, Beraud JJ, Mion C (1988) Pump-assisted continuous venovenous hemofiltration for treating acute uremia. Kidney Int 33 Suppl 24: 154–156
14. Zobel G, Ring E, Müller W (1989) Continuous arteriovenous hemofiltration in premature infants. Crit Care Med 17:534–536
15. Barzilay E, Berlot G, Kessler D, Geber D (1989) More on acute renal failure in the intensive care unit. Intensive Care Med 15:478–481
16. Mauritz W, Sporn P, Schindler I, Zadrobilek E, Roth E, Appel W (1986) Acute renal failure in abdominal infection: comparison of hemodialysis and continuous arteriovenous hemofiltration. Anasth Intensivther Nofallmed 21:212–217
17. Kierdorf H, Riehl J, Heintz B, Taya I, Sieberth HG (1992) Mortality in acute renal failure: continuous venovenous hemofiltration compared to intermittent hemodialysis. Blood Purif Perspect 2:301–305

Blood Purification by Hemofiltration in Septic Shock and Multiple Organ Dysfunction Syndrome Patients

A.F. Grootendorst and J.L.C.M. van Saase

Introduction

In 1984 and 1986 Gotloib et al. [1, 2] published their positive experiences with intermittent hemofiltration in multiple organ dysfunction syndrome (MODS) patients. The concept of blood purification by hemofiltration was received with a lot of scepticism, but nonetheless stimulated several research groups to analyze retrospective data and to perform prospective studies on this topic. Besides these clinical studies, a small number of animal experimental studies have been performed. Undoubtedly, the high expectations with which the studies on the administration of monoclonal antibodies were welcomed as the therapy of the future diminished interest in the less prestigious hemofiltration studies in MODS patients and animal models. It now seems reasonable to say that the use of monoclonals is promising and fascinating, but at the same time expensive and as yet of unproven value. The same holds for hemofiltration in this context; nonetheless, several centers have experience with this technique and use it routinely in therapy-resistant septic and cardiogenic shock. This chapter will describe the rationale for hemofiltration in shock and present an overview of the clinical and experimental studies performed so far; moreover, the limitations of the studies so far and ideas about future research will be discussed.

Rationale for Hemofiltration in Septic Shock and Multiple Organ Dysfunction Syndrome

Both septic shock and MODS are considered to result from an overreaction of the immune system, leading to a state in which the body can no longer control its own inflammatory response to several stimuli [3–6]; this response may not only be provoked by gram-negative bacteria and endotoxins, but also by gram-positive bacteria, viruses, multiple blood transfusions, splanchnic ischemia, and multitrauma.

Figure 1 schematically shows the sequence of events that are thought to lead to septic shock and MODS. Conventional therapies are aimed at killing the bacteria, increasing blood pressure, and providing optimal support to improve or replace the function of failing organs. Except for antibiotic

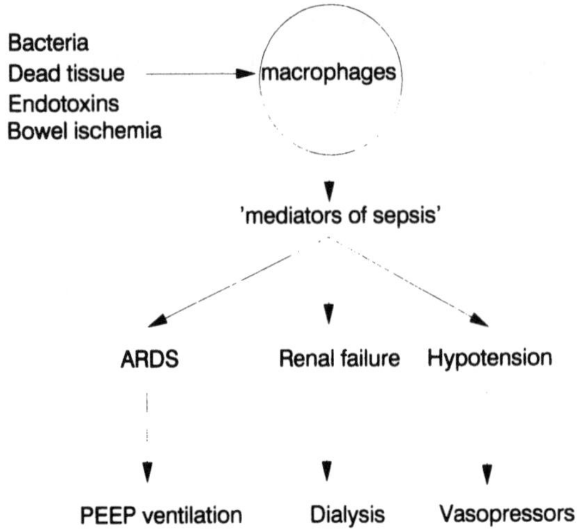

Fig. 1. Development of multiple organ dysfunction syndrome and the point at which traditional therapies influence the disease process. *ARDS*, adult respiratory distress syndrome; *PEEP*, posivitive end expiratory pressure

therapy, these therapies do not interfere with the uncontrolled response itself and therefore are only buying time for the patient to cure himself. Thus it is not surprising that mortality of septic shock and MODS patients remains alarmingly high, in spite of the huge costs and efforts that are associated with the treatment of these patients [7–9]. Newer ventilatory techniques, antibiotics, and renal replacement therapies are unlikely to further improve outcome in this group of patients. Theoretically, there are two possible ways to interrupt the complex sequence of events that leads to septic shock and MODS: one involves the removal or inactivation of proinflammatory substances – tumor necrosis factor-α (TNF-α) etc. – the other to add anti-inflammatory substances (e.g., interleukin (IL)-10, indomethacin). Inactivation of only one of the many proinflammatory substances by the administration of monoclonal antibodies has not been proven successful so far; nor has the combined administration of anti-endotoxin, anti-TNF monoclonals, and IL-1 receptor antagonists [10, 11]. Another possibility is the removal of multiple proinflammatory substances at the same time by hemofiltration in order to counteract the overstimulation of the uncontrolled immune response that is associated with septic shock and MODS. Gotloib et al. [2] recognized that many factors play a role in the clinical picture; some of these factors were shown to be present in the ultrafiltrate (UF) of MODS patients. Based on the molecular weight of these mediators, they hypothesized that they could be removed by hemofiltration and indeed were able to demonstrate their presence in the UF. At the same time, they showed improvement of hemodynamics and gas exchange in MODS patients during the hemofiltration treatment, along with a remarkably high survival in their group of MODS patients (22 of the 24 patients survived) [1, 2]. These findings raise the question whether the positive effects of hemofiltration result from convective removal of mediators or from their binding to the filter. If convective removal is the most important mechanism, the UF volume may be important and high UF volumes may be needed to achieve clinically relevant results; if binding to the filter membrane is a second important way to remove proinflammatory substances from the circulation, the choice of the filter may play an equally important role. These aspects will be addressed in the last part of this chapter.

Clinical Studies on the Effect of Hemofiltration in Septic Shock and Multiple Organ Dysfunction Syndrome Patients

Available Hemofiltration Techniques

Since the introduction of continuous arteriovenous hemofiltration (CAVH) by Kramer et al. [12], this technique has become accepted as the treatment of choice for intensive care unit (ICU) patients with acute renal failure (ARF), since it induces less hemodynamic instability than intermittent hemodialysis. Because the efficacy of CAVH is limited by its low clearance and the ultrafiltrate volume is dependent on blood pressure, metabolic control in highly catabolic patients is often difficult to achieve. Two variants of CAVH have been developed to overcome this limitation of CAVH: one comprises the addition of a diffusive component to CAVH, creating continuous arteriovenous hemodiafiltration (CAVHD) [13], the other the insertion of a pump into the arterial line, so that filter flow and ultrafiltrate volume become independent of the patient's own blood pressure, creating pumped continuous arteriovenous hemofiltration. In the latter case, a double-lumen venous catheter can replace the arterial and venous canula, creating continuous venovenous hemofiltration.

Effects of the Hemofiltration Mode on Clinical Variables

The development of ARF in ICU patients carries a poor prognosis. Initially, efforts to improve the prognosis of these patients focused on improved metabolic control, for instance by a combination of continuous and daily hemodialysis techniques. Although improved metabolic control can be achieved by this combination, survival was not affected in ARF patients [14]. Obviously, the quality of metabolic control that is achieved by continuous hemofiltration techniques will depend on the UF volume. Many clinical studies have reported mortality in ARF patients treated with one of the continuous hemofiltration techniques. A selection of these studies is shown in Table 1. In general, comparison of these studies is difficult

Table 1. Mortality rate of intensive care patients treated with hemofiltration

Author and reference	Hemofiltration mode	UF volume (l/day)/ dialysate (l/day)	Patients (*n*)	Indication for hemofiltration	Mortality (%)
Weiss et al. [15]	CAVH	12	100	MODS	55
Kramer et al. [16]	CAVH	9.6	14	ARF	64
Wendon et al. [17]	CVVH	15.2–40.8	28	ARF	46
Bellomo et al. [18]	CAVHD	n.a./19–38	12	ARF	58
Voerman et al. [19]	CAVHD	1.1–5.7/38.4	17	ARF	70
Sieberth and Kierdorf [20]	CVVH	10.7 ± 7.2 (nonsurvivors) 17.8 ± 4.9 (survivors)	79	ARF	54
Stevens et al. [21]	CAVHD	n.a./24–48	36	ARF	69
Storck et al. [22]	CAVH	6.6–7.4	48	ARF	87
	PDHF	13.6–17.8	68	ARF	68
Mauritz et al. [23]	CAVH	10.1 ± 4.6	9	ARF	89
	PDHF	25.9 ± 6.1	27	ARF	70
Macias et al. [24]	CVVH	21 ± 7.2	25	ARF	84
Klehr et al. [25]	CAVH	8.9 ± 6.3	182	ARF	78

CAVH, continuous arteriovenous hemofiltration; CVVH, continuous venovenous hemofiltration; CAVHD, continuous arteriovenous hemodiafiltration; PDHF, pump-driven hemofiltration; UF, ultrafiltrate; MODS, multiple organ dysfunction syndrome; ARF, acute renal failure; n.a., data not available.

Table 2. Effects of hemofiltration on clinical variables and inflammatory mediators in intensive care patients

Author and reference	Hemofiltration mode	Patients (n)	Indication for hemofiltration	Clinical results	Mediators
Journois et al. [26]	CAVHD/PDHF	17	ARF	Positive correlation UF volume recovery of renal function	
Gotloib et al. [2]	IHF	24	ARDS	88% survival, pH ↑ PaO_2 ↑, Qs/Qt ↓	Sieving coefficient >0.88 for PGE_2, TxB_2, beta-endorphin
Coraim et al. [27]	CAVH	36	ARDS	CI ↑, PaO_2 ↑, DO_2 ↑	[MDS] ↓, MDS in UF
Coraim et al. [28]	CAVH	29	Refractory cardiogenic shock	SVR ↑, CI ↑, MAP ↑	[MDS] ↓, MDS in UF
Garzia et al. [29]	CAVHD	14	ARDS	CI ↑, MPAP ↓, PEEP ↓ FiO_2 ↓	
Hirasawa et al. [30]	CAVH(D)	43	MSOF		Sieving coefficient C3a 0.77, TNFα 0.52
Bellomo et al. [31]	CVVHD	12	MSOF		Significant TNFα excretion in UF
Staubach et al. [32]	CAVH	66	Refractory septic or cardiogenic shock	MAP ↑, CO ↑, PaO_2 ↑	[TxB_2] ↓, TxB_2 in UF [6ketoPGF] ↓, 6ketoPGF in UF
Mauritz et al. [33]	CAVH/CVVH	36	ARF in abdominal sepsis	Positive correlation UF volume recovery of renal function	

CAVHD, continuous arteriovenous hemodiafiltration; PDHF, pump-driven hemofiltration; CVVHD, continuous venovenous hemodiafiltration; CVVH, continuous venovenous hemofiltration; ARF, acute renal failure; UF, ultrafiltrate; IHF, intermittent hemofiltration; CAVH, continuous arteriovenous hemofiltration; ARDS, adult respiratory distress syndrome; MSOF, multiple system organ failure; Qs/Qt, pulmonary shunt fraction; MAP, mean arterial pressure; CI, cardiac index; PaO_2, arterial PO_2; DO_2, oxygen transport; SVR, systemic vascular resistance; MDS, myocardial depressant factor; UF, ultrafiltrate; PGE_2, prostaglandin E_2; TxB_2, thromboxane B_2; 6keto PGF, 6-keto-prostaglandin; [ ], serum concentration; TNF-α, tumor necrosis factor-α.

because no severity score of the patients is available, the fluid balance is not mentioned, the filters that are used differ, or filter and UF flows are not mentioned. Although CAVHD can be expected to be associated with better metabolic control than CAVH, mortality in CAVHD-treated patients does not seem to differ from that in CAVH-treated patients. Some authors, however, suggest a correlation between UF volume and survival, while others fail to show this relation. Importantly, in all these studies renal replacement was started after ARF development. It may well be that *irreversible* organ damage is present in these later stages of MODS and that the choice of renal replacement therapy no longer affects outcome. The question therefore arises whether hemofiltration techniques should be used earlier in the disease, as a means to remove mediators of sepsis. This would require the early start of hemofiltration treatment in ICU patients without ARF. A summary of clinical studies on the effects of hemofiltration in non-ARF patients is given in Table 2. As can be seen from this table, hemofiltration can improve cardiac performance, gas exchange, and possibly accelerate recovery of renal function in selected patients, possibly by convective removal of mediators of sepsis into the UF. This may imply that hemofiltration techniques with high UF volume are more effective in these patients, as larger amounts of mediators of sepsis are removed into the UF.

Effects of Hemofiltration in Experimental Shock

Several studies have evaluated the effect of hemofiltration on hemodynamic variables of experimental shock in animals. The studies differ in species, the way shock was induced, UF volume, and the hemofilter that was used, making comparison difficult. Gomez et al. [34] showed that hemofiltration can remove factors responsible for reduced left ventricular contractility in dogs with *Escherichia coli* shock. Stein et al. [35, 36] showed that low-volume, zero-balanced CAVH (UF flow, 0.6 l/h) slightly improved both cardiac output and lung mechanics in pigs with endotoxic shock. In a similar model, Grootendorst et al. [37, 38] studied the effect of high-volume, zero-balanced hemofiltration (UF flow, 6.0 l/h) on global hemodynamics and right ventricular ejection fraction. In addition, they studied the potential effects of binding of mediators of sepsis to the filter membrane by including a group that was hemofiltered while clamping the UF line. They concluded that high-volume hemofiltration markedly improved global hemodynamics and right ventricular ejection fraction, while the filter itself had a negative effect on these variables. This suggests that the net positive effect of hemofiltration results from the negative hemodynamic effects of the hemofilter itself and the positive effects of convective removal of the responsible substances. This may also explain why the positive hemodynamic effects in Stein's study were less pronounced than in the study of Grootendorst et al. To further test the hypothesis that the positive effects of

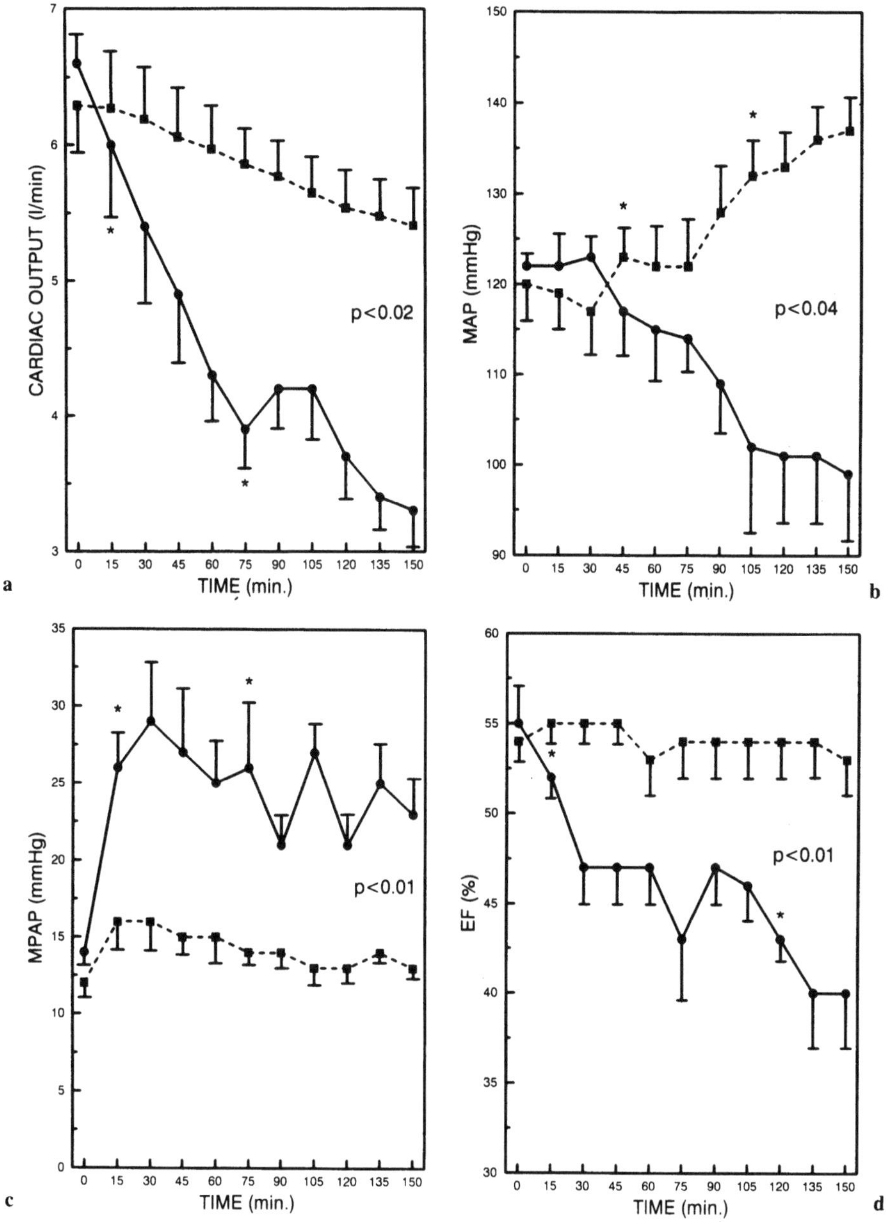

Fig. 2a–d. Course of cardiac output (**a**), mean arterial pressure (*MAP*; **b**), mean pulmonary artery pressure (*MPAP*; **c**), and right ventricular ejection fraction (*EF*; **d**), after the infusion of 2 l ultrafiltrate from endotoxic shock pigs (*closed circles*, $n = 6$) or healthy pigs (*closed squares*, $n = 6$). The mean ± SEM values are shown. The *p* value results from the overall test of profiles. *Occurrence of a new significant difference between groups ($p < 0.05$), using the antedependence method. (From [39], with permission)

hemofiltration result from convective removal of substances responsible for the hemodynamic effects of endotoxin infusion, Grootendorst et al. [39] infused UF from endotoxic shock pigs into healthy pigs and compared their hemodynamics to those of pigs infused with UF from healthy donor pigs. The results are shown in Fig. 2 and demonstrate that UF from endotoxic shock pigs contains factors that increase pulmonary artery pressures and have a negative hemodynamic effect. Recently, Lee et al. [40] showed that the reduction in performance after *Staphylococcus aureus* sepsis in pigs can partially be reversed by hemofiltration as well; the infusion of UF from these pigs into healthy pigs was shown to reduce their cardiac output. Limitations in the extrapolation of these experimental data to the clinical setting are caused by differences in species, different mechanisms of human septic shock and animal experimental shock, and the question whether the short-term hemodynamic effects that were observed correlate to long-term effect and survival. To meet some of these limitations of the experimental studies so far, Grootendorst et al. [41] induced shock in pigs by inducing bowel ischemia and subsequent reperfusion in the pig. In this model it was also shown that intermittent, high-volume hemofiltration not only improves short-term hemodynamics, but also reduces bowel damage and improved 24-h survival. Further animal studies are seriously impaired by the fact that no assays for most mediators of sepsis of animals are available.

Future of Hemofiltration in Septic Shock and Multiple Organ Dysfunction Syndrome Patients

In spite of all the experimental work and the patient series published so far, the removal of proinflammatory mediators by hemofiltration is still experimental in the treatment of septic shock and MODS patients. Once these patients have developed ARF, mortality remains high in spite of hemofiltration, though several studies indicate that high-volume hemofiltration is associated with lower mortality and more rapid recovery of renal function than low-volume hemofiltration. This may indicate that the high volumes used in these studies are not high enough to reduce the load of mediators of sepsis; in that case, higher UF volumes (100 l/day) or even higher might be necessary to achieve adequate reduction in the level of these mediators. The other possibility is that once the patients have developed ARF, structural (as opposed to functional) and irreversible changes have developed in several organs, making recovery impossible. This raises the question whether HF should be started earlier, before ARF has developed. It is unfeasible to start HF in all patients at risk for MODS, because many patients would have to be treated who would make an uneventful recovery anyway. In several Dutch hospitals high-volume hemofiltration is started in patients with therapy-resistant septic or cardiogenic shock. In the majority of these patients, a substantial improvement in gas exchange and

Table 3. Concentrations of tumor necrosis factor (TNF)-α and interleukin (IL)-6 in serum and ultrafiltrate (UF) of two patients before and after 4-h high-volume hemofiltration (HF)

	Before HF in serum	After 4 h HF	
		Serum	UF
Patient 1 (PAN filter)			
TNFα (pg/ml)	322	146	44
IL-6 (pg/ml)	1535	532	699
Patient 2 (polyamide) filter			
IL-6 (pg/ml)	1603	1598	22

Ultrafiltrate flow, 6 l/h.
PAN, polyacrylonitrile.

hemodynamics is observed within hours after the start of hemofiltration, while the amount of inotropic drugs and vasopressors can be reduced drastically. Table 3 shows data from a 32-year-old woman who was transferred to our hospital with therapy-resistant septic shock, secondary to Beta-hemolytic *Streptococcus* infection of the right arm. During necrotectomy she was reanimated twice because of cardiac arrest. Within 4 h after starting HF, gas exchange and hemodynamics strongly improved, vasopressors were discontinued, and inotropic drugs were reduced. After 3 days hemofiltration was discontinued as well; the patient was extubated and made an uneventful recovery within 2 weeks. The problem with these experiences is that they are impressive but do not prove anything. The use of hemofiltration in cardiogenic shock may seem even more obscure. As early as 1986, hemofiltration was described to improve hemodynamics and gas exchange of patients on cardiopulmonary bypass. Endotoxins, originating from the bowel, can frequently be demonstrated in these patients; in addition, myocardial depressant factors were shown to be reduced by this treatment, although the nature of these substances is subject to much debate. Experimental data show that reductions in cardiac output lead to disproportionally large reductions in splanchnic flow; the resultant bowel ischemia not only leads to the translocation of endotoxins, but also to the release of factors that have a negative effect on cardiac performance. Recent experimental work shows that the reduction in cardiac performance, caused by bowel ischemia and reperfusion, can be significantly diminished by high-volume hemofiltration. Possibly, the positive effect of HF in cardiogenic shock patients can be explained in this way.

Choice of Filter

Many filter materials (polyamide, polyacrylonitrile, polysulphon) and filter structures (hollow fiber, multilayer flat plate) are available today. The membranes have been optimized for chronic renal failure patients, but hardly any data are available on the capability of hemofilters to remove proinflammatory mediators from the circulation by either binding to the filter membrane or convective removal into the ultrafiltrate. Table 3 shows that the polyacrylonitrile filter reduces TNF-α levels, while little TNF-α can be shown in the UF. In contrast, interleukin (IL)-6 levels are reduced by removal into the UF. It also shows that IL-6 is cleared much more effectively by the polyacrylonitrile filter than by the polyamide filter. Apparently, mediators differ in their behavior during hemofiltration. Filters that seem to be equally effective in chronic renal failure patients differ in septic shock patients. Possibly, different mediators need different filters for optimal clearance. This shows that several questions have to be solved to further develop the concept of blood purification by hemofiltration in sepsis: the mediators that have to be removed need to be identified, their quantity assessed, and the filter and/or UF flow chosen accordingly. Remarkably, very few data are available today on the mediator profile of patients in the later stages of sepsis and MODS. It is unknown whether these profiles differ from patient to patient or whether uniform patterns exist. If the profiles differ markedly, rapid assays will be needed to optimize the HF treatment; if uniform patterns emerge, standard treatments may be defined. In either case, we need much more knowledge on the ability of hemofilters to clear mediators of sepsis.

Practical Aspects of High-Volume Hemofiltration in Septic Shock and Multiple Organ Dysfunction Syndrome

The evaluation of hemofiltration in septic shock and MODS patients is hindered by the fact that few intensive care clinicians have experience with high-volume hemofiltration, while high UF volumes may be required to achieve clinically relevant results. In addition, few clinicians are willing to use hemofiltration in the absence of ARF. Evaluation of hemofiltration is further made difficult by our incomplete understanding of the interaction between mediators of sepsis and MODS; MODS cannot simply be considered as an excess of mediators, as some mediators (for instance IL-4 and IL-13) have anti-inflammatory properties and their removal might in fact harm the patient. The absence of rapid assays for some of these mediators makes it difficult to select patients that might benefit from hemofiltration and to monitor the response of the hemofiltration treatment. The choice of the optimal filter is important, as filters differ in their capacity to bind or remove mediators via the UF. The practical consequence may be that a patient with septic shock and high TNF-α levels will benefit most from filter A, while later in the disease the patient needs filter B, as IL-6 levels are elevated and TNF-α levels have returned to normal levels. All these uncertainties might lead us to the conclusion that it is too early to use high-volume hemofiltration in septic patients; however, most of the current therapies in septic patients are incompletely understood, often fail to work or treat symptoms, and have not been shown to reduce mortality. Several inotropic drugs have been registered on the evidence that they improve cardiac output or blood pressure in septic shock patients. If hemofiltration in acute septic shock were judged as a drug, it would probably be registered. Unfortunately, most new therapies are judged by their capability to improve survival, in contrast to almost any currently available therapy, none of which has been shown to improve survival. Yet we know that thanks to these therapies, ICU outcome has improved over the years, although reliable data is lacking.

Given the available animal data and clinical experience, it seems to be the right time for prospective clinical trials on the hemodynamic and outcome effects of high-volume hemofiltration in high-risk ICU patients with therapy-resistant septic shock and early MODS. Further research is needed to identify the mediator profile of different phases of septic shock and MODS patients, from the first day of their disease on, so that the optimal hemofiltration volume and the optimal hemofilter can be chosen. These results could also direct the producers of filter membranes to modify membranes in such a way that optimal removal of specific mediators can be achieved. Based on the results of the studies so far, it seems important that high UF volumes are used in these studies and that serial measurements of mediators of sepsis are performed in serum, UF, and the filter membrane surface.

The use of hemofiltration in ICU patients poses logistic problems, especially when high-volume, continuous hemofiltration is used. In CVVH, three pumps (blood flow, UF flow, and substitution fluid flow) are interlinked and require continuous monitoring. As the continuous presence of a renal unit nurse in the ICU is unfeasible, monitoring of the treatment will partially have to be performed by ICU nurses. In four centers in the Netherlands, high-volume CVVH (100 l UF/day) has been implemented in this way successfully. In all these centers a CVVH device (Sartorius, Boebingen, Germany) is used; for ICU nurses these CVVH machines are easier to monitor than the more complicated all-round dialysis apparatus that are used in renal units. The knowledge and skills of nephrologists and renal nurses are a prerequisite for safe and successful hemofiltration treatment in ICU patients; with close cooperation between nephrologists and intensive care specialists, high-volume CVVH can be performed safely in ICU patients.

References

1. Gotloib L, Barzilay E, Shustak A et al. (1984) Sequential hemofiltration in non-oliguric high capillary permeability pulmonary edema of severe sepsis. Crit Care Med 12:997–1000
2. Gotloib L, Barzilay E, Shustak A et al. (1986) Hemofiltration in septic ARDS. The artificial kidney as an artificial lung. Resuscitation 13:123–132
3. Shoemaker WC (1987) Circulatory mechanisms of shock and their mediators. Crit Care Med 15:787–794
4. Bone RC (1991) The pathogenesis of sepsis. Ann Intern Med 115:457–469
5. Rackow EC, Astiz ME (1991) Pathophysiology and treatment of septic shock. JAMA 266:548–554
6. Fiddian-Green RG (1989) Studies in splanchnic ischemia and multiple organ failure. In: Marston A, Bulkley GB, Fiddian-Green RG et al. (eds) Splanchnic ischemia and multiple organ failure. Arnold, London, pp 349–363
7. Pine RW, Wertz MJ, Lennard ES et al. (1983) Determinants of organ malfunction or death in patients with intra-abdominal sepsis. A discriminant analysis. Arch Surg 118:242–249
8. Knauss WA, Wagner DP (1989) MSOF: epidemiology and prognosis. Crit Care Clin 5:221–226
9. Knauss WA, Draper EA, Wagner DP et al. (1985) APACHE II: a severity of disease classification system. Crit Care Med 13:818–823
10. Hoffman WD, Natanson C (1993) The role of endotoxin in bacterial septic shock. In: Vincent JL (ed) Yearbook of intensive care and emergency medicine 1993. Springer, Berlin Heidelberg New York, pp 49–63
11. Fisher C (1992) Clinical trials of immunotherapy for sepsis. Crit Care Med 20:721–723
12. Kramer P, Wigger P, Reiger J et al. (1977) Arteriovenous hemofiltration: a new and simple method for treatment of overhydrated patients resistant to diuretics. Klin Wochenschr 55:1121–1122
13. Geronemus R, Schneider N (1984) Continuous arteriovenous haemodialysis: a new treatment modality for acute renal failure. ASAIO Trans 30:610–613
14. Simpson HK, Allison ME, Telfer AB (1987) Improving the prognosis in acute renal and respiratory failure. Ren Fail 10:45–54
15. Weiss L, Danielson BG, Wikstrom B et al. (1987) Continuous arteriovenous hemofiltration in the treatment of 100 critically ill patients with acute renal failure: report on clinically outcome and nutritional aspects. Clin Nephrol 31:184–189
16. Kramer P, Kaufhold G, Grone HJ (1980) Management of anuric intensive care patients with arteriovenous hemofiltration. Int J Artif Organs 3:225–230
17. Wendon J, Smithies M, Sheppard M et al. (1989) Continuous high volume veno-venous hemofiltration in acute renal failure. Intensive Care Med 15:358–363
18. Bellomo R, Ernest D, Love J et al. (1990) Continuous arteriovenous hemodiafiltration: optimal therapy for acute renal failure in an intensive care setting? Aust N Z J Med 20:237–242
19. Voerman HJ, Strack van Schijndel RJM, Thijs LG (1990) Continuous arteriovenous hemodiafiltration in critically ill patients. Crit Care Med 18:911–914
20. Sieberth HG, Kierdorf H (1989) Is continuous hemofiltration superior to intermittent dialysis and hemofiltration treatment? Adv Exp Med Biol 260:181–192
21. Stevens PE, Davies SP, Brown EA et al. (1988) Continuous arteriovenous haemodialysis in critically ill patients. Lancet 2:150–152
22. Storck M, Harte WH, Zimmerer E et al. (1990) Comparison of pump-driven and spontaneous continuous hemofiltration in postoperative acute renal failure. Lancet 337:452–455
23. Mauritz W, Sporn P, Schindler I et al. (1986) Acute renal failure in abdominal infection. Comparison of haemodialysis and continuous arteriovenous hemofiltration. Anasth Intensivther Notfallmed 21:212–217

24. Macias WL, Mueller BA, Scarim SK et al. (1991) Continuous venovenous hemofiltration: an alternative to continuous arteriovenous hemofiltration and hemodiafiltration in acute renal failure. Am J Kidney Dis 18:451–458
25. Klehr HU, Kaschell HJ, Kuckenbecker CH et al. (1985) Clinical results of continuous arteriovenous hemofiltration. In: Sieberth HG, Mann H (eds) Continuous arteriovenous hemofiltration. Karger, Basel, pp 159–165
26. Journois D, Chanu D, Safran D (1991) Pump-driven hemofiltration (Letter). Lancet 1:985
27. Coraim FJ, Coraim HP, Ebermann R et al. (1986) Acute respiratory failure after cardiac surgery: clinical experience with the application of continuous arteriovenous hemofiltration. Crit Care Med 14:714–718
28. Coraim F, Pauser G, Stellwag F et al. (1985) Positive modification of hemodynamics in postcardiac surgery patients by hemofiltration. Improved method for the demonstration of myocardial depressant factor in hemofiltrate. Anaesthesist 34:236–240
29. Garzia F, Todor R, Scalea T (1991) Continuous arteriovenous hemofiltration-counter current dialysis in acute respiratory failure. J Trauma 31:1277–1285
30. Hirasawa H, Sugai T, Ohtake Y et al. (1991) Continuous hemofiltration and hemodiafiltration in the management of multiple organ failure. Contrib Nephrol 93:42–46
31. Bellomo R, Tipping P, Boyce N (1991) Tumor necrosis factor clearances during continuous veno-venous hemodiafiltration. ASAIO Trans 37:322–323
32. Staubach KH, Rau HG, Hohlbach G et al. (1987) Continuous arteriovenous hemofiltration in shock: a new strategy to lower eicosanoids. Artif Organs 11:A336
33. Mauritz W, Sporn P, Schendler I et al. (1986) Acute renal failure in abdominal infection. Comparison of haemodialysis and continuous arteriovenous hemofiltration. Anasth Intensivther Notfallmed 21:212–217
34. Gomez A, Wang R, Unruh H et al. (1990) Hemofiltration reverses left ventricular dysfunction during sepsis in dogs. Anesthesiology 73:671–685
35. Stein B, Pfenninger E, Grunert A et al. (1990) Influence of continuous hemofiltration on hemodynamics and central blood volume in experimental endotoxic shock. Intensive Care Med 16:494–499
36. Stein B, Pfenninger E, Grunert A et al. (1991) The consequences of continuous hemofiltration on lung mechanics and extravascular lung water in a porcine endotoxic shock model. Intensive Care Med 17:293–298
37. Grootendorst AF, van Bommel EFH, van Leengoed LAMG et al. (1994) High volume hemofiltration improves hemodynamics and survival of pigs exposed to gut ischemia and reperfusion. Shock 1:1–8
38. Grootendorst AF, van Bommel EFH, van der Hoven B et al. (1992) High volume hemofiltration improves right ventricular function of endotoxin induced shock in the pig. Intensive Care Med 18:235–240
39. Grootendorst AF, van Bommel EFH, van Leengoed LAMG et al. (1993) Infusion of ultrafiltrate from endotoxemic pigs depresses myocardial performance in normal pigs. J Crit Care 8:161–169
40. Lee PA, Matson JR, Pryor RW et al. (1993) Continuous arteriovenous hemofiltration therapy for Staphylococcus aureus induced septicemia in immature swine. Crit Care Med 21:914–924
41. Grootendorst AF, van Bommel EFH, van Leengoed LAMG et al. (1994) High volume hemofiltration improves hemodynamics and survival of pigs exposed to bowel ischemia and reperfusion. Shock 1(5):1–8

Nutrition in Acute Renal Failure

R. Bellomo

Introduction and Historical Background

The therapy of patients with acute renal failure (ARF) has undergone major changes over the last 30 years, and these changes have also profoundly affected its nutritional management. In the following chapter these changes will be reviewed and a modern approach to nutrition in critically ill patients with ARF will be discussed. The clinical and laboratory research underpinning the concept of a more aggressive nutritional approach in these patients will also be reviewed in an attempt to provide a full understanding of its rationale.

The major nutritional concern for physicians treating ARF in the predialysis era was directed at avoiding uncontrolled uremia. Nutrition, therefore, consisted mainly of basic caloric support (up to 800 kCal/day) and a protein-free diet [1, 2]. This approach was based on nutritional data on the protein-sparing effects of small amounts of carbohydrates when administered to fasting volunteers [3]. Later, the concept of a chronic renal failure diet containing a small amount of protein directed at meeting the essential amino acid requirements of the average young adult was developed. This dietary approach was subsequently taken up for the nutritional therapy of ARF patients [4].

The advent of more easily available hemodialysis facilities translated into easier control of uremia and increased administration of nutrients [5, 6]. The simultaneous development of modern techniques of intravenous alimentation led to their progressive application to patients with ARF. In the late 1960s and early 1970s a number of clinical reports began to highlight the benefits of adequate caloric support and greater protein supplementation [7, 8]. Such reports led to the performance of a widely quoted clinical study by Abel and coworkers in 1973 [9]. This study showed that the addition of essential amino acids (approximately 16 g/day) to the diet of patients with ARF was associated with a greater rate of recovery and survival, particulary in the most critically ill patients. Other subsequent studies have supported the use of amino acids in ARF patients [10–12], leaving it unclear, however, what the role of essential versus nonessential amino acids should be and whether such therapy did in fact reduce mortality. Such studies went hand in hand with a change in the epidemiology of ARF, with close to 50% of cases now being seen in the intensive care unit (ICU). They also took the debate into the last decade, a decade which has seen important changes in the style of renal replacement therapy and the severity of illness seen in the ICU. In order to take the issue of nutrition and ARF further, one needs to first consider some basic clinical nutritional concepts as they more broadly affect critically ill patients in general.

Nutrition in the Critically Ill

As the ARF of critical illness becomes more frequent, all major nutritional issues that apply to critically ill patients are pertinent to its management.

The first important issue is whether critically ill patients should be fed at all. The evidence is close to overwhelming that they should [13–26] and will not be discussed further.

The second important issue concerns the amount of calories that should be administered to critically ill patients. The issue is not easily resolved. A reasonable principle should be that caloric administration should match energy expenditure. This, however, is not so easily achieved because of problems inherent to the accurate measurement of energy expenditure in such patients [27]. For this reason, a number of formulae have been developed to easily calculate such expenditure with a clinically acceptable degree of accuracy [28]. Many clinicians, however, prefer to administer a fixed caloric regimen of 30–35 kCal/kg per day as this represents a very easily calculated amount which seems to achieve a reasonable degree of approximation. At this stage, despite documented differences between calculated and measured energy expenditure [29, 30], it appears unlikely that randomized controlled studies will demonstrate major benefits of caloric therapy based on indirect calorimetry versus therapy based on knowledgeable approximation.

Having achieved broad agreement on energy replacement, a third important issue pertains to the composition (lipids versus carbohydrates) of the nonprotein component of the diet. Once again, there are no controlled randomized trials to provide us with an answer. Current evidence, however, indicates that, in sepsis, there is a shift in fuel preference to lipids [31–34]. This information gained from experimental and human studies has led to a progressive increase in the use of intravenous lipid emulsions and to the common prescription of ICU nutritional regimens with a 1:1 ratio of lipid- and carbohydrate-derived calories. Despite experimental evidence suggesting that hepatic steatosis may be associated with high intravenous carbohydrate intake [35], very few clinicians administer most of their calories in the form of lipids. These general statements, of course, have exceptions in patients who develop hypertriglyceridemia requiring a switch to a predominantly glucose-based nutrition or patients who have high ventilatory requirements and are marginal candidates for weaning from the ventilator, therefore requiring a switch to lipids in order to diminish CO_2 production.

There is now broad agreement that nitrogen administration is necessary and beneficial in critically ill patients [36–39]. What remains unclear is how much nitrogen constitutes optimal therapy [40] and how caloric requirements may affect protein nitrogen requirements [41]. Presently available evidence [36] suggests that in healthy adults at least 1 g protein/day is needed and that, as the severity of illness increases, the need for nitrogen replacement also increases [40]. Furthermore, in acutely ill patients, the administration of increasing amounts of protein nitrogen is associated with a major progressive reduction in the amino acid release from muscle commonly seen in this situation. This reduction continues as nitrogen administration reaches up to 400 mg/kg per day (Fig. 1). In patients with major burns, the administration of large amounts of protein (>2.5 g/kg per day) has been shown to achieve a sufficient effect on protein synthesis and catabolism which could not be improved by the addition of carbohydrates. It remains, however, unclear whether increasing protein administration to these levels in other critically ill patients would have a clinically meaningful beneficial impact.

There is even more uncertainty in the field of mineral and vitamin therapy during critical illness. While the effects of zinc or selenium deficiency are well known [42–44], as are those of vitamin deficiency, there is little information on the requirements for these factors during critical illness.

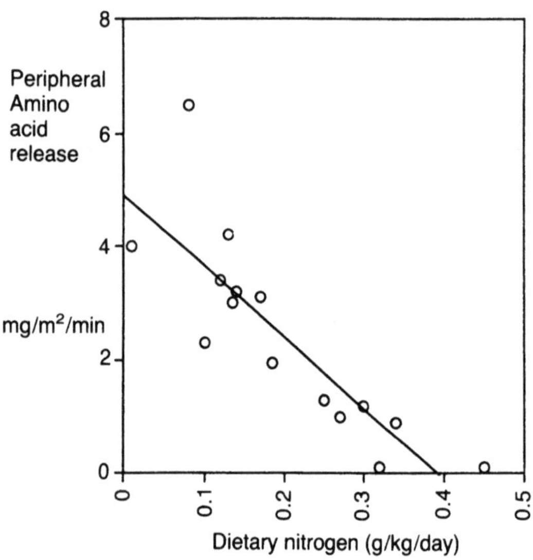

Fig. 1. Consequences of the administration of increasing amounts of nitrogen on amino acid release from muscle in acutely ill patients. As can be see, a progressive increase in protein nitrogen administration is associated with a progressive fall in amino acid release from muscle. (Modified from data in [141])

As a consequence, it is generally recommended that daily allowances be administered and, in some cases, be increased under these circumstances [45]. Once a decision has been made on the caloric amount, the protein content, the lipid to carbohydrate ratio, and the mineral and vitamin content of the diet, the next major decision concerns the route of administration of the planned diet. The general consensus is that the enteral route is both physiologically superior and safer [46, 47]. Enteral alimentation may also have other important advantages over parenteral nutrition such as better protection of the gastrointestinal mucosa and diminished bacterial translocation [48, 49]. Many critically ill patients, however, have had recent abdominal surgery and have impaired gastrointestinal motility; under these circumstances, a number of clinicians choose the parenteral route because of its easy implementation and control. Furthermore, the pursuit of enteral feeding in an aggressive fashion requires insertion of a feeding tube beyond the pyloric sphincter, a time-consuming procedure and, once again, one with no controlled randomized studies to support its widespread use.

Beyond the above essentials of critical care nutrition, experimental and clinical evidence is now emerging that other selected nutrients may be of importance during critical illness [50]. The use of medium-chain triglycerides, for instance, may diminish the deleterious effects of lipid solutions on the reticuloendothelial system [51]. The addition of arginine may significantly improve the depressed immunological response seen in the recovery phase of critical illness [52], and the addition of glutamine, an amino acid not found in standard total parenteral nutrition (TPN) solutions, appears to have major beneficial effects on gastrointestinal mucosal integrity and immunological competence [53, 54].

Impact of Uremia on Metabolism

It is unclear how well the preceeding basic concepts of nutrition in the critically ill patients apply to patients with ARF. There has been a strong belief in the literature that acute uremia is a unique metabolic situation which requires a change in the standard nutritional approach. A large body of laboratory and clinical research supports the concept that acute renal failure induces multiple changes in metabolism and that these changes are pervasive, involving protein catabolism, changes in amino acid utilization, resistance to the action of insulin, increased gluconeogenesis, and various hormonal derangements. The major metabolic abnormalities associated with acute uremia include:

1. Increased hepatic amino acid uptake and ureagenesis (E) [55]
2. Increased hepatic glucose, urea, and branched amino acid release (E) [56]
3. Increased gluconeogenesis and protein degradation (E) [56]

4. Increased hepatic and cardiac protein synthesis but increased protein degradation in muscle (E) [57–59]
5. Reduced circulating essential amino acids (H) [60]
6. Reduced tyrosine, increased cystine, and histidine clearance (H) [60]
7. Decreased muscle glycogen and increased glucagon (H) [61, 62]
8. Insulin resistance (H) [63] and glucose intolerance (E) [12]
9. Increased steroid and parathyroid hormone levels (H) [68, 69]
10. Increased serum proteolytic activity (H) [64]
11. Resistance to insulin-induced glucose uptake (E) [66]
12. Decreased insulin clearance (E) [70]
13. Abnormal insulin secretion (E) [71]

where (E) denotes data from experimental studies and (H) data from human studies.

In addition to these changes, which are associated with ARF per se, renal replacement therapies such as hemodialysis and peritoneal dialysis also lead to major metabolic consequences. Hemodialysis, for instance, is associated with the loss of 6–7 g free amino acid per treatment session [72, 73] (Fig. 2) as well as enchanced amino acid release from muscle [74] (Fig. 3). Oxygen consumption is also significantly increased [75]. If amino acids and glucose are infused for nutritional therapy, as is typically the case in the ICU, their levels are better maintained but their losses increase to more than 12 g/session [76].

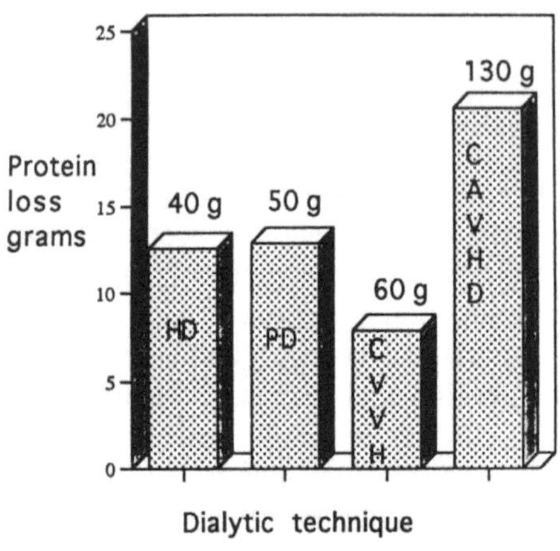

Fig. 2. Typical degree of amino acid/protein loss with different renal replacement therapy at protein administration rates as reported in the literature. As can be seen, continuous arteriovenous hemodiafiltration (*CAVHD*) appears to lead to the loss of about 15 g amino acids/day if 130 g/day of protein is administered. This loss, however, is proportionately no greater than that seen during continuous venovenous hemofiltration (*CVVH*) or during hemodialysis (*HD*) or peritoneal dialysis (*PD*)

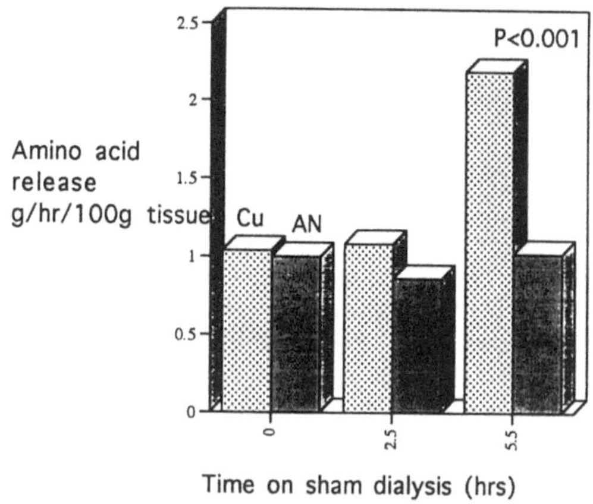

Fig. 3. Increase in amino acid release from muscle seen after 5 h of exposure of blood to a cuprophane (*Cu*) hemodialysis membrane. No such increase in amino acid release is seen if a biocompatible polyacrylonitrile (*AN*) hemofiltration-type membrane is used. (Modified from data in [74])

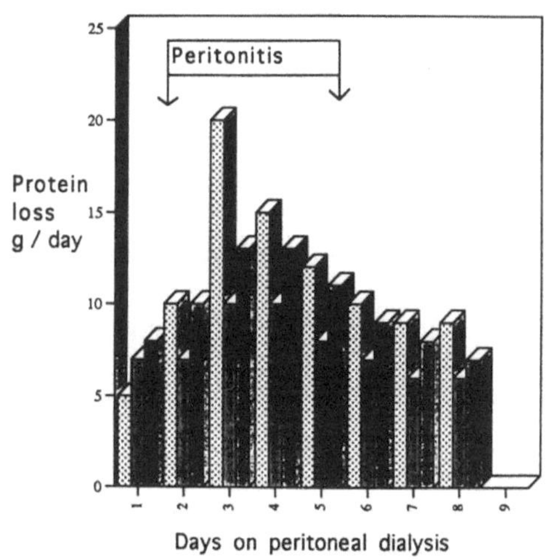

Fig. 4. Serious worsening in protein loss induced by the development of peritonitis in three patients receiving peritoneal dialysis. (From data in [79])

Peritoneal dialysis is also associated with significant protein loss (Figs. 2, 4) and, when high glucose concentrations are required, with a major degree of glucose resorption and attendant hyperglycemia [77–79].

The novel forms of continuous renal replacement therapy are also associated with significant metabolic consequences, which include the loss of 7 g or 10%–12% of infused amino acids/day (Fig. 2) and the absorption of large quantities of glucose, if glucose-based dialysate fluid is used to combine

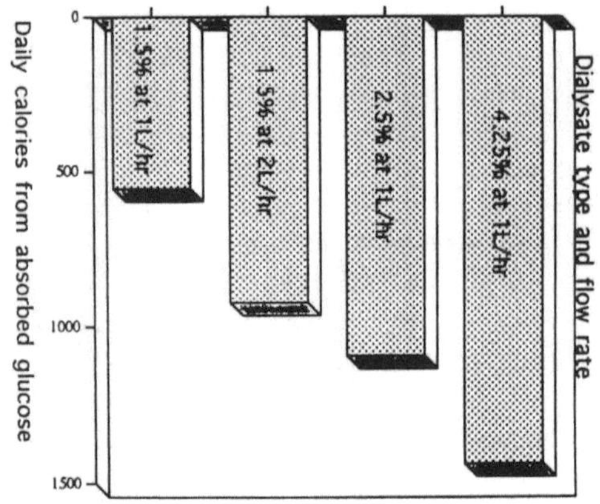

Fig. 5. Progressive increase in carbohydrate absorbtion seen with continuous arteriovenous hemodiafiltration if different amounts of dialysate glucose or dialysate flows are used. A total of 1000 calories of carbohydrates are delivered to the patient if a dialysate flow rate of 2 l/h and a 1.5% dialysate glucose concentration are use. (From data in [40])

diffusive and convective clearance (Fig. 5) [40, 80–83]. It appears, however, that these techniques, given their use of biocompatible membranes, do not lead to loss of insulin or increased release of amino acids from muscle (Fig. 3) [84, 85].

Effect of Uremia on Energy Requirements

The issue of the effect of uremia on energy requirements has been addressed in a number of studies. Schneeweiss et al. looked at the effect of acute uremia in the the presence of absence of sepsis [86] and found no effect on energy expenditure. The increase in energy expenditure seen in septic patients could be accounted for by fever and inflammation, and the presence of renal failure had no impact on resting energy requirements in patients without sepsis. Furthermore, the degree of uremia had no correlation with resting energy expenditure. The mean resting energy expenditure in a 70-kg man with sepsis and ARF was found to be approximately 1900 kCal/day. Bouffard et al. [87] investigated resting expenditure over a period of 2 h prior to hemodialysis in mechanically ventilated patients with ARF. They found that mean energy expenditure was close to 1700 kCal/day. In the absence of sepsis, the caloric expenditure of these acute renal failure patients was 1.19 times that predicted by the Harris-Benedict equation. However, their caloric expenditure was 1.31 time the predicted value in the presence of sepsis. These data highlight once again the fact that ARF per se is most unlikely to have a major effect on energy requirements and that the accompanying state of sepsis and inflammation is their major determinant.

Miller et al. [88] studied caloric expenditure in critically ill surgical patients with ARF and found that energy needs were nearly identical to those of a similar group of seriously ill patients without ARF [89]. Their overall caloric requirements were approximately 47 kCal/kg per day. Intermittent hemodialysis, however, has been shown to significantly increase oxygen consumption in critically ill patients [90]. This increase was in the range of 15%–20% of baseline values and did not depend on the use of an acetate or bicarbonate bath. Return to baseline oxygen consumption occurred with cessation of dialysis. Finally, Soop and colleagues [91] more recently reported on indirect calorimetry studies in critically ill patients with ARF. They found that the presence of ARF was associated with a close to 15% diminution in energy expenditure when compared to critically ill control patients. Furthermore, caloric requirements were close to 30 kCal/kg per day. These patients received close to twice as much dietary nitrogen as patients in Miller's study. Available evidence, therefore, strongly supports the concept that the presence of ARF does not significantly add to energy expenditure. It also confirms that the major determinant of increases in caloric needs for these patients is the underlying severity of illness with which ARF happens to be associated.

Impact of Acute Renal Failure on Nutrient Delivery

Quite apart from the metabolic derangements associated with acute uremia, its presence also poses problems related to the ability to deliver nutrients to the patient. This difficulty stems from the dangers associated with the fluid accumulation and poorly controlled uremia often seen with the application of conventional dialysis. Attempts to deal with such problems invariably lead to restrictions being placed on dietary fluid administration and, in particular, on the dietary administration of nitrogen [4–6, 10, 12]. Many authors emphasize the usefulness of frequent hemodialysis (daily treatment) in allowing easier administration of calories, but, most of all, of amino acids [5, 6, 91]. Such frequent application, however, is not so easily carried out in hemodynamically unstable and critically ill patients requiring vasopressors (now a majority of those with ARF in ICU) and may aggravate an already negative nitrogen balance (Fig. 6) Hemodialysis in this setting is a source of further hemodynamic and respiratory instabiliy [90, 92–95] and may result in life-threatening arrhythmias or death [90, 96].

The consequence of such side effects is that either daily hemodialysis is performed despite the patient's precarious cardiovascular state, with the attendant risks of major further instability and arrhythmias and the possible benefits of close to adequate caloric and nitrogen administration, or performed when clinically expedient (i.e., during periods of greater cardiovascular stability) or when inevitably needed to control uremia. This latter approach diminishes the patient's exposure to the ill effects of

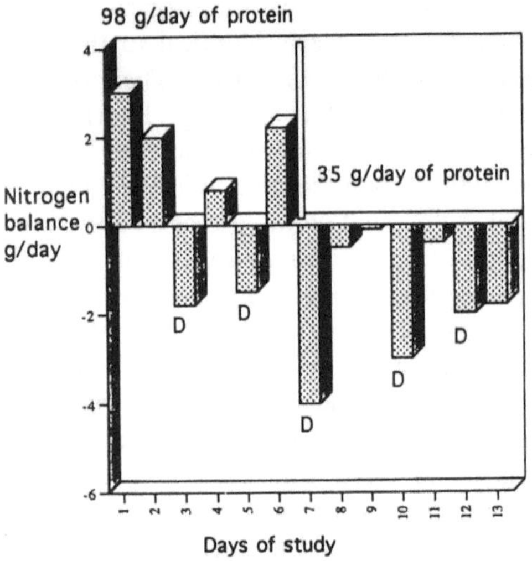

Fig. 6. Effect of hemodialysis on nitrogen balance at two different levels of daily protein intake. At a protein intake of 98 g/day, nitrogen balance is negative only on dialysis days (*D*). At a protein intake of 35 g/day, nitrogen balance is always negative and markedly so during dialysis days. (From data in [97])

hemodialysis, but invariably results in less than optimal nutrition. The study by Bouffard and colleagues [87] clearly demonstrates the shortcomings of this approach: while their patient's caloric needs appeared to have been met, nitrogen balance was markedly negative with a daily loss of body nitrogen close to 12 g. This would lead to the loss of about 1 kg body protein over a 2-week period. A strongly negative nitrogen balance in ARF patients has been described by many groups [10, 12, 88, 97–99] in this or similar contexts.

The consequences of such a persistent severely negative nitrogen balance are likely to be important in adversely affecting respiratory function and immunological competence, [15, 52, 100, 101] increasing the risk of nosocomial infection, and leading to gastrointestinal mucosal atrophy and endotoxin translocation [102–104].

The development and clinical application of continuous hemofitration techniques [105–108] fortunately appears to have provided a solution to the limitations imposed upon nutrition by intermittent hemodialysis or peritoneal dialysis. Its ability to deliver predictable water and solute removal, steady control of azotemia, and hemodynamic stability [109–111] has resulted in the ability to administer nitrogen-rich diets with a daily protein adminstration which was previously almost unthinkable. Such protein adminstration has now been shown to result in a marked improvement in nitrogen balance [40, 112–114] and the achievement of a positive nitrogen balance in several critically ill patients with multiorgan and renal failure [40]. Clinical studies also clearly demonstrate that the use of continuous hemofiltration techniques permits the administration of planned/ideal nutritional supplementataion to essentially all patients, while the use of conventional dialytic techniques does not. The difference between the two is statistically significant in retrospective studies [96–111] and represents another major advantage associated with the use of hemofiltration and its technical derivations.

Effect of Nutrition on Renal Recovery

An important question that arises with regard to nutritional therapy in ARF is whether different approaches result in speedier or delayed renal recovery. This is an issue of obvious clinical relevance as the earlier resolution of renal failure simplifies therapy and is likely to have a beneficial impact on systemic metabolic function and overall rate of recovery. There is no data to support the preferential administration of calories in the form of glucose or lipids once energy expenditure has been met. ARF, therefore, does not imply the need for alterations of the principles determining lipid and carbohydrate balance in the diet of critically ill patients.

On the other hand, much research has been devoted to the effect of amino acid administration in this setting. The impact of amino acids on the kidney is complex. It is well established, for instance, that protein ingestion causes marked changes in renal hemodynamics with an increase in renal blood flow and glomerular filtration rate between 25% and 60% [115–119]. This effect is not seen with carbohydrates or lipids [120] and is presumably an appropriate adaptive phenomenon to help the kidney deal with the increased nitrogen load associated with protein metabolism [121]. While this concept is well established in normal organs or in the setting of chronic renal failure, there is no data on the effect of amino acid infusion on renal plasma flow in ARF or in organs recovering from ARF [121]. In such organs, this phenomenon, which is probably dependent on a tubuloglomerular feedback mechanism, is likely to be markedly blunted. On the other hand, ARF is associated with a close to 25% fall in the elimination half-time of several amino acids, leading to elevated concentrations of several amino acids [122]. The effect of such an elevation on renal hemodynamics is unknown.

With regards to the potential effect of amino acids on renal recovery, there is a substantial body of experimental data showing that intravenous amino acid infusions enhance recovery after acute tubular necrosis [123], stimulate the biosynthesis of phospholipids [124], and increase protein synthesis [125]. Furthermore, the infusion of alanine was shown to offer protection from anoxic injury to rabbit proximal tubules as does glycine, a structurally related amino acid [126]. Such optimistic experimental findings, however, have been contradicted by other experimental work showing that lysine can induce ARF in rats [127] and that dietary protein prior to renal ischemia seriously aggravates its effects in the same animal [128].

This paradox has been reviewed by Zager [129], who has also shown that postischemic injury is aggravated by amino acid infusion. The mechanism for this effect remains unclear, but direct nephrotoxicity seems unlikely. It is possible that the infusion of amino acids during periods of relative oxygen deprivation might worsen its effects by increasing tubular metabolic work (amino acid uptake). Such effects could further be exacerbated by any hypotensive episodes, such as those seen during standard hemodialysis in critically ill patients. The significance of the above experimental findings in relation to the course of ARF in the critically ill remains unknown.

Effect of Nutrition on Outcome

There has not been any study demonstrating a survival advantage of a particular dietary approach to acute renal failure since Abel et al.'s work in 1973 [9]. Twenty years later, however, much has changed: most severe ARF is now seen in the ICU and in the context of multiorgan failure, therapeutic modalities have markedly changed with the advent of continuous hemofiltration, and the control of uremia has become easier and more complete [130]. Abel's findings and those of others have made the administration of some nitrogen to critically ill patients part of the accepted best clinical practice in the 1990s, and it is highly unlikely that a trial of nitrogen-free versus nitrogen-rich nutritional therapy in critically ill patients with severe ARF would either be of interest or be approved by any institutional ethics committee.

The question has clearly shifted from whether protein nitrogen should be given to how much should be given and whether any restrictions of protein nitrogen administration should apply to critically ill patients if severe ARF is present. If a controlled randomized study of these issues were performed (and unlikely event for a single institution), appropriate intermediate outcome measure should be used as end points, as survival to hospital discharge is most likely determined by other more powerful physiological and therapeutic variables. Clinically important intermediate variables could include time on the ventilator, time to recovery of urinary output, and time to cessation of artificial renal support. Even these would be unlikely to yield significant findings given the fact that they imply survival, that survival is in the 20%–40% range, and that about only 20–30 such patients would be expected in an average combined medical–surgical ICU with a yearly patient flow of about 1000 patients.

Other measures of therapeutic success may then be appropriate. Kierdorf and colleagues analyzed daily nitrogen balance in their severe ARF patients. They found that increasing protein nitrogen administration from 0.7 g amino acids/kg per day to 1.5 g/kg per day improved nitrogen balance from −8.1 g/day to −3.4 g/day [131]. These results, achieved in ARF treated by continuous venovenous hemofiltration, confirm data from patients receiving

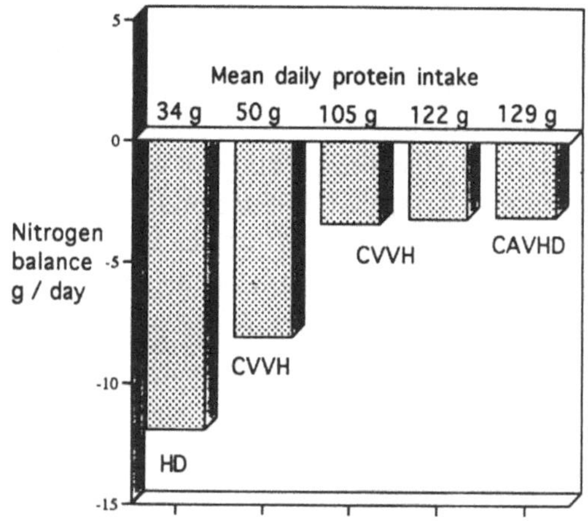

Fig. 7. Nitrogen balance in critically ill patients receiving either intermittent hemodialysis (*HD*), continuous venovenous hemofiltration (*CVVH*), or continuous arteriovenous hemodiafiltration (*CAVHD*). For each technique, the daily amount of dietary protein is reported at the top (in grams) as obtained from the literature. It is obvious that a near neutral nitrogen balance can only be achieved if in an average 70-kg man approximately 1.5 g protein/kg per day is administered. (From data in [40, 87, 112])

standard hemodialysis (negative daily nitrogen balance greater than 11 g/day) [87] and data from our own ICU in patients receiving continuous arteriovenous hemodiafiltration and approximately 1.5 g protein/kg per day (Fig. 7). We have further explored the impact of aggressive nitrogen supplementation (2.5 g protein/kg per day) in patients with multiorgan failure, sepsis, and ARF receiving continuous venovenous hemodiafiltration by studying their total body nitrogen state upon ICU discharge.

Nitrogen balance was studied by means of the technique of neutron activation [132]. With this technique, patients are irradiated bilaterally with neutrons from a sealed tube neutron generator. The neutrons generate in the body short-lived radioisotopes which are specific for various body elements and which decay with the emission of gamma rays of characteristic energies. The radiation emitted from the patient is measured in a whole-body radiation counter and the complex spectrum is analyzed by a least squares technique to give the counting rates due to ^{13}N (a short-lived reaction product of N), as well as those of other radionucleides of Na, Cl, Ca, K etc. These counting rates are corrected for decay and variations in output of the neutron generator, and the total body contents of the element of interest are calculated by multiplying the counting rates by apporpriate calibration factors. The accuracy and precision of the measurements are in the range of 1%–2%, with a coefficient of variation being a function of the radiation dose and ranging between 1.3% and 22%

Four patients were studied. These patients' total nitrogen losses had been studied at random times during their stay in ICU and had been found to be more than 25 g/day. Despite a very high rate of catabolism, their total body nitrogen after more than 7 days of anuria, multiorgan failure, and sepsis was found to be within the normal range in three cases and only mildy diminished in one. We have, thus, been able to demonstrate that an accepted nutritional end point (the preservation of lean body mass) is achievable if aggressive nitrogen therapy is administered and that this goal can be achieved while maintaining control of azotemia at all times. More data is needed in this direction, but the evidence so far suggests that aggressive nitrogen administration in these patients is safe and achieves planned nutritional goals.

New Developments

The area of nutrition in critical illness is undergoing further evaluation as new data emerge that adequate nutritional therapy not only significantly modulates immunological function, but has important implications with regard to the restoration of minute ventilation and ventilatory drive [133]. More recently, the development of techniques for the production of recombinant hormones has made it possible to diminish catabolism by hormonal manipulation [134]. Growth hormone in supraphysiological doses has now been clearly shown to promote positive nitrogen balance in the critically ill [135, 136], probably mostly by preserving protein in skeletal muscle [136]. Experimental studies have also shown improved diaphragmatic recovery [137] with its obvious implications in the setting of prolonged mechanical ventilation. Finally, in critically ill patients, growth hormone has been shown to preserve body cell mass and thus attenuate the abnormal distribution of body water so typically seen in this population [138]. Growth hormone, however, has no stimulatory impact in septic patients on insulin-like growth factor-I (IGF-I), the major mediator of its metabolic effects. This suggests a degree of resistance to its anabolic effects which may be bypassed by the direct administration of IGF-I. Early evidence indicates that this may be both feasible and safe [139]. There are presently no specific studies of patients with renal failure and of the effects of such manipulations on the rate of renal recovery or other oucome measures, but they are likely to come in the near future.

Less futuristic but relatively new is the powerful implication of having dialytic techniques (continuous hemofiltration) which permit the removal of fluid and offer excellent and steady control of uremia even in highly catabolic patients. These novel techniques make it possible to treat patients with ARF with the same nutritional approach used for other critically ill patients. Furthermore, it is now possible to use dialysates containing amino acids (C. Ronco, personal communication). These amino acids will diffuse from dialysate to blood, achieving a degree of continuous nutritional dialysis.

More data are likely to accumulate on the consequences of these changed philosophies.

Overview and Approach to Nutrition in Severe Acute Renal Failure

As previously emphasized, there have not been any controlled, randomized studies comparing different nutritional approaches to patients in ARF since Abel et al.'s work in 1973 [9], which established the need for the administration of amino acids. The amount administered to their patients (<20 g/day) would be considered grossly inadequate for a critically ill patient with multiorgan failure. .Hence we are really left with no specific data for ICU patients with ARF. This has unfortunately generated a great deal of cynicism. Furthermore, the lack of evidence showing that aggressive nutritional strategies improve outcome when compared to conservative ones in critical illness has led to a "free for all" attitude in clinical behavior. In ICU's around the world, critically ill patients will randomly receive either a low-protein diet, sometimes a "nephrologically" tailored one, and dialysis only when inevitable, or aggressive nitrogen supplementation and continuous renal replacement therapy according to the bias of the clinicians.

In the view of the author, however, there is now sufficient evidence to support the following statements:

1. A positive or neutral nitrogen balance is a worthwhile and clinically meaningful goal.
2. Maintenance of a near neutral nitrogen balance results in the preservation of lean body mass and respiratory muscle function.
3. The preservation of lean body mass requires the administration of an adequate amount of calories and of protein nitrogen (30 kCal/kg per day and 1.5 – 2 g protein/kg per day).
4. There is no new major metabolic derangement that the development of ARF in the setting of sepsis and critical illness will impose if uremia is adequately controlled.
5. Continuous renal replacement therapies permit the administration of nutritional fluids without fear of fluid overload.
6. Continuous renal replacement therapies permit the reliable and steady control of uremia in all patients with ARF, no matter what the amount of protein nitrogen admininstered is, as their effective urea clearance can be increased on demand.
7. Aggressive nitrogen administration in critically ill patients with severe ARF results in near neutral nitrogen balance and presevation of lean body mass.

Based on the above concepts, we hold that ARF patients should be fed no differently from other critically ill patients. Calories should be administered according to an estimate (direct or calculated) of energy expenditure. Protein nitrogen should be initially administered in the range of 1.5–2.5 g protein/kg per day and the amount adjusted according to nitrogen balance calculations with the aim of achieving a near neutral nitrogen balance. If this results in a rise in serum urea, the intensity of continuous renal replacement can be modified either by increasing ultrafiltrate production or by increasing countercurrent dialysate flow.

If glucose-based dialysate is used, glucose will be absorbed into the circulation in a predictable way [40] and adjustments in the rate of or need for supplemental intravenous glucose will have to be made. If hyperglycemia results, it should be treated aggressively with an intraveous infusion of insulin aimed at keeping the serum glucose level below 12 mmol/l. This approach can be expected to further diminish protein catabolism [140]. Daily trace element and vitamin administration should also take place.

The initial approach to nutrition in critically ill patients with ARF can be summarized as follows:

1. Start nutrition as soon as possible (day 1).
2. Use enteral route if possible and feed via nasojejunal tube.
3. Administer calories according to either estimated or measured caloirc expenditure.
4. Remember that ARF per se does not increase caloric needs.
5. Administer calories at a carbohydrate to lipid ratio of 1 : 1 unless specific issues contraindicate one or the other.
6. Administer protein nitrogen at 300 mg/kg per day initially and follow nitrogen balance regularly for adjustments.
7. Control azotemia by keeping plasma urea levels below 30 mol/l (blood urea nitrogen below 84 mg/dl) with the use of appropriate dialytic approach (preferably hemofiltration based).
8. Administer vitamins and trace elements daily.
9. Consider adding glutamine if preparations available lack it.
10. Monitor electrolytes and nutritional parameters on a regular basis.

We have shown this strategy to successfully maintain near neutral nitrogen balance in many critically ill patients with ARF and to do so predictably and safely. Further studies are needed, however, to compare the nutritional, immunological, and clinical consequences of this approach with one based on a conventional opproach involving low-nitrogen dialysis every second day. Future studies should also attempt to provide further insight into the consequence of adequate nitrogen adminstration by comparing the rate of infection or bacteremia, by using cellular markers of immunological competence, and by providing a follow-up of such competence under different nutritional regimens. Furthermore, studies of gut permeability and the influence on its persistence and severity in patients with low- versus high-nitrogen therapy would be of great clinical value. Such studies will likely be very difficult to perform because of the need to control for illness severity and for the degree of uremic control. They will further be hindered by the difficulty of recruiting a sufficient number of patients over short periods of time as well as the infinite other variables which operate in critically ill patients. Noneheless, if critical care support is to become more biologically sophisticated and the nutritional therapy of critically ill patients is to have a strong scientific basis, these goals must be pursued by all physicians involved in the care of critically ill patients with ARF.

References

1. Borst JGG (1948) Protein catabolism in uremia. Effects of protein-free diet, infections and blood transfusions. Lancet 1:824–827
2. Bull GM, Joekes AM, Lowe KG (1949) Conservative treatment of anuric uremia. Lancet 2:229–234
3. Gamble JL (1946–1947) Physiological information from studies on the life-raft ration. Harvey Lect 42:247–258
4. Berlyne GM, Bazzard FJ, Booth EM et al. (1967) The dietary treatment of acute renal failure. Q J Med 141:59–65
5. Teschan PE, Baxter CR, O'Brien TF et al. (1960) Prophylactic hemodialysis in the treatment of acute renal failure. Ann Intern Med 53:992–997
6. Kleinknecht D, Junkers P, Chanard J, Barbancel C, Ganeval D (1972) Uremic and non-uremic complications in acute renal failure: evaluation of early and frequent dialysis on prognosis. Kidney Int 1:190–194
7. Lee HA, Sharpstone P, Ames AC (1967) Parenteral nutrition in renal failure. Postgrad Med J 43:81–85
8. Dudrick SJ, Steiger E, Long JM (1970) Renal failure in surgical patients – treatment with intravenous essential aminoacids and hypertonic glucose. Surgery 68:180–185
9. Abel RM, Beck CH Jr, Abbot WM et al. (1973) Improved survival in acute renal failure after treatment with intravenous essential L-amino acids and glucose. N Engl J Med 288:695–699
10. Leonard C, Luke RG, Siegel RR (1975) Parenteral essential amino acids in acute renal failure. Urology 6:154–157
11. Se-Min Baek, Makabali GG, Bryan-Brown CW, Kusek J, Shoemaker WC (1975) The influence of parenteral nutrition on the course of acute renal failure. Surg Gynecol Obstet 141:405–408
12. Feinstein EI, Blumenkrantz J, Healy M et al. (1981) Clinical and metabolic responses to parenteral nutrition in acute renal failure. Medicine (Baltimore) 60:124–137
13. Weissman C, Hyman AI (1987) Nutritional care of the critically ill patient with respiratory failure. Crit Care Clin 3:185–203
14. Rochester DF, Esau SA (1984) Malnutrition and the respiratory system. Chest 85:411–415
15. Pingleton SK, Harmon GS (1987) Nutritional management in acute respiratory failure. JAMA 257:3094–3099
16. Doekel RC, Zwillich CW, Scoggin CH, Krygger M, Weil JV (1976) Clinical semistravation:
depression of hypoxic ventilatory response. N Engl J Med 295:358–361
17. Radrizzani D, Iapichino G, Cambisano M, Bonetti G, Ronzoni G, Colombo A (1988) Peripheral, visceral and body nitrogen balance of catabolic patients, without and with parenteral nutrition. Intensive Care Med 14:212–216
18. Elwyn DH (1980) Nutrional requirements of adult surgical patients. Crit Care Med 8:9–20

19. Iapichino G, Radrizzani D, Solca M et al. (1984) The main determinants of nitrogen balance during total parenteral nutrition in critically ill injured patients. Intensive Care Med 10:251–254
20. Daly JM, Reynolds J, Thom A et al. (1988) Immune and metabolic effects of arginine in the surgical patient. Ann Surg 208:512–523
21. Iapichino G, Radrizzani D, Schecini A et al. (1988) Essential and non-essential amino acid requirement in injured patients receiving total parenteral nutrition. Intensive Care Med 14:399–405
22. Cerra FB (1987) Hypermetabolism, organ failure and metabolic support. Surgery 101:1–6
23. Kirkpatrick J, Donn M, Haynes M (1981) The therapeutic advantages of a balance nutrition support system. Surgery 89:370–376
24. Seba TM, Dillon BC, Lausen ME (1983) Fibronectin and phagocytic host defense: relationship to nutritional support. JPEN J Parenter Enteral Nutr 7:62–66
25. Jeejeebhoy KN (1992) Nutrition in critical illness. In: Civetta JM, Taylor RW, Kirby RR (eds) Critical care, 2nd enn. Lippincott, Philadelphia, pp 1093–1117
26. Christman JW, Mc Cain RW (1993) A sensible approach to the nutritional support of mechanically ventilated critically ill patients. Intensive Care Med 19:129–136
27. Barison RD (1990) The measurement of energy ependiture: instrumentation, practical considerations, and clinical application. Respir Care 35:640–659
28. Harris JA, Benedict FG (1919) A biometric study of basal metabolism. Carnegie Institute of Washington, Washington (Publ no 279)
29. Mann S, Westenskow DR, Houtchens BA (1985) Measured and predicted caloric expenditure in the acutely ill. Crit Care Med 13:173–177
30. Liggett SB, Renfro AD (1990) Energy expenditure of mechanically ventilated nonsurgical patients. Chest 98:682–686
31. Askanazi J, Carpentier YA, Elwyn DH et al. (1980) Influence of total parenteral nutrition on fuel utilization in injury and sepsis. Ann Surg 191:40–46
32. Frayn KN (1986) Hormonal control of metabolism in trauma and sepsis. Clin Endocrinol (Oxf) 24:577–599
33. Romanosky AJ, Bagby GJ, Bockman EL et al. (1980) Free fatty acid utilization by skeletal muscle after endotoxin administration. Am J Physiol 239:E391–E395
34. Spitzer JJ, Bagby GJ, Meszaros K, Lang CH (1988) Alterations in lipid and carbohydrate metabolism in sepsis. JPEN J Parenter Enteral Nutr 12:553–558
35. Sax HC, Talamini MA, Brackett K, Fischer JE (1986) Hepatic steatosis in total parenteral nutrition: failure of fatty infiltration to correlate with abnormal serum hepatic enzyme levels. Surgery 100:697–703
36. Colloway DH, Spector H (1954) Nitrogen balance as related to caloric and protein intake in active young men. Am J Clin Nutr 2:405–411
37. Richardson DP, Wayler AH, Scrimshaw NS et al. (1979) Quantitative effect of an isoenergetic exchange of fat for carbohydrate on dietary protein utilization in healthy yound men. Am J Clin Nutr 32:2217–2225
38. Bozzetti F (1976) Parenteral nutrition in surgical patients. Surg Gynecol Obstet 142:1–4
39. Greenberg GR, Jeejeebhoy KN (1979) Intravenous protein sparing therapy in patients with gastrointestinal disease. JPEN J Parenter Enteral Nutr 3:427–433
40. Bellomo R, Martin H, Parkin G, Love J, Boyce N (1991) Continuous arteriovenous haemodiafiltration in the critically ill. Influence on major nutrient balances. Intensive Car Med 17:399–402
41. Burke JF, Wolfe RR, Mullany CJ et al. (1979) Glucose requirements following burn injury. Ann Surg 190:274–279
42. Golden MHN, Golden BE, Jackson AA (1980) Skin breakdown in kwashiorkor responds to zinc. Lancet 1:1256–1258
43. Golden MHN, Golden BE, Harland PSEG et al. (1978) Zinc and immuno competence in protein-energy malnutrition. Lancet 1:1226–1229

44. Johnson RA, Baker SS, Fallon JT et al. (1981) An accidental case of cardiomyopathy and selenium deficiency. N Engl J Med 304:1210–1212
45. Berger R, Adams L (1989) Nutritional support in the critical care setting. Chest 96:139–150
46. Heymsfield SB, Bethel RA, Ansley JD, Nixon DW, Rudman D (1979) Enteral hyperalimentation: an alternative to central venous hyperalimentaion. Ann Intern Med 90:63–71
47. McArdle AH, Palmason C, Mozency I, Brown RA (1981) A rationale for enteral feeding as the preferable route for hyperalimentation. Surgery 90:616–623
48. Kudsk KA, Crose MA, Fabian TC et al. (1991) Enteral versus parenteral feeding. Effects on septic morbidity after blunt and penetrating abdominal trauma. Ann Surg 215:503–513
49. Zaloga GP (1991) Bedside method for placing small bowel feeding tubes in critically ill patients. A prospective study. Chest 100:1643–1646
50. Bagley JS, Wan JMF, Georgieff M, Forse RA, Blackburn GL (1991) Cellular nutrition in support of early mulitple organ failure. Chest 100:1825–1885
51. Sobrado J, Moldawer LL, Pomposelli JJ et al. (1985) Lipids emulsions and reticuloendothelial system function in healthy and burned guinea pigs. Am J Clin Nutr 9:559–565
52. Daly JM, Reynolds J, Thom A et al. (1988) Immune and metabolic effects of arginine in the surgical patient. Ann Surg 208:512–523
53. Tamada H, Nezu R, Imamura I et al. (1992) The dipeptide alanylglutamine prevents intestinal mucosal atrophy in parenterally fed rats. JPEN J Parenter Enteral Nutr 16:110–116
54. Van der Hulst R, van Kreel BK, van Meyersfeldt MF et al. (1993) Glutamine and the preservation of gut integrity. Lancet 341:1363–1365
55. Lacy WW (1969) Effect of acute uremia on amino acid uptake and urea production by perfused rat liver. Am J Physiol 216(6):1300–1305
56. Frolich J, Sholmerich J, Hoppe-Seyler G et al. (1974) The effect of acute uremia on gluconeogenesis in isolated perfused rat liver. Eur J Clin Invest 4:453–458
57. McCormick GJ, Shear L, Barry KG (1966) Alteration of hepatic protein synthesis in acute uremia. Proc Soc Exp Biol Med 122:99–103
58. Shear L (1969) Internal redistribution of tissue protein synthesis in uremia. J Clin Invest 48:1252–1257
59. Flugel-Link RM, Salusk IB, Jones MR, Koppel JD (1983) Protein and amino acid metabolism in posterior hemicorpus of acutely uremic rats. Am J Physiol 244:E615–E623
60. Druml W, Burger U, Kleinberger G et al. (1986) Elimination of aminoacids in acute renal failure. Nephron 42:62–67
61. Bergstrom J, Hultman E (1969) Glycogen content of skeletal muscle in patients with renal failure. Acta Med Scand 186:177–182
62. Bilbrey GL, Faloona GR, White MG (1974) Hyperglucagonemia of renal failure. J Clin Invest 58:841–846
63. De Fronzora, Tobin JD, Rowe JW, Andres R (1978) Glucose intolerance in uremia. Quantification of pancreatic beta cell sensitivity to glucose and tissue sensitivity to insulin J Clin Invest 62:425–434
64. Horl HW, Heidland A (1980) Enhanced proteolytic activity – cause of protein catabolism in acute renal failure. Am J Clin Nutr 33:1423–1429
65. Mitch WE (1981) Amino acid release from the hindquarter and urea appearance in acute uremia. Am J Physiol 241:E415–E419
66. Mondon CE, Dolkans CB, Reaven GM, Alto P, Field M (1978) Ths site of insulin resistance in acute uremia. J Am Diabetes Assoc 27:571–576
67. Heidland A, Hoerl WH, Heller N, Heine H, Neumann S, Heidbreder E (1983) Proteolytic enzymes and catabolism: enhanced release of grannulocyte proeinases in uremic intoxication and during hemodialysis. Kidney Int 24 Suppl 16:S27–S36

68. Teschner M, Heidland A (1989) Hypercatabolism in acute renal failure – mechanisms and therapeutic approaches. Blood Purif 7:16–27
69. Massry SG, Arieff AI, Coburn JW, Palmieri G, Kleeman CR (1974) Divalent ion metabolism in patients with acute renal failure: studies on the mechanism of hypocalcemia. Kidney Int 5:437–445
70. Perez G, Carteni G, Ungaro B, Saccà L (1980) Influence of nephrectomy on the glucoregulatory response to insulin administration in the rat. Can J Physiol Pharmacol 58:301–305
71. Cianciaruso B, Saccà L, Terracciano V et al. (1987) Insulin metabolism in acute renal failure. Kidney Int 32:S109–S112
72. McGale EHF, Pickfor JC, Aber GM (1972) Quantitative changes in plasma amino acids in patients with renal disease. Clin Chim Acta 38:395–400
73. Kopple JD, Swendseid ME, Shinaber JH, Umezawa CY (1973) The free and bound amino acids removed by hemodialysis. Trans Am Soc Artif Intern Organs 14:309–311
74. Alverstrand A, Gutierrez A, Wahren J, Bergstrom J (1987) Protein catabolism in sham hemodialysis: the effect of different membranes. Blood Purif 5:269–275
75. Mault JR, Bartlett RU, Dechert RE, Swartz RD, Ferguson SK (1982) Oxygen consumption during hemodialysis for acute renal failure. Trans Am Soc Artif Intern Organs 28:514–516
76. Wolfson M, Jones MR, Kopple JD (1982) Amino acid losses during hemodialysis with infusion of aminoacids and glucose. Kidney Int 21:500–506
77. Nolph KD, Rosenfield PS, Pwell JV, Danforth E Jr (1970) Peritoneal glucose transport and hyperglycemia during peritoneal dialysis. Am J Med Sci 259:272–276
78. Manji N, Shikora S, McMahon M, Blackburn GL, Bistrian BR (1990) Peritoneal dialysis for acute renal failure: overfeeding resulting from dextrose absorbed during dialysis. Crit Care Med 18:29–31
79. Blumenkrantz MJ, Gahl GM, Kopple JD et al. (1981) Protein losses during peritoneal dialysis. Kidney Int 19:593–602
80. Davenport A, Roberts NB (1990) Amino acid losses during conitnuous high-flux hemofiltration in the critically ill patients. Crit Care Med 17:1010–1014
81. Davenport A, Roberts NB (1989) Amino acid losses during hemofiltration. Blood Purif 7:192–196
82. Davies SP, Realveley DA, Brown EA, Kox WJ (1991) Amino acid clearances and daily losses in patients with hemodialysis. Crit Care Med 19:1510–1515
83. Bonnardeaux A, Pichette V, Ouimet D, Geadah D, Habel F, Cardinal J (1992) Solute clearances with high dialysate flow rates and glucose absorption from the dialysate in continuous arteriovenous hemodialysis. Am J Kid Dis 19:31–38
84. Bellomo R, Colman PG, Caudwell J, Boyce N (1992) Acute continuous hemofiltration with dialysis: effect on insulin concentrations and glycemic control in critically ill patients. Crit Care Med 20:1672–1676
85. Gutierrez A, Alvestrand A, Wahren J, Bergstroem J (1990) Effect of in vivo contact between blood and dialysis membranes on protein catabolism in humans. Kidney Int 38:487–494
86. Schneeweiss B, Graninger W, Stockbuber F et al. (1990) Energy metabolism in acute and chronic renal failure. Am J Clin Nutr 52:596–601
87. Bouffard Y, Viole JP, Annat G, Delafosse B, Guillame G, Motin J (1987) Energy expenditure in the acute renal failure patient mechanically ventiated. Intensive Care Med 13:401–404
88. Miller RL, Taylor WR, Gentry W, Day AT, Gazzaniga AB (1983) Indirect calorimetry in postoperative patients with acute renal failure. Am Surg 401:494–499
89. Gazzaniga AB, Polacheck JR, Wilson AF, Day AT (1978) Indirect calorimetry as a guide to caloric replacement during total parenteral nutrition. Am J Surg 136:128–132

90. Mault JR, Dechert RE, Bartlett RH, Swartz RD, Ferguson SK (1982) Oxygen consumption during hemodialysis for acute renal failure. Trans Am Soc Artif Intern Organs 28:510–513
91. Soop M, Forsberg E, Thoerne A, Alverstrand A (1989) Energy expenditure in postoperative multiple organ failure with acute renal failure. Clin Nephrol 31:139–145
92. Korchik WP, Brown DC, De Master EG (1978) Hemodialysis induced hypotension. Int J Artif Organs 1:151–155
93. Kjellstrand CM, Rosa AA, Shidemann JR (1980) Hypotension during hemodialysis: osmolality fall is an important pathogenic factor. Am Soc Artif Intern Organs 3:11–15
94. Aurigemma NM, Feldman NT, Gottlieb M, Ingram RH, Lazarus JM, Lowrie EG (1977) Arterial oxygenation during hemodialysis. N Engl J Med 297:871–875
95. Ronco C, Fabris A, Chiaramonte S et al. (1988) Comparison of four different short dialysis techniques. In J Artif Organs 3:169–174
96. Bellomo R, Mansfield D, Rumble S, Shapiro J, Parkin G, Boyce N (1992) Acute renal failure in critical illness: conventional dialysis (CD) vs. acute continuous hemodiafiltration (ACHD). ASAIO J 38:M654–M657
97. Borah MF, Schoenfeld PY, Gotch FA, Sargent GJ, Wolfson M, Humphreys MH (1978) Nitrogen balance during intermittent dialysis therapy of uremia. Kidney Int 14:491–496
98. Pelosi G, Proietti R, Arcangely A, Magalini SI, Bondoli A (1981) Total parenteral nutrition infusate. An approach to its optimal composition in post trauma acute renal failure. Resuscitation 9:45–51
99. Proietti R, Pelosi G, Santori A et al. (1983) Nutrition in acute renal failure. Resuscitation 10:159–166
100. Weissman C, Askanazi J, Rosenbaum S, Hyman A, Milic-Emili J, Kinsey JM (1983) Amino acids and respiration. Ann Intern Med 98:41–44
101. Daly JM, Reynolds J, Sigal RK, Shou J, Liberman MD (1990) Effect of dietary protein and amino acids on immune function. Crit Care Med 18:S86–S93
102. Deitch EA, Dazhong X, Qi L, Specian RD, Berg RD (1992) Protein malnutrition alone and in combination with endotoxin impairs systemic and gut-associated immunity. JPEN J Parenter Enteral Nutr 16:25–31
103. Chandra RK (1983) Nutrition, infection and immunity: present knowledge and future directions. Lancet 1:688–691
104. Deitch EA, Winterton J, Li M et al. (1987) The gut as a portal of entry for bacteremia: role of protein malnutrition. Ann Surg 205:681–692
105. Ronco C (1993) Continuous renal replacement therapies for the treatment of acute renal failure in intensive care patients. Clin Nephrol 40:187–198
106. Ronco C (1985) Arteriovenous hemodiafiltration (AVHDF): a possible way to increase urea removal during CAVH. J Int Soc Artif Organs 8:61–62
107. Geronemus R, Schneider N (1984) Continuous arteriovenous hemodialysis: a new modality for treatment of acute renal failure. Trans Am Soc Artif Intern Organs 30:610–613
108. Bellomo R, Parkin G, Love J, Boyce N (1992) Management of acute renal failure in the critically ill with continuous veno-venous haemodiafiltration. Ren Fail 14:183–186
109. Bellomo R, Parkin G, Love J, Boyce N (1992) The use of continuous haemodiafiltration: an approach to the management of acute renal failure in the critically ill. Am J Nephrol 12:240–245
110. Barton IK, Hilton PJ, Taub NA et al. (1993) Acute renal failure treated by haemofiltration: factors affecting outcome. Q J Med 86:81–90
111. Bellomo R, Boyce N (1993) Continuous venovenous haemodiafiltration compared with conventional dialysis in critically ill patients with acute renal faiulre. ASAIO J 39:M794–M797
112. Kierdorf H (1991) Continuous versus intermittent treatment: clinical results in acute renal failure. Contrib Nephrol 93:1–12

113. Mault JR, Kresowik TF, Deckerk RE, Arnolidi DK, Swartz RD, Bartlett RH (1984) Continuous arteriovenous haemofiltration: the answer to starvation in acute renal failure. Trans Am Soc Artif Intern Organs 30:203–208
114. Kierdorf H, Kindler J, Sieberth HG (1986) Nitrogen balance in patients with acute renal failure treated by continuous arteriovenous haemofiltration. Nephrol Dial Transplant 1:72–77
115. Bergstroem J, Ahlberg M, Alverstrand A (1985) Influence of protein intake on renal haemodynamics and plasma hormone concentrations in normal subjects. Acta Med Scand 217:189–196
116. Bosch JP, Lew S, Glabman S, Lauer A (1986) Renal haemodynamic changes in humans. Response to protein loading in normal and diseased kidneys. Am J Med 81:809–815
117. Pullman TN, Alving AS, Dern RJ, Landowne M (1954) The influence of dietary protein intake on specific renal functions in norman man. J Lab Clin Med 44:320–332
118. Graf H, Stummvoll HK, Luger A, Prayer R (1983) Effect of amino acid infusion on glomerular filtration rate. N Engl J Med 308:159–160
119. Woods LL, Mizelle HL, Montani J-P, Hall JE (1986) Mechanisms controlling renal haemodynamics and electrolyte excretion during amino acids. Am J Physiol 251:F303–F312
120. Shannon JA, Joliffe N, Smith HW (1932) The excretion of urine in the dog. IV. The effect of maintenance diet, feeding, etc, upon the quantity of glomerular filtrate. Am J Physiol 101:625–638
121. Woods L (1993) Mechanisms of renal haemodynamic regulation in response to protein feeding. Kidney Int 44:659–675
122. Druml W, Buerger U, Kleinberger G, Lenz K, Laggner A (1986) Elimination of amino acids in acute renal failure. Nephron 42:62–67
123. Toback FG (1977) Amino acid enhancement of renal regeneration after acute tubular necrosis. Kidney Int 12:193–198
124. Toback FG, Teegarden DE, Havener LJ (1979) Amino acid-mediated stimulation of renal phospholipid biosynthesis after acute tubular necrosis. Kidney Int 15:542–547
125. Toback FG, Dadd RC, Maier ER, Havener LJ (1983) Amino acid administration enhances
renal protein metabolism after acute tubular necrosis. Nephron 33:238–243
126. Garza-Quintero R, Ortega-Lopez J, Stein JH, ven Katachalam MA (1987) Alanine protects rabbit proximal tubules against anoxic injury in vitro. Am J Physiol 258:F1075–F1083
127. Racusen LC, Finn WF, Whelton A, Bolez K (1985) Mechanisms of lysine-induced acute renal failure in rats. Kidney Int 27:517–522
128. Andrews PM, Bates SB (1987) Dietary protein prior to renal ischemia and postischemic kidney function. Kidney Int 32:576–580
129. Zager RA (1987) Amino acid hyperalimentation in acute renal failure. Kidney Int 32:S72–S75
130. Paganini E (1993) Continuous renal replacement is the preferred treatment for all acute renal failure patients receiving intensive care. Semin Dial 6:176–179
131. Kierdorf H (1991) Continuous versus intermittent treatment: clinical results in acute renal failure. Contrib Nephrol 93:1–12
132. Hill GL, King RFG, Smith RC (1979) Multi-element analysis of the living body by neutron activation analysis-application to critically ill patients receiving intravenous nutrition. Br J Surg 66:868–872
133. Weissman C, Askanazi J, Rosenbaum S, Hyman AI, Milic-Emili J, Kimmey J (1983) Amino acids and respiration. Ann Intern Med 98:41–44
134. Ross RJM, Rodriguez-Arnao J, Bentham J, Cokley JH (1993) The role of insulin, growth hormone and IGF-I as anabolic agents in the critically ill. 19:S54–S57
135. Ward HC, Halliday D, Sim JW (1978) Protein and energy metabolism with biosynthetic human growth hormone after gastrointestinal surgery. Ann Surg 206:56–61

136. Hammarqvist F, Stromberg C, Decken A, Vinnars E, Wernerman J (1992) Biosynthetic human growth hormone preserves both muscle protein synthesis and decrease in muscle free glutamine and improves whole-body nitrogen economy after operation. Ann Surg 216:184–191
137. Lanz JK, Donahoe M, Rogers RM, Ontell M (1992) Effects of growth hormone on diaphragmatic recovery from malnutrition. J Appl Physiol 73:801–805
138. Gatzen C, Scheltinga MR, Kimbrough TD, Jacobs DO, Wilmore DW (1992) Growth hormone attenuates the abnormal distribution of body water in critically ill surgical patients. Surgery 112:181–187
139. Miell JP, Taylor AM, Jones J et al. (1992) Administration of human recombinant insulin-like growth factor-I to patients following gastrointestinal surgery. Clin Endocrinol (Oxf) 37:542–551
140. Woolfson AMJ, Heatley RV, Allison S (1979) Insulin to inhibit protein catabolism after injury. N Engl J Med 300:14–17
141. Clowes GHA, Heideman M, Lindberg B et al. (1980) Effect of parenteral alimentation on amino acid metabolism in septic patients. Surgery 88:531–543

Immunology of Acute Renal Failure in the Critically Ill

N. Boyce

Introduction

Acute Renal Failure (ARF) has traditionally been viewed as predominantly a consequence of renal hypoxia or ischaemia, with much clinical and laboratory research in ARF focusing on renal haemodynamics and the functional consequences of renal hypoperfusion [1–3]. It is recognized that the immune system may rarely participate directly in the induction of an acute cessation of renal function (e.g., in systemic or renal-limited vasculitis, acute glomerulonephritis or acute interstitial nephritis). However, the immune system is not typically regarded as a significant contributor in the pathogenesis of the majority of cases of ARF [4, 5].

Despite much disciplined endeavour, our knowledge of the pathophysiology of ARF still has significant limitations. It is likely that ARF represents a common functional deficit capable of being initiated by a broad range of primary insults. A variety of mediator systems presumably contribute, with much investigative interest in seeking "final common pathways" of injury mediation [3–5]. Many of the experimental model systems of ARF are of limited relevance to studies of ARF in the critically ill, as they represent circumstances in which ARF occurs unassociated with other organ system dysfunction [1–5]. Indeed, the heterogeneity of experimental model systems of ARF makes extrapolation from observations in a single-model system difficult. It is probable that the ARF which accompanies critical illness will share common pathophysiological processes with other organ systems affected by multiple organ failure (MOF) or multiple organ dysfunction (MOD) syndromes [6–10]. The immune system may well contribute to the induction of ARF in the critically ill, in addition to exacerbating established renal injury and perpetuating ARF [6–10]. This review will focus on evidence suggesting a role for the immune system in the pathogenesis of the ARF of critical illness and discuss the functional immunological deficit invariably seen in this clinical context.

Role of the Immune System in the Mediation of Acute Renal Failure Injury in the Critically Ill

Recently we have seen a focus on the cellular biology of a syndrome now known as the systemic inflammatory response syndrome (SIRS), which incorporates circumstances previously encompassed by the term "sepis syndrome". Two decades ago "sequential systems failure was attributed to the cumulative impact of the initial insult and subsequent infective, haemorrhagic and toxic complications [6–10]. Currently SIRS is viewed as a consequence of the triggering of a common inflammatory mediator cascade by a variety of inciting agents [6–10]. This mediator cascade has numerous potential entry points and complex control systems (Fig. 1). The mediator cascade may be accessed at any time point, and its activation status can be modified by antecedent events [6–10]. Hence, although a single overwhelming insult may result in SIRS leading to MOF, repeated subinjurious insults feeding into this medatior cascade may result in SIRS (Fig. 2). No overt injury would occur if these subinjurious insults were suffered individually or perhaps even if the time course of exposure to injury-invoking insults was different (Fig. 2). These concepts of the inflammatory mediator

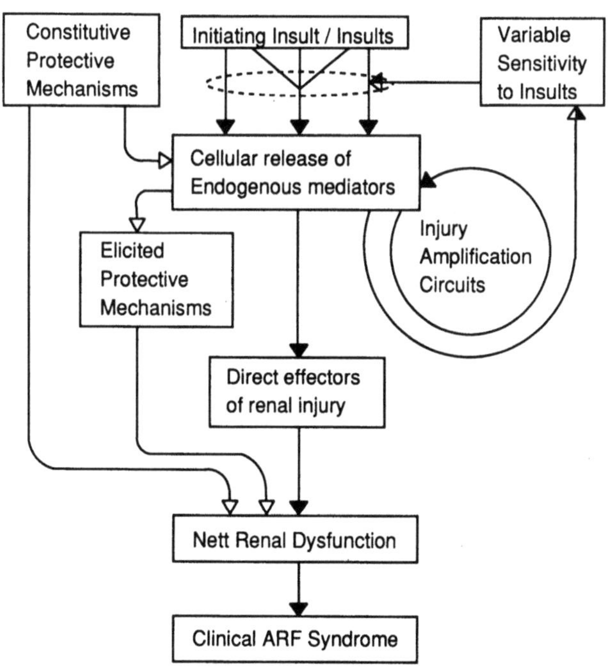

Fig. 1. Essential components of the complex, interlocking mediation processes intrinsic to the development of acute renal failure (*ARF*). The system contains the ability to both amplify or inhibit responses to subsequent potentially noxious insults

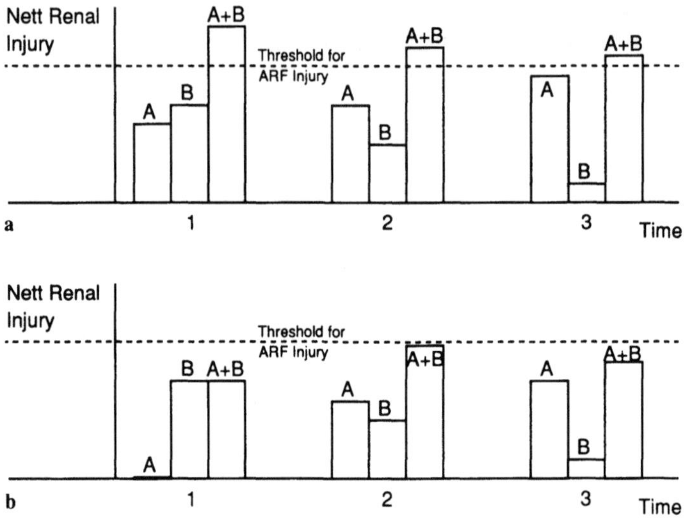

Fig. 2. a Outcome following synchronous exposure to two noxious stimuli. All three time points represented demonstrate a clinically detected acute renal failure (*ARF*) syndrome following insults *A* and *B*, although either stimulus itself would have produced insuffıcent renal injury to result in ARF. **b** Noxious stimulus *A* has been delayed such that its injurious course begins a single time point later. Noxious stimulus *B* is unchanged. Now no clinically apparent renal injury occurs at any of the time points illustrated

cascade as a complex, multicompartment, interactive process with a time course are important tools for reconciling apparently contradictory reports of research studies of ARF in critical illness. Clearly nett renal injury at any given time point is an integral of deleterious and repair processes set in train. The relative contribution of any individual injury mediation system will vary with time, as will the ability to influence outcome by interference with any particular mediation system (Fig. 3). Studies demonstrating a role for a given mediator system – or apparently negative results of intervention studies – must always be qualified with the caveat "in this model system at this time point". Given these principles and cautions, what evidence exists for a role of the immune system in the ARF of critical illness?

Cellular Mediators

Various models of acute renal injury resulting in ARF are characterized by infiltration of renal parenchyma with leucocytes [11–16]. Although the degree of leucocytic infiltration varies between model systems, the predominant leucocyte influx is focused within the interstitium, with a particular peritubular concentration [11, 12, 16]. In the few studies which have examined the immunophenotype of these infiltrating leucocytes, the

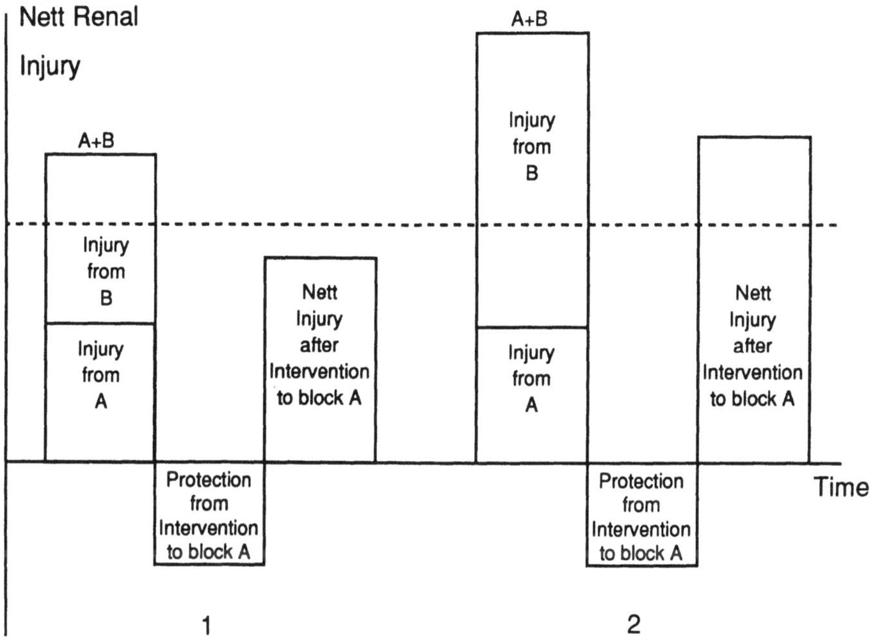

Fig. 3. Despite an identical contribution to nett renal injury and equal protection provided by inhibition of mediator system *A*, intervention at two different time points in the course of an acute renal failure (*ARF*) model produce appparently contradictory conclusions regarding the role of mediator system *A* in ARF injury. *1*, Mediator *A* crucial in ARF injury. *2*, Mediator *A* uninvolved in ARF injury

majority (two thirds) have been T lymphocytes bearing the CD8 marker [12, 16]. The remainder of these infiltrating leucocytes consist of macrophages and polymorphonuclear leucocytes (PMN), with the relative balance between these phagocytic cells differing dependent upon the time from initiation of injury (an initial PMN influx followed by a monocyte/macrophage prescence) [11, 12, 16]. The functional roles of infiltrating leucocytes in ARF remain uncertain. Theoretically, they may be important in the mediation of injury and the remodelling and repair processes. Alternatively, they may be recruited to a site of established injury and be of little functional relevance. The potential roles for infiltrating lymphocytes in ARF have effectively not yet been addressed. The roles of PMN in ARF remain a source of controversy. There is clear-cut evidence for a significant contribution of PMN and their reactive oxygen species (ROS), enzyme and leukotriene products in the mediation of ischaemic renal injury and ischaemia reperfusion injury more generally [13, 14, 17–20]. In addition PMN have been demonstrated to play a crucial role in mediating ARF injury in the acute ureteric obstruction model of ARF [21] and in the ARF accompanying experimental endotoxaemia [13]. Although apparently contradictory experimental reports exist [22, 23], it appears probable that PMN are capable of directly contributing to renal injury mediation in ARF. Their predominant roles are in association with the reperfusion phase of ischaemia/reperfusion injury [14–16, 19]. Presumably a synergism between soluble and cell surface signals results in the recruitment of circulating leucocytes into the kidney seen in ARF. At least some of this recruitment of leucocytes is likely to be mediated by CD11b–CD18-dependent cell adhesion mechanisms up-regulated by ischaemic injury, as is the case in other tissue models of ischaemia reperfusion injury [24–27].

Renal endothelial cells, epithelial cells and interstitial fibroblasts have the capacity of produce and respond to a broad range of cytokines. They also alter their expression of cell surface molecules, thereby modulating homotypic and heterotypic cell–cell interactions [28–30]. Indeed it has been proposed that alterations in integrin expression by renal tubular epithelial cells are central to the pathogenesis of acute tubular necrosis [28–30]. Infiltrating leucocytes may modulate renal parenchymal cell function and thus contribute to overall renal injury. Such interactions may contribute to the induction and maintenance of renal injury early in the course of ARF and to the processes of renal regeneration and repair in the recovery phase of ARF.

During ARF circulating leucocyte populations, including lymphocytes, macrophages and PMN populations, demonstrate clear evidence of either "priming" or frank "activation". Such cells show increased basal and elicited cytokine and mediator release and/or enhanced expression of cell surface molecular markers associated with functional activation. Whilst the significance of these changes in activation status within leucocyte populations remains unknown, it has been proposed that such primed or activated cells may contribute to the perpetuation of established renal injury [31].

Complement

It is uncertain whether complement activation per se contributes directly to injury mediation in ARF. Systemic complement activation is associated with an influx of PMN into the kidney, the lung and other vascular beds [32, 33]. It is probable that such leucocytic infiltrates contribute to the mediation of observed tissue injury in ARF (see above). The role of the interacting cascade of soluble factors that make up the complement system has been particularly examined in the maintenance phase of ARF. This interest in complement and the maintenance of ARF relates to the potential for adverse consequences from blood–membrane interactions during haemodialysis support in established ARF [34, 35]. Conventional cuprophane haemodialysis membranes are associated with significant systemic complement activation [34, 35]. Such activation of the complement system by blood–membrane interactions has been shown to delay the resolution of ARF in an exper-

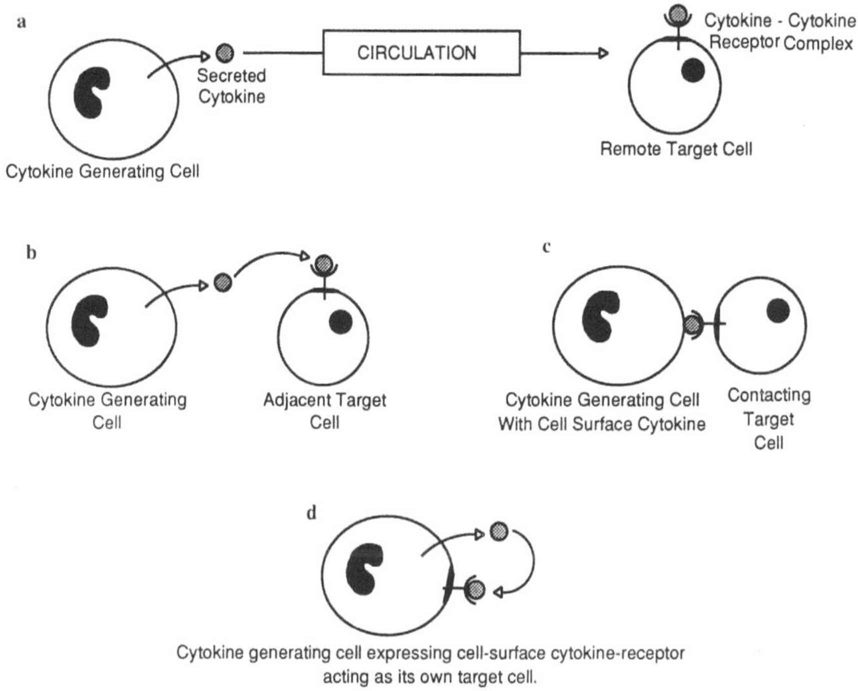

Fig. 4. Different spheres of influence – endocrine (**a**), paracrine (**b**), juxtacrine (**c**) and autocrine (**d**) – of a synthesized cytokine. ●, Recently generated cytokine; cytokine–cytokine receptor interaction; cytokine receptor.

imental model system [32]. These detrimental effects from blood–membrane interactions were not seen when more biocompatible membranes were substituted for cuprophane, raising the possibility that the use of membranes which minimally activate the complement system and/or adsorb activated complement components may facilitate recovery from established ARF [32].

Cytokines

A potential role for a wide range of cytokines in the pathogensis of ARF can be postulated. These protein mediators may act in either an endocrine, paracrine, juxtacrine or autocrine fashion (Fig. 4). They exert their actions by binding to specific cell surface receptors on target cells. These cytokine–receptor interactions open the way to several potential mechanisms for inhibiting the mediator cascade responsible for critical illness in SIRS:

1. Anticytokine strategies (all examples use tumour necrosis factor alpha, TNF-α, as the model cytokine)

   a) Block secretion, e.g., pentoxifylline, amrinone, cyclosporin A, interleukin-10 (IL-10), glucocorticoids, granulocyte colony-stimulating factor (G-CSF), leucocyte-inhibiting factor (LIF), prostaglandin E_2
   b) Enhance removal, e.g., plasma exchange, haemoabsorption, haemofiltration, antibodies
   c) Neutralize bioactivity, e.g., antibodies, soluble receptors, soluble receptor immunoglobulin (IG) fusion, proteins, antagonists
2. Antireceptor strategies
   a) Antibodies
   b) Receptor antagonists
3. Negate effects of cytokine–receptor binding
   a) Inhibitory cytokines, e.g., transforming growth factor (TGF)
   b) Inhibit secondary mediators, e.g., IL-6, interferon gamma, platelet-activating factor (PAF), nitric oxide, eicosanoids

Most studies to date of the role of cytokines in SIRS have been in the endotoxaemia model. Here the production and release of endogenous cytokine mediators from cells of haematopoietic lineage have been demonstrated to be essential for the induction of the widespread endothelial inflammation and increased vascular permeability which are the final common pathways of SIRS following endotoxaemia [10, 33, 36]. These studies in C3H/HeJ mice (which lack a functional cell surface receptor for lipopolysaccaride (LPS)/endotoxin on mononuclear leucocytes and hence produce no cytokines on exposure to LPS/endotoxin) unequivocally demonstrate the primacy of haemopoietic cell-derived cytokines in the lethality of SIRS associated with endotoxaemia [36]. They do not rule out a contributory role for cytokines derived from non-haematopoietic cells in the mediation of SIRS, nor do they establish which of the multitude of potential cytokine mediators are crucial in inducing fatal tissue injury [10, 33].

Tumour Necrosis Factor Alpha

TNF-α is produced in excess in critical illness [37–44] and is believed to contribute to the pathophysiology of SIRS, including the ARF which accompanies this syndrome [45–48]. TNF-α causes direct renal injury when infused [47, 48]. Antibodies to TNF-α and other strategies which inhibit effective TNF-α–receptor interaction protect against renal injury in the LPS/endotoxin model of SIRS [49–52]. These lines of evidence support a pivotal role for TNF-α in the mediator cascade of SIRS [37, 45, 46]. Whilst it is known that the lethality of endotoxaemia is dependent on haemopoietic cell-derived cytokines [36], in vivo TNF-α is derived from a range of non-haematopoietic cells [53–56]. It is difficult to identify the tissue sources of TNF-α in ARF, largely because TNF-α synthesis is controlled at a post-translational level [40, 57, 58]. Hence TNF-α mRNA detection in tissues does not, of itself, provide evidence for TNF-α protein production. Using a stable reporter minigene, it has been possible to model TNF-α synthesis in vivo [59]. This technique, when applied to the LPS/endotoxin model of SIRS, reveals that the kidney is a major source of TNF-α production with most of the renal TNF-α originating from glomeruli [59]. Such studies raise the intriguing possibility that local production of cytokines such as TNF-α by renal parenchymal cells and/or infiltrating leucocytes may play a dominant role in mediating the organ dysfunction seen in the ARF of SIRS [57]. TNF-α also apparently contributes to the pathophysiology of MOF/MOD injury, via either local and/or endocrine mechanisms, in patients critically ill with severe burns, trauma, haemorrhagic shock or severe pancreatitis [60–64]. The details of the pathogenic roles of TNF in these models of SIRS have yet to be addressed.

Interleukin-1

IL-1, in both its IL-1A and IL-2B isoforms, seemingly plays a pivotal role in the mediation of SIRS [33, 57, 65–69]. IL-1 production is increased in critical illness and, as for TNF, strategies which inhibit IL-1 production or prevent the interaction of IL-1 with its specific cellular receptors attenuate issue injury in SIRS [70, 71]. Such encouraging experimental observations stimulated clinical trials of a recombinant IL-1 receptor antagonist (IL-1Ra) in humans with SIRS [72, 73]. Whilst the initial reports of such endeavours were encouraging [72], the more definitive description failed to demonstrate clinically significant benefits [73]. Clearly IL-1 contributes to the production of tissue injury in the ARF accompanying SIRS [65–71]. It is believed that IL-1, TNF and other cytokines work synergistically in vivo in the production of SIRS seen in clinical practice [8–10, 33]. Because of the pleiotropy and redundancy characteristic of cytokine actions [74, 75], it may prove difficult to demonstrate a substantive clinical benefit from interuption of any single cytokine system, hence the interest in disruption of multiple components of the mediator cascade responsible for SIRS [10, 57].

Interleukin-2

As is the case for TNF and IL-1, the infusion of IL-2 is associated with the development of a capillary leak syndrome/SIRS [75–78]. IL-2 administration has been associated with the development of ARF in a significant proportion of patients receiving IL-2-containing anti-cancer protocols [77]. For some time the loss of renal function seen was attributed to systemic haemodynamic changes. Recent studies, however, have clearly indicated that IL-2 has an intrinsic injurious effect on the kidney, over and above any deleterious effects from systemic haemodynamic compromise [76]. It is uncertain what molecular mechanism/s underlie the mediation of renal injury following IL-2 exposure. The demonstration of this potential for injury induction raises the possibility that IL-2 may contribute to ARF injury mediation in other clinical circumstances.

Growth Factors

Many growth factors have been shown to be produced by renal tubular epithelial cells, including epidermal growth factor (EGF), insulin-like growth factors (IGF), platelet-derived growth factor (PDGF), fibroblast growth factors (FGF), hepatocyte growth factor (HGF) and TGF, and have been implicated in the processes of repair and recovery from renal injury [79]. Other renal parenchymal cells and infiltrating leucocytes have the capacity to either produce growth factors or respond to them [80–82]. The administration of the growth factors EGF or TGF-α facilitates recovery of renal function in ARF model systems [83, 84]. The role of endogenous growth factor production in the kidney in ARF remains uncertain, however, as although growth factor receptors may be up-regulated in ARF [79, 85], most studies indicate a reduction rather than an enhancement of the renal production of growth factors in the recovery phase of ARF [79, 85].

Other Soluble Mediators

A complex interaction between a variety of soluble mediator systems occurs in ARF. In addition to the factor discussed above, a significant role in injury mediation has been shown for reactive oxygen species (derived from sources other than infiltrating leucocytes), PAF, kinins, histamine, serotonin, the coagulation cascade, eicosanoids, nitric oxide, endothelin, angiotensin and catecholamines [86–95]. These factors variably stimulate the release of additional mediators, modify the activation status of the inflammatory mediator cascade or act as effectors of renal injury (e.g., by inducing vasoconstriction and modifying cellular permeability or other cellular functions). The inherent complexity of the system has rendered the identification of dominant mediator systems difficult. Many soluble mediators are products of cells of the immune system or modify immunological function [74, 75]. Their roles in ARF are dealt with individually in considerable detail elsewhere in this volume.

Immunological Consequences of Acute Renal Failure

The immune system is profoundly altered both by critical illness and by renal failure. The relative contributions of the initiating insult, concomitant organ dysfunction, the acute cessation of renal function and our therapeutic interventions to immunological dysregulation are unknown. Much descriptive research has catalogued the aberrant immune function seen in critical illness complicated by ARF. The paradox of these observations is that whilst many indices suggest apparent activation of the immune system, the overwhelming nett functional alteration is a deficiency of immunological function [96–98]. This immune deficiency manifests primarily at a clinical level as an increased incidence of infection in critically ill patients with ARF [1, 99]. The incidence of infective complications is variously estimated at between 30% and 70% [1, 99]. These include infections of the respiratory tract, at operative sites, urinary tract infection and septicaemia without apparent primary focus [1, 99]. Although the physical disruption of primary defence barriers contributes to these infections, so too does a significant functional immunodeficiency [96–98]. Infections account for 30%–40% of mortality in ARF and are responsible for a disproportionately large number of deaths in younger patients with ARF [1, 99]. The litany of observed alterations in immune function in ARF include abnormalities in every component of the primary and secondary immune system.

ARF in the critically ill is associated with profound inhibition of leucocyte phagocytosis, a reduction in antibody production and a functional T cell deficiency (manifesting as cutaneous anergy, a decreased ability to reject skin allografts and a decreased response to viral challenge) [100, 101]. There may also be a temporary disappearance of established autoimmunity [96]. The molecular bases for these functional cellular deficiencies remain incompletely understood. Neutrophils demonstrate impaired chemotaxis, chemokinesis, adherence, oxidative function and glycolytic metabolism after phagocytosis in uraemia [102–105]. Macrophages also demonstrate impaired phagocytosis and Fc gamma receptor function [96, 103–106]. Haemodialysis triggers a phenotypic change in both neutrophils and monocytes/macrophages, with an ex vivo increase in leucocyte enzyme production, an increased expression of adhesion molecules (CD11/CD18), an increased cytokine generation and increased ex vivo reactive oxygen species production [105, 107–112]. Despite these indices of immunological stimulation following the introduction of renal replacement therapy, the in vivo functional immunodeficiency remains, albeit with some improvement in overall immune function [96, 102, 105, 113]. The failure to reverse the observed immunodeficiency with dialysis may indicate that other non-dialyzable humoral factors are substantive contributors to the functional immunodeficiency. Alternatively, the incomplete reversal may reveal some inadequacies of the renal replacement schedule, toxicities due to bioincompatibility or even the removal by dialysis of immunological stimulants.

Studies of critical illness per se would indicate that a broad variety of critical illness syndromes have discernable immunodeficiencies accompanying them, independent of the degree of renal impairment. The observed changes in immune function in critical illness, listed below, frequently mimic those reported in uraemia [114–131]:

- Impaired leucocyte phagocytosis
- Impaired leucocyte oxidative metabolism
- Impaired leucocyte glycolytic metabolism
- Reduced leucocyte chemotaxis and chemokinesis
- Reduced intracellular killing by phagocytes
- Deficient opsonic function
- Altered balance of TH1 and TH2 lymphocytes
- Cutaneous anergy
- Reduced skin allograft rejection
- Reduced antigen-presenting function of macrophages
- Reduced major histocompatibility complex (MHC) class II antigen presentation on macrophages
- Reduced T cell proliferative responses to mitogens
- Enhanced T suppressor function
- Diminished natural killer (NK) cell activity
- Reduced numbers of antigen-specific B cells
- Reduced mass of mucosal-associated lymphoid tissue
- Reduced antibody production by plasma cells
- Failure of secondary immune responses

Presumably many of these alterations in immune function are direct or indirect consequences of the activation of the inflammatory mediator cascade by critical illness, with the immune system effectively participating in mediation of a dysregulated state. A major future challenge will be to identify which of the multitude of immunological alterations in critically ill patients with ARF function are central to the observed functional immunodeficiency and to design therapies that redress this immunological compromise. At present, meticulous attention to the preservation of physical barrier defences, adequate dialysis and optimal nutritional support remain the cornerstones of therapy for the immunodeficiency of ARF. The role of prophylactic antibiotics, cytokine and CSF administration awaits more rigorous assessment of their clinical utility before gaining widespread acceptance.

Summary

ARF is often initiated by a reduction in effective renal blood flow. The maintenance phase of ARF and the return of renal function involve sequential pathophysiological processes that are substantially independent of renal blood flow. The processes set in train following an ischaemic renal insult initially perpetuate and enhance renal injury and eventually orchestrate recovery of renal function. The immune system is undoubtedly involved in the mediation of ARF injury, the maintenance of ARF and the recovery of renal function. It plays a particularly important role in the ARF accompanying critical illness, because of the primacy of the immune system in the inflammatory mediator cascade responsible for SIRS. A clinically significant immunodeficiency is evident in patients with ARF complicating critical illness. Both the mediation of the ARF syndrome and the observed immunocompromise are complex, heterogeneous, interdependent, multifactorial processes. This inherent complexity should not deter continuing efforts for dissection of these processes with a view to enhancing our understanding of their interactions and seeking measures which either prevent ARF, promote recovery of renal function or abrogate the accompanying immunological compromise.

References

1. Lazarus JM, Brenner BM (eds) (1993) Acute renal failure, 3rd edn. Churchill Livingstone, New York
2. Levinsky NG, Alexander EA (1976) Acute renal failure. In: Brenner BM, Rector JR (eds) The kidney. Saunders, Philadelphia, pp 806–814
3. Myers BD, Moran SM (1986) Haemodynamically mediated acute renal failure. N Engl J Med 314:97–105
4. Dixon BS, Anderson RJ (1985) Nonoliguric acute renal failure. Am J Kidney Dis 6(2):71–80
5. Jennette JC, Charles L, Falk RJ (1991) Antineutrophi/cytoplasmic autoantibodies: disease associations, molecular biology and pathophysiology. Int Rev Exp Pathol 32:193–221
6. Glauser MP, Zanetti G, Baumgartner JD, Cohen J (1991) Septic shock: pathogenesis. Lancet 138:732–739
7. Braquet P, Paubert-Braquet M, Bourgain R, Hosford D, Bussolino (1989) PAF/cytokine autogenerated feedback networks in microvascular immune injury. Consequences in shock, ischaemia and graft rejection. J Lipik Med 1:75–122
8. Dal Nogare AR (1991) Septic shock. Southwestern Internal Medicine Conference. Am J Med Sci 302:50–65
9. Koltai M, Hosford D, Braquet P (1992) The role of PAF and cytokines in microvascular tissue injury. J Lab Clin Med 19:461–466
10. Shapiro L, Gelfand JA (1993) Cytokines and sepsis: pathophysiology and therapy. New Horizons 1:13–22
11. Sole ZK (1993) The morphology of acute renal failure. In: Lazarus JM, Brenner BM (eds) Acute renal failure, 3rd edn. Churchill Livingston, New York, pp 33–51
12. Schreiner G, Harris KPG, Parkersen ML, Klahr S (1988) The immunological aspects of acute ureteral obstruction: characterization and kinetics of the immune cell infiltrate in the kidney. Kidney Int 34:487–493
13. Linas SL, Whittenberg D, Repine JE (1991) Role of neutrophil derived oxidants and elastase in LPS-mediated renal injury. Kidney Int 38:618–623
14. Klausner JM, Paterson IS, Goldman G, Kobzik L, Rodzen C, Lawrence R, Valeri CR, Shepro D, Hechtmann HB (1989) Postischaemic renal injury is mediated by neutrophils and leukotrienes. Am J Physiol 256:F794–F802
15. Hellberg POA, Kallskog TOK (1989) Neutrophil-mediated post-ischaemic tubular leakage in the rat kidney. Kidney Int 36:555–561
16. Willinger C, Schramek H, Pfaller K, Pfaller W (1992) Tissue distribution of neutrophils in post-ischaemic acute renal failure. Virchows Arch [B] 62:237–243
17. Paller MS, Hoidal JR, Ferris TF (1984) Oxygen free radicals in ischaemic acute renal failure in the rat. J Clin Invest 74:1156–1164

18. Bird JE, Mihhoan K, Wilson CB, Young SG, Mundy CA, Parthasarthy S, Blantz R (1988) Ischaemic acute renal failure and antioxidant therapy in the rat. J Clin Invest 81:1630–1638
19. Vedder NB, Fouty BW, Winn RK (1989) Role of neutrophils in generalized reperfusion injury associated with resuscitation from shock. Surgery 106:509–516
20. Tate RM, Repine JE (1983) Neutrophils and the adult respiratory distress syndrome. Am Rev Respir Dis 128:552–559
21. Harris PPG, Schreiner G, Klahr S (1989) Effect of leukocyte depletion on the function of the post-obstructed kidney in the rat. Kidney Int 36:210–215
22. Paller MS (1989) Effect of neutrophil-depletion on ischaemic renal injury in the rat. J Lab Clin Med 113:379–386
23. Thornton MA, Winn R, Alpers CE, Zager RA (1989) An evaluation of the neutrophil as a mediator of in-vivo renal ischaemia-reperfusion injury. Am J Physiol 135:509–519
24. Sims HH, D'Amico R (1991) Increased PMN CD11b/CD18 expression following post-traumatic ARDS. J Surg Res 50:362–367
25. Horgan MJ, Wright SD, Malik AB (1990) Antibody against leucocyte intergrin (CD18) prevents reperfusion-induced lung injury. Am J Physiol 259:L315–L319
26. Horgan MJ, Ge M, Gu J, Rothlein R, Malik AB (1992) Role of ICAM-1 in neutrophil-mediated lung vascular injury following reperfusion. Am J Physiol 261:H1578–H1584
27. Lo SK, Everitt JE, Gu J, Malik AB (1992) TNF mediates pulmonary oedema by ICAM-1 and CD-18 dependent mechanisms. J Clin Invest 89:981–1005
28. Goligorsky M, Lieberthal W, Racusen L, Simon E (1993) Integrin receptors in renal tubular epithelium: new insights into pathophysiology of acute renal failure. Am J Physiol 264:F1–F8
29. Galit J, Colflesh D, Rabiner I, Simone J, Goligorsky MS (1993) Redistribution and dysfunction of integrins in cultured renal epithelial cells exposed to oxidative stress. Am J Physiol 264:F149–F157
30. Goligorsky MS, DiBona GF (1993) Pathogenetic role of Arg-Gly-Asp recognizing integrins in acute renal failure. Proc Natl Acad Sci USA 90:5700–5704
31. Linas S, Wittenberg D, Parsons P, Repine J (1992) Mild renal ischaemia activates primed neutrophils to cause acute renal failure. Kidney Int 42:610–616
32. Schulman G, Fogo A, Gung A, Badr K, Hakim R (1991) Complement activation retards resolution of acute ischaemic renal failure in the rat. Kidney Int 40:1069–1074
33. Bone RC (1991) The pathogenesis of sepsis. Ann Intern Med 115:457–469
34. Wegmuller E, Montandon A, Nydegger U, Descoeudres C (1986) Biocompatibility of different hemodialysis membranes: activation of complement and leucopaenia. Int J Artif Organs 9:85–92
35. Hakim RM (1993) Clinical implications of hemodialysis membrane bioincompatibility. Kidney Int 44:484–494
36. Michalek SM, Moore RN, McGhee JR, Rosenstreich DL, Mergenhagen SE (1980) The primary role of lymphoreticular cells in the mediation of host responses to bacterial endotoxin. J Infect Dis 141:55–63
37. Tracy KJ, Lowry SF, Cerami A (1988) Cachectin/TNF in septic shock and septic adult respiratory distress syndrome. Am Rev Respir Dis 138:1377–1379
38. Bird GLA, Sheron N, Goka AKJ, Alexander FJ, Williams RS (1990) Increased plasma tumour necrosis factor in severe alcoholic hepatitis. Ann Intern Med 112:917–920
39. Levine B, Kalman J, Mayer L, Fillit HM, Packer M (1990) Elevated circulating levels of tumour necrosis factor in severe chronic heart failure. N Engl J Med 323:236–241
40. Kunkel SL, Remick DG, Strieter RM, Larrick JW (1989) Mechanisms that regulate the production and effects of tumour necrosis factor alpha. Crit Rev Immunol 1:439–447
41. Basha G, Meyer S, Kunkel SL, Strieter RM (1991) Presence of tumour necrosis factor in humans undergoing cardiopulmonary resuscitation with return of spontaneous circuation J Crit Care 6:185–189

42. Damas P, Reuter A, Gysen P, Demonty J, Lamy M, Franchimont P (1989) Tumour necrosis factor and interleukin-1 serum levels during severe sepsis in humans. Crit Care Med 17:975–978
43. Marano MA, Fong Y, Moldawer LL, Weitl, Calvano SE, Tracey KJ, Barie PS, Manogue K, Cerami A, Shires GT (1990) Serum cachectin/tumour necrosis factor in critically ill patients with burns correlates with infection and mortality. Surg Gynecol Obstet 170:32–38
44. Roten R, Markert M, Feihl F, Schaller MD, Tagan MC, Perret C (1991) Plasma levels of tumour necrosis factor in the adult respiratory distress syndrome. Am Rev Respir Dis 143:590–592
45. Tracey KJ, Cerami A (1993) Tumour necrosis factor: an updated review of its biology. Crit Care Med 21:S415–S422
46. Tracey KJ (1991) Tumour necrosis factor (cachectin) in the biology of septic shock syndrome. Circ Shock 35:123–128
47. Tracey KJ, Beutler B, Lowry SF, Merryweather J, Wolpe S, Milsark I, Hariri R, Fahey T, Zantella A, Albert J, Shires T, Cerami A (1986) Shock and tissue injury induced by recombinant human cachectin. Science 234:470–474
48. Remick DG, Kunkel RG, Larrick JW, Kunkel SL (1987) Acute in vivo effects of human recombinant tumour necrosis factor. Lab Invest 56:583–590
49. Ashkenazi A, Marsters SA, Capon DJ (1991) Protection against endotoxic shock by a tumour necrosis factor receptor immunoadhesion. Proc Natl Acad Sci USA 88:10535–10539
50. Tracey KJ, Fong Y, Hesse DG, Manogue KR, Lee AT, Kuo GC, Lowry S, Cerami A (1987) Anticachectin/TNF monoclonal antibodies prevent septic shock during lethal bacteraemia. Nature 330:662–664
51. Hinshaw L, Olson P, Kuo G (1989) Efficacy of post-treatment with anti-TNF monoclonal antibody in preventing the pathophysiology and lethality of sepsis in the in the baboon. Circ Shock 27:362–269
52. Emerson TE, Lindsey DC, Jesmok GJ (1992) Efficacy of monoclonal antibody against TNF in an endotoxaemic babaoon model. Circ Shock 38:75–84
53. Chung LY, Bienveniste EN (1990) Tumour necrosis factor production by astrocytes: induction by lipopolysaccaride, LFN gamma and IL1 beta. J Immunol 144:2999–3007
54. Jaattela M, Kuusela P, Saksela E (1988) Demonstration of tumour necrosis factor in human amniotic fluids and supernatants of placental and decidual tissues. Lab Invest 58:48–52
55. Ohno I, Tanno Y, Yamauchi K, Takishima T (1990) Production of tumour necrosis factor by mastocytoma P815 cells. Immunology 69:312–315
56. Gowen M, Chapman K, Littlewood A, Hughes D, Evans D, Russel G (1990) Production of tumour necrosis factor by human osteoblasts is modulated by other cytolines, but not by osteotrophic hormones. Endocrinology 126:1250–1255
57. Beutler B (1993) Endotoxin, tumour necrosis factor and related mediators: new approaches to shock. New Horizons 1:3–12
58. Tovey MG, Cantent J, Gresser I, Gugenheim J, Blanchard B, Guymarho J, Poupart P, Giopum, Shaw A, Fiers W (1988) Genes for IFN2 (IL-6), tumour necrosis factor and IL-1 are expressed at high levels in the organs of normal individuals. J Immunol 141: 3106–3110
59. Giroir BP, Brown T, Beutler B (1992) Constitutive synthesis of tumour necrosis factor in the thymus. Proc Natl Acad Sci USA 89:4864–4868
60. Giroir BP, Johnson JH, Brown T, Allen GL, Beutler B (1992) The tissue distribution of TNF biosynthesis during endotoxaemia. J Clin Invest 90:693–698
61. Keogh C, Fong Y, Marano MA, Seniuk S, He W, Barber A, Minei JP, Felsen D, Lowry SF, Moldawer LL (1990) Identification of a novel tumour necrosis factor/cachectin from the livers of burned and infected rats. Arch Surg 125:79–85

62. Cannon JG, Friedberg JS, Gelfand JA, Tompkins RG, Burke JF, Dinarello CA (1992) Circulating interleukin-1-beta and tumour-necrosis-factor-alpha concentrations after burn injury in humans. Crit Care Med 20:1414–1419
63. Zapata-Sirvent RL, Hansbrough JF, Cox MC, Carter WH (1992) Immunologic alterations in a murine model of haemorrhagic shock. Crit Care Med 20:508–517
64. Rinderknecht H (1988) Fatal pancreatitis: a consequence of excessive leucocyte stimulation? Int J Pancreatol 3:105–112
65. Cannon JG, Tompkins RG, Gelfand JA, Michie HR, Stanford GG, Vander Meer JW, Endres S, Lonnemann G, Chernoyw B (1990) Circulating interleukin-1 and tumour necrosis factor in septic shock and experimental endotoxin fever. J Infect Dis 161:79–84
66. Smith J, Urba W, Steis R (1990) Interleukin 1 alpha: results of a phase 1 toxicity and immunomodularity trial. Am Soc Clin Oncol 9:717
67. Dinarello CA (1984) Interleukin 1 and the pathogenesis of the acute phase response. N Engl J Med 311:1413–1418
68. Kaplan E, Dinarello C, Gelfand JA (1989) Interleukin-1 and the response to injury. Immunol Res 8:118–129
69. Okusawa S, Gelfand JA, Ikejima T, Connolly RJ, Dinarello CA (1988) Interleukin-1 induces a shock-like state in rabbits. Synergism with tumour necrosis factor and the effects of cycloxygenase inhibition. J Clin Invest 81:1162–1172
70. Ohlsson K, Bjork P, Bergenfeldt M, Hageman R, Thompson R (1990) Interleukin-1 receptor antagonist reduces mortality from endotoxic shock. Nature 348:550–552
71. Wakabayashi G, Gelfand JA, Burke JF, Thompson RC, Dinarello CA (1991) A specific receptor antagonist for interleukin-1 prevents Escherichia Coli-induced shock. FASEBJ 5:338–343
72. Fisher CJ Jr, Dhainaut JF, Pribble JP et al. (1993) A study evaluating the safety and efficacy of human recombinant interleukin-1 receptor antagonist in the treatment of patients with sepsis syndrome (Abstr). Clin Intensive Care 4:8S
73. Fischer CJ, Slotman GJ, Opal SM, Pribble JP, Bone R, Emmanuel G, Ng D, Bloedow DC, Catalano MA (1994) Initial evaluation of human recombinant interleukin-1 receptor antagonist in the treatment of sepsis-syndrome. A randomized, open-label, placebo-controlled multicentre trial. Crit Care Med 22:12–21
74. Tracey KJ, Lowry SF (1990) The role of cytokine mediators in septic shock. Adv Surg 23:21–56
75. Cohen S (1986) Physiologic and pathologic manifestations of lymphokine action. Hum Pathol 17:264–270
76. Ponce P, Cruz J, Travassos J, Moreira P, Oliveria J, Melo-Gomez E, Gouvera J (1993) Renal toxicity mediated by continuous infusion of recombinant interleukin 2. Nephron 64:114–118
77. Shalmi CL, Dutcher J, Feinfield D, Chun K, Saleemi K (1990) Acute renal dysfunction during interleukin-2 treatment. J Clin Oncol 8:1839–1846
78. Walker J, Cumming A, Lindsey R, Solez K, Linton A (1986) The renal response produced by non-hypotensive sepsis in a large animal model. Am J Kidney Dis 8:88–97
79. Toback G (1992) Regeneration after acute tubular necrosis. Kidney Int 41:226–246
80. Veis JH, Yamashita W, Liu YJ, Ooi BS (1990) The biology of mesangial cells in glomerulonephritis. Proc Soc Exp Biol Med 195:160–167
81. Weinberg JM (1991) The cell biology of ischaemic renal injury. Kidney Int 39:476–500
82. Kujubu DA, Fine LG (1989) Physiology and cell biology update: polypeptide growth factors and their relation to renal disease. Am J Kidney Dis 14:61–73
83. Humes HD, Cieslinski DA, Coimbra TM, Messana JM, Galvao C (1989) Epidermal growth factor enhances renal tubule cell regeneration and repair and accelerates the recovery of renal function in post-ischaemic acute renal failure in post-ischaemic acute renal failure. J Clin Invest 84:1757–1761

84. Reiss R, Funke AJ, Cieslinski DA, Humes MD (1990) Transforming growth factor-alpha accelerates renal repair and recovery following ischaemic injury to the kidney. Kidney Int 37:492
85. Safirstein R, Zelent AZ, Price PM (1989) Reduced renal prepro-epidermal-growth-factor mRNA and decreased EGF excretion in ARF. Kidney Int 36:810–815
86. Kon V, Yoshioka T, Fogo A, Ischikawa I (1989) Glomerular actions of endothelin in-vivo. J Clin Invest 83:1762–1767
87. Tolins JP, Vercellotti GM, Wilkowske M, Ha B, Jacobs HS, Raij L (1989) Role of platelet activating factor in endotoxemic acute renal failure in the male rat. J Lab Clin Med 113:316–324
88. McCord JM (1985) Oxygen-derived free radicals in post-ischaemic tissue injury. N Engl J Med 312:159–163
89. Henrich WL, Hamasaki Y, Said SL, Campbell WB, Cronin RE (1982) Dissociation of systemic and renal effects of endotoxemia. Prostaglandin inhibition uncovers an important role for renal nerves. J Clin Invest 69:691–699
90. Badr KF, Kelley VE, Rennke HG, Brenner BM (1986) Role for thromboxane A2 and leukotrienes in endotoxin-induced acute renal failure. Kidney Int 30:474–480
91. Hurland H, Augustin HJ, Engels T (1981) The influence of angiotensin II antagonists on postischaemic acute renal failure. Urol Int 36:15–22
92. Hansson R, Jonsson O, Lundstam S (1983) Effects of free radical scavengers on renal circulation after ischaemia in the rabbit. Clin Sci 65:605–610
93. Shaw SG, Weidemann P, Hodler J, Zimmermann A, Paternostro A (1987) Atrial natriuretic peptide protects against acute ischaemic renal failure in the rat. J Clin Invest 1987; 80:1232–1237
94. Lelcuk S, Alexander FA, Kobzik L, Valeri CR, Shepro D, Hechtman HB (1985) Prostacyclin and thromboxane A2 moderate post-ischaemic renal failure. Surgery 98: 207–212
95. Vadei K, Brunner LJ, Luke DR (1989) Effects of pentoxifylline in experimental acute renal failure. Kidney Int 36:466–470
96. Chatenoud L, Jungers P, Descamps-Latscha B (1994) Immunological considerations of the uraemic and dialyzed patient. Kidney Int 45 Suppl 44:S92–S96
97. Wilson WEC, Kirkpatrick CH, Talmage DW (1965) Suppression of immunological responsiveness in uraemia. Am Intern Med 62:1–12
98. Newberry WM, Sanford JP (1971) Defective cellular immunity in renal failure: depression of reactivity of lymphocytes to phytohaemagglutinin by renal failure serum. J Clin Invest 50:1262–1269
99. Mailloux LU, Bellucci AG, Wilkes BM, Napolitano B, Mossey RT, Lesser M, Bluestone PA (1991) Mortality in dialysis patients: analysis of the causes of death. Am J Kidney Dis 3:326–335
100. Dammin GJ, Couch NP, Murray JE (1957) Prolonged survival of skin homografts in uraemic patients. Ann NY Acad Sci 64:967–976
101. Montgomerie JZ, Kalmanson GM, Guze LB (1968) Renal failure and infection. Medicine (Baltimore) 47:1–14
102. Chatenoud L, Herbelin A, Beauran G, Descamps-Latscha B (1990) Immune deficiency of the uraemic patient. Adv Nephrol 19:259–274
103. Vanholder R, Ringoir S, Dhondt A, Hakim R (1991) Phagocytosis in uraemic and haemodialysis patients: a prospective and cross-sectional study. Kidney Int 39:320–327
104. Lewis SL, Van Epps DE (1987) Neutrophil and monocyte alterations in chronic dialysis patients. Am J Kidney Dis 9:381–395
105. Deschamps-Latshca B, Herbelin A (1993) Long term dialysis and cellular immunity: a critical review. Kidney Int 43 Suppl 41:S135–S142
106. Ruiz P, Gomez F, Schreiber AD (1990) Impaired function of macrophage FC-gamma receptors in end-stage renal disease. N Engl J Med 322:717–722

107. Himmelfarb J, Zaoui P, Hakim R (1992) Modulation of granulocyte LAM-1 and MAC-1 during dialysis – a prospective, randomized controlled trial. Kidney Int 41:388–395
108. Ritchey EE, Wallin JD, Shah SV (1981) Chemiluminescence and superoxide anon production by leucocytes from chronic haemodialysis patients. Kidney Int 19:349–358
109. Nguyen AT, Lethias C, Zingraff J, Herbelin A, Naret C, Descamps-Latcha B (1985) Haemodialysis membrane-induced activation of phagocyte oxidative metabolism detected in-vivo and in-vitro within microamounts of whole blood. Kidney Int 28:158–167
110. Tielemans CL, Delville JP, Husson CP, Madhoun P, Lambrechts AM, Goldman M, Vanherweghem JL (1993) Adhesion molecules and leucocyte common antigens on monocytes and granulocytes during haemodialysis. Clin Nephrol 39(3):158–165
111. Zaoui P, Hakim RM (1993) Natural killer-cell function in haemodialysis patients: effect of the dialysis membrane. Kidney Int 43:1298–1305
112. Vanholder R, Dell'Aquila R, Jacobs V, Dhont A, Veys N, Waterloss MA, Van Landschoot N, Van Biesen W, Ringoir S (1993) Depressed phagocytosis in haemodialysis patients: in-vivo and in-vitro mechanisms. Nephron 63(4):409–415
113. Tetta C, Camussi G, Mariano F, Triolo G, Vercellone A (1993) Immunomodulation and biomaterials. Biomater Artif Cells Immobil Biotechnol 21(2):253–265
114. Baxevanis CN, Papilas K, Dedoussis GV, Pavlis T, Papamichail M (1994) Abnormal cytokine serum levels correlate with impaired cellular immune responses after surgery. Clin Immunol Immunopathol 71:82–88
115. Quattrocchi KB, Frank EH, Miller CH, MacDermott JPA, Hein L, Frey L, Wagner FC Jr (1990) Suppression of cellular immune activity following severe head injury. J Neurotrauma 7:77–87
116. Salo M (1992) Effects of anaesthesia and surgery on the immune response. Acta Anaesthesiol Scand 36:201–220
117. Akiyoshi T, Koba F, Arinaga S, Miyazaki S, Wada T, Tsuji H (1985) Impaired production of IL2 after surgery. Clin Exp Immunol 59:745–749
118. Ertel W, Faist E, Salmen B, Huber P, Heberer G (1989) Influence of cyclooxygenase inhibition on interleukin-2 receptor expression after major trauma. Surg Res Commun 5:17–23
119. Livingston DH, Appel SH, Wellhausen SR, Sonnenfeld G, Polk HC Jr (1988) Depressed interferon gamma production and monocyte HLA-DR expression after severe injury. Arch Surg 123:1309–1312
120. Nishijima MK, Takezawa J, Hosotsubo KK, Takahashu H, Shimida Y, Yoshiya I (1986) Serial charges in cellular immunity in septic patients with multiple-organ system failure. Crit Care Med 14:87–91
121. Padova FD, Pozzi C, Tondrem J, Tritapepe R (1991) Selective and early increase in IL-1 inhibitors and IL-6 and cortisol after elective surgery. Clin Exp Immunol 85:137–142
122. Hack E, de Groot ER, Felt-Bersma JF, Nuijens JH, van Schijndel RJMS, Erenberg-Belmer AJM, Thijs LG, Aarden AL (1989) Increased plasma levels of interleukin 6 in sepsis. Blood 74:1704–1710
123. Prochazka M, Vyhnanek F, Jira SM, Strejcek J (1987) Effect of interleukin-2 on peripheral blood monoculear cells in severely injured patients. Acta Chir Scand 153:401–404
124. Dinarello CA, Gelfand JA, Wolff SM (1993) Anticytokine strategies in the treatment of the systemic inflammatory response syndrome. JAMA 269:1829–1835
125. Giroir BP (1993) Mediators of septic shock: new approaches for interrupting the endogenous inflammatory cascade. Crit Care 21:780–789
126. Abrahams E (1989) Host defense abnormalities after haemorrgage, trauma and burns. Crit Care Med 17:934–939
127. Abraham E, Freitas AA (1989) Haemorrhage produces abnormalities in lymphocyte function and lymphokine generation. J Immunol 142:899–906
128. Abraham E, Regan RF (1984) The effects of haemorrhage and trauma on interleukin-2 production. Arch Surg 120:1341–1345

129. Ayala A, Perrin MM, Chaudry H (1990) Defective macrophage antigen presentation following haemorrhage is associated with the loss of MHC Class II (Ia) antigens. Immunology 70:33–39
130. Kupper TS, Green DR (1984) Immunoregulation after thermal injury: sequential appearances of I-J positive, Ly-1 T suppressor-inducer and Ly-2 T suppressor-effector cells following thermal trauma in mice. J Immunol 135:3047–3053
131. Robinson A, Abraham E (1993) Effects of haemorrhage on bacterial antigen specific pulmonary plasma cell function. Clin Exp Immunol 88:124–128

Adequacy of Renal Replacement Therapy

C. Ronco and R. Bellomo

Basic Principles

An important issue for intensive care unit (ICU) patients with acute renal failure (ARF) is the adequacy of prescription and delivery of renal replacement therapy.

Individualization is generally done in an attempt to optimize renal replacement and to adjust the treatment dose to the size of the patient. In general, the parameter used is the volume of distribution of urea (i.e., total body water, TBW), since urea is employed as a marker molecule [1].

There are two major drawbacks to this approach: (1) TBW is frequently assumed to be 58% of body weight. This is unlikely to be the case in the critically ill. TBW may also be calculated or measured with bioimpedance, but these measurements are often inaccurate; (2) urea is taken as a reference molecule; however, other molecules are probably important and their volume of distribution can differ significantly. Thus, the therapy required for adequate blood purification for various molecules will also differ [2–7].

Current practice in ARF patients is based on experience from the area of chronic renal failure. In the chronic renal failure patient, we assume treatment to be adequate when the product of clearance × time (Kt) divided by TBW is 1 in a single session of dialysis and three sessions per week are performed. Adequacy is defined by low statistical risk of morbidity and mortality and by maintenance of uremic toxins within an "acceptable" range [1]. This biochemical and kinetic definition of adequacy is more popular in the USA than in Europe, where adequacy is seen more as a clinical, and general concept involving patient rehabilitation, correction of hypertension, and control of acidosis, overhydration, and other metabolic derangements [8].

In the acute patient, no criteria are yet available to define the adequacy of dialysis. We propose, however, that a combination of biochemical and clinical parametes should be used to guide renal replacement therapy. Such guidelines are necessary to compare the efficacy of different therapies and improve our understanding of how renal replacement therapy can increasingly approach its therapeutic goals. From the clinical and biochemical point of view the patient should be stable and maintained in balance in the following areas:

1. **Urea and protein metabolism.** Urea accumulation is a mirror of protein intake and catabolism, while urea removal is a mirror of the efficiency of blood purification.
2. **Clearance of other molecules.** It is known that various molecules may act as toxins or mediators of sepsis, and these molecules must be cleared adequately.
3. **Acid-base homeostasis.** Daily acid production is high in the critically ill and exceeds the amount of 1 mmol/kg per 24 h encountered in normal subjects. Acids are often infused parenterally (for example saline solution, Ca chloride etc). Such acids can be buffered either by buffer-containing dialysate or by replacement solutions which contain bicarbonate or other buffers [8].
4. **Electrolyte homeostasis.** The impact of parenteral nutrition, fluids, and medications must be counterbalanced by dialytic- or hemofiltration-based therapies.
5. **Body weight and hydration.** Since these patients are anuric, TBW should be maintained by the balance between extracorporeal ultrafiltration, extrarenal fluid losses, and fluid infusion. This must be done with maximal cardiovascular and respiratory stability.

Given these goals, for an adequate dialytic prescription and implementation of therapy, there are several factors that may induce a discrepancy between the prescription and true delivery of renal replacement therapy. A description of these factors will clarify why therapy prescription and delivery correlate only when continuous therapies are delivered, while intermittent treatments are unphysiologic and unlikely to achieve a delivery to prescription ratio of 1. In addition, while in the chronic patient a compromise is necessary to ensure the shortest period of time spent in dialysis by the patient (maximal rehabilitation is achieved when the patient is out of hospital), in the acute patient in the ICU, dialysis-free time is not needed, and treatment can be continuous, as is the case for normal renal function [9, 10].

Dialysis Delivery Versus Dialysis Prescription (High-Efficiency Dialysis)

Renal replacement therapy by hemodialysis seeks to achieve adequate blood purification from metabolic waste products, prevention and correction of electrolyte and acid-base disorders, and maintenance of dry body weight. Such aims must be obtained with the best level of clinical tolerance to treatment in order to effectively rehabilitate the patient [9].

Recent advances in technology have permitted the clinical application (in chronic renal failure) of highly efficient dialysis treatment with solute clearances and ultrafiltration rates that are significantly higher than those of standard hemodialysis. These developments have made reduction of dialysis treatment time possible without reducing the quantity of treatment delivered.

However, the successful application of high-efficiency therapy requires a comprehensive approach and a recognition of the underlying clinical principles and technical aspects of the extracorporeal circuit. Reduction of dialysis treatment time must take place without a parallel reduction in quantity of treatment. Therefore, in highly efficient treatments of short duration, the efficiency of treatment must be proportionally increased per unit of time. Furthermore, strict control must be exerted on the effective amount of treatment delivered per session.

In summary, the clinical application of high-efficiency treatment requires an accurate prescription of the quantity of therapy and the definition of reliable criteria to define treatment adequacy and the guidelines necessary to ensure that prescribed therapy is delivered. Morbidity and mortality will, of course, finally define whether treatment prescription and delivery were really adequate as initially hypothesized.

Guidelines for Prescription

Several approaches have been taken in the past to define adequacy of dialysis therapy. In a general sense, in the chronic renal failure patient, the treatment is considered adequate if uremic solutes are maintained within acceptable ranges in the presence of sufficient dietary protein intake and if the interdialytic weight gain is corrected with the lowest possible incidence of side effects. These requirements are somewhat narrow and simplistic and may not apply to acutely ill patients. They are time independent and therefore treatment time may be adapted to the solute removal (clearance) and the ultrafiltration capacity of the dialyzer. Since highly efficient treatments are now available and clearance and ultrafiltration no longer represent limiting factors, the treatment time must be set according to the patient's cardiovascular tolerance to fluid withdrawal per unit of time and to the speed of solute equilibration between the different compartments of the body. When similar results are to be obtained in the acute patient, short treatment time is not a primary requirement and 24-h treatments can be scheduled.

The clinical application of renal replacement therapies both in the acute and chronic patient with renal failure thus requires accurate prescription of the quantity of therapy, practical recommendations regarding the implementation of the clinical dialysis procedure, and guidelines to ensure that prescribed therapy has actually been delivered, achieving the desired clinical results.

Treatment Prescription Models

Several approaches have been suggested in the past to define a common view for dialysis adequacy and therefore for therapy prescription.

Babb et al. [11] proposed the *square meter/hour and dialysis index model* in 1971 to define the amount of dialysis required. The dialysis index (DI) was obtained and defined by the sum of the dialyzer clearance of vitamin B_{12} plus the patient's residual renal function, normalized per body surface area. According to Babb's DI, the amount of weekly dialysis clearance plus residual renal clearance should be about 30 l in a normal-size patient.

In 1972, Kjellestrand et al. [12] proposed a different index, *Nkj*, to approach dialysis quantification, based on the product of clearance and treatment time divided by body weight. They pointed out that the concentration of urea at the end of the dialysis session was exponentially correlated with the initial concentration by a factor including the product clearance × time and the solute distribution space.

Teschan et al. [13] proposed a similar *index for urea* in 1977. According to this index, the ratio between the volume of cumulative urea clearance per week (dialysis plus residual renal function) and the volume of TBW had to equal a value of 3 in order to achieve blood purification comparable to 10% of the normal glomerular filtration rate (GFR) and sufficient to maintain the patient in a stable metabolic state.

The American National Cooperative Dialysis Study [14] demonstrated that the probability of high morbidity and treatment failure was related to patients' blood urea nitrogen (BUN) levels. The mechanistic analysis of this study proposed a domain map of dialysis prescription (clearance × time) based on daily protein intake, midweek predialysis BUN, and the patient's TBW. Prescription was defined with an index called Kt/V, where K is the dialyzer clearance in ml/min, t is the treatment time, and V is the patient's TBW (assuming an equal value for the urea distribution space). Patients with a Kt/V of 1 or more per dialysis session had low morbidity and mortality, and the probability of treatment failure was lower compared to patients with a Kt/V of less than 1 [15].

In the acute patient, the higher degree of catabolism together with the critical illness of the patients call for a more efficient degree of blood purification and a specifically designed form of renal support. We have noted, for instance, that a better survival rate correlates with higher amounts of ultrafiltration per day. This leads us to the hypothesis that when the volume of daily ultrafiltration approaches that of TBW, efficient blood purification is achieved even in the most hypercatabolic patient.

Is it possible to describe an adequacy index for acute patients? A description of the actual adequacy indexes for the chronic patient is necessary in order to familiarize the reader with the terms and then to provide a description of a possible approach to the concept of dialytic adequacy in the acute patient.

Urea Kinetic Modeling and Formulas to Calculate Kt/V *in Intermittent Treatments*

Urea kinetic models are based on the assumption that residual renal function is absent and urea generation during treatment is negligible. (It is important to note that neither may apply in the ICU). In the presence of low ultrafiltration, the concentration of urea at the end of a single dialysis session (C_t) will depend on the inital concentration (C_o) and the treatment efficiency (Kt/V):

$$C_t = C_o e^{-Kt/V}$$

where K is clearance in ml/min, t is time on dialysis in min, and V is the volume of TBW in l.

This equation defines the postdialytic urea concentration as a function of the fractional clearance of urea distribution space [16]. Accordingly the following equations can be derived:

$$Kt/V = \text{Ln}(C_o/C_t)$$

$$K = \text{Ln}(C_o/C_t) \times Vt$$

$$V = Kt/\text{Ln}\ (C_o/C_t)$$

where Ln is natural logarithm.

These simple equations permit the evaluation at the bedside of either the value of Kt/V or the overall clearance of the treatment. According to a simple mathematical calculation, when $Kt/V = 1$, the final pool of urea will be 37% of the initial pool. In the original urea kinetic model, Gotch [16] defined K_d or the dialyzer clearance as a necessary input in order to derive other parameters G (urea generation) and V (distribution volume). When a value of V different from that expected is obtained, errors in dialysis delivery can be suspected. This can also be the case when V is utilized as the initial input. Assuming a certain V according to anthropometric tables [17], the initial pool of urea can be established ($C_o \times V_o$). Once variations of V during dialysis have been defined, the final pool will be measurable from the final urea concentration ($C_t \times V_t$). In this case the overall clearance achieved in a single session will be described.

The various formulas proposed to calculate Kt/V at the bedside are shown in Table 1 [18–23]. All these formulas may introduce some errors in the calculation of Kt/V and therfore the value found in a single dialysis session has to be critically evaluated and matched with the expected efficiency of the treatment.

In the acute patient treated with continuous therapy, the Kt/V calculation is much easier because of the continuous treatment and because of the possibility of exact body clearance and not just extracorporeal clearance achieved by the system.

There is now a general consensus that, in the chronic patient, weekly dialysis prescription in l urea clearance, should be three times the patient's

Table 1. Formulas to calculate Kt/V at the bedside

Reference	Formula	Comments
Lowrie [18]	$Kt/V = \mathrm{Ln}(C_o/C_t)$	Neglects the urea generation rate (G) during treatment and possible variations of V due to ultrafiltration and residual renal function (K_r)
Jindal et al. [19]	$Kt/V = (0.04 \times \mathrm{PUR\%}) - 1.2$	Also takes Qf, G, and K_r to be zero; since urea concentration is measured in whole blood and not in plasma water, this calculation leads to an overestimation of about 15%
Barth [20]	$Kt/V = (C_o - C_t)C_{mid}$	K_r, G, and Qf are taken as zero
Daugirdas [23]	$Kt/V = -\mathrm{Ln}((C_t/C_o) - 0.03 - (\mathrm{UF} \times t/w)$	$K_r = 0$ and G is constant (0.03). Required inputs are C_o and C_t and the ratio UF/W (total ultrafiltration/dry body weight)
Calzavara et al. [21]	$Kt/V = (C_o - C_t)/((C_o + C_t)/2)$	Simplification of a formula proposed by Barth, since C_{mid} is calculated approximately
Keshaviah et al. [34]	$Kt/V = 1.162 \times \mathrm{Ln}(C_o/C_t)$	Permits the calculation of Kt/V and normalized PCR thanks to the specific nomogram; in this case UF is considered to be a fixed value (15 ml/min), while G and K_r are neglected

K, dialyzer clearance in ml/min; t, treatment time; V, patient's total body water; C_o, initial urea concentration; C_t, urea concentration after single dialysis session; PUR%, percentage urea reduction ratio = $((C_o - C_t)/C_o) \times 100$; C_{mid}, blood urea nitrogen (BUN) concentration at midtreatment time; Ln, natural logarithm; PCR, protein catabolic rate.

urea distribution space or TBW. This means an average of 126 l clearance per week in a 70-kg patient or 144 l in an 80-kg patient. This value must take into account the residual renal function. This concept holds for a standard 4-hour dialysis treatment, while the value must be increased in highly efficient short treatments (average treatment duration, 150–180 min). In this cases the Kt/V index must be increased up to 1.4–1.5 [24]. In acute hypercatabolic patients treated with daily intermittent hemodialysis, a minimim Kt/V of 1 per daily session is generally required.

In the acute patient treated with continuous treatments, a Kt/V of 0.7–0.8/day is sufficient for most patients [25]. Higher values may be required in specific patients with hypercatabolic states, poor solute equilibration between body compartments (cardiopulmonary recirculation), or severe cardiovascular instability. In these cases a Kt/V of 1 per day is only apparently at this level, because the actual volume of distribution to which the treatment had access may in reality be smaller [10].

Finally', it should be noted that this concept of adequacy is substantially biochemical. A true index should include other aspects of dialytic therapy such as fluid, electrolyte, and acid-base balance as well as hemodynamic stability. Urea represents a good marker for adequacy of blood purification, but it does not represent the whole meaning of chronic renal replacement therapy.

Problems Related to Intermittent Treatments

Once agreement on the concept of adequacy of dialysis has been reached, prescription for blood purification must be made by determining the optimal product of efficiency × time. The same dialytic dose (for example 48 l clearance per treatment in an 80-kg patient) can be delivered both with a low clearance over a rather long time period (200 ml/min × 240 min) or with a higher clearance in a shorter time (270 ml/min × 180 min).

While the arithmetical product of the above-mentioned approaches is the same, when short, highly efficient treatments are planned, some technical requirements must be fulfilled and the patient's clinical and pathophysiologic state must be considered to avoid overestimation of the delivered dialytic dose. To achieve better clearances, several dialysis treatment parameters must be adjusted to a higher operational level. There is, for example, a linear correlation between blood flow and urea clearance in hemodialysis over a wide range of values. The function reaches a plateau at different levels according to the dialyzer surface area. The maximal efficiency achievable in a given dialyzer corresponds to the product Ko*A*, where *A* is the dialyzer surface area and Ko is the mass transfer coefficient of urea. For example blood flows higher than 300 ml/min and dialyzers with a surface area larger than 1.3 m^2 must be used to achieve significantly higher clearances and highly efficient treatments.

When the urea clearance is higher thant 150 ml/min, acetate must also be replaced with bicarbonate in order to prevent a massive loss of CO_2 that will not be compensated for by acetate backdiffusion from the dialysate [8].

When high blood flows are utilized, large needles should be employed in order to reduce the pressure variation inside the extracorporeal circuit, and frequent calibration of the blood pump becomes necessary [26–28]. These problems are aggravated by higher hematocrits, since the resistance of the venous needle to blood flow may cause a significant increase in hydrostatic pressure inside the dialyzer, resulting in high ultrafiltration rates (whose values are dependent on the membrane utilized). The use of machines with ultrafiltration control systems is strongly advised. Increases in dialysate flow rates to up to 800 ml/min can be achieved with modern dialysis machines, although this parameter is not as critical for efficiency as blood flow. In such cases, however, the accuracy of mixing, degassing, and heating and the microbiological purity of the dialysate must be carefully checked [29, 30].

Nurses must be aware that errors in procedure or a temporary reduction in blood pump speed may result in a significant decrease in the amount of delivered treatment and therefore cause treatment failure.

All these technical requirements are important in achieving efficient blood purification, but several other factors may interfere with the accuracy of dialysis delivery and may reduce the amount of treatment given compared to the prescribed dose.

Factors Affecting Treatment Delivery and *Kt/V* Estimation

As previously mentioned, a number of factors may be responsible for underdialysis in patients undergoing highly efficient treatments. These factors are responsible for incorrect estimations of the *Kt/V* index, resulting in a treatment delivery which is only apparently adequate.

Kt/V may be incorrectly calculated because of errors in the evaluation of urea clearance, real treatment time, and total body water. Urea clearance is frequently assumed to be constant throughout the treatment and equal to the values reported by the industry for a given dialyzer. This is a major source of error, and direct clearance measurements are strongly recommended in the dialysis routine.

Furthermore, we must consider that clearance measurements in the extracorporeal circuit made with the classical formulas, both from the blood and the dialysate, only describe a phenomenon occurring in the dialyzer and poorly describe what is happening in the patient's body. In other words, we must distinguish the extracorporeal clearance measured at the dialyzer level from the overall treatment clearance which is measured from the final effects achieved in the patient at the end of the dialysis session.

Factors Affecting Extracorporeal Clearance

The extracorporeal clearance value k is extemporarily measured at a given moment of the treatment and is not a stable function throughout the entire length of the session. Clearance is commonly measured by the following formulas:

$$K = Q_{\mathrm{bi}} \times \frac{C_{\mathrm{bi}} - C_{\mathrm{bo}}}{C_{\mathrm{bi}}} + Q_{\mathrm{f}} \times \frac{C_{\mathrm{bo}}}{C_{\mathrm{bi}}} = Q_{\mathrm{di}} \times \frac{C_{\mathrm{do}} - C_{\mathrm{di}}}{C_{\mathrm{bi}}} + Q_{\mathrm{f}} \times \frac{C_{\mathrm{do}}}{C_{\mathrm{bi}}}$$

$$= \frac{Q_{\mathrm{do}} \times C_{\mathrm{do}}}{C_{\mathrm{bi}}}$$

where C is concentration, b is blood, d is dialysate, i is inlet, o is outlet, Q is flow rate, and f is filtrate and a precise measurement requires a mass balance error lower than 5%. Clearance in this case is influenced by several factors, which are summarized below.

Extracorporeal Blood Flow Rate

It has been demonstrated that mature, well-functioning arteriovenous fistulas can provide blood flows up to 600 ml/min. The increase in blood flow rate, however, must take into account some aspects peculiar to the extracorporeal circuit. Arterial line and needle provide remarkable resistance, creating a negative pressure in the blood tubing prior to the blood pump [26, 27]. The value of such pressure is proportional to the blood flow, hematocrit, blood viscosity, and needle size. When blood flows up to 500 ml/min are utilized, the pressure in this segment may reach values of about −300 mmHg. This pressure may negatively affect the accuracy of the blood pump, leading to an overestimation of the blood flow really delivered. This aspect leads to overestimation of dialyzer clearance if clearance is calculated on the basis of programmed blood flow. Periodic accurate calibration of the blood pump and pressure measurements in the circuit are therefore useful to avoid such errors in clearance measurements.

The importance of slightly higher blood flows, and therefore the substitution of continuous arteriovenous hemofiltration (CAVH) with continuous venovenous hemofiltration (CVVH) has been demonstrated in several cases. The rates of ultrafiltration are stable and the permeability of the membrane is better if a lower filtration fraction is achieved in the filter. This reduces the magnitude of the concentration polarization phenomenon due to protein cake formation and eliminates the condition of filtration pressure equilibrium that leads to easy filter clotting.

Extracorporeal Recirculation

One important cause of overestimation of treatment delivery is related to the amount of extracorporeal blood recirculation. Recirculation is the fractional amount of blood entering the arterial line that originates from the venous line returning to the circulation from the dialyzer. Higher blood flows may provoke higher amounts of recirculation, and recirculation may affect the overall treatment dose. When recirculation exceeds 15%, the final treatment delivered may be 10% lower than that originally prescribed. For this reason frequent measurements of blood recirculation using the stop-flow technique are strongly recommended. In highly efficient treatments, the classical technique using the controlateral arm vein as a peripheral blood sample may not be accurate, since BUN equilibration between different districts of the body may not have occurred. We will discuss later in this paper the impact of intracorporeal distribution of the blood and its possible recirculation inside systemic vasculature.

Dialysate Flow Rate

Dialysate flow rates have been maintained at 500 ml/min for a long time. The use of high-surface area dialyzers and higher blood flows has permitted the useful increment of dialysate flow rates to 800 ml/min or more, with a significant increase in dialysis efficiency. As in the case of blood flow, dialysate flow rate must be accurately checked to avoid an overestimation of the real delivery. High pressure in the circuit as well as limitations imposed by the heating system, degassing procedures, and dialysate mixing may sometimes significantly reduce the dialysate flow rate actually delivered and/or the quality of the dialysis fluid. Recently developed machines have been equipped with appropriate systems to make a real increase in dialysate flow rate possible. In case of high dialysate flow rates, the distribution of dialysate in the dialysate path may sometimes be limited to parts of the fiber bundle without a complete uniform utilization of the exchange surface area available. In these cases the observed efficiency will be lower than that expected. In continuous hemodialysis, the dialysate flow is maintained between 10 and 100 ml/min, and this reduces at minimum the above problems.

Ultrafiltration Volumes

Ultrafiltration volumes clearly affect the efficiency of both intermittent and continuous treatments. In particular in hemofiltration, where the ultrafiltrate to plasma concentration ratio for solutes is 1, the clearance value equals the ultrafiltration rate.

It should be noted that solute extraction is proportional to the product (clearance × plasma concentration): in rapid treatments plasma concentrations rapidly fall and clearance is acting on a blood extremely poor in solutes. Therefore, high filtration rates in intermittent hemofiltration only remove high quantity of solutes in the first few minutes, but in the long run, if solutes do not equilibrate from tissues into the blood, the efficiency is reduced. In continuous treatments, ultrafiltrate volumes are lower or similar depending on the technique of choice; however, the removal of solutes is much higher because the plasma concentrations are at constant levels and a continuous intravascular refilling constantly occurs. Therefore, urea and other toxins generated are rapidly distributed into the whole TBW, and the volume to which the treatment has access is the body water of the patient.

Ultrafiltration Control Systems

The use of high flow rates and highly permeable dialyzers in short, intermittent treatments necessitate ultrafiltration control systems in order to avoid uncontrolled patient weight loss. Some of these systems, however, may cause a small amount of dialysate recirculation or intermittent delivery of dialysate. These aspects must be considered as a possible source of reduction in the final treatment efficiency. On the other hand the rise in dialysate pressure to achieve ultrafiltration control produces significant amounts of backfiltration. This aspect must be taken into account when a complete evaluation of treatment biocompatibility is carried out [29–31].

Filter Permeability and Clearance

The use of large, highly permeable dialyzers has permitted ultrafiltration rates and clearances significantly higher than those achieved in the past with standard cellulosic dialyzers. Therefore, the interdialytic fluid gain can be removed from the patient in a shorter period of time with an effective reduction of dialysis treatment time and no reduction in the amount of blood purification. Fluid withdrawal rate, however, must be adapted to the clinical tolerance of the patient. The amount of ultrafiltration can be equal to the patient's fluid gain or it can be in excess of it, as in the case of highly convective therapies (hemofiltration or hemodiafiltration). In these cases reinfusion of replacement solutions is required. As a compromise, in high-flux dialysis, highly convective transport takes place in the proximal side of the dialyzer, but fluid balance is maintained thanks to a significant amount of backfiltration in the distal part of the dialyzer. In all these cases, the concentration polarization phenomenon due to high ultrafiltration rates may lead to a significant protein cake formation at the blood–membrane interface, thus reducing the permeability of the membrane. This phenomenon, together with a possible clotting of groups of fibers and reduction of the effective surface area of the dialyzer, may lead to a significant reduction in clearance throughout the length of the dialysis session. Therefore, the average clearance during the session will be lower than that expected under ideal conditions. This aspect must be considered in continuous therapies when the filter is in use for long periods of time.

Clearance might also be influenced at the beginning of a session by washing and rinsing procedures. Trapping of air bubbles inside the fiber bundle or inside groups of hollow fibers may significantly reduce the effective exchange surface area for several minutes at the beginning of the session. When reuse procedures are utilized, the permeability of the reprocessed dialyzer cannot be precisely foreseen and accurate measurements are needed.

Finally, we must consider the possibility of variation of performance from one filter to another, depending on assembly and sterilization procedures.

Accuracy of Nursing Procedures

The role of nurses in the accurate delivery of the prescribed dialytic dose is critical. The continuous monitoring of the dialysis machine, with early corrections of possible problems occurring in the extracorporeal circulation, permits safe and continuous maintenance of the scheduled efficiency. Any temporary reduction of blood flow rate, dialysate flow rate, or ultrafiltration rate may produce a significant reduction in the filter performance and in the final average efficiency. In such cases, the amount of time lost during treatment must be added at the end of the session with a critical evaluation of the effective efficiency delivered during treatment. It is clear that the percentual impact of errors or complications occurring in short dialysis treatments will be significantly higher compared to that observed in standard dialysis treatments [10].

Factors Affecting Overall Treatment Efficiency

As above mentioned, the ideal condition of efficiency is achieved when the scheduled value of extracorporeal clearance is maintained constant for the entire length of the dialysis session and the desired amount of body water is completely cleared. It must be observed, however, that several factors may contribute to a potential reduction of this overall efficiency of treatment or to an erroneous calculation of the volume cleared in a given session.

Overall clearance is generally calculated from the percentage reduction in urea concentration during the dialysis session. Some factors, however, may contribute to an artificially high ratio of C_t to C_0 and to a significant overestimation of treatment efficiency.

We have already described the possibility of error using the dialyzer clearance K_d as a fixed input. This may lead to a false value of $K \times t$ and to a nonreliable calculation of the treatment efficiency.

We have also described the potential error due to an imprecise definition of the time spent by the patient on dialysis. This parameter is frequently overestimated and the final efficiency will therefore be overestimated as well. The accuracy of nursing procedures is a critical factor for the effective delivery of the scheduled treatment time.

V can also be a source of error, since anthropometric tables do not precisely define the patient's TBW [17]. In acutely ill patients who have received fluid resuscitation, TBW estimates are particularly inaccurate. In addition, studies carried out with bioimpedance have demonstrated the high variability of the percentual water content of the body from one patient to another. The volume apparently cleared as determined by the ratio of C_t to C_0 may be an overestimate and may often require correction by taking into account the postdialysis urea concentration rebound.

Using the C_t to C_0 ratio, we may find two conditions in which the calculated treatment efficiency is different from the expected one. In one case, C_t to C_0 is lower than expected and this can be due to significant extracorporeal recirculation, to poor dialyzer performance, or to a treatment duration shorter than the time scheduled. In the other case, we may observe a lower than expected postdialysis urea concentration and then remarkable concentration rebound a few minutes after dialysis. This suggests that the achievement of the total number of liters of clearance prescribed may be limited by the slow transport and equilibration of solutes between body compartments.

Urea kinetics has been studied with single-pool models in standard hemodialysis, showing a good correlation between estimated urea distribution space and liters of body water cleared. In high-efficiency hemodialysis, most of the urea removal is achieved in the first hour of treatment, followed by a plateau. Such behavior, confirmed by a significant rebound in plasma urea concentration after treatment (20%–30% after 30 min), demonstrates that single-pool analysis is inaccurate in high-efficiency treatments [27]. Therefore, the effective limitation to the achievement of the prescribed amount of clearance per treatment in liters is likely secondary to slow equilibration between different body compartments and an apparently smaller urea distribution space. Although the treatment achieves a high instantaneous clearance, solutes have limited access to the blood entering the dialyzer because of slow equilibration and removal from compartments different from the fraction of blood entering the extracorporeal circuit. For this reason the value of instantaneous clearance cannot be extrapolated to the overall clearance achieved during treatment, and different methods must be utilized to determine the effective amount of clearance (in l) delivered.

A possible explanation for this phenomenon is that remarkable resistance to solute transfer exists among different compartments or that systemic blood flow is nonuniform during dialysis (intracorporeal recirculation).

It has been demonstrated by Colton [32] that transcellular equilibration of urea is faster than that of other solutes and takes place within a few minutes or seconds. We have also observed a rapid equilibration of urea from the intracellular space into the extracellular fluid (Fig. 1). Therefore, it is unlikely that the transcellular mass transfer coefficient represents an effective limitation for solute equilibration or plays a role in the rebound phenomenon. Other mechanisms might be proposed, and we favor the hypothesis of a "functional" rather than "anatomic" resistance to urea equilibration in the body (Fig. 2).

Some patients tolerate ultrafiltration rates up to 0.7 ml/min per kg body weight (i.e., 3000 ml/h in a 70-kg patient), but the average patient presents with symptomatic hypotensive episodes during treatment when ultrafiltration exceeds 0.5 ml/min per kg [33]. Studies on patients' intravascular refilling made by on-line hemoglobin concentration measurements have shown that when plasma volume is reduced below 20% of normal, hypotension occurs unless ultrafiltration is stopped and intravascular refilling from the interstitial space is allowed. Some patients are "faster refillers" than others, and this might be related to myocardial efficiency and circulatory compensation. It is clear, however, that during treatment a significant vasoconstriction will occur in some areas of the body with a remarkable fall in tissue perfusion.

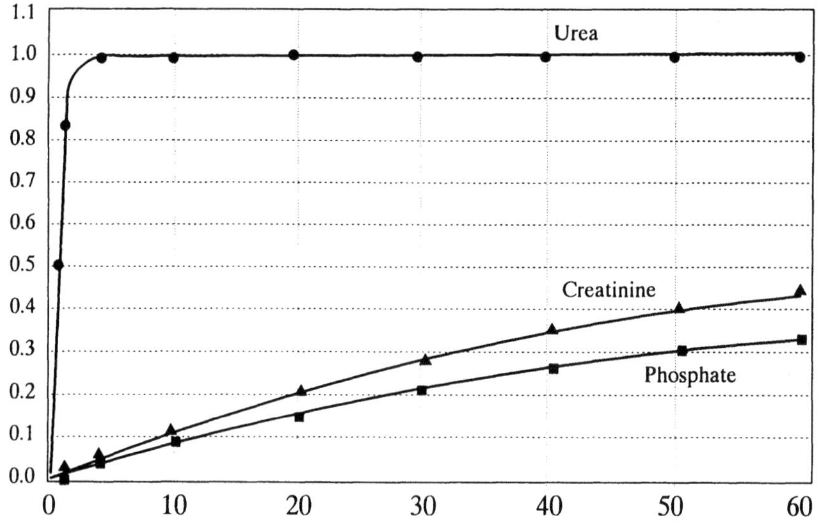

Fig. 1. Equilibration times for different solutes from the intracellular compartment to the extracellular compartment (uremic red cells)

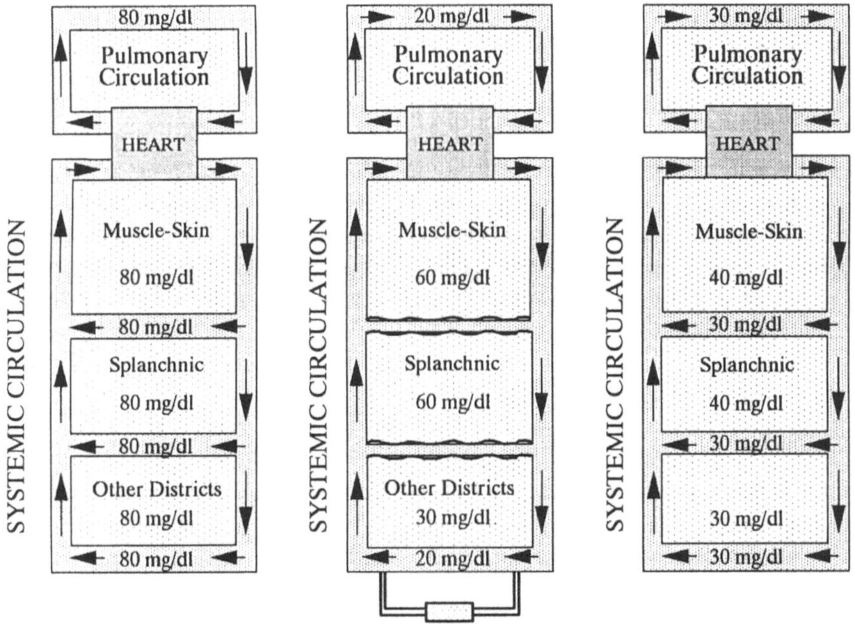

Fig. 2. Circulation before (*left*), during (*middle*), and after (*right*) hemodialysis. Before dialysis all compartments have the same concentration of urea nitrogen. During dialysis urea nitrogen concentration falls inside the intravascular space, while it is maintained at higher levels in poorly perfused areas. The insufficient perfusion is also worsened by sympathetic stimuli that create a further vasoconstriction in some areas. After dialysis these stimuli diminish and urea nitrogen is drained at higher speeds from the previously sequestrated compartments. The result is a postdialysis rebound in concentration

Such a phenomenon will obviously be much greater in the critically ill patient and will lead to a limited drainage of urea from such compartments as the muscles or splanchnic territory. The final result will be a disequilibrium between plasma and tissue concentration, with artificially low concentrations in systemic blood. As long as this blood is not refilled with urea from poorly perfused areas, the volume cleared will appear artificially low.

After dialysis, when the vasoconstricting stimuli are diminished and further time has elapsed, tissues are further perfused and a larger drainage of urea takes place from the areas previously excluded from the systemic circulation. This leads to a remarkable rebound in urea concentration. Our clinical observations led us to conclude that in patients with dialytic intolerance and cardiovascular instability, this mechanism is more important and the volume cleared is artificially low with apparently high *Kt/V* values (in these patients the postdialysis rebound can reach values of up to 50%–60%). Treatment time and efficiency must therefore be adapted to the clinical tolerance to ultrafiltration during treatment. When treatment time is reduced below 180 min, a *Kt/V* value of 1 may not be sufficient to guarantee efficient blood purification.

Continuous Versus Intermittent Treatments

From this analysis of the factors influencing dialysis delivery versus dialysis prescription, we conclude that materials, nursing procedures, and treatment time must be accurately checked and standardized in order to achieve the desired level of efficiency. In intermittent treatments, however, several factors interfere with a correct delivery of the prescribed therapy. In continuous treatments, a lower efficiency is needed to achieve similar goals.

With CAVH-CVVH, weekly urea *Kt/V* is in the range of 4–5, while with daily hemodialysis weekly *Kt/V* generally ranges from 7 to 8. The question arises as to why a lower *Kt/V* is adequate in continuous therapies, but not for intermittent daily dialysis.

In the critically ill patient with ARF, the removal of urea nitrogen follows various pathways and may be distributed in variable amounts among such elimination routes. In addition to renal losses, urea nitrogen is lost in the stool, breath, and sweat. Due to constantly slightly higher plasma levels in continuous therapies, these alternative pathways of urea loss may become more important. It is evident that residual renal function may strongly affect the capacity of urea nitrogen elimination in a given patient. The lower percentage removal of urea nitrogen observed in the ultrafiltrate or dialysate of patients with residual renal function is dependent on the fixing of the blood concentration at a lower level, and it is compensated by the elimination of the solute in the urine. According to this observation, the efficiency index should be $K_{pr}t/V$, as proposed by Gotch [5], where K_{pr} represents the overall dialytic and renal clearance.

It should also be remembered that hemofiltration is more physiologic than dialysis, since it creates isotonic ultrafiltration that can hardly be achieved in dialysis even with high sodium. In dialysis, a rapid fall in plasma osmolality may create a water shift into the cells with a consequent reduction of the circulating volume greater than the scheduled on the basis of the ultrafiltration programmed; diuresis is consequently frequently suppressed just after the first session of intermittent dialysis. Clearly the time of application is a major factor in determining adequacy, and when continuous therapies are used the total amount of urea removed over 1 week may be a more appropriate way of assessing blood purification than Kt/V.

Thus, equal scales cannot be used for different treatments. It is evident that clearance (K) per se does not represent the real efficiency of the treatment, describing only the instantaneous ratio between the solute removal and its concentration in the blood entering the system. Only when the clearance value is multiplied by the time in which that clearance is applied to the patient does the result obtained offer a reliable measure of the obtained blood purification. Therefore, while instantaneous clearance K (10–15 ml/min in CAVH, 200–300 ml/min in hemodialysis, HD) represents the efficiency of the dialytic system at a given moment, the product Kt gives the number of liters of blood cleared by the dialytic treatment in a given period. Finally, if we normalize this product according to the volume of distribution of the studied solute in the body, we will achieve a fractional clearance value that represents the ratio between the liters of clearance obtained and the liters that should be cleared in the body (Kt/V).

We could also consider the overall amount of urea removed from the body by the treatment. However, to make two different treatments comparable, this parameter must assume identical volumes of distribution for the solute, similar predialysis blood levels, and similar rates of ultrafiltration. Since clearance can also be considered as the ratio between solute removal over time and the solute concentration in blood (plasma for the solutes confined to the extracellular fluid), the rate of removal (R) can therefore be identified by the formula

$$R \text{ (mg/min)} = K \text{ (ml/min)} \times P \text{ (mg/ml)}$$

While in CAVH clearance and removal are proportional and linearly correlated since the solute concentration in blood is constant, in hemodialysis this may not be the case, since the solute concentraion in blood declines exponentially during treatment. Therefore, in hemodialysis, the removal rate is maximal at the beginning of the treatment, while it is much lower at the end of the session. In such a condition the efficiency of the system characterizes the profile of concentration of the solute in blood during treatment, and the solute concentration at the end of the session will be governed by the formula

$$C_t = C_o \times e^{(-Kt/V)}$$

where C_t is the final concentration of the solute in blood after dialysis, C_o is the concentration at the beginning, and *Kt/V* is the exponential term representing the fractional clearance. However, while identical *Kt* products lead to equal amounts of clearance in the patient, they do not necessarily lead to identical amounts of solute removal. The decline in concentration of the solute in blood may be different according to the different efficiency of the system. Similar *Kt* products may produce different amounts of solute removal. For example, as the time is reduced, the solute mass transfer between body compartments may be too low to permit a complete equilibration. Therefore, as previously argued, when time is short and clearance is high, the treatment may not have access to the real volume of distribution of the solute and an apparently smaller volume is cleared. In such a condition, a sudden decrease in blood concentration is observed after a short time from the beginning of the session, and even high clearances will only remove small amounts of solute [34]. This may partially explain why intermittent treatments such as hemodialysis may require higher *Kt/V* values to achieve the same amount of solute removal and the same degree of patient blood purification as continuous therapies. It becomes clear that *t* may be a critical factor in evaluating the efficiency of a given treatment and intermittent treatments can hardly be compared with continuous treatments using the same parameters and the same scale.

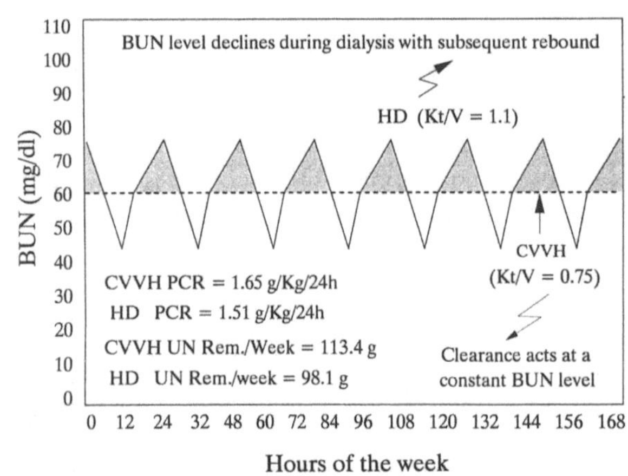

Fig. 3. Urea nitrogen levels in hemodialysis (*HD*; daily, 210 min/day) and continuous venovenous hemofiltration (*CVVH*; 27 l/day) in a 62-kg patient. A typical intermittent treatment regimen is compared with a continuous one. Despite a lower *Kt/V*, CVVH permits the removal of higher quantities of urea nitrogen, maintaining the blood concentration at a stable value. In HD, the high efficiency permits rapid removal of urea nitrogen in a short time with a consequent fall in blood concentrations. When dialysis ends, a concentration rebound takes place and the patient spends several hours of the week with a higher level of uremic intoxication. *BUN*, blood urea nitrogen; *PCR*, protein catabolic rate

In continuous hemofiltration, the evaluation of the ultrafiltrate to plasma equilibration behavior for solutes such as urea and creatinine is critical in ensuring that the clearance (ultrafiltration) and solute removal are strictly correlated (in a typical stable treatment, the permeability of the membrane is maintained for up to 24 h) [35, 36].

In conclusion, a certain amount of solute removal per week should be the real target of treatment. Different *Kt* producs may lead to the same amount of solute removals because of the different kinetics of the solute concentration in the blood and body compartments. At the same time, similar *Kt* products do not always lead to the same amount of solute removals and time becomes the critical factor for the adequacy of treatment. In intermittent hemodialysis, clearance and *Kt*/*V* may therefore be incorrect parameters to identify an adequate prescription, since the amount of solute removed will depend on the time for which clearance has been applied, on the blood concentration profile during treatment, on the mass transfer rate between body compartments, and on the average blood concentration to which the clearance is applied. In contrast, in continuous therapies clearance can be safely used for prescription, since it perfectly correlates with the amount of solute removal at a given stable concentration of the solute in blood (Fig. 3). Therefore we suggest that *Kt*/*V* can be used only as a marker of treatment efficiency of small molecules.

Daily creatinine removal may also be much greater in continuous therapies than in intermittent treatments because of the slow equilibration of creatinine among the body compartments.

Several authors have shown various degrees of correlation between the protein catabolic rate (PCR) and *Kt*/*V* both in hemodialysis and peritoneal dialysis in chronic patients. Nobody has investigated whether the nitrogen balance can be affected by the dialytic dose in the acute patient. As an example, in a well-dialyzed patient the degree of catabolism could be reduced and the impact of parenteral nutrition may be different (higher degree of anabolism).

Discussion

The aim of renal replacement therapies is to achieve a blood purification from metabolic waste products sufficient for patient rehabilitation, control of dry body weight, and correction of acid-base and electrolyte derangements. Among these effects, the correction of derangements derived from the initial renal disease would also be required. However, this objective is difficult to achieve and the majority of substitutive therapies such as hemodialysis or peritoneal dialysis are mostly focused on blood purification and fluid and electrolyte homeostasis.

For this reason the optimization of dialytic therapy is directed towards improved removal of metabolic waste products. Therefore, *adequacy of renal support* has been selected to describe a renal replacement therapy that can overcome most of the uremic symptoms and allow sufficient patient well-being. This means that even the most adequate treatment may be far from being a complete and ideal substitution of lost kidney function. Furthermore, we should probably consider the possibility that adequate renal support should also aim at removing the causes of ARF. Therefore, modulation of the immune response and clearance of specific mediators is probably desirable in the phase of the disease when kidney function is not yet lost and treatment may contribute to kidney protection.

In critically ill patients with ARF, it is clear that the concept of dialytic adequacy must be broader that simple control of azotemia. While this chapter focuses on important issues of urea kinetics and traditional concepts of clinically applied hemodialysis, it must not be forgotten that in the ICU avoidance of hemodynamic instability, hypoxemia, electrolyte imbalances and acidosis, arrhythmias, activation of inflammatory mediators, and adequate control of edema with the associated ability to administer full nutritional support may be much more significant determinants of dialytic adequacy than mathematical determinations of urea kinetics. Both, however, must be understood in order to provide optimal care from a nephrological point of view.

Finally, the nature and kinetics of different molecules to be cleared with extracorporeal treatments must be carefully analyzed in order to define the most adequate form of therapy for each substance. Molecules with low serum concentrations may require prolonged continuous treatments, while life-threatening concentrations of some substances may require rapid and efficient dialysis treatments.

References

1. Lowrie EG, Laird NM, Parker TF, Sargent JA (1981) Effect of the hemodialysis prescription on patient morbidity. N Engl J Med 305:1176–1181
2. Nolph KD, Keshaviah P, Popovich R (1991) Problems in comparison of clearances prescription in hemodialysis and continuous ambulatory peritoneal dialysis. Perit Dial Int 11:298–300
3. Nolph KD (1991) Quantitating peritoneal dialysis delivery: a required standard of care. Semin Dial 4:139–141
4. Bergstrom J, Lindholm B (1993) Nutrition and adequacy of dialysis: how do hemodialysis and CAPD compare? Kidney Int 43 Suppl 40:S39–S50
5. Keshaviah P, Nolph KD, Prowant BF (1990) Defining adequacy of CAPD with urea kintetics. Adv Perit Dial 6:173–177
6. Gotch FA (1991) The application of urea kinetic modeling to CAPD. In: La Greca G, Feriani M, Chiaramonte S et al. (eds) Peritoneal dialysis. Wichtig, Milan, pp 47–51
7. Gotch FA (1993) Dependence of normalized protein catabolic rate on Kt/V in continuous ambulatory peritoneal dialysis: not a mathematical artifact. Perit Dial Int 13:173–175
8. La Greca G, Fabris A, Feriani M, Chiaramonte S, Ronco C (1989) Acid-base homeostasis in clinical dialysis. In: Maher JF (ed) Replacement of renal function by dialysis. Nijhoff, Dordrecht, pp 808–826

9. Maher JF (ed) (1989) Replacement of renal function by dialysis. Nijhoff, Dordrecht
10. Ronco C (1993) Dialysis delivery vs dialysis prescription. Int J Artif Organs 16:628–635
11. Babb AL, Popovich RP, Christopher TJ, Scribner BH (1971) The genesis of the square meter-hour hypothesis. ASAIO Trans 17:81–86
12. Kjellestrand CM, Evans RI, Peterson RJ (1972) Considerations of the middle molecule hypothesis. Proc Clin Dial Transplant Forum 2:127–132
13. Teschan PE, Ginn HE, Bourne JR, Ward JW (1977) Neurobehavioral probes for adequacy of dialysis. Trans Am Soc Artif Intern Organs 23:556–561
14. Lowrie EG, Laird NM (1983) The National Cooperative Dialysis Study. Kidney Int 23 Suppl 13:S1–S5
15. Gotch FA, Sargent JH (1985) A mechanistic analysis of the national cooperative dialysis study. Kidney Int 28:526–533
16. Gotch FA (1990) Kinetic modeling in hemodialysis. In: Nissenson AR, Fine RN, Gentile DE (eds) Clinical dialysis, 2nd edn. Appleton and Lange, Norwalk, pp 118–146
17. Watson PE, Watson ID, Batt RD (1980) Total body water volumes for adult males and females estimated from simple anthropometric measurements. Am J Clin Nutr 33:27–39
18. Lowrie EG, Tehean BP (1983) Principles of prescribing dialysis therapy. Implementing recommendations from the National Cooperative Dialysis Study. Kidney Int 23 Suppl 13:S113–S122
19. Jindal KK, Manuel A, Goldstein MB (1987) Percent reduction of the blood urea concentration during hemodialysis (PUR). A simple and accurate method to estimate Kt/V urea. ASAIO Trans 33:286–288
20. Barth RH (1988) Direct calculation of Kt/V: a simplified approach to monitoring of hemodialysis. Nephron 50:191–195
21. Calzavara P, Vianello A, daPorto A, Gatti PL, Bertolone G, Caenaro G, Dalla Rosa C (1988) Comparison between three mathematical models of Kt/V. Int J Artif Organs 11:107–110
22. Keshaviah P, Hanson GL, Berkeseth RO, Collins AJ (1988) A simplified approach to monitoring in vivo therapy prescription. ASAIO Transactions 34 (abstr 57)
23. Daugirdas JT (1989) Bedside formulas for urea kinetic modeling. Contemp Dial Nephrol 10:23–25
24. Miller JH, Von Albertini B, Gardner PW, Shinaberger JH (1984) Technical aspects of high flux hemodiafiltration for adequate short (under two hours) treatment. Trans Am Soc Artif Intern Organs 30:377–381
25. Ronco C, Burchardi H (1993) Management of acute renal failure in the critically ill patient. In: Dhainaut JF, Pinsky, M (eds) Pathophysiologic foundations of critical care. Williams and Wilkins, Baltimore, pp 630–676
26. Keshaviah P, Luehmann D, Ilstrup K, Collins A (1987) Technical requirements for rapid high efficiency therapies. Artif Organs 3:189–194
27. Von Albertini B, Miller JH, Gardner PW, Shinaberger JH (1984) High flux hemodiafiltration under six hours/week treatment. ASAIO Trans 30:227–231
28. Ronco C, Brendolan A, Bragantini L et al. (1988) Technical and clinical evaluation of different short dialysis techniques. Contrib Nephrol 61:46–68
29. Ronco C (1988) Backfiltration in clinical dialysis: nature of the phenomenon and possible solutions. J Artif Organs 2:69–74
30. Bommer J, Ritz E (1987) Water quality: a neglected problem in hemodialysis. Nephron 46:1–6
31. Ronco C, Fabris A, Feriani M, Chiaramonte S, Brendolan A, Bragantini L, Milan M, Dell'Aquila R, Conz P, Frigato G, Borra M, von Albertini B, La Greca G (1988) Technical and clinical evaluation of a new system for ultrafiltration control during hemodialysis. ASAIO Trans 34(3):613–616
32. Colton CK (1987) Analysis of membrane processes for blood purification. Blood Purif 5:202–251

33. Ronco C, Feriani M, Chiaramonte S et al. (1990) Impact of high blood flows on vascular stability in hemodialysis. Nephrol Dial Transplant 1 Suppl 5:109–114
34. Keshaviah PR, Nolph KD, Van Stone JC (1989) The peak concentration hypothesis: a urea kinetic approach to comparing the adequacy of continuous ambulatory peritoneal dialysis (CAPD) and hemodialysis. Perit Dial Int 9:257–260
35. Kjellestrand C, Skroder R, Cederlof IO, Eriksson F, Kjellestrand P, Jacobson S (1994) Patient related factors leading to slow urea transfer in the body during dialysis. ASAIO J 40:164–170
36. Frankenfield D, Reynolds HN, Wiles CE, Badellino MM, Siegel JH (1994) Urea removal during continuous hemodiafiltration. Crit Care Med 22:407–412

Acute Renal Failure in the Intensive Care Unit: Which Treatment Is Best?

R. Bellomo and C. Ronco

Introduction

Since the clinical application of continuous hemofiltration techniques to the management of acute renal failure in critical illness, there has been persistent controversy as to which therapy (continuous hemofiltration or intermittent hemodialysis) constitutes the best form of renal replacement in the intensive care unit (ICU). Some of this controversy stems from a relative lack of interdisciplinary collaboration between critical care physicians and nephrologists, the former being ambivalent about their role in the management of acute renal failure and the latter often unwilling to accept the concept that critically ill patients with acute renal failure profoundly differ from those seen in nephrology wards. As a consequence, an adversarial relationship sometimes develops instead of the desirable collaboration directed at implementing "state of the art" care and innovative dialytic approaches. In addition, in some centers overburdened dialysis and intensive care facilities and physicians often do not have sufficient time and resources to tackle the complex problems related to acute renal failure management in the critically ill. In this chapter, we will analyze in detail the major aspects related this issue. We will also seek to provide a series of practical suggestions which we hope will guide clinicians as they face real clinical choices in their daily practice.

Acute Renal Failure: A Definition

Acute renal failure is not easily defined. Large epidemiological studies have used the criterion of a sudden rise in serum creatinine to more than 500 μmol/l [1]. Studies on the incidence of this disorder in the ICU, however, have used different criteria: the doubling of serum creatinine levels, a rapid increase in serum creatinine to a level greater than 280 μmol/l [2], or a 20% increase from the baseline serum creatinine value [3].

Clearly, these values are quite variable and only partly reflect issues of clinical practice. An increase in serum creatinine from 80 to 280 μmol/l has very different clinical implications from a similar rise in serum creatinine from 350 to 550 μmol/l, particularly if the latter is associated with progressive oliguria. The advantages of such division lines lie in the fact that they are clear and not dependent on the vagaries of subjective clinical judgement. What these definitions ignore, however, is that, apart from the obvious clinical implications (removal of nephrotoxins and maintenance of adequate renal perfusion), a serum creatinine of 300 μmol/l in the absence of severe oliguria often does not have any major implications in terms of therapeutic complexity. It could be argued, in fact, that one is dealing with acute renal impairment, not failure. We consider that the word "failure" is best used to describe another level of renal impairment: the need for renal replacement therapy. Thus we are dealing in sequence with normal renal excretory function, acute renal impairment, and acute renal failure, the latter requiring either hemofiltration or hemodialysis. It is this state that we will concern ourselves with in this chapter.

Once again, however, even this definition has pitfalls, because the timing for the initiation of renal replacement therapy and the indications for its implementation are not objectively established. Many physicians would agree with the classical criteria for dialysis in acute renal failure: difficult to control, progressive hyperkalemia, uremic complications, severe metabolic acidosis, and refractory fluid overload, although even these criteria are poorly defined. The degrees of hyperkalemia or acidosis or fluid overload that should trigger the use of dialysis are different under different circumstances and under the care of different physicians. Furthermore, in 1994, it seems highly undesirable to wait for complications to develop before appropriate therapies are implemented. This is particularly true as we gain insight into the role of the kidney as a modulator and excretor of some of the humoral mediators of sepsis and as evidence accumulates that some forms of renal replacement therapy may have clinically important beneficial effects on the systemic inflammatory reaction seen with the multiorgan dysfunction syndrome. At a more practical, yet clinically subtle level, it is also not established what degree of azotemia/uremia is severe enough to require artificial renal support (is a plasma urea of more than 35 mmol/l too high in the absence of other complications? Or is 40 mmol/l acceptable?). In this way, acute renal failure is not dissimilar from acute respiratory failure, with which the intensive care specialist is very familiar. It has gradations of severity of available therapies and, just as the decision to initiate mechanical ventilation has a subjective judgement component, so does the decision to implement renal replacement therapy. Furthermore, as in the case of respiratory failure, the premorbid functional state of the organ is of great importance. Acute injuries of similar severity will have quite different consequences in a healthy kidney compared with a chronically impaired organ. In particular, recovery from such an injury will likely follow a very different course. However, in the ICU most patients who develop acute renal failure do so in association with oliguria and the dysfunction of multiple other organs. In this setting, the severity of injury is substantial and the need for renal replacement clear, although the timing may be a source of disagreement.

We propose a series of criteria that define the need for renal replacement therapy in the ICU and consequently the presence of acute renal failure:

1. Oliguria (urinary output less than 500 ml/day)
2. Anuria (no urinary output for more than 12 h)
3. Plasma urea concentration greater than 35 mmol/l; blood urea nitrogen (BUN) greater than 100 mg/dl)
4. Serum creatinine greater than 500 μmol/l (greater than 5.6 mg/dl)
5. Hyperkalemia (serum potassium greater than 6.5 mmol/l)
6. Pulmonary edema not responsive to diuretics
7. Metabolic acidosis (pH less than 7.2)
8. Uremic encephalopathy
9. Uremic pericarditis
10. Uremic neuropathy

The presence of one of the above criteria constitutes sufficient grounds for the initiation of renal replacement therapy in critically ill patients. The presence of two of these criteria makes its implementation mandatory.

Epidemiology

The incidence of acute renal failure requiring renal replacement in the ICU is not established. Recent data on the incidence of the condition in the community [1] provide useful insights. This analysis of two health districts in the UK (population studied > 400000) found that there was an acute dialysis/hemofiltration rate of 18 cases per million population per year. Although no specific information was given on the incidence of ICU admission for these patients, it can be gleaned from the manuscript that a minimum of ten patients were dialyzed in ICU during the study period, giving an overall rate of combined critical illness and acute renal failure in the range of 12 cases per million per year.

Given a Western European population of about 350 million people, close to 4000 such patients are probably treated every year in European ICU. Similarly, about 3000 such patients would be treated in North America and close to 2000 in Australasia. At an approximate cost of at least US$3000–4000 for renal replacement alone during their stay, close to US$40 million may be spent each year worldwide on renal replacement for acute renal failure in the ICU. This is probably a conservative estimate. If the ICU perspective is used, the development of renal failure requiring dialysis has been calculated at around 3% of all admissions to a medical ICU [4] or up to 10% of all admissions [2].

In the institution of one of the authors (R.B.) its incidence over a period of 5 years has been around 5% of all admissions. It is important to realize that these figures will be altered by therapeutic strategies which may pursue different hemodynamic goals, for instance, in the presence of septic shock. A therapeutic approach directed at avoiding pulmonary edema at all costs by avoiding higher pulmonary occlusion pressures may be expected to result in a higher incidence of acute renal failure than one in which aggressive fluid resuscitation is persistently pursued over time to maintain urinary output. Such considerations, however, have not yet been tested in prospective controlled studies. A further observation is that acute renal failure in the ICU may be seen either as part of the multiorgan failure syndrome or in patients who originally presented with isolated renal failure and who have then gone on to develop sepsis or other complications requring their admission to intensive care. These subpopulations may have different outcomes, but no studies have yet addressed this issue. Whatever the path to the ICU, it is now increasingly rare to find patients in the ICU who have isolated renal failure. In a consecutive series of 150 critically ill patients from the ICU of one of the authors' institution (R.B.), only eight (5.3%) had isolated renal failure (single organ failure).

Historical Background

In the 1950s, hemodialysis was mostly considered an emergency treatment for desperate situations and was used in life-threatening acute renal failure (e.g., in the Korean War). In the 1960s, chronic dialysis programs were developed, but the limited availability of these developing dialysis facilities meant that acute renal failure was often treated conservatively. The absence of widespread structured ICU also meant that critical illness and multiorgan failure, as we know them today, were not as much part of the common clinical background for the development of acute renal failure. The patterns of the 1960s progressively changed over the following decade, as the introduction of ICU around the world meant that sicker and older patients were now requiring renal replacement therapy [5]. As a consequence, despite remarkable improvements in medical care, the overall mortality associated with acute renal failure did not appear to fall [6, 7]. As sicker and older patients were being treated with either peritoneal dialysis or hemodialysis and required vasopressor drugs to sustain the circulation, mechanical ventilation to maintain oxygenation, and total parenteral nutrition to support metabolism, the shortcomings of conventional dialytic therapy became more obvious.

Peritoneal dialysis exposed patients to a high risk of peritonitis, was often unable to provide sufficient urea clearances, caused diaphragmatic splinting, unpredictable swings in serum glucose, protein loss, and, more importantly, often failed to provide the ultrafiltration necessary to maintain a neutral fluid balance [8–10]. As a consequence, pulmonary and peripheral edema could not be aggressively treated, resulting in prolonged ventilator dependence with its attendant morbidity and mortality.

Intermittent hemodialysis was the dominant form of renal replacement throughout the 1970s. Its use, however, was and still is associated with a plethora of undesirable side effects. Acute hypotension is the most common side effect of intermittent hemodialysis [11], and it is particularly problematic in patients who already require pressor treatment. Furthermore, the need for aggressive ultrafiltration to deal with concomitant extravascular fluid overload aggravates this phenomenon [12]. Hypoxemia is another of its deleterious side effects and is probably due to the induction of hypoventilation [13] and an increase in oxygen consumption [14]. Cardiac arrhythmias can be triggered by rapid electrolyte shifts [15], particularly in the presence of a strong adrenergic drive. In addition, rapid changes in extracellular tonicity can promote the development of cerebral edema [16, 17]. A great deal of morbidity results from these shortcomings, especially when conventional hemodialysis is applied to a population of critically ill patients [18, 19]. These shortcomings have provided a strong stimulus towards the development of newer forms of renal replacement therapy that would be better suited to the care of critically ill patients. Kramer and colleagues [20] first desribed continuous arteriovenous hemofiltration (CAVH) in 1977. This novel therapy provided the first real alternative to intermittent hemodialysis. It was technically simple and did not induce hemodynamic instability. Fluid or electrolyte shifts were avoided, as were cerebral edema and hypoxemia. Ample fluid removal become easy. Azotemia could slowly be decreased and nutritional fluids, blood, and blood products could now be administered without concern for the development of fluid overload. Even this therapy, however, had its shortcomings: relatively low urea clearances and the need for arterial and venous access. It held so much promise, however, that the following years saw its increasing application in the clinical arena and multiple attempts to improve it [21–24]. A major step in the right direction was the addition of diffusive clearance to the convective clearance achieved with hemofiltration. The development of continuous arteriovenous hemodialysis [25] and continuous arteriovenous hemodiafiltration [26] permitted the achievement of urea clearances of the order of 23–26 ml/min, which, in turn, allowed full control of azotemia in all patients without the need for the occasional supplemental hemodialysis. The arrival of dual-lumen catheters and the application of simple peristaltic pumps eventually resulted in the development of techniques which did not require arterial cannulation, such as continuous venovenous hemofiltration (CVVH) and continuous arteriovenous hemodiafiltration (CVVHD) [27, 28]. Continuous hemofiltration therapies had moved from an experimental approach to acute renal failure in the critically ill to one that could challenge the role of intermittent hemodialysis.

Controversy

The technical simplicity of continuous hemofiltration techniques and their increasing use have led to the inevitable question of which treatment constitutes the renal replacement therapy of choice in critically ill patients with acute renal failure in the 1990s [29, 30]? Over the last 5 years, multiple debates have taken place with advocates of continuous hemofiltration and supporters of hemodialysis clashing over this question. One of the major reasons this issue has not yet been resolved lies in the lack of clearcut comparative data and in the difficulty of mounting a prospective randomized study comparing intermittent hemodialysis and continuous hemofiltration/hemodiafiltration in the management of acute renal failure in the ICU [31]. Another lies in the fact that no meaningful retrospective comparisons can be made with previously published series of patients in the absence of illness severity scoring. Such lack of illness severity assessment has characterized almost all outcome studies of acute renal failure in the ICU. It appears, however, that the use of hemofiltration is increasing [32] in ICU around the

Table 1. Clinical series of critically ill patients treated with intermittent hemodialysis

Reference	Patients (*n*)	Survivors		Comments
		(*n*)	(%)	
Kierdorf [33]	73	5	6.9	No illness severity scores No details about ICU type
McDonald and Mehta [34]	10	3	30	No illness severity scores Most patients appeared to have multiorgan failure
Schaefer et al. [4]	134	58	43.3	Medical ICU 74.6% incidence of sepsis Mean APACHE II score approximately 24
Berisa et al. [35]	59	25	42.4	All following surgery for abdominal aortic aneurysm No illness severity scores
Spiegel et al. [36]	43	5	11.6	From surgical and medical ICU No illness severity scores 31 required mechanical ventilation
Ishitani et al. [37]	33	20	60.6	All following liver transplantation All treated with biocompatible membranes
Bellomo et al. [18]	80	24	30	Mean APACHE II score approximately 26 Combined medical and surgical ICU Mean number of failing organs, 4
Frost et al. [38]	50	27	54	All with bacteremia No illness severity scores Unclear whether all patients in ICU
Total	482	167	34.6	

ICU, intensive care unit; APACHE, Acute Physiology and Chronic Health Evaluation.

Table 2. Clinical series of critically ill patients treated with continuous hemofiltration

Reference	Patients (*n*)	Survivors (*n*)	Survivors (%)	Treatment	Comments
Pataca et al. [39]	33	18	54.5	CAVHD	All required mechanical ventilation No illness severity scores
Alarabi et al. [40]	43	26	60.5	CAVHD	No illness severity scores
Badouin et al. [41]	35	6	17	CVVH	All with renal failure after coronary surgery Most patients had failure of three organs
Tominaga et al. [42]	26	9	34.6	CAVHD	All trauma patients No illness severity scores
Vesconi et al. [43]	18	8	44.4	CVVH	Multiorgan failure SAPS used for illness severity score (mean, 17.2)
Reynolds et al. [44]	28	5	17.9	CAVHD	Most patients had multiorgan failure
Barton et al. [45]	250	132	52.8	CVVH	General ICU No illness severity scores
Storck et al. [46]	120	20	16.7	CAVH/ CVVH	Surgical ICU
Bellomo and Boyce [47]	110	42	38.2	CAVHD/ CVVHD	General ICU Mean APACHE II score, 27.7 Mean number of failing organs, 3.4
Bagshaw et al. [48]	13	3	23.1	CAVH	–
Macias et al. [49]	25	4	16	CVVH	General ICU No illness severity scores
Voerman et al. [50]	17	5	29.4	CAVHD	General ICU
Alarabi et al. [51]	112	58	51.2	CAVH	General ICU
Sluiter et al. [52]	89	39	43.8	CAVH	General ICU
Schaefer et al. [53]	62	22	35.5	CAVHD/ CVVHD	–
Hirasawa et al. [54]	43	26	60.5	CVVH/ CVVHD	–
Canaud et al. [55]	32	5	15.6	CVVH	General ICU All patients had multiorgan failure
Keller et al. [56]	26	4	15.4	CAVHD	General ICU No illness severity scores
Keusch et al. [57]	49	18	36.7	CAVH/ CVVH	All with multisystem organ failure No illness severity scores 18 patients discharged from hospital
Total	1131	450	39.8		

CAVHD, continuous arteriovenous hemodiafiltration; CVVH, continuous venovenous hemofiltration; CAVH, continuous arteriovenous hemofiltration; CVVHD, continuous venovenous hemodiafiltration; ICU, intensive care unit; SAPS, Simplified Acute Physiology Score; APACHE, Acute Physiology and Chronic Health Score.

world, suggesting that slowly this debate will become obsolete due to the obvious practical advantages of using continuous hemofiltration techniques in the ICU. In Tables 1 and 2 we have summarized the results and features of studies published since the beginning of the decade. In these studies, patients were either treated with continuous hemofiltration techniques or with intermittent dialysis. The tables highlight several important points. First, since the beginning of the decade, the use of continuous hemofiltration has seen an exponential growth. Second, it appears that, at least in Europe and Australia, continuous hemofiltration techniques are now the most common form of renal replacement therapy in the ICU. This impression is confirmed by recent evidence [32, 58]. Third, in the absence of validated forms of illness severity scoring, clinical series will never allow any meta-analysis or meaningful comparisons of data or advancement in our understanding of whether we are indeed moving forward in this area.

The ideal approach to this controversy would be to perform a controlled randomized study. Such a study, however, will not only be impeded by the sheer cost, the need for large numbers of patients, and for uniformity of technique, but also by the fact that more severely ill patients with hemodynamic instability will not tolerate intermittent hemodialysis and will, therefore, have to be switched over to continuous hemofiltration (Mehta, personal communication). As a consequence, there will not be true randomization and all that we are likely to learn is that continuous hemofiltration is associated with much greater hemodynamic stability than intermittent hemodialysis. This we already know. A different approach to the issue of which therapy is the treatment of choice in critically ill patients is to analyze the problem from a theoretical point of view by describing what the features of an ideal form of renal replacement would be and then assessing how intermittent hemodialysis and continuous hemofiltration compare to this ideal form of therapy.

Ideal Form of Renal Replacement

The major requirement for any form of renal replacement therapy is that it maintain homeostasis in the absence of endogenous renal function. This may seem straightforward but there are, in fact, many areas of physiologic control the kidney is at least in part responsible for. They include the excretion of toxic metabolites and drugs, the maintenance of dry body weight, the fine regulation of cardiovascular stability, the maintenance of acid-base homeostasis, the regulation of erythropoiesis, the maintenance of calcium balance, the regulation of total body sodium and potassium as well as that of other electrolytes, and, possibly, even the modulation of cytokine metabolism by excretion [59–63]. The ideal replacement therapy, therefore, should be able to perform all the above tasks safely, effectively, and simply.

Toxin and Metabolite Excretion

A number of toxic substances accumulate following the onset of renal failure. Their nature is yet undefined, but taken together they are responsible for a toxic state known as uremia, of which an elevated plasma urea concentration is a marker. If allowed to proceed unabated, this condition leads to profound derangements of body function and, eventually, death. A number of theories have been put forward concerning the molecular weight of these uremic toxins. For a time, as hemodialysis appeared to provide adequate patient well-being, it was assumed that "small molecules" were mostly responsible for this toxic state. More recent evidence indicates that "middle molecules" (molecular weight 0.5–20 kDa) are also important in the mediation of the uremic state [64]. While there is little doubt concerning their long-term toxic effects, little is known about their short-term toxicity. Among them, however, are a number of cytokines which have been increasingly shown to play a pivotal role in the pathogenesis of septic shock [65–68]. More realistically, in fact, the pathogenesis of uremia is extremely complex, reflecting deranged homeostasis and blood intoxication at various levels by a multitude of processes and molecules. Their clearance may be of importance in the management of septic acute renal failure. The question arises as to how conventional intermittent hemodialysis performs the task of blood purification necessary for the optimal management of uremia. The answer is probably that it does so barely adequately. There is no doubt that small molecules are effectively cleared by the technique but, even with regard to these, the intermittent nature and the short time of application (3–5 h) of this therapy mean that the extracellular compartment may be better purified than the intracellular one. This phenomenon will be particularly true in septic and hemodynamically unstable patients, in whom the distribution of regional blood flow may be poor and is always highly variable. As a consequence, effluent from, for instance, the gastrointestinal tract may be quantitatively suboptimal. Intracellular toxin extraction from this body compartment, therefore, cannot proceed adequately over a short period of time. That compartmental intracellular solutes concentrations do not reach equilibrium with extracellular solute concentration is evidenced by the disequilibrium syndrome and the development of various degrees of cerebral edema during and after hemodialysis [16, 17]. The intermittent nature of the therapy is clearly unphysiologic and is reflected in the fact that the peak and trough of uremic intoxication result in a greater overall uremic load than that seen during continuous therapies (Fig. 1). Continuous hemofiltration, on the other hand, overcomes these problems by providing control of azotemia 24 h a day at a steady state level (Fig. 1). The clinical consequences of different degrees of uremic intoxication in critically ill patients with acute renal failure are unknown at present. It is important to note, however, that neutrophils from uremic patients exhibit a number of defects in chemotaxis, adherence, oxidative metabolism, and metabolic glycolysis in response to

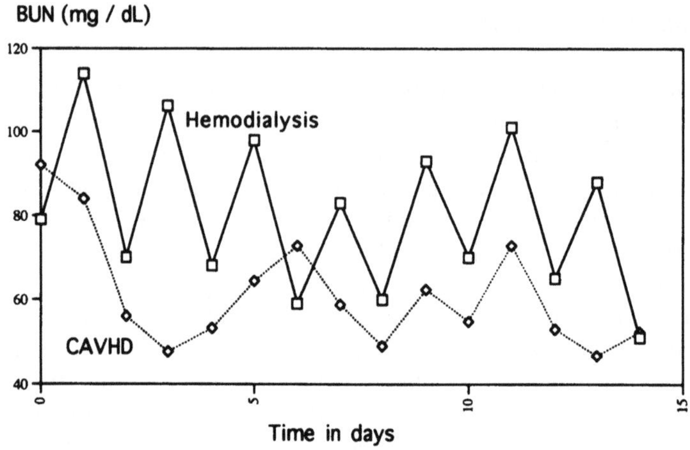

Fig. 1. Differences in azotemic control with hemodialysis and continuous arteriovenous hemodiafiltration (*CAVHD*). Two actual patients have been used. Second daily dialysis (as can be seen here) leads to large swings in plasma urea levels and to an area under the curve which is much larger than that seen with continuous treatment and which indicates suboptimally treated uremic intoxication. *BUN*, blood urea nitrogen

phagocytosis [68–71]. These deficits may have clinical implications by impairing the patient's defenses against infection and, thereby, predisposing critically ill patients to infectious complications. Better control of uremia may lessen the severity of these immunological derangements. Furthermore, the use of cuprophane membranes for intermittent hemodialysis has a number of side effects which are of themselves the source of important deleterious changes in homeostais. They will be discussed further below (see "Biocompatibility").

Maintenance of Dry Body Weight

The importance of maintaining intra- and extravascular fluid homeostasis in the critically ill cannot be overemphasized. One of the major management problems encountered in patients with oliguric renal failure is, in fact, that of fluid overload. This almost invariably results in the development of interstitial edema and, in some cases, in the development of organ (lung) edema with the obvious associated morbidity. Furthermore, critically ill patients have ongoing fluid requirements: nutritional fluids, blood and blood products, vehicular fluids for the administration of antibiotics, and drug infusions (vasopressors, sedatives, muscle relaxants). It is not uncommon for the average patient to require at least 2 l fluid/day. Many of these patients may already be significantly fluid overloaded from the effect of prior aggressive fluid resuscitation directed at averting the development of acute renal failure. In the vast majority of these patients, therefore, the removal of adequate amounts of fluid in order to maintain the desired state of intravascular and extravascular filling is a major clinical priority. In this regard, intermittent hemodialysis falls short of the ideal requirements for renal replacement. With this technique, in fact, fluid removal has to happen over a short period of time and is limited by its deleterious hemodynamic impact. In order to avoid hypotension, smaller amounts of volume are often removed than originally prescribed. This results in the progressive aggravation of fluid overload. If, on the other hand, aggressive fluid removal is pursued at all costs, severe hypotension commonly develops. Such hypotension likely aggravates ischemic renal injury and may exacerbate multiorgan failure by inducing gut ischemia. The opposite is true for continuous hemofiltration techniques [72]. Fluid removal is constant and can be regulated at whim to achieve desired targets. Because it occurs slowly and steadily, it does not induce hemodynamic instability and often, by improving the myocardial tension–volume relationship, it results in improved cardiac indices [73]. There is no problem of volume overload and any pulmonary edema that may have developed during resuscitative efforts can be easily treated. Finally, the risk of inducing changes in brain cell size with increased intracranial pressure and its attendant morbidity is dramatically diminished, making continuous hemofiltration the technique of choice in any patient with, or at risk of, intracranial hypertension [74].

Regulation of Acid-Base Balance

The development of renal failure leads to metabolic acidosis. The clinical significance of this phenomenon is unclear, though experimental work suggests that acidosis may have important effects on myocardial excitability and contractility [75, 76]. The ideal renal replacement therapy would allow correction of acidosis as desired without adverse clinical consequences. If acetate-based intermittent hemodialysis is used, however, a number of problems may develop. First, bicarbonate extraction may outpace acetate metabolism, leading to an immediate worsening of metabolic acidosis [77]. Second, hypoventilation is induced in up to 90% of patients by an acetate-induced fall in $PaCO_2$. This in turn induces the development of hypoxemia [78, 79]. In the presence of liver dysfunction, these problems are likely to be more severe. Finally, acetate infusion induces vasodilatation and hypotension [80, 81], an undesirable side effect in most critically ill patients. The use of bicarbonate dialysis may improve the way in which hemodialysis achieves its acid-base goals [82], particularly with regard to hemodynamic stability [83]. Even this area of nephrological practice, however, remains controversial [84].

Continuous hemofiltration, on the other hand, leads to slow bicarbonate extraction and therefore requires the administration of bicarbonate with the replacement fluids. This can be easily done to both compensate for losses and correct metabolic acidosis to desired target values. Severe lactic acidosis, for instance, has been treated successfully with hemofiltration and bicarbonate-based replacement fluid [85]. Some authors, however, have reported hyperlactatemia and a paradoxical increase in acidosis in liver failure patients treated with lactate-based replacement fluids [86]. While an increase in serum lactate levels is to be expected, it is unclear whether the associated acidosis is in any way related to it. This kind of hyperlactatemia has been found to bear no relationship to hydrogen ion concentration in a group of critically ill patients without liver disease [87]. In summary, a number of serious problems are associated with the correction of metabolic acidosis by intermittent hemodialysis. With hemofiltration the control is not episodic and is achieved slowly and with ease. It appears advisable, however, at this stage to use bicarbonate-based replacement fluids in patients with severe liver disease.

Anemia of Renal Failure

There is no data on the effect of different modes of renal replacement on residual erythropoietin production by the kidney and on the severity of acute renal failure-associated anemia. There is also no data on therapy-associated blood loss (change of filter or dialyzer etc.). The only thing that can be stated confidently is that blood and blood product administration is markedly facilitated by the removal of fluid associated with continuous hemofiltration.

Electrolyte and Water Homeostasis

There is also no comparative data on the degree of electrolyte control and stability achieved with each of the major forms of renal replacement therapy. A number of anecdotal reports, on the other hand, suggest that the rapid electrolyte shifts seen in association with intermittent hemodialysis may be responsible for cardiac arrhythmias or disturbances in neurological function [88]. Furthermore, as dialysis is only applied intermittently and nutritional fluids are typically hypotonic, a degree of hyponatremia typically develops which is then temporarily corrected during therapy, only to return to its previous value over 24 h or so. The consequences of such swings are unknown. Typically, no matter what the total body water may be, all these patients are total body sodium overloaded. The impact of this is also unknown. Continuous hemofiltration allows full control of tonicity and total body sodium by regulation of the sodium concentration in the replacement fluid and the amount of negative fluid balance aimed for. If countercurrent dialysate is administered (CAVHD/CVVHD), the serum sodium equilibrates with sodium concentration in the dialysate reaching a servocontrolled state of mild hyponatremia (serum Na of approximately, 135 mmol/l). The clinical impact of this phenomenon is unknown. The same concepts described for sodium apply to other electrolytes, from potassium to magnesium, from calcium to chloride.

Cytokine Excretion

Given that the kidney is involved in the final disposition of cytokines, an ideal form of renal replacement ought to do the same. This is clearly not the case for intermittent hemodialysis. This technique has been shown to induce the production of cytokines, thereby achieving the opposite of the physiologic task normally performed by the kidney [89, 90]. In contrast to this effect, the highly porous membranes used for continuous hemofiltration allow the ultrafiltration and excretion of these molecules [91, 92]. Although the clinical consequences of this phenomenon are still unclear, the consensus of opinion is that downmodulation of the cytokine response to sepsis is desirable and that, in this regard, once again the effect of continuous hemofiltration is in accordance rather than discordance with the general goals of therapy in sepsis. These differences in the handling of cytokines are but one component of the wider issue of biocompatibility.

Biocompatibility

Cellulose-based membranes used in standard hemodialysis are bioincompatible [90]. During contact between these membranes and blood, several normally homeostatic mechanisms become overactivated. This activation is pervasive at a humoral and cellular level and involves a cascade of interrelated events that range from upregulation of neutrophil adhesion receptors [93] to the release of reactive oxygen species [94], from the activation of monocytes to produce more cytokines [95] to the release of leukotrienes [96], from the activation of platelets to release thromboxane B_2 [97] to the activation of the complement cascade [98] and of other contact systems. The multiple effects of this interaction are summarized in Fig. 2. At a clinical level these events translate into a variety of adverse effects which include thrombocytopenia, leukopenia, fever, electrocardiogram (ECG) changes, chest pain, dyspnea, and acute changes in pulmonary artery pressures [90]. These complications highlight the severe shortcomings of conventional hemodialysis. This bioincompatibility may also translate into a delay in recovery from acute renal failure, as inflammatory activation aggravates the consequences of the original insult [99]. In this regard, the intermittent hemodialysis of the future may abandon traditional membranes and be performed with the same biocompatible membranes now used for continuous hemofiltration [100].

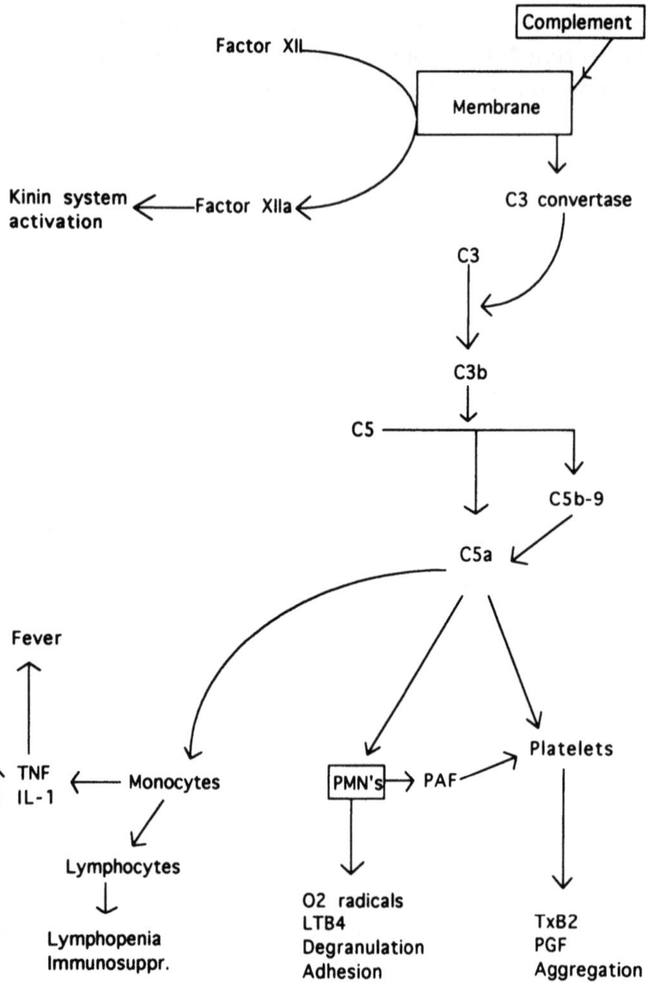

Fig. 2. Major consequences of blood–membrane interaction when a nonbiocompatible membrane is used. As can be seen, multiple humoral inflammatory mediators are activated, while the cellular component of the immune system is also affected. *TNF*, tumor necrosis factor; *IL*, interleukin; *PMN*, polymorphonuclear neutrophil; *PAF*, platelet-activating factor; *PGF*, prostaglandin F; *TXB2*, thromboxane B_2; *LTB4*, leukotriene B4

Other clinically important consequences may involve the induction of catabolism (discussed in detail in the chapter by Bellomo on "Nutrition in Acute Renal Failure", this volume) and a shortening in red cell survival [90]. These adverse consequences are either eliminated or substantially diminished by the use of biocompatible membranes. Once again, these data support the preferential use of continuous hemofiltration over standard intermittent hemodialysis in critically ill patients.

Blood Purification in Sepsis

Over the last decade, another aspect of continuous hemofiltration has emerged as important when choosing a modality of renal replacement in critically ill patients with acute renal failure: its blood purification effect. First remarked upon in the mid-1980s [101, 102], its significance has grown remarkably over the last 10 years, supported by growing evidence that the systemic manifestations of sepsis may be ignited and fueled by a number of powerful humoral mediators of injury whose molecular weight would theoretically allow removal from the circulation during continuous hemofiltration procedures. A number of experimental and clinical studies support the concept that continuous hemofiltration does, in fact, achieve a degree of clinically significant blood purification in septic states. Gomez et al. [103], for instance, have shown that CAVH can reverse the left ventricular dysfunction seen in dogs following the infusion of live *Escherichia coli* into the circulation. These beneficial effects on the cardiovascular system have been confirmed by Grootendorst et al. [104] in a porcine model of endotoxemia using high-volume hemofiltration. Even more interestingly, this author was able to demonstrate that the infusion of ultrafiltrate obtained from endotoxemic pigs treated by continuous venovenous hemofiltration could induce hemodynamic changes similar to those triggered by endotoxin itself [105]. Others have demonstrated the removal of a myocardial depressant factor in patients with cardiogenic shock [106] and a beneficial effect on endotoxin-induced lung injury [107]. The blood-purifying effect of CAVH has also been demonstrated in experimental staphylococcal sepsis [108]. In this latest study, once again, the infusion of ultrafiltrate from septic animals had remarkably adverse consequences in the recipient pigs. These experimental data have inevitably led to some clinical studies which, although partly flawed, are consistent with the above experiments [109]. Taken together, this body of research adds yet another important rationale for the selection of continuous hemofiltration over intermittent hemodialysis.

Conclusions

In the preceding pages we have reviewed the clinical evidence pertaining to renal replacement strategies in acute renal failure in the ICU. We have tried to offer some perspective to the clinical studies so far available and have sought to explain some of the difficulties inherent to trying to demonstrate a mortality advantage for one technique over another. Given the lack of clear-cut clinical studies, we have analyzed how each therapy compares to an ideal system of renal replacement and how they perform in achieving important therapeutic goals in this setting. It is obvious from the preceding discussion that we feel that continuous hemofiltration techniques are the renal replacement therapy of choice in critically ill patients. In these patients, standard hemodialysis is obsolete. Those who wish to oppose this change in outlook will choose to ignore the evidence we have just presented and will focus on the fact that continuous hemofiltration has yet to be proven to diminish mortality and that it is more expensive. To use an analogy that relates to critical care medicine, this reasoning is similar to one that would stop the use of the now available highly sophisticated volume-cycled ventilators because they have never been shown to decrease the mortality of acute respiratory failure when compared to pressure cycled ventilators! The issue of cost is equally to be dismissed. A recent analysis [29] of the costs associated with intermittent hemodialysis compared to those of continuous hemofiltration showed that hemodialysis costs US$751 per week and hemofiltration US$1369 per week. Even if this were true (and it is not), the additional cost for hemofiltration over dialysis would be less than 3% of total ICU care charges or approximately equal to the cost of a third-generation cephalosporin.

A rapid review of how these costs were arrived at shows that if CVVH instead of CVVHD were considered there would be no cost difference at all. Furthermore, the critical care nurse-related costs are often, in truth, minimal as the patient often already requires one-to-one nursing. If the cost of buying a dialysis machine is also factored in, hemofiltration is cheaper. Many of these issues do not apply to some countries in Europe or to Australia, where one-to-one nursing is often the norm in the ICU and where ready-made low-cost replacement fluids are available.

The only remaining issue, then, is which continuous hemofiltration technique is best. The answer is simple: the one for which there are both local expertise and facilities. The present authors both have the availability of peristaltic pumps. These allow them to use single-venous cannulation and to perform either CVVH or CVVHD. Clearly this approach will reduce the morbidity inevitably associated with arterial cannulation. In the absence of such resources, however, an arteriovenous circuit is perfectly adequate. Whatever the technique, we have outlined a set of practical suggestions, summarized below, that we hope will assist clinicians in successfully implementing these techniques in their institution:

1. Provide full theoretical and practical training in continuous hemofiltration for all nurses in the ICU.
2. Develop strict protocols for the setting up, maintenance, and cessation of hemofiltration in the ICU.
3. All patients on hemofiltration should receive one-to-one nursing.
4. Aim for a steady plasma urea level of 20–25 mmol/l (BUN, 55–70 mg/dl).
5. Monitor filter and patient anticoagulation with either whole-blood clotting time or partial thromboplastin time on a regular basis.
6. If arterial cannula has been in situ for more than 3 days and is no longer needed, consider removal under direct surgical vision.

7. Frequently reassess the patient's fluid status and adjust fluid replacement rate accordingly.
8. Have an experienced physician available for consultation and advice 24h a day.
9. If control of azotemia is inadequate with the technique in use, consider adding countercurrent dialysate flow or increasing its flow rate.
10. Develop and maintain a quality assurance program with prospective documentation, regular review of all cases treated, and an acute renal failure mortality and morbidity meeting.

We believe that, with a clear understanding of what an ideal form of treatment should be, the view that treatment should be tailored to the needs of the patient, the knowledge of local resources and expertise, and the use of these guidelines, continuous hemofiltration will be made safer and more effective and future improvements easier.

Future Prospects

Both hemodialysis and continuous hemofiltration will certainly undergo significant changes in the next few years. Hemodialysis wil be improved in the setting of critical illness by becoming more like hemofiltration. New biocompatible membranes will be used to minimize its side effects. Hemodialysis machines will be made more sophisticated and able to rapidly detect changes in hemoconcentration such as signals of excessive fluid removal or to respond to changes in automatically and continuously monitored serum electrolyte concentrations by servocontrol of dialysate/water mixing. As dialysis becomes safer, it will be applied for longer periods and more frequently (e.g., 6h a day each day) almost as a form of intermittent hemodiafiltration or continuous high-flux dialysis [110]. In this guise, it may make a comeback in the ICU.

Hemofiltration is also likely to move forward in two directions. The first will be towards further technical improvements with the introduction of sophisticated and automated fluid replacement systems and with the development of heparin-bonded membranes which will make therapy without anticoagulation a daily routine. The second will be towards ever increasing levels of blood purification. In this regard, and with modifications, continuous hemofiltration may become part of a broad armamentarium available to the intensive care specialist in the management of sepsis. Such modifications may include the binding of anticytokine antibodies to the filtering membrane or the creation of complex circuits which add, in series, other modalities of blood purification such as plasmapheresis, polymixin-bound matrices [111], resin columns, and charcoal cartridges [112].

References

1. Feest TG, Round A, Hamad S (1993) Incidence of severe acute renal failure in adults: results of a community based study. Br Med J 306:481–483
2. Groeneveld ABJ, Tran DD, van der Meulen J, Nauta JJP, Thijs LG (1991) Acute renal failure in the medical intensive care unit: predisposing, complicating factors and outcome. Nephron 59:602–610
3. Menashe PI, Ross SA, Gottlieb JE (1988) Acquired renal insufficiency in critically ill patients. Crit Care Med 16:1106–1109
4. Schaefer H, Jochimsen F, Keller F, Wegscheider K, Distler A (1991) Outcome prediction of acute renal failure in medical intensive care. Intensive Care Med 17:19–24
5. Abreo K, Moorthy VA, Osborne M (1986) Changing pattern and outcome of acute renal failure requiring hemodialysis. Arch Intern Med 146:1338–1341
6. Butkus DE (1983) Persistent high mortality in acute renal failure. Arch Intern Med 143:209–212
7. Stott RB, Cameron JS, Ogg CS et al. (1972) Why the persistently high mortality in acute renal failure? Lancet 2:75–79
8. Maher JF, Chackrabarti E (1984) Ultrafiltration by hyperosmotic peritoneal dialysis fluid excludes intracellular solutes. Am J Nephrol 4:169–174
9. Cameron JS, Ogg C, Trounce JR (1967) Peritoneal dialysis in hypercatabolic acute renal failure. Lancet 1:1118–1121
10. Tzamaloukas AH, Garella S, Chazan JA (1973) Peritoneal dialysis for acute renal failure after major abdominal surgery. Arch Surg 106:639–645
11. Korchik WP, Brown DC, De Master EG (1978) Hemodialysis induced hypotension. Int J Artif Intern Organs 1:151–156
12. Ronco C, Fabris A, Chiaramonte S et al. (1988) Comparison of four different short dialysis techniques. Int J Artif Intern Organs 3:169–174
13. Aurigemma NM, Feldman NT, Gottlieb M, Ingram RH, Lazarus JM, Lowrie EG (1977) Arterial oxygenation during hemodialysis. N Engl J Med 279:871–875
14. Mault JR, Dechert RE, Bartlett RH, Swartz RD, Ferguson SK (1982) Oxygen consumption during hemodialysis for acute renal failure. Trans Am Soc Artif Intern Organs 28:510–515
15. Koshariah P, Ilstrup A, Constantini I, Berkseth R, Shapiro F (1980) The influence of ultrafiltration and diffusion on cardiovascular parameters. Trans Am Soc Artif Intern Organs 26:328–333
16. La Greca G, Dettori P, Biasioli S et al. (1980) Brain density changes during hemodialysis. Lancet 2:582–584
17. La Greca G, Dettori P, Biasioli S et al. (1981) Study on morphological and densitometrical changes in the brain after hemodialysis and peritoneal dialysis. Trans Am Soc Artif Intern Organs 27:40–44
18. Bellomo R, Mansfield D, Rumble S, Shapiro J, Parkin G, Boyce N (1992) A comparison of conventional dialytic therapy and acute continuous haemodiafiltration in the management of acute renal failure in the critically ill. ASAIO J 38:M654–M657
19. Bellomo R, Boyce N (1993) Continuous venovenous hemodiafiltration compared with conventional dialysis in critically ill patients with acute renal failure. ASAIO J 39:M794–M797
20. Kramer P, Wigger W, Rieger J, Matthaei D, Scheler F (1977) Arteriovenous hemodiafiltration: a new and simple method for treatment of overhydrated patients resistant to diuretics. Klin Wochenschr 55:1121–1122
21. Lauer A, Saccaggi A, Ronco C, Belledonne M, Glabman S, Bosch JP (1983) Continuous arteriovenous hemofiltration in the critically ill patient. Ann Intern Med 99:445–460
22. Kaplan AA, Longnecker RE, Folkert VW (1984) Continuous arteriovenous hemofiltration – a report of six months' experience. Ann Intern Med 100:358–367

23. Kaplan AA (1983) Predilution versus postdilution for continuous arteriovenous haemofiltration. Trans Am Soc Artif Intern Organs 31:2832–2833
24. Kaplan AA, Longnecker RE, Folkert VW (1983) Suction assisted continuous arteriovenous hemofiltration. Trans Am Soc Artif Intern Organs 29:408–423
25. Geronemus, R, Schneider N (1984) Continuous arteriovenous hemodialysis: a new modality for treatment of acute renal failure. Trans Am Soc Artif Intern Organs 30:610–613
26. Ronco C, Brendolan A, Bragantini L et al. (1986) Arteriovenous hemofiltration associated with continuous arteriovenous hemodiafiltration: a combined therapy for acute renal failure in hypercatabolic patients. In: La Greca G, Fabris A, Ronco C (eds) Proceedings of the international symposium on continuous arteriovenous hemofiltration. Wichtig, Milan, pp 171–183
27. Canaud B, Garred LJ, Christol JP, Anbas S, Beraud JJ, Mion C (1988) Pump assisted continuous venovenous hemofiltration for treating acute uremia. Kidney Int 33:S154–S156
28. Bellomo R, Parkin G, Love J, Boyce N (1992) Management of acute renal failure in the critically ill with continuous venovenous hemofiltration. Ren Fail 14:183–186
29. Heinrich WL (1993) Arteriovenous or venovenous continuous therapies are not superior to standard hemodialysis in all patients with acute renal failure. Semin Dial 6:174–176
30. Paganin E (1993) Continuous renal replacement is the preferred treatment for all acute renal failure patients receiving intensive care. Semin Dial 6:176–179
31. Bellomo R, Boyce N (1993) Does continuous hemodiafiltration improve survival in acute renal failure? Semin Dial 6:16–19
32. Firth JD (1993) Renal replacement therapy on the intensive care unit. Q J Med 86:74–77
33. Kierdorf (1991) Continuous versus intermittent treatment: clinical results in acute renal failure. Contrib Nephrol 93:1–12
34. McDonald BR, Mehta RL (1991) Decreased mortality in patients with acute renal failure undergoing continuous arteriovenous hemodialysis. Contrib Nephrol 93:51–56
35. Berisa F, Beaman M, Adu D et al. (1990) Prognostic factors in acute renal failure following aortic aneurysm surgery. Q J Med 76:689–698
36. Spiegel DM, Ullian ME, Zerbe GO, Berl T (1991) Determinants of survival and recovery in acute renal failure patients dialyzed in intensive-care units. Am J Nephrol 11:44–47
37. Ishitani M, Wilkowski M, Stevenson W, Pruett T (1993) Outcome of patients requiring hemodialysis after liver transplantation. Tranplant Proc 25:1762–1763
38. Frost L, Pedersen RS, Hansen HE (1991) Prognosis in septicemia complicated by acute renal failure requiring dialysis. Scand J Urol Nephrol 25:307–310
39. Pataca MI, Ramesh BR, Parmer A, Rifkin I, Ware RJ, Parsons V (1992) Continuous arteriovenous haemodialysis in severe combined renal and respiratory failure. Blood Purif 10:262–628
40. Alarabi AA, Danielson BG, Wikstroem B (1993) Continuous arteriovenous hemodialysis: outcome in intensive care acute renal failure patients. Nephron 64:58–62
41. Baudouin SV, Wiggins J, Keogh BF, Morgan CJ, Evans TW (1993) Continuous venovenous haemofiltration following cardiopulmonary bypass. Intensive Care Med 19:290–293
42. Tominaga GT, Ingegno M, Ceraldi C, Waxman K (1993) Vascular complications of continuous arteriovenous hemofiltration in trauma patients. J Trauma 35:285–289
43. Vesconi S, Sicignano A, De Pietri P et al. (1993) Continuous venovenous hemofiltration in critically ill patients with multiple organ failure. Int J Artif Organs 16:592–598
44. Reynolds HN, Borg U, Belzberg H, Wiles CE (1991) Efficacy of continuous arteriovenous hemofiltration with dialysis in patients with renal failure. Crit Care Med 19:1387–1394
45. Barton IK, Hilton PJ, Taub NA et al. (1993) Acute renal failure treated by hemofiltration: factors affecting outcome. Q J Med 86:81–90
46. Storck M, Hartl WH, Zimmerer E, Inthorn D (1991) Comparison of pump driven and spontaneous continuous haemofiltration in post operative acute renal failure. Lancet 1:452–455

47. Bellomo R, Boyce N (1993) Acute continuous hemodiafiltration: a prospective study of 110 patients and a review of the literature. Am J Kidney Dis 21:508–518
48. Bagshaw ONT, Anaes FRC, Hutchinson A (1992) Continuous arteriovenous hemofiltration and respiratory function in multiple organ system failure. Intensive Care Med 18:334–338
49. Macias WL, Mueller BA, Scarim SK, Robinson M, Rudy DW (1991) Continuous venovenous hemofiltration: an alternative to continuous arteriovenous hemofiltration and hemodiafiltration in acute renal failure. Am J Kidney Dis 18:451–458
50. Voerman HJ, Strack van Schijndel RJ, Thijs L (1990) Continuous arterial-venous hemodiafiltration in critically ill patients. Crit Care Med 18:911–914
51. Alarabi AA, Brendolan A, Danielson BG, Raimondi F, Ronco C, Wikstroem B (1991) Outcome of continuous arteriovenous hemofiltration in acute renal failure. Contrib Nephrol 93:17–19
52. Sluiter HE, Froberg L, van Dijl J, Go JG (1991) Mortality of high-risk intensive care patients with acute renal failure treated with continuous arteriovenous hemofiltration. Contrib Nephrol 93:20–22
53. Schaefer GE, Doering C, Sodemann K, Russ A, Schroeder HM (1991) Continuous arteriovenous and veno-venous hemodialysis in critically ill patients. Contrib Nephrol 93:23–28
54. Hirasawa H, Sugai T, Ohtake Y (1991) Continuous hemofiltration and hemodiafiltration in the management of multiple organ failure. Contrib Nephrol 93:42–46
55. Canaud B, Cristol JP, Berthelemy C, Klouche K, Beraud JJ, Mion C (1991) Acute renal failure associated with multiple organ failure: pump-assisted continuous venovenous hemofiltration, the ultimate treatment modality. Contrib Nephrol 93:32–38
56. Keller E, Reetze-Bonorden P, Luecking H-P, Boehler J, Schollmeyer P (1991) Continuous arteriovenous hemodialysis: experience in twenty-six intensive care patients. Contrib Nephrol 93:47–50
57. Keusch G, Schreier P, Binswanger U (1991) Outcome in critically ill patients with acute renal failure treated by continuous hemofiltration. Contrib Nephrol 93:57–60
58. Harris D (1990) Acute renal replacement – which treatment is best. Aust N Z J Med 20:197–200
59. Bocci V (1991) Interleukins. Clinical pharmacokinetics and practical implications. Clin Pharmacokinet 21:274–284
60. Ferraiolo BL, McCabe J, Hollenbach S et al. (1989) Pharmacokinetics of recombinant human tumor necrosis factor-alpha in rats: effects of size and number of doses and nephrectomy. Drug Metab Dispos 17:369–372
61. Pessina GP, Pacini A, Bocci V, Maioli E, Naldini A (1987) Studies on tumor necrosis factor. II. Metabolic fate and distribution of recombinant TNF. Lymphokine Res 6:35–43
62. Kudo S, Mizuno K, Hirai Y, Shimizu T (1990) Clearance and tissue distribution of recombinant human interleukin 1 beta in rats. Cancer Res 50:5751–5755
63. Konrad MW, Hemstreet G, Hersh EM et al. (1990) Pharmacokinetics of recombinant interleukin 2 in humans. Cancer Res 50:2009–2017
64. Hakim RA (1990) Assessing the adequacy of dialysis. Kidney Int 37:822–832
65. Lowry SF (1993) Anticytokine therapies in sepsis. New Horizons 1:120–126
66. Fong Y, Moldawer LL, Shires GT et al. (1990) The biological characteristics of cytokines and their implication in surgical injury. Surg Gynecol Obstet 170:363–378
67. Ohlsson K, Bjork P, Bergenfeldt M et al. (1990) Interleukin-1 receptor antagonist reduces mortality from endotoxin shock. Nature 348:550–552
68. Chatenoud L, Herbelin A, Beauran G, Descamps-Latscha B (1990) Immune deficiency of the uremic patients. Adv Nephrol 19:259–274
69. Lewis SL, van Epps DE (1987) Neutrophil and monocyte alterations in chronic dialysis patients. Am J Kidney Dis 9:381–395
70. Vanholder R, Ringoir S, Dhont A, Hakim R (1991) Phagocytosis in uremic and hemodialysis patients: a prospective and cross-sectional study. Kidney Int 39:320–327

71. Descamps-Latscha B, Herbelin A (1993) Long-term dialysis and cellular immunity: a critical survey. Kidney Int 43:S135–S142
72. Bosch JP, Ronco C (1989) Continuous arteriovenous hemofiltration (CAVH) and other continuous replacement therapies: operational characteristics and clinical use. In: Maher (ed) Replacement of renal function by dialysis, 3rd edn. Kluwer, Dordrecht, pp 347–359
73. Biasioli S, Barbaresi F, Barbiero M et al. (1992) Intermittent venovenous hemofiltration as a chronic treatment for refractory and intractable heart failure. ASAIO J 38:M658–M663
74. Davenport A, Will EJ, Davison AM et al. (1989) Changes in intracranial pressure during hemofiltration in oliguric patients with grade IV hepatic encephalopathy. Nephron 53: 142–146
75. Campbell TJ, Wyse KR, Hemsworth PD (1991) Effects of hyperkalemia, acidosis, and hypoxia on the depression of maximum rate of depolarization by class I antiarrhythmic drugs in guinea pig myocardium: differential actions of class Ib and Ic agents. J Cardiovasc Pharmacol 18:51–59
76. Zhou HZ, Malhotra D, Shapiro JI (1991) Contractile dysfunction during metabolic acidosis: role of impaired energy metabolism. Am J Physiol 261:H1481–H1486
77. Kveim M, Nesbakken R (1975) Utilization of exogenous acetate during hemodialysis. Trans Am Soc Artif Intern Organs 21:138–142
78. Niessenson AR, Kraut JA, Shinaberger JH (1984) Dialysis associated hypoxemia: pathogenesis and prevention. Trans Am Soc Artif Intern Organs 7:1–9
79. Bouffard Y, Viale JP, Annat G et al. (1986) Pulmonary gas exchange during hemodialysis. Kidney Int 30:920–927
80. Bauer W, Richards JW (1928) A vasodilatory action of acetate. J Physiol 66:371–384
81. Kirkendol PL, Devia CJ, Bower JD, Holbert RD (1977) A comparison of the cardiovascular effects of sodium acetate, sodium bicarbonate and other potential sources of fixed base in hemodialysate solutions. Trans Am Soc Artif Intern Organs 23:399–403
82. Graefe U, Milutinovich J, Follette WC, Vizzo JB, Babb AL, Scribner BH (1978) Less dialysis-induced morbidity and vascular instability with bicarbonate in dialysate. Ann Intern Med 88:332–340
83. Borges H, Fryd DS, Rosa AA, Kjellstrand CM (1981) Hypotension during acetate and bicarbonate dialysis in patients with acute renal failure. Am J Nephrol 1:24–31
84. Eiser AR, Jayammane D, Kokseng C, Che H, Slifkin RF, Neff MS (1982) Contrasting alterations in pulmonary gas exchange during acetate and bicarbonate hemodialysis. Am J Nephrol 2:123–129
85. Barton IK, Streather CP, Hilton PJ, Bradley RD (1991) Successful treatment of severe lactic acidosis by hemofiltration using a bicarbonate-based replacement fluid. Nephrol Dial Transplant 6:368–370
86. Davenport A, Will EJ, Davison AM (1990) Paradoxical increase in arterial hydrogen ion concentration in patients with hepatorenal failure given lactate based fluids. Nephrol Dial Transplant 5:342–346
87. Nimmo GR, MacKenzie SJ, Walker S, Nicol M, Grant IS (1993) Acid-base responses to high volume haemofiltration in the critically ill. Nephrol Dial Transplant 8:854–857
88. Sieberth H, Mann H, Kierdorf H (1993) Acute complications in patients with chronic renal failure. In: Pinsky MR, Dhainaut A (eds) Pathophysiologic foundations of critical care. Williams and Wilkins, Baltimore, pp 677–695
89. Dinarello CA (1990) Cytokines and biocompatibility. Blood Purif 8:208–213
90. Hakim R (1993) Clinical implications of hemodialysis membrane bioincompatibility. Kidney Int 44:484–494
91. Bellomo R, Tipping P, Boyce N (1993) Continuous venovenous hemofiltration with dialysis removes cytokines from the circulation of septic patients. Crit Care Med 21:522–526
92. Tonnessen E, Hansen MB, Hoehndorf K et al. (1993) Cytokines in plasma and ultrafiltrate during continuous arteriovenous haemofiltration. Anaesth Intensive Care 21:752–758

93. Arnout MA, Hakim RM, Todd RF, Dana N, Colten HR (1985) Increased expression of an adhesion promoting glycoprotein in the granulocytopenia of hemodialysis. N Engl J Med 312:457–462
94. Himmelfarb J, Lazarus M, Hakim R (1991) Reactive oxygen species production by monocytes and polymorphonuclear leukocytes during dialysis. Am J Kidney Dis 3:271–276
95. Luger A, Kovarik J, Stummvoll HK, Urbanska A, Luger TA (1987) Blood membrane interaction in hemodialysis leads to increased cytokine production. Kidney Int 32:84–88
96. Strasser T, Schiffl H (1991) Generation of leukotriene B4 by hemodialyzer membranes: a novel index of biocompatibility. Klin Wochenschr 69:808–812
97. Hakim RM, Schafer AI (1985) Hemodialysis associated platelet activation and thrombocytopenia. Am J Med 78:575–580
98. Chenoweth DE, Cheung AK, Ward DM, Henderson LW (1983) Anaphylatoxin formation during hemodialysis: effect of different dialyzer membranes. Kidney Int 24:770–774
99. Conger JD (1990) Does hemodialysis delay recovery from acute renal failure? Semin Dial 3:146–148
100. Hakim R, Wingard RL, Lawrence P, Parker RA, Schulman G (1992) Use of biocompatible membranes improves outcome and recovery from acute renal failure (Abstr). J Am Soc Nephrol 3:367
101. Gotloib L, Barzilay E, Shustak A, Wais Z, Jaichenko J, Lev A (1986) Hemofiltration in septic ARDS. The artificial kidney as an artificial endocrine lung. Resuscitation 13:123–132
102. Ossenkoppele GJ, van der Meulen J, Bronsveld W, Thijs LG (1985) Continuous arteriovenous hemofiltration as an adjunctive therapy for septic shock. Crit Care Med 13:102–104
103. Gomez A, Wang R, Unruh H et al. (1990) Hemofiltration reverses left ventricular dysfunction during sepsis in dogs. Anesthesiology 73:671–685
104. Grootendorst AF, van Bommel EFH, van der Hoven B, van Leengoed LAMG, van Osta ALM (1992) High volume hemofiltration improves right ventricular function in endotoxin induced shock in the pig. Intensive Care Med 18:235–240
105. Grootendorst AF, van Bommel EFH, van Leengoed LAMG, van Zanten ARH, Huipen HJC, Groeneveld ABJ (1993) Infusion of ultrafiltrate from endotoxemic pigs depresses myocardial performance in normal pigs. J Crit Care 8:161–169
106. Coraim F, Trubel W, Ebermann R, Wolner E (1991) Elimination of myocardial depressant substances by hemofiltration in patients with cardiogenic shock (Abstr). Circ Shock 34:117
107. Stein B, Pfenninger E, Gruenert A, Schmitz JE, Deller A, Kocher F (1991) The consequences of continuous haemofiltration on lung mechanics and extravascular lung water in a porcine endotoxic shock model. Intensive Care Med 17:293–298
108. Lee P, Matson JR, Pryor RW, Hinshaw LBH (1993) Continuous arteriovenous hemofiltration therapy for staphylococcus aureus-induced septicemia in immature swine. Crit Care Med 21:914–924
109. Barzilay E, Kessler D, Berlot G, Gullo A, Geber D, Ben Zeev I (1989) Use of extracorporeal supportive techniques as additional treatment for septic-induced multiple organ failure patients. Crit Care Med 17:634–637
110. Ronco C, Burchardi H (1993) Management of acute renal failure in the critically ill patient. In: Pinsky, Dhainaut (eds) Pathophysiologic foundations of critical care. Williams and Wilkins, Baltimore, pp 630–676
111. Cheadle W, Hanasawa K, Gallinaro RN, Nimmanwudipong T, Kodama M, Polk AC (1991) Endotoxin filtration and immune stimulation improve survival from gram negative sepsis. Surgery 100:785–792
112. Nagaki M, Hughes RD, Keane HM, Lau JYN, Williams R (1992) In vitro plasma perfusion through adsorbent and plasma ultrafiltration to remove endotoxin and cytokines. Circ Shock 38:182–188

Drug Use in Critically Ill Patients with Acute Renal Failure

T.A. Golper, H.H. Vincent, and U.F. Kroh

Introduction

Patients with acute renal failure (ARF) who are critically ill are too sick to tolerate pharmaceutical errors. Therefore, an understanding of proper drug management in this setting is mandatory. The three major renal replacement therapies are peritoneal dialysis (usually long dwell after an initial short-dwell phase), hemofiltration, and hemodialysis. The purpose of this chapter is to review factors related to drug usage during renal insufficiency and drug handling during these therapies.

Pharmacokinetic Background

Drug Distribution Volume

The apparent volume of distribution of a drug at steady state (V_d) is the amount of drug in the body (mg/kg) divided by the plasma concentration (mg/l) at plasma and tissue equilibrium. Its units are (mg/kg)/(mg/l) or l/kg. V_d does not correspond to a particular anatomic compartment or fluid space, but denotes a mathematical relationship which assumes the body is a homogeneous reservoir of water. A drug highly bound to certain tissues (e.g., digoxin, tricyclic antidepressants, metoclopramide) will frequently have a large V_d, while drugs highly bound to circulating proteins (e.g., oxacillin, phenytoin) will be restricted to the vascular space and thus will have a small V_d. Certain disease states (such as uremia) change the V_d, but this becomes clinically important only when the V_d is small (less than 0.7 l/kg). During changing rates of fluid gain and loss, as in ARF, V_d is likely to vary, especially for drugs whose V_d is predominantly the extracellular fluid space, e.g., aminoglycosides. There are no studies specifically investigating the V_d of drugs during continuous hemofiltration. However, Matzke et al. [1] have described a rebound in serum vancomycin concentration following high-flux hemofiltration, reflecting redistribution. In addition, Morse et al. [2] have shown that peritonitis alters the V_d of vancomycin.

Elimination Half-Life

Most drugs are eliminated from the body by first-order kinetics, which means that a constant *fraction* of the drug is eliminated per unit time. When the elimination process is saturated, zero-order kinetics apply, wherein a constant *amount* is eliminated per unit time. Very few drugs are metabolized this way. In practical clinical terms, a drug following first-order kinetics will have its plasma concentration drop by a constant fraction per unit time. Drug removal rate is conventionally expressed as the elimination half-life ($T_{1/2}$), the time required for the total body drug burden and plasma level to decrease by half. The $T_{1/2}$ for any drug is dependent on its clearance (renal, hepatic, dialytic, hemofilter, other) and its V_d by the formula

$$T_{1/2} = \frac{0.693 \times V_d}{\text{clearance}} \tag{1}$$

Thus for a given clearance, the larger the V_d, the longer the $T_{1/2}$. Conversely, a reduction in clearance prolongs $T_{1/2}$. When *maintenance doses* are administered, steady state plasma levels are achieved after three to five half-lives. If a *loading dose* is administered, a steady state level is reached within minutes. Without further doses, after five half-lives only 3% of the drug remains.

Clearance

Total body clearance is the sum of all regional clearances which include renal, hepatic, other endogenous clearances, and any exogenous techniques such as hemofiltration or dialysis. A procedure which improves uremia may alter endogenous clearance. For example, correcting uremia can improve hepatic function. On the other hand, uremia can induce some hepatic enzymes such that drug clearance is enhanced (e.g., anticonvulsants). The acuity of the renal dysfunction also may impact on the metabolism of a drug [3]. Clearance units (ml/min) are awkward and of limited use in the acute clinical setting. Absolute drug removal per unit time (usually 6- to 24-h increments) is more useful in ARF. If clearance is the preferred concept, steady state serum concentrations are necessary for proper comparisons (see above). For example during continuous renal replacement therapy (CRRT) with a clearance of 20 ml/min (28.8 l/day), 28.8 l plasma is completely cleared of the steady state solute or drug. However, during a once-daily 4-h intermittent hemodialysis procedure, a clearance of 100 ml/min cannot be extrapolated to be 240 min × 100 ml/min or 24 l/day. The reason is that the plasma concentration falls dramatically during the 4 h of hemodialysis, which is the only actual clearance period over the course of the day. Any extrapolation assumes a steady state plasma concentration. Thus, while the clearance term is technically correct, it is very misleading. The traditional clearance unit (ml/min) is applicable when totaling regional clearances to determine total body clearance. Generally speaking, a regional clearance of 30% or greater of the total body clearance is considered substantial enough to appreciate clinically [4, 5].

When discussing "regional" clearances (e.g., renal, hepatic, extracorporeal device etc.) in ARF, several confounding factors must be considered. In the critically ill patient with ARF extrarenal (nonrenal) clearance may be altered by the ARF itself. Nonrenal imipenem clearance is increased in this setting, hence its aggressive dosing recommendations (see Table 1). This altered elimination has been discussed in detail by Kroh et al. [6–8]. For example, the nonrenal clearance of cefotaxime, piperacilin, and theophylline are reduced by multiorgan failure.

Protein Binding

Drugs have the potential to reversibly bind to circulating nonultrafilterable plasma proteins, especially, but not exclusively, albumin. Only the free or unbound fraction of drug is pharmacologically distributed, active, metabolized, and excreted. Protein-bound drug is unavailable for removal by renal replacement therapies with the possible exception of certain sorbents. Other exceptions are discussed below. Drug levels measured in serum, blood, or plasma are almost always totals of the bound and free fractions and are thus potentially misleading regarding drug activity.

Many factors affect protein binding including uremia, acidosis, the presence of elevated free fatty acids (FFA), the molar ratios of drug to protein, temperature, and the presence of displacing substances such as drugs, organic acids, bilirubin, and heparin [9–20]. The clinical significance will vary from drug to drug and patient to patient. Subsequently, protein-binding alterations in uremia are not necessarily predictable [20]. The possibility clearly exists that during hemofiltration or dialysis, drug displacement will occur and ultrafiltrative and diffusive losses will be increased. Furthermore, when displacement occurs, the drug's clinical effect will be enhanced. Altered protein binding may become clinically important in the setting of highly bound drugs with a low therapeutic index. To further point out the complexity of the issue of drug–protein binding, it has been shown that elevated FFA may displace cefamandole, but may actually enhance the binding of another cephalosporin (e.g., cephalothin or cefoxitin) [15]. The effects of FFA are particularly relevant in ARF when intravenous fat emulsions are used during hyperalimentation. In addition to this exogenous administration of fatty acid, heparin produces a rapid increase in FFA through activation of the enzyme lipoprotein lipase. Gulyassy and Depner have extensively reviewed drug–protein binding in uremia [16]. Drug protein

Table 1. Drugs frequently used in the intensive care unit (ICU)

Drug/toxicity notes	Half-life in uremia (h)[a]	Plasma protein binding (%)	Volume of distribution (l/kg)	Dose for normal renal function	Method	GFR		Supplement		
						10–50 ml/min	<10 ml/min	Hemo	CEPD	CRRT
Antiarrythmics										
Adenosine	10 s	0	Unknown	3–6 mg i.v. bolus	D	100%	100%	None	None	nd
Amiodarone	14–120 days	96	70–140	800–2000 mg load 200–600 mg q day	D	100%	100%	None	None	nd
Bretylium	16–32	6	8.2	5–30 mg/kg load 5–10 mg i.v. q 6 h	D	25%–50%	25%	None	None	nd
Disopyramide	10–18	54–81	0.8–2.6	100–200 mg q 6 h	I	q 12–24 h	q 24–40 h	None	None	nd
Encainide	1.5–9	75–81	2–2.7	25 mg q 8 h to 50 mg q 6 h	D	75%	50%	nd	nd	nd
Flecainide	19–26	52	8.4–9.5	100 mg q 12 h to 350–400 mg prn	D	100%	50%–75%	None	None	nd
Lidocaine	1.3–3	60–66	1.3–2.2	50 mg over 2 min repeat q 5 min × 3 then 1–4 mg/min	D	100%	100%	None	None	nd
Lorcainide	Unknown	80–85	10	100 g b.i.d.	D	100%	100%	nd	nd	nd
Mexilitine	16	70–75	5.5–6.6	100–300 mg q 6–12 h	D	100%	50%–75%	None	None	None
Moricizine	3	95	>5	200–300 q 8 h	D	100%	100%	None	None	nd
N-Acetyl-procainamide	42–70	10–20	1.5–1.7	500 mg q 6–8 h	D/I	50% q 8–12 h	25% q 12–18 h	None	None	Replace by blood level
Procainamide	5.5	15	2.2	350–400 mg q 3–4 h	I	q 6–12 h	q 8–24 h	200 mg	None	Replace by blood level

Propafenone	Unknown	>95	3	150–300 mg q 8 h	D	100%	100%	None	None	nd
Quinidine	4–14	70–95	2–3.5	200–400 mg q 4–6 h	D	100%	75%	100–200 mg	None	nd
Tocainide	22–27	10–20	3.2	200–400 g q 4–6 h	D	100%	50%	200 mg	None	nd
Antibacterial antibiotics										
Aminoglycosides										
Amikacin	17–150	<5	0.22–0.29	5 mg/kg q 8 h	D/I	30%–70% q 12–18 h	20%–30% q 24–48 h	Two thirds normal dose after dialysis	15–20 mg/l per day	Dose for GFR of 10–50 ml/min measure levels
Gentamicin	20–60	<5	0.23–0.26	1 mg/kg q 8 h	D/I	30%–70% q 12 h	10%–20% q 24–48 h	Two thirds normal dose after dialysis	3–4 mg/l per day	Dose for GFR of 10–50 ml/min measure levels
Netilmicin	35–72	<5	0.16–0.30	5 mg/kg q 8 h	D/I	20%–60% q 12 h	10%–20% q 24–48 h	Two thirds normal dose after dialysis	3–4 mg/l per day	Dose for GFR of 10–50 ml/min and measure levels
Tobramycin	27–60	<5	0.22–0.33	1 mg/kg q 8 h	D/I	30%–70% q 12 h	20%–30% q 24–48 h	Two thirds normal dose after dialysis	3–4 mg/l per day	Dose for GFR of 10–50 ml/min
Cephalosporins										
Cefaclor	3	25	0.24–0.35	250–500 mg t.i.d.	D	50%–100%	50%	250 mg after dialysis	250 mg q 8–12 h	na
Cefadroxil	22	20	0.31	0.5–1.0 g q 12 h	I	q 12–24 h	q 24–48 h	0.5–1.0 g after dialysis	0.5 g/day	na

D, dose reduction method (the numbers that follow "D" refer to the fraction of the normal dose which should be administered); I, the interval extension method where the usual dose is administered, but at an extended interval between doses (the numbers that following "I" refer to the dosing interval); Hemo, conventional hemodialysis; CEPD, continuous equilibrium peritoneal dialysis; CRRT, continuous renal replacement therapy (arteriovenous or venovenous filtration, dialysis, or diafiltration); nd, no data; na, not applicable; GFR, glomerular filtration rate; q hs, delivered at bedtime.

[a] In hours unless stated otherwise.

Table 1. *Continued*

Drug/toxicity notes	Half-life in uremia (h)[a]	Plasma protein binding (%)	Volume of distribution (l/kg)	Dose for normal renal function	Method	GFR		Supplement		
						10–50 ml/min	<10 ml/min	Hemo	CEPD	CRRT
Cefamandole	6–11	75	0.16–0.25	0.5–1.0 g q 4–8 h	I	q 6–8 h	q 12 h	0.5–1.0 g after dialysis	0.5–1.0 g q 12 h	Dose for GFR of 10–50 ml/min
Cefazolin	40–70	80	0.13–0.22	0.5–1.5 g q 6 h	I	q 12 h	q 24–48 h	0.5–1.0 g after dialysis	0.5 g q 12 h	Dose for GFR of 10–50 ml/min
Cefmenoxime	6–12	43–75	0.27–0.37	1 g q 6 h	D/I	0.75 g q 8 h	0.75 g q 12 h	0.75 g after dialysis	0.75 g q 12 h	Dose for GFR of 10–50 ml/min
Cefmetazole	21	75	0.18	2 g q 6–12 h	I	q 24 h	q 48 h	Dose after dialysis	Dose for GFR <10 ml/min	Dose for GFR of 10–50 ml/min
Cefonicid	17–59	96	0.09–0.18	1 g q 24 h	D/I	0.1–0.5 g q day	0.1 g q day	None	None	None
Cefoperazone	2.9	90	0.14–0.20	1–2 g q 12 h	D	100%	100%	1 g after dialysis	None	None
Ceforanide	25	80	0.17	0.5–1.0 g q 12 h	I	q 12–24 h	q 24–48 h	0.5–1.0 g after dialysis	None	1 g q 24 h
Cefotaxime	15	37	0.15–0.55	1 g q 6 h	I	q 8–12 h	q 24 h	1 g after dialysis	1 g q day	1 g q 8–12 h
Cefotetan	13–25	85	0.15	1–2 g q 12 h	D	50%	25%	1 g after dialysis	1 g q day	750 mg q 12 h
Cefoxitin	13–23	41–75	0.2	1–2 g q 6–8 h	I	q 8–12 h	q 24–48 h	1 g after dialysis	1 g q day	Dose for GFR of 10–50 ml/min

Cefpodoxime	26	26	0.6–1.2	200 mg q 12 h	I	q 16 h	q 24–48 h	200 mg after dialysis only	Dose for GFR <10 ml/min	na
Cefsulodin	13	15–30	0.25	0.5–1.0 g q 6 h	I	q 12–24 h	q 24 h	Dose after dialysis	Dose for GFR <10 ml/min	Dose for GFR of 10–50 ml/min
Ceftazidime	13–25	17	0.28–0.4	1–2 g q 8 h	I	q 24–48 h	q 48 h	1 g after dialysis	0.5 g q day	1 g q 12 h
Ceftizoxime	35	28–50	0.26–0.42	1–2 g q 8–12 h	I	q 12–24 h	q 24 h	1 g after dialysis	0.5–1.0 g q day	Dose for GFR of 10–50 ml/min
Ceftriaxone	12–24	90	0.12–0.18	0.2–1.0 g q 12 h	D	100%	100%	Dose after dialysis	750 mg q 12 h	Dose for GFR of 10–50 ml/min
Cefuroxime sodium	17	33	0.13–1.8	0.75–1.5 g q 8 h	I	q 8–12 h	q 24 h	Dose after dialysis	Dose for GFR <10 ml/min	1 g q 12 h
Cephalothin	3–18	65	0.26	0.5–2.0 g q 6 h	I	q 6–8 h	q 12 h	Dose after dialysis	1 g q 12 h	1 g q 8 h
Cephapirin	2.5	45–60	0.22	0.5–2.0 g q 6 h	I	q 6–8 h	q 12 h	Dose after dialysis	1 g q 12 h	1 g q 8 h
Moxalactam (Latamoxef)	18–23	35–59	0.18–0.40	1–2 g q 8–12 h	I	q 12–24 h	q 24–48 h	Dose after dialysis	Dose for GFR <10 ml/min	Dose for GFR of 10–50 ml/min
Miscellaneous										
Aztreonam	6–8	55	0.1–2.0	1–2 g q 8–12 h	D	50%–75%	25%	0.5 g after dialysis	Dose for GFR <10 ml/min	Dose for GFR of 10–50 ml/min
Chloramphenicol	3–7	45–60	0.5–1.0	12.5 mg/kg q 6 h	D	100%	100%	None	None	None

D, dose reduction method (the numbers that follow "D" refer to the fraction of the normal dose which should be administered); I, the interval extension method where the usual dose is administered, but at an extended interval between doses (the numbers that following "I" refer to the dosing interval); Hemo, conventional hemodialysis; CEPD, continuous equilibrium peritoneal dialysis; CRRT, continuous renal replacement therapy (arteriovenous or venovenous filtration, dialysis, or diafiltration); nd, no data; na, not applicable; GFR, glomerular filtration rate; q hs, delivered at bedtime.

[a] In hours unless stated otherwise.

Table 1. *Continued*

Drug/toxicity notes	Half-life in uremia (h)[a]	Plasma protein binding (%)	Volume of distribution (l/kg)	Dose for normal renal function	Method	GFR		Supplement		
						10–50 ml/min	<10 ml/min	Hemo	CEPD	CRRT
Clavulanic acid	3.5	30	0.3	100 mg q 4–6 h	D	100%	50%–75%	Dose after dialysis	Dose for GFR <10 ml/min	Dose for GFR of 10–50 ml/min
Clindamycin	4	60–95	0.6–1.2	150–300 mg q 6 h	D	100%	100%	None	None	None
Erythromycin	5.5	60–95	0.78	250–500 mg q 6–12 h	D	100%	50%–75%	None	None	None
Imipenem	4	13–21	0.17–0.3	0.25–1.0 g q 6 h	D	50%	25%	Dose after dialysis	Dose for GFR <10 ml/min	500 mg q 8 h
Meropenem	7	Low	0.35	500–1000 mg q 6 h	D/I	250–500 mg q 12 h	250–500 mg q 24 h	Dose after dialysis	Dose for GFR <10ml/min	Dose for GFR of 10–50 ml/min
Metronidazole	7–21	20	0.25–0.85	7.5 mg/kg q 6 h	D	100%	50%	Dose after dialysis	Dose for GFR <10 ml/min	Dose of GFR of 10–50 ml/min
Pentamidine	118	69	55–462	4 mg/kg per day	I	q 24–36 h	q 48 h	None	None	None
Rifampin	9.2	30	0.9	600 mg q 6 h	D	50%–100%	50%	None	Dose for GFR <10 ml/min	Dose for GFR <10 ml/min
Sulbactam	10–21	30	0.25–0.50	0.75–1.5 g q 6–8 h	I	q 12–24 h	q 24–48 h	Dose after dialysis	0.75–1.5 g q 24 h	750 mg q 12 h
Sulfamethoxazole	20–50	50	0.28–0.38	1.0 g q 8 h	I	q 18 h	q 24 h	1 g after dialysis	1 g q 24 h	Dose for GFR of 10–50 ml/min
Tazobactam	7	22	0.21	1.5–2.25 g/day	D	75%	50%	One third of dose after dialysis	Dose for GFR <10 ml/min	Dose for GFR of 10–50 ml/min

Teichoplanin	62–230	60–90	0.5–1.2	6 mg/kg per day	I	q 48 h	q 72 h	Dose for GFR <10 ml/min	Dose for GFR <10 ml/min	Dose for GFR of 10–50 ml/min
Trimethoprim	20–49	30–70	1–2.2	100–200 mg q 12 h	I	q 18 h	q 24	Dose after dialysis	q 24 h	q 18 h
Vancomycin	200–250	10–50	0.47–1.1	500 mg q 6 h or 1 g q 12 h	D/I	500 mg q 24–48 h	500 mg q 48–96 h	Dose for GFR <10 ml/min	Dose for GFR <10 ml/min	Dose for GFR of 10–50 ml/min
Penicillins										
Amoxicillin	5–20	15–25	0.26	250–500 mg q 8 h	I	q 8–12 h	q 24	Dose after dialysis	250 mg q 12 h	na
Ampicillin	7–20	20	0.17–0.31	250 mg–2 g q 6 h	I	q 6–12 h	q 12–24 h	Dose after dialysis	250 mg q 12 h	Dose for GFR of 10–50 ml/min
Azlocillin	5.5	30	0.18–0.27	2–3 g q 4 h	I	q 6–8 h	q 8 h	Dose after dialysis	Dose for GFR <10 ml/min	Dose for GFR of 10–50 ml/min
Methicillin	4	35–60	0.31	1–2 g q 4 h	I	q 6–8 h	q 8–12 h	None	None	None
Mezlocillin	2.6–5.4	20–46	0.18	1.5–4.0 g q 4–6 h	I	q 6–8 h	q 8 h	None	None	None
Nafcillin	1.2	85	0.35	1–2 g q 4–6 h	D	100%	100%	None	None	None
Penicillin G	6–20	50	0.3–0.42	0.5–4 million U q 6 h	D	75%	20%–50%	Dose after dialysis	Dose for GFR <10 ml/min	Dose for GFR of 10–50 ml/min
Piperacillin	3.3–5.1	30	0.18–0.30	3–4 g q 4 h	I	q 6–8 h	q 8 h	Dose after dialysis	Dose for GFR <10 ml/min	Dose for GFR of 10–50 ml/min
Ticarcillin	11–16	45–60	0.14–0.21	3 g q 4 h	D/I	1–2 g q 8 h	1–2 g q 12 h	3 g after dialysis	Dose for GFR <10 ml/min	Dose for GFR of 10–50 ml/min

D, dose reduction method (the numbers that follow "D" refer to the fraction of the normal dose which should be administered); I, the interval extension method where the usual dose is administered, but at an extended interval between doses (the numbers that following "I" refer to the dosing interval); Hemo, conventional hemodialysis; CEPD, continuous equilibrium peritoneal dialysis; CRRT, continuous renal replacement therapy (arteriovenous or venovenous filtration, dialysis, or diafiltration); nd, no data; na, not applicable; GFR, glomerular filtration rate; q hs, delivered at bedtime.

[a] In hours unless stated otherwise.

Table 1. *Continued*

Drug/toxicity notes	Half-life in uremia (h)[a]	Plasma protein binding (%)	Volume of distribution (l/kg)	Dose for normal renal function	Method	GFR		Supplement		
						10–50 ml/min	<10 ml/min	Hemo	CEPD	CRRT
Tetracyclines										
Doxycycline	18–25	80–93	0.75	100 mg q 24 h	D	100%	100%	None	None	None
Minocycline	12–18	70	1.0–1.5	100 mg q 12 h	D	100%	100%	None	None	None
Tetracycline	57–108	55–90	>0.7	250–500 mg q.i.d.	I	q 12–24 h	q 24 h	None	None	None
Quinolones										
Ciprofloxacin	609	20–40	2.5	500–750 mg q 12 h	D	50%–75%	50%	250 mg q 12 h	250 mg q 8 h	200 mg i.v. q 12 h
Fleroxicin	21–28	20	1.1–2.4	400 mg q 12 h	D	50%–75%	50%	400 mg after hemodialysis	400 mg q day	na
Norfloxacin	8	14	<0.5	400 mg q 12 h	I	q 12–24 h	Avoid	na	na	na
Ofloxacin	28–37	25	1.5–2.5	400 mg q day	D	50%	25%–50%	100 mg b.i.d.	Dose for GFR <10 ml/min	300 mg q day
Pefloxacin	15	25–43	2	400 mg q day	D	100%	100%	None	None	None
Antifungals										
Amphotericin	24	90	4	20–40 mg q 24 h	I	q 24 h	q 24–36 h	None	Dose for GFR <10 ml/min	Dose for GFR of 10–50 ml/min
Fluconazole	Unknown	12	0.7	200–400 mg q 24 h	I	q 24–48	q 48–72 h	200 mg after dialysis	Dose for GFR <10 ml/min	Dose for GFR of 10–50 ml/min
Flucytosine	75–200	<10	0.6	37.5 mg/kg q 6 h	I	q 16 h	q 24 h	Dose after dialysis	0.5–1.0 g q 24 h	Dose for GFR of 10–50 ml/min

Itraconazole	25	99	10	100–200 mg q 12 h	D	100%	50%–100%	100 mg q 12–24 h	100 mg q 12–24 h	100 mg q 12–24 h
Ketoconazole	3.3	99	1.9–3.6	200 mg q 24 h	D	100%	100%	None	None	None
Miconazole	22	90	Large	200–1200 mg q 8 h	D	100%	100%	None	None	None
Antivirals										
Acyclovir	20	15–30	0.7	5 mg/kg q 8 h	D/I	5 mg/kg q 12–24 h	2.5 mg/kg q 24 h	Dose after dialysis	Dose for GFR <10 ml/min	3.5 mg/kg per day
Amantadine	500	60	4–5	100 mg q 12 h	I	q 48–72 h	q 7 days	–	–	–
Didanosine	Unknown	Unknown	1.0	100–300 mg q 12 h	I	q 24 h	q 48 h	Dose after dialysis	Dose for GFR <10 ml/min	Dose for GFR <10 ml/min
Foscarnet	Prolonged	17	0.3–0.6	60 mg/kg q 8 h Induction doses only	D/I	15 mg/kg q 8 h	6 mg/kg q 8 h	Dose after dialysis	Dose for GFR <10 ml/min	Dose for GFR of 10–50 ml/min
Ganciclovir	30	Unknown	0.47	5 mg/kg q 12 h	I	q 24–48 h	q 48–96 h	Dose after dialysis	Dose for GFR <10 ml/min	2.5 mg/kg per day
Zidovudine (AZT)	1.4–3	10–30	1.4–3	200 mg q 4 h	D/I	200 mg q 4 h	100 mg q 6 h	100 mg after dialysis	Dose for GFR <10 ml/min	100 mg q 4 h
Anticonvulsants										
Carbamazepine	24 single dose 4–6 chronic dosing	75	0.8–1.6	200 mg b.i.d. to 1200 mg q day	D	100%	100%	None	None	None
Ethosuximide	45	10	0.6–0.9	500–1500 mg q day	D	100%	100%	None	Unknown	Unknown
Phenytoin	24	90	1.0	1000 mg load then 300–400 mg q day	D	100%	100%	None	None	None
Primidone	10	20–30	0.4–1.0	250–500 mg q.i.d.	I	q 8–12 h	q 12–24 h	One third of dose	Unknown	Unknown

D, dose reduction method (the numbers that follow "D" refer to the fraction of the normal dose which should be administered); I, the interval extension method where the usual dose is administered, but at an extended interval between doses (the numbers that following "I" refer to the dosing interval); Hemo, conventional hemodialysis; CEPD, continuous equilibrium peritoneal dialysis; CRRT, continuous renal replacement therapy (arteriovenous or venovenous filtration, dialysis, or diafiltration); nd, no data; na, not applicable; GFR, glomerular filtration rate; q hs, delivered at bedtime.

[a] In hours unless stated otherwise.

Table 1. *Continued*

Drug/toxicity notes	Half-life in uremia (h)[a]	Plasma protein binding (%)	Volume of distribution (l/kg)	Dose for normal renal function	Method	GFR		Supplement		
						10–50 ml/min	<10 ml/min	Hemo	CEPD	CRRT
Sodium valproate	6–15	90	0.19–0.23	15–60 mg/kg q day	D	100%	100%	None	None	None
Antihistamines										
H-1 Antagonists										
Diphenhydramine	Unknown	80	3.3–6.8	25 mg t.i.d.–q.i.d.	D	None	None	None	None	None
Promethazine	Unknown	93	13.5	12.5–25 mg q day–q.i.d.	D	None	None	None	None	None
H2-Antagonists										
Cimetidine	5	20	0.8–1.3	400 mg b.i.d. or 400–800 mg q hs	D	50%	25%	None	None	Unknown
Famotidine	12–19	15–22	0.8–1.4	20–40 mg q hs	D	25%	10%	None	None	None
Ranitidine	6–9	15	1.2–1.8	150–300 mg q hs	D	50%	25%	Half dose	None	Unknown
Barbiturates										
Phenobarbital	117–160	40–60	0.7–1	50–100 mg b.i.d.–t.i.d.	I	q 8–12 h	q 12–16 h	Dose after dialysis	Half of normal dose	None
Benzodiazepines										
Diazepam	20–90	94–98	0.7–3.4	5–40 mg q day	D	100%	100%	None	Unknown	Unknown
Lorazepam	32–70	87	0.9–1.3	1–2 mg b.i.d.–t.i.d.	D	100%	100%	None	Unknown	Unknown
Bronchodilators										
Albuterol	4	7	2.0–2.5	2–4 mg t.i.d. to q.i.d.	D	75%	50%	Unknown	Unknown	Unknown

Ipratropium	Unknown	Unknown	4.6	2 inhalations q.i.d.	D	100%	100%	None	None	None
Metaproterenol	Unknown	10	7.6	2–3 inhalations q 3–4h	D	100%	100%	Unknown	Unknown	Unknown
Terbutaline	Unknown	15–25	0.9–1.5	2.5–5 mg t.i.d.	D	50%	Avoid	Unknown	Unknown	Unknown
Theophylline	4–12	55	0.4–0.7	6 mg/kg load then 9 mg/kg per day	D	100%	100%	Half dose	Unknown	Unknown
CA Channel blockers										
Nifedipine	6	97	1.4	10–20 mg q 6–8 h	D	100%	100%	None	None	nd
Verapamil	2.4–4	83–93	3–6	80 mg q 8 h	D	100%	100%	None	None	nd
Cardiac glycosides										
Digitoxin	210	94	0.6	0.1–0.2 mg q day	D	100%	50%–75%	None	None	nd
Digoxin	80–120	20–30	5–8	1–1.5 mg load 0.25–0.5 mg q day	D/I	25%–75% q 36 h	10%–25% q 48 h	None	None	0.5 mg q 12 h
Ouabain	65	40	Unknown	0.25 mg load 0.1 mg q 12 h	I	q 24–36 h	q 36–48 h	None	None	None
Miscellangeous cardiac drugs										
Amrinone	Unknown	20–40	1.3–1.6	5–10 μg/kg per min; Daily dose <10 mg/kg	D	100%	50%–75%	nd	nd	nd
Dobutamine	Unknown	Unknown	0.25	2.5–15 μg/kg per min	D	100%	100%	nd	nd	nd
Milrinone	1.5–3	Unknown	0.25–0.35	15–75 ng/kg i.v. as load, then 2.5–15 mg q 6 h p.o.	D	100%	50%–75%	nd	nd	nd
Nitroglycerine	3 min	Unknown	2–3	Many methods and routes of dosing	–	100%	100%	nd	nd	nd

D, dose reduction method (the numbers that follow "D" refer to the fraction of the normal dose which should be administered); I, the interval extension method where the usual dose is administered, but at an extended interval between doses (the numbers that following "I" refer to the dosing interval); Hemo, conventional hemodialysis; CEPD, continuous equilibrium peritoneal dialysis; CRRT, continuous renal replacement therapy (arteriovenous or venovenous filtration, dialysis, or diafiltration); nd, no data; na, not applicable; GFR, glomerular filtration rate; q hs, delivered at bedtime.

Table 1. *Continued*

Drug/toxicity notes	Half-life in uremia (h)[a]	Plasma protein binding (%)	Volume of distribution (l/kg)	Dose for normal renal function	Method	GFR		Supplement		
						10–50 ml/min	<10 ml/min	Hemo	CEPD	CRRT
Miscellaneous drugs										
N-Acetyl-cysteine	Unknown	50	0.33–0.47	140 mg/kg load then 70 mg/kg q 4 h for 17 doses	D	100%	75%	Unknown	Unknown	Unknown
Pentoxifylline	0.8	None	2.4–4.2	400 mg t.i.d.	D	100%	100%	Unknown	Unknown	Unknown
Neuromuscular agents										
Tubocurarine	5.5	30–50	0.22–0.39	0.1–0.2 mg/kg	D	50%	Avoid	Unknown	Unknown	Unknown
Vecuronium	0.5–1.3	30	0.18–0.27	0.08–0.1 mg/kg load then 0.01–0.05 mg/kg q 12–15 min	D	100%	100%	Unknown	Unknown	Unknown
Phenothiazines										
Chlorpromazine	11–42	91–99	8–160	300–800 mg q day	D	100%	100%	None	None	Unknown
Promethazine	Unknown	Unknown	Large	20–100 mg q day	D	100%	100%	Unknown	Unknown	Unknown
Sedatives										
Haloperidol	Unknown	90–92	14–21	1–2 mg b.i.d.–t.i.d.	D	100%	100%	None	None	Unknown
Tricyclic antidepressants										
Amitriptyline	24–40	96	6–36	25 mg t.i.d.	D	100%	100%	None	None	Unknown
Doxepin	10–20	95	9–33	25 mg t.i.d.	D	100%	100%	None	None	Unknown

D, dose reduction method (the numbers that follow "D" refer to the fraction of the normal dose which should be administered); I, the interval extension method where the usual dose is administered, but at an extended interval between doses (the numbers that following "I" refer to the dosing interval); Hemo, conventional hemodialysis; CEPD, continuous equilibrium peritoneal dialysis; CRRT, continuous renal replacement therapy (arteriovenous or venovenous filtration, dialysis, or diafiltration); nd, no data; na, not applicable; GFR, glomerular filtration rate; q hs, delivered at bedtime.

[a] In hours unless stated otherwise.

binding is utilized below to determine the absolute amount of drug removed during hemofiltration.

Peritoneal Dialysis

Continuous equilibrium peritoneal dialysis (CEPD) is similar to continuous ambulatory peritoneal dialysis (CAPD) except that the patients are not ambulatory [21]. For purposes of drug removal it is appropriate to review the data from the CAPD experience. Factors affecting peritoneal drug clearance include the following:

1. Drug properties:
   a) Molecular weight
   b) Charge
   c) Lipid or water solubility
   d) V_d (tissue binding)
   e) Protein binding
   f) Other forms of steric hindrance
   g) Rapid excretion by another pathway
   h) Red cell partitioning
2. Intrinsic peritoneal membrane properties:
   a) Surface blood flow
   b) Surface area
   c) Loculation
   d) Sclerosis
   e) Pore size
   f) Vascular disease
   g) Fluid films
3. Dialysate properties:
   a) Flow rate
   b) Volume
   c) Chemical composition
   d) Distribution
   e) Temperature
4. Miscellaneous:
   a) Ultrafiltration
   b) Clearance additives to blood or dialysate

Several reviews cite specific drugs and their handling during peritoneal dialysis. CEPD is considered a long-dwell type of peritoneal dialysis [22–24]. Short-dwell peritoneal dialysis will increase clearances of all sizes of molecules, as compared to CEPD. The reviews cited above suggest that there does not appear to be substantial drug removal during either CAPD or CEPD.

A reasonable and practical generalization is that if hemodialysis does not remove a drug, then CEPD is unlikely to remove that drug either. Lasrich et al. [25] describe an inverse semilogarithmic relationship between peritoneal dialysis clearance and molecular weight. Another generalization is that unless there are very unusual physiochemical characteristics to the drug, the peritoneal dialysis clearance of the unbound drug can be estimated by multiplying urea clearance (20 ml/min for a 1-hour dwell, 8 ml/min for a 4-h dwell, or 4 ml/min for an 8-h dwell) by the ratio of the square root of the mass of urea (60 Da) over the square root of the drug's molecular weight [26].

If one wants to calculate the clearance of a drug by peritoneal dialysis, it is done in the following manner.

$$\text{clearance} = \boldsymbol{D/P} \times \frac{\text{effluent volume}}{\text{exchange time}} \tag{2}$$

where D and P are dialysate and plasma drug concentrations, respectively, volume of effluent is the dialysate drained (in ml), and exchange time is the total time of the exchange (in min) including inflow, dwell, and drainage.

Hemofiltration

Convective Transport: Plasma Water Versus Whole Plasma

Hemofiltration removes solutes by convection, i.e., solutes dissolved in the water component of plasma are removed with the plasma water. Since plasma water constitutes 92%–97% of plasma, for clinical purposes they will be considered synonymous.

Sieving Coefficient

The sieving coefficient (S) of a solute is the concentration in the ultrafiltrate (UF) divided by the concentration in the water component of the retentate [24]. A solute that freely passes has an S of 1.0 and if completely rejected has an S of 0. Colton and associates [27] have shown that the rigorous expression can be reasonably approximated to

$$S = \frac{\text{UF}}{(A + V)/2} \quad \text{or} \quad \frac{2\text{UF}}{(A + V)} \tag{3}$$

where A is the plasma water concentration at the filter inlet and V is the plasma water concentration at the filter outlet. Kroh et al. [28] have shown that for drugs an accurate definition of S is $\text{AUC}_f/\text{AUC}_p$, where AUC_f and AUC_p represent the areas under the time–drug concentration curves for filtrate (f) and plasma (p), respectively.

For a particular membrane and solute under conditions of continuous hemofiltration, S will generally be constant [29–31]. Major changes in the transmembrane pressure can decrease the sieving of large solutes [32, 33], presumably by generating retarding protein layers (protein concentration polarization) or protein–membrane interactions. Solute sieving is generally independent of blood flow [30–32].

Clearance

The clearance of a solute (drug) across a hemofilter is the sieving coefficient times the ultrafiltration rate (UFR). Thus, clearance is linearly dependent on the UFR when fluid replacement is in a postdilutional mode. Therefore, the important way to describe a drug's convective movement across a hemofilter is to define its S.

Drug Removal During Hemofiltration: Theory

Factors affecting drug removal during hemofiltration include the following:

1. Delivery of drug to hemofilter membrane
   - Volume of distribution
   - Blood flow (macro)
   - Blood flow (micro)
   - Protein concentration polarization
2. Unique ultrafiltration properties of the drug
   - Drug–protein binding
   - Drug–membrane interaction
   - Drug charge
   - Molecular size
   - Sieving coefficient
3. Ultrafiltration rate
   - Hydrostatic pressure (blood pressure, blood flow, blood access, UF column height, UF suction)
   - Oncotic pressure
   - Viscosity
   - Length and width of blood lines
   - Venous resistance
   - Filter surface area and intrinsic membrane properties

An adequate blood flow to the filter is necessary for maximum performance. Furthermore, the delivery of drug to the filter is dependent on the drug's V_d. Protein concentration polarization may decrease UF flux by increasing the osmotic pressure at the membrane and/or by offering an additional resistance

Table 2. Drug-sieving coefficients during hemofiltration

Sieving coefficients	Observed[a]	Expected[b]
Antibiotics		
Amikacin	0.95	0.95
Amphotericin B	0.35	0.10
Ampicillin	0.69	0.80
Cefoperazone	0.27	0.10
Cefotaxime	0.85	0.62
Cefoxitin	0.83	0.59
Ceftazidime	0.90	0.83
Ceftriaxone	0.82	0.15
Cephapirin	1.48	0.55
Cilastin	0.75	0.56
Ciprofloxacin	0.69	0.60
Clindamycin	0.49	0.40
Doxycycline	0.40	0.20
Erythromycin	0.37	0.30
Gentamicin	0.81	0.95
Imipenem	0.90	0.80
Metronidazole	0.84	0.80
Mezlocillin	0.71	0.68
Nafcillin	0.55	0.20
Netilmicin	0.93	0.95
Oxacillin	0.02	0.05
Pefloxacin	0.80	0.80
Penicillin	0.68	0.50
Piperacillin	0.82	0.80
Streptomycin	0.30	0.65
Sulfamethoxazole	0.30	0.60
Tobramycin	0.90	0.95
Vancomycin	0.80	0.90
Miscellaneous		
Bromide	1.00	1.00
Chlorodiazepoxide	0.05	0.05
Cisplatin	0.10	0.10
Clofibrate	0.06	0.04
Cyclosporine	0.58	0.10
Diathybarbital	1.00	0.90
Diazepam	0.02	0.02
Digoxin	0.70	0.80
Digitoxin	0.15	0.05
Famotidine	0.73	0.85
Glibenclamide	0.60	0.01
Glutethimide	0.02	0.50
Lidocaine	0.14	0.36
Metamizole	0.40	0.40
N-acetyl procainamide	0.92	0.90
Nitrazepam	0.08	0.10

Table 2. *Continued*

Sieving coefficients	Observed[a]	Expected[b]
Nomifensin	0.70	0.40
Oxazepam	0.10	0.10
Phenobarbital	0.80	0.60
Phenytoin	0.45	0.10
Procainamide	0.86	0.86
Theophylline	0.80	0.47

[a] Some of these data represent a mean of as many as 20 observations and others may represent one observation. Adsorption to the membrane decreases sieving coefficients and could be occurring. See text.
[b] Sieving coefficient assuming that protein binding is the *sole* determinant of drug sieving and that protein binding is as stated in Aronoff et al. [22], i.e., in healthy subjects. See text for explanations challenging the validity of these assumptions.

barrier [27, 34]. Its effects on convective solute transport are real, but minor [30, 32].

In the absence of confounding circulating proteins, there are drug–membrane interactions during continuous arteriovenous hemofiltration (CAVH) [31, 35, 36]. Sieving coefficients for several drugs through polyacrylonitrile and polyamide membranes were significantly different from those through polysulfone [30, 35, 37]. Among the explanations offered was an effect of drug charge–membrane interaction, retarding sieving. Also a Gibbs-Donnan effect of circulating proteins contributes to the retention of small cations [38–40]. From the limited observations in vivo the anionic drugs cephapirin and cefotaxime have an S greater than 1 [41] (Table 2; also see below). However, these data have been challenged by in vitro studies [37]. Obviously the effect of drug charge on sieving is worthy of further investigation.

The role of drug binding to membranes can be significant. Gentamicin and doxycycline binding to polyacrylonitrile is pH dependent [42–44]. Twenty milligrams of tobramycin bind to Hospal's PAN filter, suggesting that a substantial fraction of the drug can be removed from the circulation by this process [45, 46]. The introduction of a negative charge on macromolecules can decrease sieving during hemofiltration [47]. Thus, drug charge–membrane interactions occur. The clincial significance of these observations has yet to be determined.

Protein binding is affected by the molar ratios of drug and protein [18, 19]. At the inner surface of the membrane these ratios are dramatically altered. If that should decrease protein binding, then the newly freed drug could diffuse down its diffusion gradient into the filtrate. Henderson has suggested a related situation for presumably unbound solute [48]. There are no data to support this, except that drug sieving is not always as one would expect from known protein binding data [6–8, 28, 41]. The finding clinically of a drug's S greater than 1 could be explained by this scenario.

A drug's binding to large, nonultrafilterable circulating plasma proteins will play the dominant role in determining its sieving. Protein-bound drug will not be filtered. As discussed above, many factors affect drug–protein binding. The unbound drug is the pharmacologically active fraction. If there is displacement from protein, the pharmacologic effect, the metabolism, and the removal will be enhanced (see above).

The role of molecular size on membrane transport has been extensively studied [27, 32–34, 49], but for most drugs molecular size will not be an issue for removal during filtration. The molecular weight cutoffs of filtration membranes are much greater than the molecular weight of the drugs.

Drug Removal During Hemofiltration: Approach Using Arterial Levels and Presumed Ultrafiltrate Levels

Inulin readily traverses hemofilter membranes [32, 34, 50, 51]. Since virtually all therapeutic agents have a molecular weight less than that of inulin, one can reasonably assume that these drugs will permeate these membranes limited mostly by the extent of their protein binding. Only the unbound fraction is ultrafilterable. Aronoff et al. [22] have provided protein binding data, usually from studies of healthy subjects. Therefore, some discrepancies may arise when comparing those data to observations in critically ill patients. This is discussed again.

For practical purposes, one can measure the removal of drug during hemofiltration by multiplying the UF drug concentration by the UFR. Since (arterial) plasma levels are usually required for clinical management, one could calculate the UF concentrations from the arterial concentration (A) by the formula

$$\mathrm{UF} = A \times \text{unbound fraction} \tag{4}$$

where the protein binding is assumed to be as stated in Aronoff et al. [22].

The technique used to determine drug removal during hemofiltration, using the plasma arterial level exclusively, and to calculate the UF concentration from it can be summartized as follows:

1. Determine steady state arterial concentration (A).
2. Determine fraction *not* bound to protein [22].
3. Determine UFR from flow sheet.
4. Amount removed = A × unbound fraction × UFR.

If this approach is used, the arterial sample should represent a steady state level (see above). The ideal time to obtain such a sample is halfway between maintenance doses after at least three half-lives. Aronoff et al. [22] also recorded $T1_{/2}$ data.

Clinical Observations

For practical purposes, clinically with therapeutic agents the difference between plasma water and plasma can be ignored. During CAVH, defining a drug's S as UF/A rather than as 2UF/(A + V) does not introduce appreciable error [41]. Table 2 lists drug sieving coefficients observed during hemofiltration and the "expected" sieving coefficients from known protein binding data. Differences between the observed S and that expected may be due to displacement, altered binding affinity, the affect of drug charge, and the possible effects of drug binding to membranes. Nonetheless, from Table 2 protein binding appears to be the major factor affecting drug sieving (r = 0.74, $p < 0.001$).

Hemodialysis

Drug Removal by Diffusion

Diffusion dialysis (peritoneal or hemodialysis) solute removal is driven by the concentration gradient from blood to dialysate, but protein binding and volume of distribution play a role. Protein-bound drugs or drugs with a large V_d will not be appreciably dialyzed. Factors affecting the hemodialyzability of a drug include the following:

1. Drug properties:
   a) Molecular weight
   b) Charge
   c) Lipid or water solubility
   d) V_d (tissue binding)
   e) Red cell pratitioning
   f) Protein binding
   g) Other forms of steric hindrace
   h) Membrane binding
   i) Rapid excretion by another pathway
2. Hemodialyzer properties:
   a) Blood flow
   b) Surface area
   c) Membrane permeability
   d) Pore size
   e) Fluid films (membrane geometry)

3. Dialysate properties:
   a) Folw rate
   b) Solute concentration
   c) pH
   d) temperature
4. Miscellaneous
   a) Convective transport during ultrafiltration

Hemodialysis membrane pores act as cylinders of uniform diameter. As the molecular volume increases, a drug's diffusiveness decreases. There is a negative linear relationship between the log of dialysance and the log of molecular weight [52]. A drug or solute approaching a molecular mass of 500 Da will be poorly hemodialyzed using conventional cellulosic membranes. The dialyzer clearance of a molecule of less than 500 Da is significantly dependent upon the blood and dialysate flows and dialyzer surface area [53]. As molecular mass increases, dialyzer clearance becomes less dependent on flow rates and more dependent on surface area and convective mass transfer (ultrafiltration). Maher has suggested that when the transport properties are unknown, the hemodialysis clearance of an unbound solute can be estimated by multiplying the urea clearance by the ratio of urea molecular mass (60 Da) to the other solute's molecular mass [26]. This approach seems reasonable if the urea clearance is predominantly by diffusive transport. Vincent and associates [54] have shown that a drug's diffussive mass transfer coefficient through "open" membranes during continuous arteriovenous hemodiafiltration (CAVHD) is dependent on molecular weight according to the formula

$$K_d/K_{dc} = (MW/113)^{-0.42} \quad (5)$$

where K_d and K_{dc} are the diffusive mass transfer coefficients for the drug and creatinine, respectively, and MW is the drug's molecular weight.

Hemodiafiltration and CAVHD

Henderson and associates [55–57] demonstrated that convection removes larger molecules more readily than does diffusion. Most drugs will be larger than creatinine and smaller than macromolecules. Furthermore, the solute losses during combined convection and diffusion are less than the simple sum of convective losses and diffusive losses, because convection impairs diffusive losses [58, 59]. The presence of convectively derived solute on the dialysate side of the membrane decreases the concentration gradient necessary for diffusion [59, 60]. This is particularly evident for unbound solutes. For protein-bound solutes, ultrafiltration leads to the high concentration of solute against the membrane as protein concentration polarization occurs. This contributes to a high concentration gradient from blood to dialysate, albeit of highly protein-bound species. Nonetheless, this concentration gradient may play a factor in solute removal during combined convection and diffusion [42].

Small-solute clearance during CAVHD is the simple sum of diffusive and convective clearance when dialysate flow rate is as low as 16.6 ml/min [59]. The diffusive component is limited by dialysate flow rate [61] and the convective component is equal to the UFR. Increasing dialysate flow rate disrupts this simple relationship [60]. Drugs behave like other solutes in that their clearance is dialysate flow rate limited [62]. These interactions have been described in several mathematical models and corroborative in vitro studies [54, 63, 64].

As molecular weight increases, dialyzer clearance becomes less dependent on blood and dialysate flow rates and more dependent on the convective component [41]. The membrane and transport process both are important. During high-flux hemodiafiltration netilmicin (500 Da), clearance was twice that of comparably performed diffusion dialysis [65]. Thus, both dialysate flow rate and molecular size affect the prediction of combined diffusive and convective transport.

Protein concentration polarization could form a barrier potentially retarding diffusion, but even in high-flux hemodiafiltration this effect appears to be small [58, 66]. It is possible that UFR will be shown to be a complicating variable. Large volumes of filtrate will decrease the concentration gradient unless there is a commensurate increase in dialysate flow rate.

Despite this background theory and speculations, we need more primary data. Pauls et al. [67] attempted to compare drug removal by various blood cleansing techniques and concluded that there were too many confounding variables. Keller et al. [17] felt that drug removal by dialysis was clearly complicated by convective losses. Thus, there is much yet to accomplish in this area of study.

Supplemental Doses

Drug Levels

Drug levels are a valuable tool when clinicians know what level they wish to achieve. Both loading and maintenance doses can be determined. The amount of drug administered can be calculated, as shown in the examples below:

1. Tobramycin loading:
   Tobramycin V_d = 0.23 l/kg
   1 μg/ml = 1 mg/l

Desired level (peak)	6 mg/l
– Present level	*0*
Difference level	$6 \times V_d \times \text{BW} = 6 \times 0.23 \times \text{BW} = 1.4$ mg/kg

2. Tobramycin maintenance:
   Desired level (peak) 6 mg/l
   – *Present level (trough)* *2 mg/l*
   Difference level 4 mg/ml × V_d × BW = 0.92 mg/kg

The presently observed level (present level) is subtracted from the level one wishes to achieve (desired level) leaving the difference level (all in the same units). The difference level times the V_d times the body weight (BW) in kg will give the amount of drug needed to boost the present level to the desired level.

For loading doses, the present level is zero and the difference level is the desired level. For maintenance doses, the trough level is the present level. This method is useful for administering any drug whose level is available and whose V_d is known. It is especially applicable to the setting of ARF when the amount of drug removed by the renal replacement therapy is not clearly known and the clinician has only drug levels to assess the pharmacologic status of the patient. V_d data are given in Aronoff et al. [22].

Combining Steady State Levels and Clearances

Bickley [68] has applied standard dosing principles to the setting of CRRT. This approach utilizes the steady state serum concentration (C_{ss}, see "Elimination Half-Life" above), the total plasma clearance (comprised of the device clearance plus any endogenous clearance), the dosing interval, and bioavailability. If the drugs are administered intravenously, then bioavailability is unity and the term can be discarded. The calculation of the dose is then:

$$\text{dose} = C_{ss} \times \text{clearance} \times \text{dosing interval} \qquad (5)$$

As mentioned, the clearance term is total plasma clearance. When the entire clearance is by hemofiltration, then clearance is as defined above in "Clearance," namely filter clearance = $S \times \text{UFR}$. One may find this approach difficult because of the necessity to measure clearance. Thus, the approach discussed above in "Drug Levels" utilizing desired, peak, and trough levels and volume of distribution is preferred. However, this approach is vulnerable to the problems of altered V_d during disease, as discussed above in "Drug Distribution Volume."

Conclusion

Drugs frequently utilized in the intensive care unit (ICU) are listed in Table 1: the drug's half-life in uremia, protein binding under normal conditions, V_d under normal conditions, the dose for normal conditions, the dose modification method for renal insufficiency, the modification for a glomerular filtration rate (GFR) between 10 and 50 ml/min, the modification for when the GFR is less than 10 ml/min, and finally the supplemental doses to make up for losses through hemodialysis, continuous equilibrium peritoneal dialysis, or continuous renal replacement therapy such as hemofiltration, hemodialysis, or hemodiafiltration are given.

References

1. Matzke GR, O'Connell MB, Collins AJ, Keshaviah PR (1986) Disposition of vancomycin during hemofiltration. Clin Pharmacol Ther 40:425–430
2. Morse GD, Nairn DK, Walshe JJ (1987) Once weekly intraperitoneal therapy for gram-positive peritonitis. Am J Kidney Dis 10:300–305
3. Mueller BA, Scarim SK, Macias WL (1993) Comparison of imipenem pharmakokinetics in patients with acute or chronic renal failure treated with continuous hemofiltration. Am J Kidney Dis 21:172–179
4. Levy G (1977) Pharmacokinetics in renal disease. Am J Med 62:461–463
5. Gibson TP (1985) Problems in designing hemodialysis drug studies. Pharmacotherapy 5:23–29
6. Kroh UF, Dehne M, El Abed K, Feussner KD, Hofmann W, Lennartz H (1991) Drug dosage during continuous hemofiltration: pharmacokinetics and practical implications. Contrib Nephrol 93:56–59
7. Kroh UF, Holl T, Feussner KD (1992) Pharmacokinetics and dosage adjustment of antibiotics during continuous extracorporeal lung assistance and hemofiltration. Artif Organs 16:457–460
8. Kroh UF, Lennartz H (1992) Evaluation and first validation study on a simplifed drug dosage algorithm for multiple organ failure patients. Ren Fail 14:579–585
9. Reidenberg MM, Affrime M (1973) Influence of disease on binding of drugs to plasma proteins. Ann NY Acad Sci 226:115–126
10. Dayton PG, Israili ZH, Perel JM (1973) Influence of binding on drug metabolism and distribution. Ann NY Acad Sci 226:172–194
11. Anton AH (1973) Increasing activity of sulfonamides with displacing agents. Ann NY Acad Sci 226:273–292
12. Reidenberg MM (1977) The binding of drugs to plasma proteins and the interpretation of measurements of plasma concentration of drugs in patients with poor renal function. Am J Med 62:466–470
13. Tillement JP, Lhoste F, Findicelli TF (1978) Diseases and drug protein binding. Clin Pharmacokinet 3:144–154
14. McNamara PJ, Lalka D, Gibaldi M (1981) Endogenous accumulation products and serum protein binding in uremia. J Lab Clin Med 98:730–740
15. Suh B, Craig WA, England AC, Elliott RL (1981) Effect of free fatty acids on protein binding of antimicrobial agents. J Infect Dis 143:609–610
16. Gulyassy PF, Depner TA (1983) Impaired binding of drugs and endogenous ligands in renal disease. Am J Kidney Dis 2:578–601
17. Keller F, Wilms H, Schultze G, Offerman G et al. (1983) Effect of plasma protein binding, volume of distribution and molecular weight on the fraction of drugs eliminated by hemodialysis. Clin Nephrol 19:201–205
18. Lunde PKM, Rane A, Yaffe SJ, Lund L, Sjoquist F (1970) Plasma protein binding of diphenylhydantoin in man: interaction with other drugs and the effect of temperature and plasma dilution. Clin Pharmacol Ther 11:846–855

19. Koch-Weser J, Sellers EM (1976) Drug therapy. Binding of drugs to serum albumin (first of two parts). N Engl J Med 294:311–316
20. Vanholder R, Van Landschoot N, De Smet R, Schoots A, Ringoir S (1988) Drug protein binding in chronic renal failure: evaluation of nine drugs. Kidney Int 33:996–1004
21. Posen GA, Luisello J (1980) Continuous equilibrium peritoneal dialysis in the treatment of acute renal failure. Perit Dial Bull 1:6–7
22. Aronoff GR, Bennett WM, Brater DC, Golper TA, Morrison G (1994) Drug prescribing in renal failure: dosing guidelines for adults, 3rd edn. American College of Physicians, Philadelphia
23. Paton TW, Cornish WR, Manuel MA, Hardy BG (1985) Drug therapy in patients undergoing peritoneal dialysis: clincial pharmacokinetic considerations. Clin Pharmacokinet 10:404–426
24. Janknegt R, Koks CHW (1984) Pharmacokinetic aspects during continuous ambulatory peritoneal dialysis: a literatire review. Pharm Weekbl [Sci] 6:229–236
25. Lasrich M, Maher JM, Hirszel P, Maher JF (1979) Correlation of peritoneal transport rates with molecular weight: a method of predicting clearances. ASAIO J 2:107–113
26. Maher JF (1984) Pharmacokinetics in patients with renal failure. Clin Nephrol 21:39–46
27. Colton CK, Henderson LW, Ford CA, Lysaght MJ (1975) Kinetics of hemodiafiltration. I. In vitro transport characteristics of a hollow fiber blood ultrafilter. J Lab Clin Med 85:355–371
28. Kroh U, Hofmann W, Dehne M, El Abed E, Lennartz H (1989) Dosisanpassung von Pharmaka während kontinuierlicher Haemofiltration. Anaesthesist 38:225–232
29. Ronco C, Brendolan A, Borin D, Bragantini L et al. (1985) Permeability characteristics of polysulfonic membranes in CAVH. In: Sieberth HG, Mann H (eds) Continuous artriovenous hemofiltration (CAVH). Karger, Basel, pp 59–63
30. Golper TA, Saad AM (1980) Gentamicin and phenytoin in vitro sieving characteristics through polysulfone hemofilters: effect of flow rate, drug concentration and solvent systems. Kidney Int 30:937–943
31. Lau AH, Kronfol NO, Barakat M (1987) Effect of blood and ultrafiltrate flow rates on drug sieving during continuous hemofiltration. Trans Am Soc Artif Intern Organs 33:297–299
32. Frigon RP, Leypoldt JK, Alford MF, Uyeji S et al. (1984) Hemofilter solute sieving is not governed by dynamically polarized protein. Trans Am Soc Artif Intern Organs 30: 486–490
33. Klein E, Holland FF, Eberle K (1978) Rejection of solutes by hemofiltration membranes. ASAIO J 1:15–23
34. Leypoldt JK, Frigon RP, Henderson LW (1983) Dextran sieving coefficients of hemofilter membranes. Trans Am Soc Artif Intern Organs 29:678–683
35. Kronfol NO, Lau AH, Colon-Rivera J, Libertin CL (1986) Effect of CAVH membrane types on drug sieving coefficients and clearances. Trans Am Soc Artif Intern Organs 32:85–87
36. Lau A, Kronfol N, Jaber N, Libertin C (1986) Determinants of drug removal by continuous arteriovenous hemofiltration. Drug Intell Clin Pharmacol 20:467
37. Lau AH, Libertin CR, Pyle K, Kronfol NO (1989) Removal of cephalosporins by continuous hemofiltration. Int J Artif Organs 12:379–383
38. Lysaght MJ (1983) An experimental model for the ultrafiltration of sodium ion from blood or plasma. Blood Purif 1:25–30
39. Kaplan AA, Longnecker RE, Folkert VW (1984) Continuous arteriovenous hemofiltration – a report of 6 months' experience. Ann Intern Med 100:358–367
40. Paganini EP, Flague J, Whitman G, Nakamoto S (1982) Amino acid balance in patients with oliguric renal failure undergoing slow continuous ultrafiltration (SCUF). Trans Am Soc Artif Intern Organs 28:615–620
41. Golper TA, Wedel SK, Kaplan AA, Saad AM et al. (1985) Drug removal during CAVH: theory and clinical observations. Int J Artif Organs 8:307–312

42. Rumpf KW, Rieger J, Doht B, Ansorg R, Scheler F (1977) Drug elimination by hemofiltration. J Dial 1:677–688
43. Rumpf KW, Rieger J, Ansorg R, Doht B, Scheler F (1978) Binding of antibiotics by dialysis membranes and its clinical relevance. Proc Eur Dial Transplant Assoc 14:607–609
44. Kraft D, Lode H (1979) Elimination of ampicillin and gentamicin by hemofiltration. Klin Wochenschr 57:195–196
45. Kronfol NO, Lau AH, Barakat MM (1987) Aminoglycoside binding to polyacrylonitrile hemofilter membranes during continuous hemofiltration. Trans Am Soc Artif Intern Organs 33:300–303
46. Ciggaran-Guldris S, Brier ME, Golper TA (1991) Tobramycin clearance in simulated continuous arteriovenous hemodialysis. Contrib Nephrol 93:120–123
47. Leypoldt JK, Frigon RP, Henderson LW (1986) Macromolecular charge affects hemofilter solute sieving. Trans Am Soc Artif Intern Organs 32:384–387
48. Henderson LW (1987) Hemofiltration. Kidney 20:25–30
49. Rockel A, Gilge U, Liewald A, Heidland A (1982) Elimination of low molecular weight proteins during hemofiltration. Artif Organs 6:307–317
50. Dodd NJ, O'Donovan RM, Bennett-Jones DN, Rylance PB et al. (1983) Arteriovenous hemofiltration: a recent advance in the management of renal failure. Br Med J 287:1008–1010
51. Kaplan AA, Golper TA (1987) Sieving characteristics of a new polysulfone hemofilter for use with continuous arteriovenous hemofiltration. Int J Artif Organs 10:357–360
52. Henderson LW (1976) Hemodialysis: rationale and physical principles. In: Brenner BM, Rector FC (eds) The kidney. Saunders, Philadelphia, pp 1643–1671
53. Maher JF (1977) Principles of dialysis and dialysis of drugs. Am J Med 62:475–481
54. Vincent HH, Vos MC, Akcahuseyin E, Goessens WHF, van Duyl WA (1993) Drug clearance by continuous haemodiafiltration (CAVHD). Analysis of sieving coefficients and mass transfer coefficients of diffusion. Blood Purif 11:99–107
55. Henderson LW, Silverstein ME, Ford CA, Lysaght MJ (1975) Clinical response to maintenance hemodiafiltration. Kidney Int Suppl 2:S58–S63
56. Hamilton R, Ford C, Colton C, Cross R et al. (1971) Blood cleansing by diafiltration in uremic dog and man. Trans Am Soc Artif Intern Organs 17:259–265
57. Henderson LW, Ford C, Colton CK, Bluemle LW et al. (1970) Uremic blood cleansing by diafiltration using a hollow-fiber ultrafilter. Trans Am Soc Artif Inern Organs 16: 107–112
58. Sprenger KGB, Stephan H, Kratz W, Huber K et al. (1985) Optimizing of hemodiafiltration with modern membranes? Contrib Nephrol 46:43–60
59. Golper TA, Ciggaran-Guldris S, Jenkins R, Brier ME (1991) The role of convection during continuous arteriovenous hemodialysis. Contrib Nephrol 93:146–148
60. Van Geelen JA, Vincent HH, Schalekamp MADH (1988) Continuous arteriovenous haemofiltration and haemodiafiltration in acute renal failure. Nephrol Dial Transplant 2:181–186
61. Sigler MH, Teehan BP (1987) Solute transport in continuous hemodialysis: a new treatment for acute renal failure. Kidney Int 32:562–571
62. Kronfol NO, Adams LJ, Powell SS, Lau AH (1988) Drug removal in continuous arteriovenous hemodialysis (Abstr). National Kidney Foundation Annual Meeting
63. Pallone TL, Hyver S, Petersen J (1988) The simulation of continuous arterio-venous hemodialysis with a mathematical model. Kidney Int 35:125–133
64. Vos MC, Akcahuseyin E, Van Duyl WA, Vincent HH (1990) Continuous A-V haemodiafiltration (CAVHD). Predicting the clearance of drugs. Intensivbehandlung 15:108
65. Basile C, DiMaggio A, Curino E, Scatizzi A (1985) Pharmacokinetics of netilmicin in hypertonic hemodiafiltration and standard hemodialysis. Clin Nephrol 24:305–309

66. Bosch T, Schmidt B, Samtleben W, Gurland HJ (1985) Effect of protein adsorption on diffusive and convective transport through polysulfone membranes. Contrib Nephrol 46: 14–22
67. Pauls A, Grigolett HG, von Herrath D, Schaefer K (1984) Comparison of drug elimination by current methods of blood purification. Blood Purif 2:14–22
68. Bickley SK (1988) Drug dosing during continuous arteriovenous hemofiltration. Clin Pharm 7:198–206

Subject Index

MIX
Papier aus verantwortungsvollen Quellen
Paper from responsible sources
FSC® C105338

If you have any concerns about our products,
you can contact us on
ProductSafety@springernature.com

In case Publisher is established outside the EU,
the EU authorized representative is:
Springer Nature Customer Service Center GmbH
Europaplatz 3, 69115 Heidelberg, Germany

Printed by Libri Plureos GmbH
in Hamburg, Germany